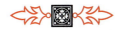

HEALTH CARE
ECONOMICS
FIFTH EDITION

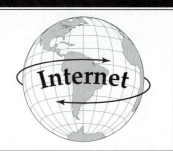

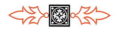

HEALTH CARE ECONOMICS

FIFTH EDITION

Paul J. Feldstein, Ph.D.
Professor
Robert Gumbiner Chair in Health Care Management
Graduate School of Management
University of California
Irvine, California

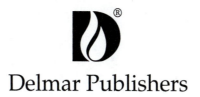

Delmar Publishers

Albany • Bonn • Boston • Cincinnati • Detroit • London • Madrid • Melbourne
Mexico City • New York • Pacific Grove • Paris • San Francisco • Singapore • Tokoyo
Toronto • Washington

Notice to the Reader

Publisher does not warrant or guarantee any of the products described herein or perform any independent analysis in connection with any of the product information contained herein. Publisher does not assume, and expressly disclaims, any obligation to obtain and include information other than that provided to it by the manufacturer.

The reader is expressly warned to consider and adopt all safety precautions that might be indicated by the activities herein and to avoid all potential hazards. By following the instructions contained herein, the reader willingly assumes all risks in connection with such instructions.

The publisher makes no representation or warranties of any kind, including but not limited to, the warranties of fitness for particular purpose or merchantability, nor are any such representations implied with respect to the material set forth herein, and the publisher takes no responsibility with respect to such material. The publisher shall not be liable for any special, consequential, or exemplary damages resulting, in whole or part, from the readers' use of, or reliance upon, this material.

Cover Graphic Design: *Christopher Oakes*
Delmar Staff
Publisher: *William Brottmiller*
Acquisitions Editor: *Cathy L. Esperti*
Production Editor: *Christopher Oakes*
Editorial Assistant: *Darcy Scelsi*

COPYRIGHT © 1999
by Delmar Publishers
an International Thomson Publishing Company

I(T)P

The ITP logo is a trademark under license.
Printed in the United States of America

For more information, contact:

Delmar Publishers, Inc.
3 Columbia Circle, Box 15015
Albany, New York 12212-5015

International Thomson Publishing Europe
Berkshire House
168-173 High Holborn
London, WC1V 7AA
England

Nelson ITP, Australia
102 Dodds Street
South Melbourne,
Victoria, 3205 Australia

Nelson Canada
1120 Birchmont Road
Scarborough, Ontario
M1K 5G4, Canada

International Thomson Publishing France
Tour Maine-Montparnasse
33 Avenue du Maine
75755 Paris Cedex 15, France

International Thomson Editores
Seneca 53
Colonia Polanco
11560 Mexico D. F. Mexico

International Thomson Publishing GmbH
Königswinterer Strasße 418
53227 Bonn
Germany

International Thomson Publishing Asia
60 Albert Street
#15-01 Albert Complex
Singapore 189969

International Thomson Publishing Japan
Hirakawa-cho Kyowa Building, 3F
2-2-1 Hirakawa-cho, Chiyoda-ku,
Tokyo 102, Japan

ITE Spain/Paraninfo
Calle Magallanes, 25
28015-Madrid, Espana

2 3 4 5 6 7 8 9 10 XXX 01 00 99 98

Library of Congress Cataloging-in-Publication Data

Feldstein, Paul J.
    Health care economics / Paul J. Feldstein. — 5th ed.
       p.   cm. — (Delmar series in health services administration)
    Includes bibliographical references and index.
    ISBN 0-7668-0699-5
    1. Medical economics.   2. Medical economics—United States.
I. Title. II. Series.
RA410.F44   1998
338.4'73621'0973—dc21   98-15358
                                      CIP

DELMAR SERIES IN HEALTH SERVICES ADMINISTRATION

Stephen J. Williams, Sc.D., Series Editor

Ambulatory Care Management, third edition
Austin Ross, Stephen J. Williams, and Ernest Pavlock, Editors

The Continuum of Long-Term Care
Connie J. Evashwick, Editor

Health Care Economics, fifth edition
Paul J. Feldstein

Health Care Management: Organization Design and Behavior, third edition
Stephen M. Shortell and Arnold D. Kaluzny, Editors

Health Politics and Policy, second edition
Theodor J. Litman and Leonard S. Robins, Editors

Introduction to Health Services, fourth edition
Stephen J. Williams and Paul R. Torrens, Editors

Motivating Health Behavior
John P. Elder, E. Scott Geller, Melbourne F. Hovell, and Joni A. Mayer, Editors

Really Governing: How Health System and Hospital Boards Can Make More of a Difference
Dennis D. Pointer and Charles M. Ewell

Strategic Management of Human Resources in Health Services Organizations,
second edition
Myron D. Fottler, S. Robert Hernandez, and Charles L. Joiner, Editors

Financial Management in Health Care Organizations
Robert A. McLean

Principles of Public Health Practice
F. Douglas Scutchfield and C. William Keck

The Hospital Medical Staff
Charles H. White

Essentials of Health Services
Stephen J. Williams

Essentials of Health Care Management
Stephen M. Shortell and Arnold D. Kaluzny, Editors

Essentials of Human Resources Management in Health Services Organizations
Myron D. Fottler, S. Robert Hernandez, and Charles L. Joiner, Editors

Health Services Research Methods
Leiyu Shi

SUPPLEMENTAL READER:

Contemporary Issues in Health Services
Stephen J. Williams

To Anna

CONTENTS

Preface to the Fifth Edition   xv

List of Tables   xvii

List of Figures   xxi

Chapter 1 An Introduction to the Economics of Medical Care   1

Trends in Medical Expenditures   1

The Contribution of Economics to Health Policy   4

Basic Choices That Must Be Made with Regard to Medical Services   6

The Applicability of Economics to the Study of Medical Care   12

The Trade-off between Quantity and Quality in the Provision of Medical Services   13

Summary   16

Chapter 2 The Production of Health: The Impact of Medical Services on Health   18

Medical Care as an Output of the Medical Services Industry and as an Input to Health   18

Determining the Allocation of Resources to Medical Care Using a Health Production Function   20

Empirical Studies of a Health Production Function   26

Applications of a Health Production Function   30

Summary   33

Chapter 3 An Overview of the Medical Care Sector   37

Description of the Medical Care Markets   37

Applications of a Model of the Medical Care Sector   44

Summary   49

Chapter 4 Measuring Changes in the Price of Medical Care   52

The Uses of a Definition of the Product of the Medical Care Industry   52

The Consumer Price Index   53

The Medical Care Component of the CPI (MCPI)   60

Summary   79

*Appendix: Health Insurance Premiums as a Measure
of the Price of Medical Care* — 79

Chapter 5   The Demand for Medical Care — 82

The Purpose of Demand Analysis — 82

Demand versus Need as a Basis for Policy and Planning — 83

A Model of the Demand for Medical Care — 86

An Application of Demand Analysis: Explaining Annual
Changes in Personal Medical Expenditures — 105

The Demand for Medical Care Faced by the Firm — 108

Summary — 110

*Appendix: The Effect of Co-insurance on the Demand
for Medical Care* — 111

Chapter 6   The Demand for Health Insurance — 117

Appropriateness of Health Insurance Coverage — 117

Health Insurance Terminology — 118

The Theory of Demand for Health Insurance — 122

An Application of the Theory of the Demand
for Health Insurance — 135

Biased Selection in Health Care Markets — 137

The Demand for Health Insurance under Conditions
of Moral Hazard — 141

Summary — 146

*Appendix 1: The Allocative Inefficiency of Blue Cross'
Service Benefit Policy* — 149

*Appendix 2: The Tax Advantage of Health Insurance
as a Fringe Benefit* — 153

*Appendix 3: The Effect on the Insurance Premium
of Extending Coverage to Include Additional Benefits* — 154

Chapter 7   The Supply of Medical Care: An Overview — 163

Determinants of Supply — 163

Evaluation of Economic Efficiency in Supply — 169

Summary — 173

**Chapter 8   The Market for Health Insurance:
Its Performance and Structure** — 175

Economic Efficiency — 175

The Demand Side of the Health Insurance Market — 176

The Supply Side of the Health Insurance Market — 179

Industry Conduct and Competitive Behavior — 183

The Performance of the Health Insurance Market — 186

Summary — 198

Chapter 9   **Market Competition in Medical Care**   205
The Emergence of Competition in Medical Care   205
Characteristics of Managed Care Plans   217
Performance of a Competitive Managed Care Market   221
Summary   233

Chapter 10   **The Physician Services Market**   239
The Structure of the Physician Services Market   242
Market Conduct   250
Performance of the Physician Services Market   266
Physician Payment under Medicare   276
Summary   286

Chapter 11   **The Market for Hospital Services**   294
Background   294
Determinants of Market Structure   297
Hospital Conduct and Behavior   311
Hospital Performance   333
Summary   339

Chapter 12   **Health Manpower Shortages and Surpluses:**
                   Definitions, Measurement, and Policies   345
Definitions of a Health Manpower Shortage   346
The Definitions of a Surplus of Health Manpower   355
The Measurement of Health Manpower Shortages
       and Surpluses   356
Empirical Estimates of Shortages and Surpluses   362
Conflicting Estimates of a Physician Surplus   369
Proposed Policies to Correct Imbalances Between
       the Demand and Supply of Physicians   372
Summary   375

Chapter 13   **The Market for Physician Manpower**   380
Entry Restrictions in Medicine   380
Barriers to Entry in Medicine   381
The Physician as a Price-Discriminating Monopolist   387
Proposed Changes in the Physician Manpower Market   395
Summary   398

Chapter 14   **The Market for Medical Education:**
                   Equity and Efficiency   401
Performance of the Medical Education Sector   401
The Economic Efficiency of the Medical Education Sector   401
Equity in the Current System of Financing Medical Education   416

Summary   423

Chapter 15   **The Market for Registered Nurses**   427
Economists' Interests Regarding the Nursing Market   427
A Framework for Understanding the Performance
    of the Market for Registered Nurses   427
The Performance of the Market for Registered Nurses   432
Market Structure and Nurse Wages and Employment   443
Federal Support for Nurse Training   447
An Economic Analysis of Comparable Worth   453
Summary   457

Chapter 16   **The Role of Government in Health
    and Medical Care**   463
Government Intervention in Medical Care   463
Market Imperfections   464
Market Failure   468
Redistribution Using In-Kind Subsidies   474
Summary   481

Chapter 17   **The Legislative Marketplace**   484
The Legislative Marketplace   484
The Public Interest View of Government   484
An Economic Theory of Government   486
The Demand for Legislation by Health Associations   491
Summary   506

Chapter 18   **National Health Insurance: An Approach
    to the Redistribution of Medical Care**   514
The Economic and Political Frameworks   514
Achieving Efficiency for Different Values Underlying
    National Health Insurance   515
Specific Criteria for Evaluating National Health
    Insurance Plans   525
The Current System for Financing Medical Services   531
National Health Insurance Proposals   537
Why the United States Has Not Had
    National Health Insurance   551
Summary   559

Chapter 19   **The Market for Long-Term Care Services**   562
Demographic Trends and Long-Term Care   562
The Demand for Long-Term Care Services   563
The Supply of Long-Term Care Services   577

Government Policy and the Nursing Home Industry 583
Financing Long-Term Care 590
Summary 593

Chapter 20 **Concluding Comments on the Economics of Medical Care** 598

Glossary 605
Index 619

PREFACE

◈

This book is an introductory text that provides an analytical approach to the study of medical services, and through the use of numerous applications, illustrates the usefulness of economics to the understanding of public policy issues affecting this sector. The material in this book presumes some familiarity with the economic concepts presented in an undergraduate microeconomics course. Several of these concepts are, however, reviewed when the applicability of economics to medical issues is discussed. Since the institutional knowledge of medical care isues is generally not uniform among students, particularly undergraduates, descriptive information and definitions are also provided.

This book is meant to be used in a one-semester course in health economics. realizing that instructor's preferences for topics to include in such a course may differ, more material in included than would normally be covered in one semester. For the interested student, both recent and historical references are provided should the student wish to pursue a particular subject in greater depth.

In writing this book I have tried to clarify those subjects that my students found most difficult and inadequately explained in the classroom. For example, as a result of student comments I became aware of the need to make explicit the relationship between economic analysis and the value judgments underlying different public policies. For this reason I have tried to stress these issues in the various subjects discussed.

The emphasis of this book is on the financing and delivery of personal medical services, rather than on the broader issues of health and health services. This narrower focus reflects the extensive emphasis of federal and state legislation and of current policy issues, such as financing medical services and concern with efficiency in the delivery of services, on personal medical services rather than health or health services, which might well be more appropriate. The relationship of personal medical services to health is discussed in an early chapter; thereafter, the text emphasizes the definition, measurement, and selection of public policies to achieve economic efficiency and equity in the financing and delivery of personal medical services.

Since the time the first edition appeared in 1979, the medical sector has undergone dramatic changes. Health policy is constantly changing. The emphasis on national health insurance, once high, has now declined; the initial concern over a shortage of physicians changed to a concern over a possible surplus of physicians. From being reimbursed on the basis of their costs, hospitals now face prospective, fixed, prices, and physician payment under Medicare has similarly undergone dramatic changes. The structure of the medical services sector has also been changing, from independent community hospitals to multi-hospital systems that are becoming vertically integrated. Managed care, which includes HMOs and PPOs, is the fastest-growing method of delivering medical services.

This latest edition provides more recent data on the medical sector, the latest information on legislative changes affecting this industry, incorporation of recent literature and research, while attempting to provide a historical perspective within which these changes are occurring. In addition to the above updating, several chapters have been extensively revised.

In writing this book and in teaching my course, I have greatly benefited from the work of other health economists. Some measure of that debt is indicated by the numerous references found throughout this book. For assistance in preparing this edition, I wish to thank Elzbieta Kozlowski and the helpful comments of the reviewers, John T. O'Connor, Ph.D., MBA, MPH of Clark University, Richard B. Dwore, Ph.D. of the University of Utah at Salt Lake City and John Troidl, MBA of the University of California at Davis. Since this edition is a continuation of previous editions, I also wish to acknowledge some of my previous research assistants: Courtand Reichman, John Goddeeris, Thomas Wickizer, Rober Miller, and Darrell Graham. A number of my colleagues also provided helpful comments on the various editions: Peter Buerhaus, Ron Vogel, Jerry German, Judy Lave, John Kuder, Carolyn Watts, and Jack Wheeler.

Paul J. Feldstein
Irvine, California

LIST OF TABLES

Table 1.1.   Trends in personal medical care expenditures, 1950–95

Table 2.1.   Cost per life saved among three programs to reduce neonatal mortality

Table 3.1.   Total private and public expenditures for personal health care services by type of expenditure and source of funds, calendar years 1965, 1980, and 1995

Table 3.2.   Amount and percent distribution of personal health care expenditures, by source of funds and type of expenditure, 1995

Table 3.3.   Percentage distribution of personal health expenditures by source in the United States, 1965, 1975, 1985, and 1995

Table 4.1.   Relative importance of major components of the CPI, selected years (percent)

Table 4.2.   CPI and major groups, 1935–96 (1982–84 = 100)

Table 4.3.   Trends in the MCPI, selected years, 1965–96 (1982–84 = 100 unless noted)

Table 4.4.   Relative weights of items in the MCPI (December 1996)

Table 4.5.   Relative weights of items in the MCPI, in consumer expenditures on health services and supplies , and in total national expenditures on health services and supplies, calendar years 1975, 1985, and 1995

Table 4.6.   Consumer expenditures on health services and supplies, and total national expenditures on health services and supplies, 1995 (billions)

Table 4.7.   Weights of medical care in CPI, in personal consumption, and in personal consumption plus government purchases, calendar years 1975, 1985, and 1995

Table 4.8.   Percentage increase in the costs of treatment of selected illnesses, 1951–81

Table 4.9.   Annual rates of change in various medical price indices, adjusted for inflation, 1983–94

Table 5.1.   Selected results on price elasticities of demand for medical care

Table 5.2.   Firm-specific price elasticities

Table 5.3.   Time-price elasticities for physician services

Table 5.4.   Estimated income elasticities of demand for medical services

Table 5.5.   Differences between plans in predicted total expenditures per person and in the probability of one or more physician visits or hospital admissions (all participants)

Table 5.6.   Price elasticities for various types of care

Table 5.7.   Factors affecting changes in personal health care expenditures

Table 6.1.   Classification of medical services by probability of occurrence, potential loss, and insurance benefits, 1957–58

Table 6.2.   Distribution of health expenditures for the U.S. population by magnitude of expenditures, selected years, 1928–87

Table 8.1.   Enrollment of persons with hospital expense protection, 1950–95

Table 8.2.   Ratio of benefit expenditures to premium income, according to type of plan, 1955–95

Table 8.3.   Plan switching by type of plan

Table 8.4.   Simulated probability of switching plans in response to various premium increases

Table 9.1.   Year-end enrollment and number of HMOs by age of plan, size of plan, profit status, and model type, 1986–96

Table 9.2.   Growth in number of HMOs and their enrollment, 1976–95

Table 10.1.   Physicians and aides employed in offices of physicians, 1970–95

Table 10.2.   Number, average size, and distribution of office–based physicians by group affiliation, selected years, 1969–95

Table 10.3.   Distribution of groups and group physicians by group size

Table 10.4.   Physicians' contractual arrangements by size of group, 1996

Table 10.5.   Distribution of expenditures on physician services by source of funds, 1950–95

Table 10.6.   Annual rate of change in total physician expenditures, the CPI, and the CPI for physicians' fees, 1960–96

Table 10.7.   Number of physician visits per person per year, number of visits per physician per week, and the mean fee for office visits for established and new patients, 1975–96

Table 10.8.   Annual percent change in professional expenses, fees, and incomes of physicians, 1982–96

Table 10.9.   Average annual percent change in pretax net income from medical practice by specialty, 1965–96

Table 11.1.   Selected data on community hospitals, 1995

Table 11.2.   Trends in selected medical technologies provided by community hospitals, 1984 and 1994

Table 11.3.   Hospital cost growth in the United States by level of managed care penetration and hospital market competitiveness, 1986–93

Table 11.4.   Selected characteristics of community hospitals, measures of hospital costs and percentage rates of increase, 1960–95

Table 12.1.   Internal rates of return to male college graduates, physicians, dentists, and ratios of internal rates of return of physicians and dentists to male college graduates, United States, 1939, 1949, and 1956

Table 12.2.   Internal rates of return, all physicians and general practitioners, 1955–91

Table 12.3.   Number of physicians and physician/population ratios, United States, 1950–96

Table 12.4.   Ratio of applicants to acceptances, 1947–48 to 1995–96

Table 14.1.   Patterns of support for general operations of public and private medical schools, 1968–69, 1979–80, and 1994–95 (millions of dollars)

Table 14.2.   U.S. medical school enrollment, first-year students and graduates, 1946–47 to 1995–97

Table 14.3.   Average family incomes, average higher education subsidies received, and average state taxes paid by families, by type of California higher education institution, 1964–65

Table 14.4.   Family income of medical students, all U.S. families, by control of medical school, 1974–75

Table 15.1.   Number and distribution of active registered nurses by place of employment, 1996

Table 15.2.   Vacancy rates in hospitals for general-duty nurses

Table 15.3.   Ratio of all registered nurses' and hospital general-duty negistered nurses' salaries to those of teachers and female professional, technical, and kindred workers

Table 15.4.   Ratio of RNs to LPNs in nonfederal short-term general and other special hospitals

Table 16.1.   Major federal government expenditures on health services, 1977

Table 17.1.   Determining the redistributive effects of government programs

Table 17.2.   Health policy objectives and interventions

Table 17.3.   Health Policy Objectives under Different Theories of Government

Table 18.1.   Medicare reimbursements for covered services under the supplementary medical insurance program and persons served, by income, 1968 and 1977

Table 18.2. Persons served and Medicare reimbursement per person served, by race, 1988 and 1995

Table 18.3. Average physician visits for the elderly, by health status and family income, adjusted for other determinants, 1969 and 1977

Table 18.4. Employer contributions to health benefit plans and employee tax benefits, 1994

Table 18.5. Health insurance coverage and employment status of the civilian noninstitutionalized population under age sixty-five, 1996

Table 18.6. Total population of workers ages sixteen to sixty-four and uninsured workers: Percent distribution by selected characteristics, United States, 1996

Table 19.1. Percent of the aged requiring long-term care services, 1987

Table 19.2. Percent increase in U.S. population for ten-year intervals by age groups: Selected years and projections, 1970–2020

Table 19.3. Percent distribution of helper days, by sex and relationship to individuals sixty-five years of age or over with limitations to activities of daily living, 1982

Table 19.4. Percent distribution of personal health care expenditures per capita for people sixty-five years of age or over, by source of funds and type of service: United States, 1987

Table 19.5. Estimates of total money income for elderly individuals and elderly families in 1995

Table 19.6. Expenditures for nursing home care, 1960–95

LIST OF FIGURES

1.1.   Marginal benefit curves of a single commodity, (A) different commodities (B).

1.2.   The quantity–quality trade-off in medical care.

2.1A   The relationship between total output and program size.

2.1B   Marginal effects on health with a change in program size.

2.2.   Average and marginal benefits from alternative health programs.

3.1.   An overview of the medical care sector.

3.2.   An economic model of the medical care sector: the market for medical care services (A); the markets for institutional services (B); the markets for health manpower (C); the markets for health professional education (D).

3.3.   The effect on prices and medical services of an increase in demand when there are different supply elasticities.

3.4.   Alternative demand and supply policies to achieve a redistribution of medical care.

5.1.   Need versus demand as the basis for planning in medical care.

5.2.   Summing individual demands to obtain market demand.

5.3.   The effect of co-insurance on the demand for medical care.

5.4.   Insurance as a shift in the aggregate demand for medical care.

5.5.   The effect of co-insurance on the aggregate demand for medical care with a rising supply curve.

6.1.   The expected distribution of family medical expenses with different types of co-payments; (A) the imposition of a deductible; (B) a co-insurance provision; (C) a maximum or limit to coverage.

6.2.   The relationship between total utility and wealth: (A) diminishing marginal utility with increased wealth; (B) expected utility.

6.3.   The amount above the pure premium an individual is willing to pay for health insurance: according to different probabilities of the event occurring (A); according to different magnitudes of the expected loss (B).

6.4.   The relationship between price of insurance and quantity demanded.

6.5.   Adverse selection.

6.6.   The demand for medical care under conditions of moral hazard.

6.7.   The effect of (A) co-insurance and (B) deductibles on the demand for medical care.

6.8.   The effect of health insurance on the expected distribution of medical expenses among families.

6.9.   The allocative inefficiency of Blue Cross's service benefit policy.

6.10. Fringe benefits versus money income.

6.11. The effect on hospital utilization of insuring out-of-hospital services: (A) hospital utilization, (B) home health visits.

7.1.   The effect of different supply elasticities on the price, quality, and cost of national health insurance.

7.2.   The industry and the firm under long-run competitive equilibrium.

8.1.   The determinants of health insurance premiums

9.1.   Allocation of HMO premiums.

10.1. The market for physician services.

10.2. Monopolistic competitive market for physician services.

10.3. The impact of insurance on physician services.

10.4. An illustration of the target-income hypothesis.

10.5. The effect of advertising on the elasticity of demand and on the firm's pricing strategy.

10.6. The effect of differences in physicians' practice styles on procedure use rates.

10.7. Physician decision whether to accept Medicare assignment.

11.1. Variations in average cost between hospitals.

11.2. Hospital concentration in metropolitan statistical areas, 1995.

11.3. Price and output policies of a profit-making hospital.

11.4. The effect of increases in hospital quality on hospital costs .

11.5. A production function for medical care.

11.6. Hospital cost-shifting.

11.7. The effects of Medicare on hospital use, by age group.

12.1. Alternative policy prescriptions based on a normative shortage of health manpower.

12.2. A shortage created by restriction of supply.

12.3. An economic shortage.

12.4. The market for physician services and for an individual physician firm.

12.5.   An increase in foreign medical graduates on physician earnings and consumer benefit.

13.1.   Determination of price and output by a profit-making monopolist.

13.2.   Determination of prices and outputs by a price-discriminating monopolist.

14.1.   The excess demand for a medical education.

14.2.   An illustration of external benefits in medical education.

15.1.   The market for registered nurses.

15.2.   A dynamic shortage in the market for registered nurses.

15.3.   RN vacancy rates, annual percent changes in real RN wages, and the national unemployment rate, 1979–96.

15.4.   An illustration of a monopsonistic market for registered nurses.

15.5.   Collective bargaining and a monopsony market for registered nurses.

15.6.   Percent distribution of nursing graduates by type of nursing school program and average annual change in total graduates, 1960–96.

16.1.   Externalities in production and consumption: (A) a case of external costs, (B) a case of external benefits.

18.1.   Demand curves of different income groups.

18.2.   Equal treatment for equal needs through a system of negative prices.

18.3.   The cost of different demand subsidies when supply of medical care is relatively inelastic.

18.4.   The burden of a tax on labor is the same regardless of who pays the tax: (A) employees pay the tax, (B) employers pay the tax.

18.5.   The burden of a tax on labor according to different elasticities of demand for labor: (A) less elastic demand for labor, (B) more elastic demand for labor.

18.6.   The burden of a tax on labor according to different elasticities of labor supply: (A) inelastic supply of labor, (B) more elastic supply of labor.

19.1.   Distribution of elderly decedents who used nursing homes.

19.2.   A model of pricing and output for private-pay and Medicaid patients by a proprietary nursing home.

19.3.   An increase in private-pay demand in a nursing home serving private-pay and Medicaid patients.

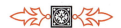

CHAPTER

An Introduction to the Economics of Medical Care

TRENDS IN MEDICAL EXPENDITURES

Expenditures on personal medical services have risen more rapidly than expenditures on most other goods and services in the economy. Annual expenditures on personal medical services increased from $35 billion in 1965 to $879 billion in 1995. In 1965, 5 percent of the gross national product (GNP) was being spent on *personal* medical services (see Table 1.1). By 1995, 12.1 percent of the GNP was being allocated to *personal* medical services. Total medical expenditures were approximately $988 billion in 1995 and comprised 13.7 percent of GNP. The difference between personal and total medical expenditures, about $110 billion, represents expenses for prepayment and administration ($48 billion), government public health activities ($31 billion), and research and construction of medical facilities ($31 billion).

While the rate of increase in personal medical expenditures has slowed during the 1990s (to approximately 9 percent per year compared to almost 13 percent annually), medical expenditures continue to increase at a faster rate than inflation and are continuing to consume an increasing portion of all goods and services produced in the United States.

Part of the increase in personal medical care expenditures is the result of increases in the population receiving such services. The population, however, has been growing at less

TABLE 1.1 Trends in Personal Medical Care Expenditures, 1950–95

Calendar Year	Total (Billions)	Average Annual % Inc. Total	% of GNP	Annual % Inc. Per Capita Total	Annual % Inc. in CPI Medical Care	Private Expend. (Billions)	Average Annual % Inc. Private	% of Total	Public Expend.	Average Annual % Inc. Public	% of Total	Federal Expend. (Billions)	Average Annual % Inc. Federal	State and Local Expend. (Billions)	Average Annual % Inc. State
1950	$10.9		3.8			$8.5		78.0	$2.4		22.0	$1.1		$1.3	
1955	15.7	8.8	3.9	6.4	3.8	12.1	8.5	77.1	3.6	10.0	22.9	1.6	9.1	2.0	10.8
1960	23.6	10.1	4.7	7.6	4.1	18.5	10.6	78.4	5.1	8.3	21.6	2.1	6.3	3.0	10.0
1965	35.2	9.8	5.1	7.7	2.6	27.9	10.2	79.5	7.3	8.6	20.8	3.0	8.6	4.3	8.7
1970	63.8	16.3	6.4	14.5	7.0	41.3	9.6	64.7	22.5	41.6	35.3	14.7	78.0	7.8	16.3
1975	114.5	15.9	7.4	14.1	7.9	69.2	13.5	60.4	45.3	50.3	39.6	30.9	22.0	14.4	16.9
1980	217.0	17.9	7.9	16.0	11.5	130.0	17.6	59.9	87.0	18.4	40.1	63.4	21.0	23.6	12.8
1985	376.4	14.7	9.3	13.1	10.3	228.5	15.1	60.7	148.0	14.0	39.3	111.3	15.1	36.7	11.1
1990	614.7	12.7	11.0	11.2	8.7	371.7	12.5	60.5	243.0	12.8	39.5	178.1	12.0	64.9	15.4
1995	878.8	8.6	12.1	7.2	7.1	486.7	6.2	55.4	392.1	12.3	44.6	303.6	14.1	88.5	7.3

Sources: U.S. Department of Health and Human Services, Health Care Financing Administration, Internet site http://www.hcfa.gov/stats/nhce96.htm, and unpublished data, 1996; U.S. Bureau of the Census, *Statistical Abstract of the United States* (Washington, D.C.: U.S. Department of Commerce), various editions: 1985, 105th ed., Table 714, 1996, 116th ed., Table 2, 691, 745.

Note: "Personal medical care expenditure" is equal to total health care expenditures less expenditures for prepayment and administration, government public health activities, and research and contruction of medical facilities.

than 1 percent (0.9) per year. Thus, when we adjust for such population increases by examining expenditures on a per capita basis, we find that the annual percentage increase in per capita medical expenditures over the past twenty-five years is still very close to the annual percentage increase in total personal medical expenditures.

Not all of the increase in medical expenditures represents an increase in the quantity of services per capita. A substantial part of the expenditure increase has been due to an increase in prices for the same services, as well as a change in the type of services and in their quality. As shown in Table 1.1, the price of medical care, as measured by the medical care component of the consumer price index, has increased quite rapidly.

To better understand the changes that have occurred in medical care it is important to have an historical perspective on this industry. There have been important economic and legislative developments that have changed demands for care, the costs of providing that care, and patient and provider incentives.

In 1966, the passage of Medicare and Medicaid produced dramatic changes in the medical sector. Medicare is a federal program for financing the medical services of the aged; Medicaid is a federal–state financing program for the medically indigent. With the enactment of these two programs, the aged and the poor had increased access to medical care. Hospitals were paid according to their costs and physicians received their usual and customary fees. As a result of Medicare and Medicaid, the price of medical care increased at a faster pace than previously. The role of government as a payer of medical services increased dramatically, from paying 20 percent of medical expenditures before 1966 to 45 percent currently, with the federal government paying three-fourths of that amount.

Adding to the removal of patient incentives to be concerned with the cost of their care was the rapid growth in private medical insurance. The rise in the rate of inflation in the economy and the high federal marginal tax brackets (up to 70 percent) provided employees with an incentive to substitute their cash income for nontaxable fringe benefits. The consequence was that the aged (Medicare), the poor (Medicaid), and middle- and high-income employees (employer-paid health insurance) increased the use of medical services and became less concerned with medical prices.

Hospital and physician prices began to increase more rapidly, as did expenditures on medical services. As both private insurance and government payments lessened the financial burden on the patient, there were few constraints on the use of services and prices charged by providers. This acceleration in medical prices continued until the early 1970s, when federal price controls (the Economic Stabilization Program) were imposed on the economy. Although the price controls were removed after a year, they remained in place for the medical sector from 1971 until 1974. After the removal of those price controls, medical prices rose rapidly. As the economy-wide rate of inflation increased in the late 1970s, so did the rise in medical prices.

The federal and state governments became alarmed as they saw their expenditures under Medicare and Medicaid exceed their budgets for these two programs. Regulatory programs, such as controls on hospital capital, were enacted to hold down the rise in medical expenditures. A number of states instituted hospital rate controls. However, by the late 1970s, it was clear that the regulatory programs were not working.

With a deep recession and consequent strong import competition in the early 1980s, business and labor also became concerned about the rapid increases in employees' health insurance premiums. And then in the 1980s, to the surprise of most health care experts, the medical care market became price-competitive.

Excess capacity among hospitals and physicians, new federal hospital payment systems, and new organizational forms for delivering medical services emerged. The structure of the medical care market changed as consolidation occurred among insurance companies, hospital mergers increased, and the size of physician groups increased. Previous concern with overutilization of medical services changed to a concern that access to care was being decreased, as providers faced new payment incentives. And as market competition became more widespread, access to medical care by the poor decreased as federal and state governments became concerned with balancing their budgets. Public policy shifted from an emphasis on redistribution in the 1960s to constraining of medical expenditures.

THE CONTRIBUTION OF ECONOMICS TO HEALTH POLICY

Government policy should be concerned with achieving two objectives: improvement of market efficiency and, based on society's values, redistribution of resources or services. Market efficiency is typically concerned with improving the performance of an industry, such as eliminating anticompetitive elements so that an industry is more competitive. It includes issues of consumer protection in a particular industry, such as when consumers have insufficient information to make informed choices. And it also includes "externalities," as when an industry produces pollution in the process of producing its product and the cost of that product does not reflect all its costs, including pollution.

The objective of redistribution of services is based on society's value judgment that those with higher incomes should be taxed to provide for those with lower incomes. The extent of redistribution is highly controversial. The economist's role with regard to redistribution policy is not to substitute her values for those of others, but to evaluate which approach is more efficient (less costly) for achieving a given set of values.

"Positive" economic analysis attempts to determine the consequences of a particular policy and which groups benefit and which groups bear the burden of that policy. "Normative" analysis states which policies should be implemented. The contribution of economics is with respect to positive analysis, which is also the emphasis of this book.

The basic premise underlying all economic analysis is the concept of rational choice. Consumers and producers are assumed to weigh the costs and benefits of different courses of action in order to choose the most preferred alternative. Choice is necessary because there are inadequate resources to satisfy all of our wants. At times the scarce resource is time itself, which forces one to choose among alternative uses of time. Since resources and time can be used in alternative ways, it becomes necessary to choose among alternative uses of those scarce resources. Implicit in the discussion of choice is that individuals, on average, are assumed to act rationally.

Problems of scarcity and, consequently, choice, are the basis for the development and use of the economist's two basic tools and a set of criteria with which to analyze issues of efficiency and distribution.

The first tool is marginal analysis, which underlies all optimization problems. Optimization techniques specify the appropriate criteria to be used when allocating scarce resources so as to minimize the cost of producing a given output or, similarly, maximize output, subject to a budget constraint. Techniques of optimization can be used, for example, to determine which set of health manpower, given their relative productivity and wages, are least costly for producing a given medical service or whether one combination of institutional settings is less costly than another for treating particular types of patients. Similarly, marginal analysis can be used by governments and other organizations to determine the most efficient allocation of medical and nonmedical resources to achieve a given objective, such as an improvement in the health status of the population.

The second economic tool is supply and demand analysis, which is used for predicting new equilibrium situations, such as predicting the effect of a change in demand for a service or in its cost of production on the price and quantity of that service. Supply and demand analysis makes it possible to understand the reasons for the rapid increases in medical care prices and expenditures; it also enables us to predict future prices and expenditures. Supply and demand analysis can also estimate the consequences, in price, quantity of service, and total expenditure, of redistributive policies to increase medical services in the population, such as through national health insurance.

These two tools, marginal analysis (optimization techniques) and supply and demand analysis (predicting new equilibrium situations), are interrelated. Demand analysis is based on the assumption that in allocating their resources, consumers try to maximize their satisfaction, subject to a budget constraint (their income and prices—including time prices). By choosing how to allocate their scarce resources (income and time) across different goods and services, given their prices, consumers attempt to "optimize." If a consumer's income or prices change, this will cause a change in the demand for particular services. Similarly, the supply of a service is based on the assumption that producers attempt to maximize their output while having to choose among using different inputs, each having different prices, subject to an overall budget constraint. A change in any aspect of the consumer's or producer's budget constraint will, because each is assumed to optimize, cause changes in the demand for and supply of different goods and services. A change in consumer preferences or in the productivity of different inputs, will, through the optimization process, also result in changes in demand and supply.

Implicit in the use of the foregoing analytical tools is a set of criteria for evaluating economic welfare. These welfare criteria are used to determine whether someone is made better or worse off as a result of a particular action or policy. These criteria also make it possible to evaluate the performance of an industry. Public policy is based on the values held by individuals and their perception of the most efficient method for achieving the given set of values. A specific set of welfare criteria provides the means by which differences in values and differences in methods for achieving a set of values can be separately evaluated.

BASIC CHOICES THAT MUST BE MADE WITH REGARD TO MEDICAL SERVICES

The economist's skill in using marginal analysis (optimization techniques) and supply and demand analysis, under conditions of scarcity, and the economist's criteria for evaluating economic performance are useful and necessary regardless of how medical care is organized and provided in a country. Given that resources are scarce, three basic decisions must be made in any medical system, regardless of whether they are made by consumers or by government.

Every country must decide (a) how much it wants to spend on medical services (and the composition of those services), (b) the best methods for producing medical services, and, (c) the method for distributing medical services among the population. The first two choices are concerned with issues of economic efficiency (in consumption and in production); the third, with equity in use of health services.

A discussion of the possible choices for each of the above decisions should clarify whether disagreement over which choice should be selected is based on differences in values or varying perspectives on the method of achieving an agreed-on set of values. In the following discussion of these three sets of medical care decisions, the economic tools discussed above will be used to illustrate the usefulness of economics both in clarifying and in making choices.

Determining the Output of Medical Services

The first set of medical care decisions to be made is referred to as the determination of output: How much should be allocated to, and what should be the composition of, medical services? In a medical system that relies on a price system for resource allocation, consumer and physician decisions determine the quantity and quality of medical services. Theoretically, the consumer selects those services which, given his income and the prices of different services, maximize satisfaction. It is assumed that consumers make such choices rationally (they consider the costs and benefits of their choices) and that they have information on both the benefits derived from different services and the prices of those services. If these assumptions are correct, consumers will allocate their scarce resources (both time and income) to those services and activities that provide them with the greatest amount of benefits. The accuracy of these assumptions with respect to medical services are discussed below.

To understand the allocation process used by consumers when selecting among various commodities, including both goods and services, and also to be able to predict changes in consumer allocation, it is necessary to understand marginal analysis, which is the basis of the optimization technique. Consumers' purchases provide them with benefits, or utility; additional purchases of those same services provide additional benefits, but these additional benefits decline as more units are purchased. The benefits derived from consuming the first unit of a commodity are high; subsequent units of that same commodity provide smaller benefits. Although total benefits increase with additional units of the same commodity, the marginal benefit of additional units declines. This relationship between marginal benefits and additional units of a service is shown in Figure 1.1A. The marginal benefit from consuming $0A$ units of the particular commodity represented in Figure 1.1A is MB_1. If additional units are consumed, the marginal benefit received from those additional units declines, from MB_1 to MB_2.

The consumer receives benefits from many different commodities. To maximize the total benefits from all commodities purchased, the consumer will allocate his limited resources to ensure that the marginal benefits received from all commodities purchased are equal.[1] This optimization rule for equating the marginal benefits of the last units of different commodities does not mean that the same number of units of each commodity will be consumed. It is more likely that when the marginal benefits of different commodities are equal, the buyer will be consuming differing quantities of the commodities purchased. The reason is that the marginal benefits decline at different rates for different commodities. The consumer is likely to purchase more units of those commodities with a gradual decline in marginal benefits than those with a very sharp decline. As shown in Figure 1.1B, the marginal benefits are equal at MB_0 for different commodities when the consumer is purchasing $0A$ units, $0B$ units, and $0C$ units of three different commodities. Any other allocation process would result in a lower total level of benefits. The consumer therefore maximizes the amount of benefits for a given income by allocating it across commodities to ensure that the marginal benefits from the last units are equal.

To allow for differences in commodity prices, the consumer must compare not only the marginal benefits of different commodities but also the ratio of the marginal benefit to the price of each commodity (MB/P). When this is done, *the marginal benefit per dollar spent will be equal for all commodities.* (It should be noted that the marginal benefits received from the purchase of a commodity vary among consumers. These differences are illustrated in Figure 1.1B. The marginal benefit curves in this case represent the marginal benefits received from the same commodity by different consumers.)

The consumer evaluates the marginal benefits of a purchase in relation to its price, or stated differently, the consumer compares the ratio of marginal benefit to marginal cost for each purchase with the ratio of every other purchase. The marginal cost to the consumer is the price she must pay for that commodity. When the consumer has equated the

---

[1]For the sake of simplicity, it is here assumed that the prices of the different commodities are equal.

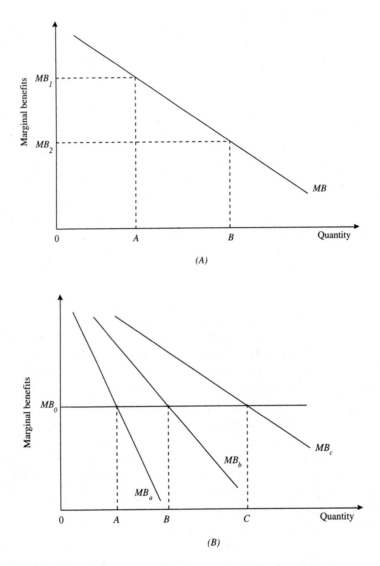

FIGURE 1-1 Marginal benefit curves of (A) a single commodity,
(B) different commodities.

marginal benefits and the marginal costs of each purchase, her scarce resources have been allocated to maximize total benefits. In an equilibrium situation, when the quantity demanded equals the quantity supplied, the equilibrium price reflects the value placed on the last units purchased by all consumers since all consumers face the same price in a given market. In a competitive market, prices represent the costs of production. The costs of production in turn reflect the value of other goods and services that might have been produced with the same resources. When an efficient price system is used for allocating resources, the marginal benefits to consumers of purchasing the last unit equal the marginal costs of the resources used to produce it.

Any of the following changes in factors affecting consumers' allocation decisions would cause a change in their purchasing behavior: a change in the price of one commodity relative to the prices of other commodities, a change in income, or a change in perception of the benefits to be derived from consuming additional units. The optimization technique (marginal analysis) enables consumers to allocate resources so as to maximize their benefits. This technique also provides the basis for understanding changes in consumer demand. It is in this way that the two tools of economics—optimization techniques and the determination of equilibrium situations—are related.[2]

The above description of the consumer choice process in a market system illustrates the importance of price in making choices. A nonmarket approach to determining the amount of resources to be allocated to medical care requires a substitute mechanism that will perform the price function—that is, will provide an incentive to consumers to limit their use of services to the point at which the cost of those services equals their value. Such a mechanism must also ration the available quantity of services among consumers and provide information to providers of changes in their demand. Although the functions that prices perform must still be performed in a nonprice system, alternative mechanisms to perform these functions have been found to be unsatisfactory.

How Best to Produce Medical Services

The second set of decisions that must be made in any health system is selection of the best method for producing the amount of medical services (of constant quality) to be provided. Medical services can be provided in different organizational settings, including health maintenance organizations (HMOs) or solo practitioners practicing under a fee-for-service arrangement. Even within a particular delivery system, the combination of health personnel and equipment can vary. If the providers of medical services have an incentive to minimize their costs, they will use the various inputs—health personnel and capital—according to their relative costs and productivity. The method of optimization used by the provider will be similar to that used by the consumer of medical services. In place of marginal benefits and relative prices on the consumer side, marginal productivity of inputs

---

[2]This discussion of marginal analysis is not meant to imply that *every* consumer continuously undertakes an exact system of calculation for purchasing all commodities. Consumers, on average, do consider such factors as marginal benefits, relative prices, and their level of income when making their purchase decisions. While economic models also include noneconomic variables, such as psychological and sociological variables, as predictors of consumer behavior, these variables do not change as frequently or rapidly as do the economic variables. Thus, to the extent that consumers have information and act to maximize their total benefits, predictions based on changes in relative prices and income will result in more accurate predictions of consumer demand than will other (e.g., psychological or sociological) models of consumer behavior that exclude such economic variables.

and their relative costs will be used by providers to determine the least costly method of providing a service. The decision rule will also be the same. When the ratio of the marginal productivity of an input to its wage is equal to that of other inputs, the firm is minimizing its costs of providing medical services.

When the provider's costs are minimized, the combination of services (hospital, physician services, and home care) and the inputs (types of health personnel and capital) used to provide medical care will be both technically and economically efficient. Technical efficiency means that the inputs used will produce the maximum quantity of medical services. However, several different combinations of inputs may be technically efficient. To minimize the cost of providing medical services, it is necessary to be not only technically but also economically efficient. The decision maker must choose among the several combinations of inputs, each of which is technically efficient, to determine which combination is also economically efficient—that is, least costly. To do so, the decision maker must consider the relative costs of the different inputs as well as their productivities.

When the economist applies the optimization tools to the set of choices governing the production of medical services, several problems of medical services delivery are brought into sharper focus. Some medical professionals have proposed the use of standards in the delivery of medical services: four hospital beds per thousand population was one such standard; specified lengths of stay, by diagnosis, for hospitalized patients is another example; and ratios of the number of registered nurses per hospitalized patients is a third. Standards such as these imply that medical services can or should be produced by only one method. If the provision of medical services was actually subject to such fixed proportions, no choice of production methods would exist, and the effectiveness of the economist's tools for minimizing medical care costs would be very limited. It is, however, unlikely that the choices for producing medical care are so limited.

Depending on the illness being treated, ambulatory care and nursing home services can be substituted for hospital care, with no decrease in the quality of treatment. Lengths of stay can be varied depending on the availability of other facilities in the community and someone to care for the patient at home. Other kinds of nursing personnel can substitute for registered nurses in the care of hospitalized patients. Presently, wide variations exist across communities in lengths of stay by diagnosis, in use of registered nurses, and in number of hospital beds per thousand population. Substituting medical services and personnel without a decrease in overall quality is more possible than some would have us believe.

Using specific standards as described above, when substitution is possible, will hinder economic efficiency in providing medical care. Using inputs without regard to their relative costs is unlikely to result in the least-cost combination. As the relative costs (and productivities) of inputs change over time, it is to be expected that the combination of inputs that is least costly for providing medical services will change also. The economist's tools of optimization can determine which combination of services and inputs is most efficient for providing medical care. Similarly, the concepts embodied in these tools provide a decision maker with vital information about the costs of different choices, which can be used to decide how best to deliver medical services.

The second of the economist's tools, the prediction of new equilibrium levels of prices and quantities, flows from the optimization technique and can be used to anticipate changes in the production of medical services. A change in the price of an input will, as discussed above, result in a change in the combination of inputs that is least costly to use in producing medical care. It is also possible to analyze the new equilibrium situation that will result from that change. An increase in the price of an input will cause a reduction in the quantity demanded of it and an increase in demand for those inputs whose prices have not changed. If the higher-priced inputs are used mainly in the provision of one type of service, such as hospital care, we would then expect to observe a reduction in the quantity demanded of that service because its price has risen as its inputs have become more costly. As the cost of medical services increases, the supply curve of medical care will shift to the left. Assuming no change in the demand for medical services, the price of medical care will increase and the quantity demanded will decrease. The extent of the actual change in prices and quantities of medical care will depend on the elasticities of supply and demand.

The tools of demand and supply can be used to trace the consequences of a change in input prices throughout the medical system. They can also be used to anticipate the effects of changes in medical technology on productivity, medical prices, and quantities of services. Such equilibrium analyses are particularly helpful in anticipating future expenditures for medical care to be borne either by patients or by the government, such as those that would occur under a system of national health insurance.

The Distribution of Medical Services

The third set of decisions that must be made in any medical system governs the distribution of the system's output. Medical services can be provided free of charge to all persons, or they can be distributed in accordance with consumers' willingness to spend their incomes for it. Subsidies can be provided to those persons whose incomes are insufficient to purchase the amount of medical care society deems appropriate and necessary.

Economics can clarify the issues involved in the distribution of medical services by using criteria for determining whether a person's welfare is improved by a particular policy. If the purpose of that policy is to improve the person's welfare, economic criteria will suggest the most efficient means for accomplishing that goal. Two value judgments govern the distribution of medical services. The first is whether consumers should determine the amount they wish to spend on medical services. The second concerns the method and size of subsidy to be extended to those low-income consumers whose use of medical services is below what society believes it should be. The economist cannot decide which set of values is preferable; however, economics can help make the process of choosing more rational by providing information on the costs and the implications of different sets of values, and also by providing criteria for determining the most efficient method for achieving a given set of values.

Chapter 18 contains a more complete discussion of the different values underlying the subsidies designed to redistribute medical services in the population. It also contains an analysis of the economic efficiency of existing methods of financing medical services as well as of those proposed under alternative approaches to national health insurance.

THE APPLICABILITY OF ECONOMICS TO THE STUDY OF MEDICAL CARE

Critics have questioned the applicability of economics to the study of medical services on two levels: first, they have questioned the accuracy of assumptions underlying economic behavior of consumers and medical providers, and second, they have challenged the implicit values, such as consumer sovereignty, that influence the goal to be achieved (i.e., consumer satisfaction). For example, critics have claimed that it is inaccurate to assume that the consumer of health services is rational and that she has sufficient information when deciding on use of services. Such critics also claim that the purchaser of medical services is not the consumer, as in nonmedical markets, but the physician, who also has a financial interest in the services purchased. With regard to economists' traditional assumptions about providers of medical services, critics claim that these providers are organized as nonprofit organizations and therefore do not have the same motivations as for-profit firms in other industries. Further, since consumers may be irreparably harmed by incompetent providers, more stringent controls must be exercised over the provision of medical services than over nonmedical goods and services. Finally, such critics claim that access to medical services is considered a right by society and its distribution cannot be left solely to the marketplace.

It is important to distinguish between criticism directed at the validity of economic assumptions and criticism of the use of economic criteria for evaluating medical system performance. If economic analyses are undertaken, they will be based on a given set of assumptions, which will lead us to predict a certain outcome. If the observed behavior is different from what would be expected in a competitive market, the assumptions are reexamined to determine whether a different assumption can explain the divergence between the expected and observed behavior.

For example, one factor affecting the performance of an industry is whether entry of new firms (providers) is permitted. An economic analysis would initially assume that there are no barriers to entry in a market, such as home care services. Based on this assumption, we expect to observe certain measures of market performance; high profits to home health agencies would lead to increased entry by new home health agencies until profits are similar to what can be earned in other industries. If what we observe is different from what we have predicted, we then examine whether the free-entry assumption (entry of new home health agencies) is accurate. Public policy prescriptions attempt to make structural changes, for example, reduce entry barriers, that will bring an industry's performance into greater conformity with its expected performance. Thus, economic analysis isolates those assumptions to be reexamined when a divergence occurs between expected and observed behaviors.

For each of the aspects of medical care to be analyzed in this book, the expected performance of consumers and providers is contrasted to observed performance. When a divergence exists, the underlying assumptions are reexamined to account for the observed behavior. The specific assumptions regarding consumer information, incentives for efficiency, and barriers to entry are examined to determine what effect they have on the economic performance of the medical care sector when they differ from their theoretical assumptions.

Medical care is acknowledged to be different from other markets because it includes a greater demand for consumer protection. However, different approaches to providing consumer protection are available. These alternative approaches, together with other, possibly unique, aspects of medical care are analyzed with respect to their impact on the performance of the medical care sector.

Criticisms of the values underlying the use of economic criteria for evaluating medical system performance are more difficult to resolve. Given a scarcity in the availability of resources for providing medical services, what criteria should society use for making the three basic medical care decisions? A medical system that values economic efficiency in consumption and production will base its choice of the amount to spend on medical services on the criterion of satisfying consumer preferences; it will base its method of providing services on the criterion of least cost; and it will base its choice of the amount and method of medical services redistribution on the criterion of consumer preference. Under this value system, medical service benefits are defined by consumer preference rather than by government or health agency perception of consumer preference.

If decision makers reject the above criteria, new criteria must be specified. The criterion of efficiency in production is more likely to be acceptable than is the criterion of satisfying consumer preferences. Some prefer a "needs" approach to the allocation of medical services, which relies on centrally determined resource allocations. However, because resources are insufficient to satisfy all medical needs, an additional decision rule must be developed that will enable the decision makers to choose which needs and which population groups will be given highest priority.

The replacement of one set of values by another does not diminish the usefulness of economics in the decision-making process; its value lies in its ability to make that process more explicit by showing what the costs of different choices are. To the extent that economic analysis can clarify the costs of alternatives and make the values underlying those alternatives explicit, it is a useful approach to the study of medical care.

THE TRADE-OFF BETWEEN QUANTITY AND QUALITY IN THE PROVISION OF MEDICAL SERVICES

The three basic choices that must be made with regard to medical services are illustrated in Figure 1.2, which represents a production possibilities curve. This curve shows the trade-off between two different goods or outputs, for example, quantity and quality of medical services. The curve is shaped as it is (concave to the origin) because the resources

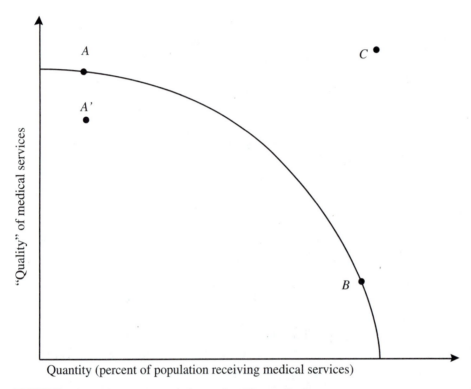

FIGURE 1.2 • The quantity–quality trade-off in medical care.

used in producing quantity and quality (each of which is a different output) are not completely substitutable for one another. As more of one combination of services is produced (as represented by point *A* or *B*), the resources are switched from producing one type of service to producing the other. The released resources are more specialized, hence more efficient, in producing their previous output. Moving those same resources into the production of a different good or service will cause them to be less efficient in the production of that new service. Thus, the costs of producing more of the new output are increased.

The first choice that must be made in any medical system is what types of medical services are to be produced, for example, what combination of quantity and quality of medical services. If the length of training of health professionals is long, and if the equipment and facilities used are the most technically advanced, fewer services will be available to the entire population. Point *A* represents a combination where quality (which actually refers to the level of training of health professionals—a process measure, not an outcome measure, of quality) is relatively high and is received by a small percentage of the population. Point *B* represents a different combination: a large percentage of the population receives some medical services, while the quality of those services is relatively low.

What criterion should determine the combination of quality and quantity of medical services that a society should choose? If the criterion were the maximizing of consumer preferences, then, assuming adequate information and proper safeguards, consumers would be the appropriate group to select the quantity–quality combination that should prevail.[3] Alternatively, health professionals can select the quantity–quality trade-off, as they have done in the United States. For example, health professionals establish the educational requirements and determine the number of educational institutions through their accreditation policies. Less emphasis on process requirements and more on outcomes and testing would provide greater assurance of quality, at lower cost, hence greater quantity.

The discussion of the quantity–quality trade-off can also be used to illustrate the second set of choices that must be made in any medical care system—namely, how best to produce medical services. Any quantity–quality combination on the production possibilities curve is assumed to be produced in the least costly manner. The amount of resources devoted to medical services is represented by the area under the curve. If, owing to the placement of restrictions on the least costly manner of production or the use of a method of provider reimbursement that removes efficiency incentives, the providers of medical services are not as efficient as they might be, then fewer medical services will be produced for the same amount of resources. This situation is shown in Figure 1.2, where A' represents the same amount of resources as used at point A but the output is less than that achieved at point A. A' is obviously inefficient in that resources are being wasted; either more medical services or medical services of higher quality could be produced with the same quantity of resources. It is important to determine whether the current medical care system is at point A or A' and, if so, the reasons why.

The third set of choices concerning medical services distribution might be illustrated by a quantity–quality analysis of the statement, "All Americans should receive the highest quality of medical care." The highest quality of medical care to all would be represented by point C in Figure 1.2, which is equivalent to 100 percent of the population (farthest to the right on the horizontal axis), and by the highest point on the quality axis. To achieve such a goal, additional resources equivalent to the distance between point C and the current production possibilities curve would be required. These additional resources would be financed either by an increase in taxes or by decreased expenditures on other programs. These choices provide differing marginal benefits. Who is to decide their relative benefits? Health professionals attach greater benefits to medical as opposed to other services; however, they do not bear the costs of their decisions. Consumers, who will bear the costs, may not share professional estimates of the relative benefits.

---

[3]The resultant quantity–quality combination would maximize consumer satisfaction because the marginal benefits of those services (to the consumer) would equal the marginal cost of resources used in their production.

SUMMARY

Economics employs the optimization technique for the allocation of scarce resources to achieve a given objective. Supply and demand analysis, the second tool of economics, enables economists to predict new equilibrium situations, such as increased prices, quantities, and expenditures. The welfare criteria used by economists provide a means to judge whether people are made better or worse off as the result of a policy change.

The economist's tools and welfare criteria clarify the consequences of how society responds to three basic decisions: how much to spend on medical services, how best to produce those services, and how to distribute them. People differ in their values as to how those choices should be made. To evaluate how the medical system performs with respect to each of those choices, it is necessary to establish criteria for what is considered good performance. The performance criteria used by economists are based upon a set of values incorporated into their definition of economic efficiency—namely, maximizing consumer satisfaction and using the least costly method of production. If decision makers disagree over these values, it is necessary to state explicitly an alternative set of values. People can then decide whether they prefer one set of values over another. For any alternative set of values, it is also necessary to state the criteria to be used for evaluating the performance of the medical system. The debate over appropriate public policy in medical care is often confused because a clear distinction is not made between differences in values and differences in the best way to achieve a particular set of values. Clarification of these differences should sharpen the debate over the most appropriate public policies for medical care.

Key Terms and Concepts

- Economic efficiency
- Market efficiency
- Redistribution
- Technical efficiency

- Criteria for cost minimization
- Criteria for maximization
- Definition of rational choice
- Interrelationship of two tools of economics
- Optimization techniques (marginal analysis)
- Production possibilities curve
- Supply and demand analysis

Review Questions

1. Every economy, as well as the medical care sector, must decide the following: what should be produced, how it should be produced, how it should be distributed, and how to allow for growth and innovation. With respect to the medical care sector, how are these choices currently made? How have they changed over time? What are the assumptions and value judgments underlying each of these choices?
2. What are the two basic tools of economics? Give an example of each with respect to health, medical services, and hospitals.
3. Explain how the two tools of economics are interrelated.
4. Prices serve various purposes. For each purpose, give an application of the use of prices, or its lack thereof, in the medical care industry.
5. What are the economic criteria for an optimal rate of output? How well are these criteria met with respect to the medical care sector?

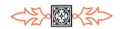

CHAPTER

The Production
of Health: The Impact
# of Medical Services
on Health

MEDICAL CARE AS AN OUTPUT OF THE MEDICAL SERVICES INDUSTRY AND AS AN INPUT TO HEALTH

The first of two alternative ways of looking at medical care is to regard it as the "output" produced by physicians, hospitals, and other providers in the medical care industry. When viewing medical care as an output, it is important to determine how efficiently it is produced. The combination of resources that can produce these services at least cost, for a given level of quality, should be used. Efficiency depends not only on the mix of inputs but also on the structure of the industry. A structural change might affect the productivity of certain inputs or their cost. For example, reorganizing physicians from solo practice into organized medical groups might make it possible to increase the productivity of physicians by producing more services with the same amount of labor. Changing the requirements for entering a health profession would affect the cost of that manpower input. Industry analyses of the factors affecting the supply of and demand for physician services, hospital care, and the various manpower markets enable us to infer the performance of the medical care industry; that is, we can compare the price and output of the industry as it now exists with the price and quantity (as well as quality) that might exist if the medical care industry underwent a structural change. When medical care is viewed as the output of the medical services industry, our understanding of the structure of that industry (and of its component industries) enables us to evaluate its performance.

The second way of looking at medical care is to view it, not as a final output, but as one input among many, all of which contribute to an output referred to as "good health." Improvements in health status may be achieved by providing medical services, undertaking medical research, instituting environmental health programs, such as those that control air pollution, or conducting health education programs aimed at changing the lifestyle of consumers.

The efficiency criterion is also important for determining the amount of resources to be allocated to the medical services sector if the objective is to increase health. It may be less costly to increase health levels by spending less on medical care and more on health education to improve diets and exercise. Viewing health levels as the output enables us to determine how resources should be allocated among different programs so as to improve health. The allocation question for improving health levels is different from determining the allocation of resources for producing medical care itself. These two ways of viewing medical care should be recognized explicitly, as each is useful for different public policies. To determine whether medical care is being produced efficiently, one must examine it as a final output; to determine the most efficient way to allocate resources to increase health, one must view medical services as one of several inputs for achieving that goal.

The second, or input, view will be adopted in the remainder of this chapter, which will first present a theoretical approach for determining how many resources should be allocated to medical care versus other inputs; second, empirical estimates of medical care's marginal contribution to increased health will be reviewed; and third, applications and implications of those findings will be discussed.

The concept of a health production function has become more relevant with the growth of health maintenance organizations and capitation-based payment systems. As HMOs seek to reduce the medical costs of their enrolled population, they have an incentive to seek the least expensive way to care for their enrollees. For example, to reduce the use of costly neonatal intensive care units for caring for low birthweight infants, HMOs have an incentive to provide prenatal care so that fewer low birthweight infants are born. Similarly, providing family planning services to their enrollees' teenagers is likely to reduce the number of pregnancies among a risk group likely to give birth to low birthweight infants.

Further, as employer coalitions place greater emphasis on their employees' health outcomes, HMOs are beginning to view medical services as only one input to produce that health outcome, and not necessarily the least costly way of doing so.

DETERMINING THE ALLOCATION OF RESOURCES TO MEDICAL CARE USING A HEALTH PRODUCTION FUNCTION

To determine the least costly input combination for achieving an increase in health levels, it is necessary to understand the concept of a "health production function." A production function describes the relationship between combinations of inputs and the resulting output. It is to be distinguished from a production possibility curve, which describes the trade-off between different outputs from a given set of resources. Health can be produced using different combinations of inputs. (It is assumed in empirical studies of health production functions that the estimated relationships are technically efficient; that is, the inputs produce the maximum possible output.) The economist and the policymaker, however, is interested in more than technical efficiency; they want to determine which combination of inputs is economically efficient—that is, least costly, for producing the output, health.

Before we can determine the least costly combination of inputs for producing a given level of health, the production function for health must be specified. Once specified, and estimates have been developed for the marginal effects of each of the inputs on health, comparisons can then be made between increasing expenditures on different inputs. The process of allocating resources to increase health can be improved once information becomes available on each program's (input's) effect on health status and on the relative cost of expanding each program.

Often the real intent of a program's expenditures may be inferred by determining the effect of its resources.

The first step in using a health production function for making allocation decisions is to state a specific function—that is, to define the output (or objective) to be achieved. Unless the desired output is explicitly defined, it will not be possible to state the alternative approaches for achieving that output, which is the second step. For example, if the objective is increased health of the population, the alternatives will also be fairly general: a better environment, improved nutrition, greater emphasis on preventive care, improved access to medical services, and better personal health habits. For policymakers and HMO managers, however, these alternative policies are not sufficiently specific to indicate which environmental, preventive, or medical care programs to undertake so as to have an impact on the health levels of specified population groups. Unless the health objective is defined by age and sex groupings (and probably location), it will not be possible to determine which project—a cancer screening program or a maternal and child health project—will have the greatest effect on health status.

Health professionals and others knowledgeable about health programs are best able to specify which programs are alternatives for increasing the health status of a particular age-sex population group. By using optimization tools (the third step), the economist can determine how to allocate limited health funds among alternative programs to achieve the largest possible increase in health status.

The discussion that follows illustrates the approach that should be used to allocate expenditures among alternative programs to achieve the maximum possible increase in the health objective.

Assume that the health objective is to decrease the infant mortality rate. On which programs should additional funds be spent? For illustrative purposes, assume that there are only two programs for reducing infant mortality rates: one is to establish additional intensive care units (ICUs) in selected hospitals for infants at high risk; the other is to increase funding for prenatal care to low-income expectant mothers. The following approach demonstrates the type of information and analysis required to determine how best to allocate limited funds between these two programs (1).

The relationship between spending additional funds on each program and their impact on infant mortality rates is assumed to be as shown in Figure 2.1A and B. The curve in Figure 2.1A represents the relationship between increased program expenditures or size of that program (on the horizontal axis) and the total effect (output) of those program inputs. When a program is relatively small, additional inputs devoted to that program are likely to result in relatively large increases in the program's output (decreased infant mortality rates). As additional resources are allocated to that program, total output will continue to increase, but at a more gradual rate. Finally, increases in output will become negligible even though the program's inputs continue to increase. The relationship between program inputs and program output is curvilinear because as additional intensive care units are established there is an insufficient number of high-risk infants to fill them. (Similar to the law of variable proportions or diminishing returns, the number of high-risk infants in a community are assumed to be the fixed factor.) Thus, with additional ICU units either the number of high-risk infants per ICU unit declines or lower-risk infants will be admitted. In either case, improvements in infant mortality rates become smaller.

Initial prenatal care programs are likely to provide care for those patients most likely to benefit from them. As more resources are devoted to prenatal care, it either becomes more costly to find recipients who will benefit most from these programs, or the program begins to include recipients whose need is not as great. In either case, the additional health improvement per unit of input begins to decline as the size of the program is increased.

It is thus inappropriate to assume that there is a constant (i.e., linear) relationship between a program's inputs and its output. Additional resources spent on health programs are unlikely to produce the same increase in output as did previous increases in the program's expenditures.

Since the relationship between total program output and program input is curvilinear, as shown in Figure 2.1A, it must be determined at which point on that total output curve a particular program is operating. If the size of the program is relatively large, as shown

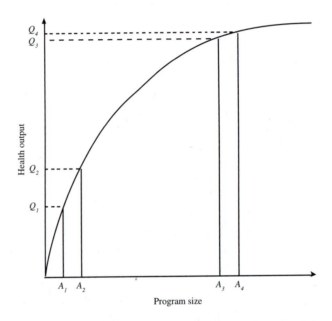

FIGURE 2.1A • The relationship between total output and program size.

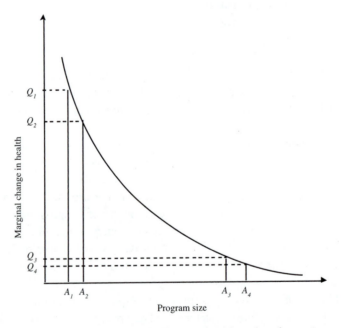

FIGURE 2.1B • Marginal effects on health with a change in program size.

by point A_3, then adding resources equivalent to A_3–A_4 will result in an increase in total output of the magnitude Q_3–Q_4. If the program is smaller-for example, at size A_1—the same increase in program resources will result in a larger increase in total program output, from Q_1 to Q_2. (For simplicity, it is assumed that both programs have the same curve as shown in Figure 2.1A. In reality, each program will have a different curve, although each curve will have the same curvilinear shape.)

Figure 2.1B is another way of showing the relationship between a program's inputs and output as the size of the program is increased. The curve shown in Figure 2.1B is the slope of the total output curve shown in Figure 2.1A; thus, it shows the marginal change in output as inputs are increased. These marginal relationships, which reflect the change in total output resulting from a unit increase in a program's inputs, eventually decline with increased program size for the same reason that the total output curve shown in Figure 2.1A increases at a decreasing rate.

Still using the simplified example, if it costs the same to increase the inputs in two health programs, but one program (e.g., the intensive care unit program) is at size A_3, while the other (i.e., the prenatal care program) is at size A_1, to which of the two programs should additional resources be allocated? Assuming the output and input relationships for both are as shown in Figure 2.1, the allocation of a given amount of resources to the program at point A_1 would result in the largest change in health output. Thus, the decision rule for allocating resources between the two programs (when the cost of changing either program is the same) is to select that program whose change in total output would be greatest.

An alternative decision rule that has been suggested is that additional resources should be allocated to those programs whose total output is the largest. Such a decision rule, however, would not necessarily result in the largest increase in output for a given expenditure. Allocating additional resources among programs does not mean that those receiving little or no increase in their resources have to close down, thereby losing their entire output. Allocation decisions are based not on the total output of competing programs, but rather on *changes* in the total output of competing programs. The total output achievable from all programs will be at its maximum only when additional resources are allocated to programs whose increase in total output (marginal change) is greatest.

Once it is understood that marginal analysis is the tool for maximizing total output, the implications of allocation decisions based on a need criterion become clear. If additional resources were devoted to intensive care units, an increase in infant health levels from Q_3 to Q_4 would result. Advocates of the "need" approach would likely favor still additional resources to expand their program beyond Q_4, since further increases in output are possible. Scarce resources, however, have a "cost." The additional resources required to increase the ICU program beyond size A_4 could be spent on programs whose change in total output would have been greater. The real cost of the resources devoted to increasing the size of the ICU program is the benefit (output) that could have been achieved if those resources had been spent on alternative programs.

Resources will be allocated in an optimal manner when the additional output produced by resources in one program equals the foregone benefits of using those same resources on alternative programs. This approach toward allocating resources differs from that of health professionals, who generally see only the unmet needs that could be eliminated by devoting still more resources to their own programs.

Since empirical studies on the relationship between total program output and program inputs are not always available, it is difficult to develop estimates of the marginal effect of increased program resources. Data are more likely to be available on the program's total output and total expenditures. Analysts are therefore able to calculate the *average* benefits of the program (total output/total inputs). Because of the greater availability of average measures, they are often used as the basis for comparing the benefits of and allocating resources to competing programs. The use of such average measures, however, can result in an incorrect allocation of resources among health programs.

The average and marginal benefits of two programs are shown in Figure 2.2. At point Z (equivalent to a certain program size) the two programs could appear to be identical because their average benefits are equal. However, at point Z, the marginal benefits of program B are greater than those of program A. Since resource allocations made on the basis of marginal benefits result in the greatest increases in total output, using average benefits (perhaps as a proxy for marginal benefits) can result in error, as this example illustrates.

In Figure 2.1 it was assumed for the sake of simplicity that the cost of increasing the size of the two programs was the same. This is generally not the case. When the costs of increasing program size are not equal, the comparison cannot simply be made between the changes in the output of the two programs. The relevant criterion for allocating resources to programs having different benefits and costs is to select those programs whose

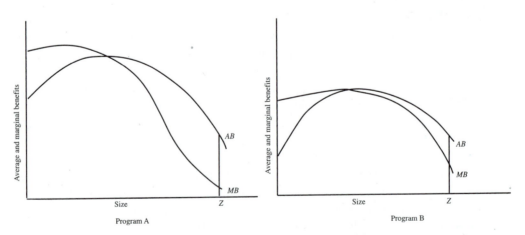

FIGURE 2.2 • Average and marginal benefits from alternative health programs.

marginal benefit per dollar spent is greatest. For example, assume that an increase in program A would result in a decrease in infant mortality of thirty infants. The marginal costs of achieving that increased benefit is $300,000. An increase in program B yields, as a marginal benefit, a decrease in infant mortality of twenty infants at a marginal cost of $100,000. Dividing the cost by the benefit (*MC/MB*) yields a cost of $10,000 per life saved in program A and $5,000 per life saved in program B. It is clear from such an analysis that additional dollars should be spent to increase program B.[1]

Based on the foregoing discussion, we can summarize the type of information needed to allocate scarce resources among alternative health programs. First, the particular population group whose health is to be affected must be specified. Second, the disease category for that given population group must also be specified so as to be able to form a health production function. Third, the marginal effect on health of each of the health programs should be empirically estimated. Unfortunately, very little information exists among health professionals or economists about the marginal impacts of alternative health programs. Thus, allocation decisions are currently being made with little or no information about the marginal effect that specific medical and other health programs have on disease-specific illness rates for particular population groups.[2]

If decision makers are to allocate scarce resources so as to produce the maximum possible increase in health levels, they must understand the economic concepts underlying their allocation; they must also generate the information needed to enable appropriate analyses to be undertaken. Program managers often avoid generating useful information because they do not want their program to be compared with competing health programs. They believe that the uncertainty of their program's effects will enhance their bargaining position.

---

[1]For the sake of simplicity, this discussion has assumed that the input–output relationship for each program is independent of changes in scale in the other programs. In actuality, this is not the case. For example, if one health program emphasizes prevention, then an increase in resources for this program is likely to affect the productivity of others, such as acute care services. These interrelationships between health programs may cause the input–output curve of particular programs to shift either to the left or to the right; that is, the marginal benefits of the affected program may be increased or decreased without changing expenditures for that program. In some cases, acute care programs may become more productive as, for example, after an increase in knowledge or technology (perhaps resulting from increased expenditures on research programs). An increase in knowledge or technology may enable a provider to see more patients or to have a more favorable effect on the outcome of the treatment provided. Alternatively, an increase in preventive programs may decrease the need for acute treatment in the population, thereby lowering the number of patients treated in existing acute care programs. The productivity of existing programs would therefore be lessened.

[2]Given the very limited data on the marginal effects of alternative health programs, only the grossest comparisons can be made. When more appropriate data become available, additional refinements can be incorporated into the comparisons. For example, differences over time in both the stream of benefits and costs of alternative programs should be discounted. However, before too great an emphasis is placed on such refinements, improvements must be made in the basic data used in the analysis. The large variability in estimates of a program's effects as a result of poor data may outweigh the consequences of these refinements.

EMPIRICAL STUDIES OF A HEALTH PRODUCTION FUNCTION

The justification often given for government intervention to provide more medical services to the population in general and to underserved population groups in particular is the desire to improve health status. If the objective of government expenditures is to increase health levels, it is important to derive empirical estimates of the net impact that medical care has on health.

Empirical studies attempting to estimate the marginal contribution of medical services to improved health have been conducted at two levels of aggregation. At the more aggregate level, counties, states, and even countries were used as the unit of observation and each of the factors affecting health, including the measure of health itself, were based on population averages (2). The less aggregate studies of health production, "microanalyses," used individuals as the unit of measurement (3). These studies attempted to estimate the independent effect that each of the various factors, including medical services, has had on health levels.

An important distinction between the macro- and microstudies of health production lies in the variables used to measure health status. No single measure of health can adequately represent the concept of health status; instead, it is described by certain of its quantifiable aspects. It is always implicitly assumed that these quantifiable measures are closely related to other aspects of health. On an aggregate level, available health measures are those collected by government agencies as part of vital statistics. These measures, such as births and deaths, also tend to be more accurate than others. Morbidity and disability measures of health are generally unavailable on an aggregate level, and they are not likely to be as reliable as mortality data. When mortality rates are used as the measure of health, the simplest such index is the crude death rate, which is the number of deaths per thousand population. More useful health indices are those that are age-sex specific. Such population-specific death rates, unlike the crude death rate, would not be affected by changes in the overall composition of the population (4).

When studies of health production use individuals as the unit of observation, mortality rates cannot be used meaningfully unless a longitudinal analysis is used. Instead, measures of health such as the number of work-loss days, the individual's own evaluation of health status, and the number of chronic conditions are used.[3] The unavailability of data needed to measure health status adequately has led to the practice of measuring health by the use of its reciprocal, such as mortality rates. These measures are obviously incomplete in their assessment of what is believed to constitute good health.

---

[3]In his study on work-loss rates, M. Silver found that work loss was positively correlated with income but negatively correlated with the earnings rate (a weekly wage measure). Although Silver acknowledges that this finding may be caused by a combination of incentives and causations—higher earnings make work loss more expensive, while higher income may carry with it some health risks—he claims that recovery at home is a "superior" good. Therefore, the positive association of income with work loss represents normal economic behavior rather than a health risk. Silver therefore concludes that work loss may be an unreliable measure of true health status because it is too greatly affected by economic behavior.

In addition to medical services, other factors affecting age-sex specific mortality rates in studies of health production include lifestyle variables, such as income, occupation, cigarette smoking, and alcohol consumption; environmental variables, such as the quality of housing and urbanization (which, in addition to capturing the effect of pollution, might also represent such offsetting factors as increased access to medical care); and an efficiency factor, measured by the number of years of formal education, which assumes that persons who are more efficient at producing health can do so at a lower cost. The better-educated person may not only be able to recognize symptoms and seek treatment earlier than others, but may also be more likely to use preventive services.

Health production studies generally measure the contribution of medical services to health in several ways: by quantities of the individual components of medical services, such as the number of physicians and hospital beds per thousand population; by the utilization of medical services, such as the number of physician visits or hospital patient days; or by aggregate expenditures on medical services, which include changes in prices, utilization of services, and differences in quality of services.

Auster, Leveson, and Sarachek (ALS) analyzed interstate differences in age-sex adjusted mortality rates for 1960 (5). Their principal purpose was to estimate the elasticity of health with respect to medical services, which is the percentage change in mortality rates that would occur as a result of a 1 percent change in medical services. The authors used multivariate analysis and included measures of medical services, as well as a number of environmental factors, believed to affect health.[4] The medical services input was measured in two ways: as expenditures on medical services and as a separate production function for medical services (which included as inputs into that production function the number of physicians per capita, the number of paramedical persons per capita, and so on).

The statistical results of the ALS study, which accounted for more than 50 percent of the interstate differences in mortality rates, indicated that environmental and personal factors had a greater effect on mortality rates than did medical services. The specific findings for some of the more important factors affecting interstate differences in mortality rates were as follows: (a) expenditures on medical care had an elasticity of approximately −0.1, meaning that a 10 percent increase in medical expenditures would lead to a 1 percent decrease in age-sex adjusted mortality rates; (b) the elasticity of mortality rates with respect to education was almost twice as large as for medical services (−0.2); and (c) cigarette consumption per capita resulted in a positive increase in mortality rates (i.e., the elasticity estimate was +0.1, meaning that a 10 percent increase in cigarette consumption per capita results in a 1 percent increase in mortality rates). In the ALS study, the total effect of environmental and personal factors (e.g., education and cigarette consumption) outweighed the marginal contribution of medical services to health status.

---

[4]An important assumption in such cross-sectional studies, of which the authors are well aware, is that the mortality rate is related only to the quantity of medical services used in the particular year for which the study was undertaken. In reality, it is likely that medical services and environmental factors will affect the population's health status over the lifetime of the population, rather than just during the current period.

Hadley estimated the impact (elasticity) of medical care, education, and income on both general and disease-specific mortality rates (6). Separate production functions were estimated for twelve age-race-sex cohorts—eight for adults forty-five years of age and over and four for infants. The data were from 1968 to 1972 and were based on counties with a minimum population size. Although the results differed somewhat from cohort to cohort, Hadley found that the elasticity of the mortality rate, from all causes, with respect to medical care expenditures is approximately − 0.15; that is, a 10 percent increase in medical care expenditures would lead to a 1.5 percent decrease in the mortality rate. The effect was much greater for white males than for black males. Income and education were also found to have a negative effect on mortality rates.

Using individuals as the unit of measurement, Michael Grossman estimated the individual's demand for healthy time. Good health, or healthy time, in Grossman's model is demanded both because it enters the individual's utility function directly for its consumption value and because, as an investment, it increases the time available for other activities. Grossman found that education increases efficiency in producing health and that the elasticity of health with respect to medical services varies between 0.1 and 0.3. Grossman also found that the income elasticity of health is negative, in spite of a positive income elasticity with respect to medical services (7).

A problem with cross-sectional studies that attempt to measure the effect of medical services on health status is that, at any point in time, greater use of medical services may represent increased use by those whose health is poor. Further, increased use of medical services may have an effect on health status over a period longer than that in which they are used. To correct for these problems in interpreting the effect of increased use of medical services on health status, Lee Benham and Alexandra Benham studied the change in health status of groups of individuals during the 1963–70 period (8). Using data from two different surveys, the authors classified individuals into twenty-eight education-age categories (consisting of four education and seven age groupings) and attempted to determine the impact that increased use of medical services had on the health status of each education-age category between 1963 and 1970. (Education was considered as a proxy measure for permanent income.)

During the period studied, two large government programs were started (Medicare and Medicaid) to finance increased use of medical services for the poor and elderly. The measures of health status used were: health status reported, the number of symptoms reported, and disability days reported during the previous year. The contribution of medical services was measured by the number of nonobstetric physician visits and nonobstetric hospital utilization.

The authors' statistical analysis related the (average) health status of each education-age group in 1970 to the (average) health status of that same group in 1963 and to changes in that group's utilization of medical services between 1963 and 1970. The authors assumed that increased utilization of medical services between 1963 and 1970 was primarily the result of an increase in government financing of medical services to the poor and elderly rather than a response to changes in that group's health status. The results of the Benham and Benham study were consistent with the previous studies. Increased use of medical services did not result in an improvement in health status during the period studied.

Results from the RAND Health Insurance Experiment provide more evidence regarding the effect of an increase in medical care on health outcomes (9). Participants were assigned to alternative health insurance plans for a period of three to five years. The plans varied in the amount that the participant had to pay out of pocket for medical care. Participants in plans with less cost sharing had higher utilization, with the highest utilization of medical services occurring in the insurance plan where the participant did not have to pay anything out of pocket. In addition to studying the effect that out-of-pocket payment has on medical use and expenditures, the study also analyzed the effect of greater use of medical services on the participants' health status.

The health of adults was compared according to whether they were in a plan in which utilization was greater (i.e., no out-of-pocket payment) or smaller (those plans where the patients paid various amounts for their medical services). General health measures, such as physical and role functioning, mental health, social contacts, and health perceptions, were used as well as measures of physiologic health, such as diastolic blood pressure and functional far vision. Of the numerous health status measures used, the health benefits of increased use of medical services were quite limited; greater use of medical services resulted in lower diastolic blood pressure for those initially diagnosed as hypertensive and improved far vision for those with initial far-vision problems. Further, increased medical use had no statistically significant impact on the general health of subgroups, which differed according to their incomes and their initial health status. The researchers concluded that, for the average participant, greater medical care use had no statistically significant effect on health habits associated with cardiovascular disease and certain kinds of cancer, nor on five general measures of health. However, "people with specific conditions that physicians have been trained to diagnose and treat (myopia, hypertension) benefit from free care."

Perhaps more persuasive than these statistical attempts to determine the contribution of additional medical services to increased health is Victor Fuchs' excellent discussion of causes of death by age (10). Fuchs examined the contribution of living standards, lifestyle, and medical services to the decline in infant mortality rates since 1900 and to causes of adult deaths. The large decline in infant mortality rates from 1900 to the present[5] has been due largely to rising living standards, the spread of literacy and education, a large decline in the birthrate, possibly chlorination of the water supply and pasteurization of milk, and the introduction of antimicrobial drugs in the 1930s. "It is important to realize that medical care played almost no role in this decline" (11). It was not until the late 1960s that maternal and infant services were extended to underserved families and intensive care units were provided for premature infants who were at high risk. Fuchs also

---

[5]For example, the U.S. infant mortality rate declined from 162 per 1,000 live births in 1900 to 26 per 1,000 in 1960. By 1993, the mortality rate had declined to 8.3 per 1,000 live births.

points out that in other developed countries with fewer medical services than the United States and a large proportion of home births delivered by a midwife, infant mortality rates are lower than in the United States. Specific medical service programs targeted to high-risk pregnancies are likely to make a larger contribution to decreases in infant mortality rates than merely making more medical services generally available to the entire population. For example, in countries where medical services are provided free, as in Great Britain, the infant mortality rate is still not as low as that achieved in other developed countries. The lowest infant mortality rates in 1993 (between 4.3 and 4.8 per thousand live births) were those of Sweden, Switzerland, Finland, and Japan.

When Fuchs examined mortality rates by cause of death for different age groups—adolescents and young adults (15–24 years of age), middle-aged persons (35–44), and late-middle-aged persons (55–64)—he again concluded that increased use of medical services has a smaller impact on health than the way in which people live. In the younger age groups, accidents (particularly from use of automobiles), suicides, and homicides are the major causes of death. In middle age, heart disease is the leading cause of death; accidents, suicides, cirrhosis of the liver (caused by alcoholism), and lung cancer are the other major contributors. Among nonwhites, homicides are the second leading cause of death. Again, the major causes of death may be attributed to behavioral factors. For persons in late middle age, heart disease is the leading cause of death; neoplasms are second.

Fuchs compares causes of death by age group in the United States and Sweden, with interesting results. The major factors explaining the lower Swedish mortality rates in each of the various age groups are again determined to be behavioral (Swedes are less violent and have fewer accidents) and attributed to lifestyle (diet, exercise, smoking, and stress). "At present . . . the greatest potential for reducing coronary disease, cancer, and the other major killers still lies in altering personal behavior." Fuchs further notes: "Given our present state of knowledge, even the most lavish use of medical care would not bring the U.S. rate more than a small step closer to the Swedish rate" (12).

The studies employing statistical techniques to estimate a health production function and the discussion by Fuchs on the leading causes of death both suggest that health status is more importantly related to lifestyle factors than to increments of medical services. Although the total benefit of medical services may be large, allocation decisions are rarely all-or-nothing decisions; instead, they are incremental. If policymakers have as their objective an increase in health status, increased provision of medical services is likely to have a relatively smaller impact on health than will alternative policies. Further, these additional expenditures on medical services are not without a cost; greater increases in health status could be achieved if these same funds were spent on other programs.

APPLICATIONS OF A HEALTH PRODUCTION FUNCTION

The decline in mortality over the past thirty years is generally attributed to two components: declines in infant mortality rates and in deaths from heart disease.

The largest declines in mortality rates during the 1970–88 period occurred in infant mortality rates, which decreased from 26.4 per 1,000 live births in 1955, to 24.7 in 1965, to 16.1 in 1975, to 8.3 in 1993. It has been suggested that this more rapid decline in infant mortality rates is, for the most part, the result of factors other than increased medical care expenditures, particularly liberalized abortion laws.

Between 1955 and 1964, the infant mortality rate declined by 0.6 percent per year. After 1964, however, the infant mortality rate fell more rapidly, approximately 4.5 percent a year. The most important portion of the decline in infant mortality (77 percent) was the decline in the neonatal death rate (i.e., infant deaths within the first 27 days of life per 1,000 live births), which is twice as large as and fell more rapidly than the post-neonatal mortality rate (i.e., infant deaths occurring between 28 and 364 days). Attempts to explain the decline in infant mortality must therefore take into account the reasons for the decline in the neonatal rate.

Grossman and others conducted several studies to determine the causes of the decline in neonatal mortality rates. In one study, using county-level aggregate data, Corman and Grossman examined the determinants of neonatal mortality rates for a three-year period centered on 1977 (13). Specifically, the authors examined the impact on neonatal mortality of the availability of neonatal intensive care, the legalization of abortion, subsidized family planning services for low-income women, community health centers, maternal and infant nutrition programs, and Medicaid. Separate analyses were conducted for white and black women to determine the effects of each of the above on the neonatal mortality rate. The various factors affecting neonatal mortality differed in their effects on white and black women.

The authors then used their estimates of a health production function to determine which programs were more cost-effective in reducing the neonatal mortality rate (14). For illustrative purposes, three of the programs analyzed—teenage family planning programs, neonatal intensive care units, and prenatal care—are presented in Table 2.1. Based on an empirical analysis, an estimate was derived of the number of lives saved per 1,000 additional participants for each of the above programs, which were, respectively, 0.6, 2.8, and 4.5. The respective costs of these programs, per 1,000 additional participants (in 1984 dollars), were $122,000, $13,616,000, and $176,000. Dividing the cost by the estimate of lives saved (e.g., $176,000/4.5) results in the following cost per life saved from each of these programs: $203 for teenage family planning, $4,778 for intensive care, and $39 for prenatal care. According to these results, prenatal care is the most cost-effective input for reducing neonatal mortality.

Policies such as teen family planning and prenatal care reduce the infant mortality rate by decreasing the number of births that are likely to be high-risk (low birthweight), which is a less expensive approach than expanding the number of ICUs that increase the survival of the high-risk infant.

The authors also used the results of their analysis to explain the decline in infant mortality between the years 1964 and 1977. During that time, the white neonatal mortality

TABLE 2.1 Cost Per Life Saved Among Three Programs to Reduce Neonatal Mortality

	Number of Lives Saved per Thousand Additional Participants	Cost of Each Program per Thousand Additional Participants	Cost per Life Saved
Teenage Family Planning[a]	0.6	$122,000	$203
Neonatal ICUs [b]	2.8	$13,616,000	$4,778
Prenatal Care[c]	4.5	$176,000	$39

Source: Theodore Joyce, Hope Corman, and Michael Grossman, "A Cost-Effectiveness Analysis of Strategies to Reduce Infant Mortality," *Medical Care,* 26 (4), April 1988: 348–360, Table 3.

[a] Percentage of women, aged fifteen to nineteen with family income less than 200% of the poverty level in 1975 who used organized family planning services in 1975.

[b] Total hospital days in neonatal intensive care units in 1979 per average number of low birthweight births.

[c] Percentage of live births for which prenatal care began in the first three months of pregnancy.

rate declined from 16.2 to 8.7 per 1,000 live births, whereas the black neonatal rate declined from 27.6 to 16.1. The authors determined that for blacks the most important factor causing a reduction in the neonatal rate was the availability of abortion; its effect, 1.2 deaths per 1,000 live births, was almost twice as large as the next most important contributor. Next in importance was availability of neonatal intensive care units and the increase in schooling, each reducing the rate by 0.7 deaths per 1,000 live births. Medicaid expenditures was fourth, at 0.5 death per 1,000 live births. For whites, schooling was most important, followed by subsidized nutrition programs, Medicaid, and the availability of neonatal intensive care units; the availability of abortion was fifth. The abortion effect on blacks was four times greater than on whites, and the effect of neonatal intensive care units was twice as large.

A cost/benefit analysis of averting deaths was not undertaken by the authors because of the problems involved in valuing a human life. However, they were able to estimate the cost/benefit ratio of decreasing the number of low birthweight infants. Considering just the hospitalization costs of caring for a low birthweight infant (which would be reduced) and dividing that cost by the program costs of decreasing the number of low birthweight infants, the authors concluded that programs that decrease low birthweight, such as prenatal care, have very favorable cost/benefit ratios. The authors concluded that to continue to achieve declines in the neonatal mortality rate, attention must be focused on reducing the number of low birthweight infants.

Grossman conducted several other studies on the determinants of health and the importance of nonmedical variables. In a study of child and adolescent health, Grossman and others found that the home environment in general and mother's schooling in particular played an extremely important role. Holding other factors constant, "children and teenagers of more-educated mothers have better oral health, are less likely to be obese, and less likely to have anemia than children of less-educated mothers. Father's schooling plays a much less important role" (15).

Reductions in mortality from heart disease have also contributed to the sharp decline in the overall mortality rate. Between 1968 and 1990, the mortality rate from coronary heart disease fell by 50 percent. According to several studies, the main contributing factors to the decline in heart disease, and in its mortality, have been changes in lifestyle factors, such as reduced smoking, lower serum cholesterol levels, control of hypertension, and improvements in the number and quality of coronary care units (16). For example, Goldman and Cook attempted to quantify the relative contribution of lifestyle changes and medical interventions in explaining the 21 percent decline in ischemic heart disease mortality that occurred between 1968 and 1976. They concluded that lifestyle changes accounted for 54 percent of the decline (reduced serum cholesterol levels contributed 30 percent and reduced cigarette smoking, 24 percent). Over the nine-year period studied, medical interventions accounted for less than 40 percent of the decline. The authors note that while the medical interventions, such as coronary care units, are expensive innovations, lifestyle changes, aside from government-financed publicity, are relatively costless and contributed more to the decline in ischemic heart disease mortality. Decreases in heart disease, however, are not uniform across the population. White males have done better than blacks, salaried workers better than hourly workers, and those with more education have benefited more, as they have reduced by greater percentages their smoking and consumption of highly saturated fats.

SUMMARY

The cost/benefit application, the explanation of mortality rates over time, and the cost-effectiveness analysis of decreasing neonatal mortality illustrate the types of analyses that could be undertaken based on knowledge of a health production function. To be useful for decision makers, specific information on health production functions, by disease categories and for different population groups, is required. Before more precise estimates of health production functions can be derived, however, it is necessary for policy analysts to understand the types of data that need to be collected and how they will be useful for decision making.

A question arises from the finding that the marginal contribution of additional medical expenditures on health is relatively small: Why have government medical expenditures increased so rapidly, particularly on some population groups (the aged) rather than others (the poor and young)? One possible explanation is that the government's objective has never really been to increase the health of the nation by allocating resources among alternative inputs; instead, government medical expenditures are a means of redistributing wealth among different population groups. Further, the criterion for such redistribution has not been medical or economic need, but has instead been provision of net benefits to those groups that are more politically powerful (17).

The remainder of this book will examine the efficiency with which medical care is produced by the medical care industry. Even though the marginal impact of medical services on health may be relatively small, the increase in private and governmental financing of medical services has been large. The contribution to health of such expenditures will be reduced even further if most of the increase in expenditures results from increased medical prices, caused by inefficiency. The efficiency of medical services and the equity of their distribution are addressed in the remaining chapters.

Key Terms and Concepts

- Allocation criteria
- Cost-effectiveness analysis
- Health production
- Health inputs
- Marginal, average, and total output effects
- Marginal costs/marginal benefits

- Declining marginal effects of health inputs
- Macro- and micro- production function studies
- Marginal contribution of medical care to health
- Relationship between inputs and output

Review Questions

1. Explain why one would or would not use the total contribution of health services as compared to the marginal contribution of health services for decision making, if the objective were to determine how to allocate a limited budget for increasing health levels.
2. Assume you are a consultant to an HMO that is being evaluated on how well it improves the health status of an enrolled population group. What information would you need and how would you use it to advise the HMO on how to allocate its resources?
3. What is a production function for health? How might it be used for allocating resources to health? How would you use it to explain changes in health status over time?
4. You have been hired by Medicaid to advise the director on how to reduce infant mortality among the population eligible for Medicaid. What are the various alternative

programs you would suggest and how would you allocate funds among them to achieve the greatest reduction in infant mortality for a given budget?

5. How can employers use the concept of a production function for health for decreasing their employees' medical expenditures?
6. Describe a production function for decreasing deaths of young adults.

REFERENCES

1. For a more complete discussion of the principles and applications of cost/benefit analysis, see Marthe Gold, Louise Russell, Joanna Siegal, and Milton Weinstein, eds., *Cost-Effectiveness in Health and Medicine* (New York: Oxford University Press, 1996).
2. Examples of health production functions using macro data are given by Richard Auster, Irving Leveson, and Deborah Sarachek, "The Production of Health, an Exploratory Study," *Journal of Human Resources*, 4, Fall 1969: 411–436; Charles T. Stewart, Jr., "The Allocation of Resources to Health," *Journal of Human Resources,* 6, Winter 1971; see also a critique of the Stewart article by Edward Meeker, "Allocation of Resources to Health Revisited," *Journal of Human Resources,* 8, Spring 1973: 257–259; and Jack Hadley, *More Medical Care, Better Health?* (Washington, D.C.: The Urban Institute, 1982).
3. Joseph P. Newhouse, "Determinants of Days Lost from Work Due to Sickness," in Herbert E. Klarman, ed., *Empirical Studies in Health Economics*, Proceedings of the 2nd Conference on the Economics of Health (Baltimore: Johns Hopkins University Press, 1970), pp. 59–70; Morris Silver, "An Economic Analysis of Variations in Medical Expenses and Work-Loss Rates," in Klarman, ed., *ibid.*, pp. 121–140; Michael Grossman, "On the Concept of Health Capital and the Demand for Health," *Journal of Political Economy*, March–April 1972; Lee Benham and Alexandra Benham, "The Impact of Incremental Medical Services on Health Status, 1963–1970," in R. Andersen, J. Kravitz, and O. Anderson, eds., *Equity in Health Services: Empirical Analysis of Social Policy* (Cambridge, Mass.: Ballinger, 1975); Joseph P. Newhouse and Lindy J. Friedlander, "The Relationship Between Medical Resources and Measures of Health: Some Additional Evidence," *Journal of Human Resources*, 15(2), 1980.
4. For a more complete review of health measures, their definitions, and attendant difficulties, see "Advances in Health Status Assessment: Conference Proceedings," *Medical Care*, 27(3) supplement, March 1989.
5. Auster, Leveson, and Sarachek, *op. cit.*
6. Hadley, *op. cit.*
7. Grossman, *op. cit.*
8. Benham and Benham, *op. cit.*
9. Robert H. Brook et al., "Does Free Care Improve Adults' Health? Results from a Randomized Controlled Trial," *New England Journal of Medicine*, 309(23), December 1983: 1426–1434 and Emmett B. Keeler et al., "Effects of Cost Sharing on Physiological Health, Health Practices, and Worry," *Health Services Research*, 22(3), August 1987: 297–306.
10. Victor R. Fuchs, *Who Shall Live?* (New York: Basic Books, 1974), pp. 30–55. The data

presented by Fuchs represent average relationships and do not indicate the relative marginal costs of achieving changes in health status. For policy purposes, it would be desirable to know the marginal effects of each of the variables on health status.

11. *Ibid.*, p. 32.

12. *Ibid.*, p. 46.

13. Hope Corman and Michael Grossman, "Determinants of Neonatal Mortality Rates in the U.S.: A Reduced Form Model," *Journal of Health Economics*, 4(3), September 1985: 213–236. For additional discussion of the reasons for the decline in infant mortality, see Jeffrey E. Harris, "Prenatal Medical Care and Infant Mortality," and Mark R. Rosenzweig and T. Paul Schultz, "The Behavior of Mothers as Inputs to Child Health: The Determinants of Birth Weight, Gestation and Rate of Fetal Growth," in Victor R. Fuchs, ed., *Economic Aspects of Health* (Chicago: University of Chicago Press, 1982).

14. Theodore Joyce, Hope Corman, and Michael Grossman, "A Cost-Effectiveness Analysis of Strategies to Reduce Infant Mortality," *Medical Care*, 26(4), April 1988: 348–360.

15. Michael Grossman, "Government and Health Outcomes," *American Economic Review*, May 1982: 192.

16. Michael Stern, "The Recent Decline in Ischemic Heart Disease Mortality," *Annals of Internal Medicine*, 91, October 1979: 630–640; Joel Kleinman, Jacob Feldman, and Mary Monk, "The Effects of Changes in Smoking Habits on Coronary Heart Disease Mortality," *American Journal of Public Health*, 69, August 1979: 795–802; Lee Goldman and Francis Cook, "The Decline in Ischemic Heart Disease Mortality Rates: An Analysis of the Comparative Effects of Medical Interventions and Changes in Lifestyle," *Annals of Internal Medicine*, 101(6), December 1984: 825–836.

17. For a more complete discussion of the redistributive aspects of government health policy, see Paul J. Feldstein, *The Politics of Health Legislation: An Economic Perspective* (Chicago: Health Administration Press, 2nd edition, 1996).

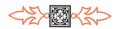

CHAPTER

An Overview of the Medical Care Sector

DESCRIPTION OF THE MEDICAL CARE MARKETS

Expenditures on the Major Components of Medical Care

As an introduction to the medical care sector, let us examine the magnitude and changing composition of expenditures on the major components of medical care. As shown in Table 3.1, the two largest components of medical care, hospital and physician services, accounted for 40 and 23 percent, respectively, of the $879 billion of total personal medical expenditures in calendar year 1995. Hospital expenditures ($350 billion) are the largest component of medical expenditures—almost twice as large as those for physician services ($202 billion). (Personal health care expenditures were approximately $110 billion less than total health care expenditures, which were $988 billion—13.7 percent of GNP. The difference between the two, in billions, were expenses for prepayment and administration [$47.7], government public health activities [$31.4], and research and construction of medical facilities [$30.7].)

The relative proportions of expenditures on hospital, physician, and other medical services have been changing over time. In 1965, hospital expenditures represented 40 percent of total personal medical expenditures, while physician services were 23 percent. By 1980, the hospital portion exceeded 47 percent and then declined to 40 percent by 1995. After the enactment of Medicare and Medicaid, and the growth in private health insurance, out-of-pocket payments for hospital care dropped sharply—on average to less than 3 percent of the bill. And, as shown in Table 3.2, the remainder was paid primarily by

TABLE 3.1 Total Private and Public Expenditures for Personal Health Care Services by Type of Expenditure and Source of Funds, Calendar Years 1965, 1980, and 1995

	1965			1980			1995		
	Total (Billions)	Percent Distribution[a]	Private Percentage	Total (Billions)	Percent Distribution	Private Percentage	Total (Billions)	Percent Distribution[a]	Private Percentage
Hospital care	$14.0	39.8	61.2	$102.7	47.3	45.6	$350.1	39.8	38.8
Physician services	8.2	23.3	92.9	45.2	20.8	71.0	201.6	22.9	68.3
Dental services	2.8	8.0	100.0	13.3	6.1	95.5	45.8	5.2	96.1
Drug/drug sundries	5.9	16.8	96.2	21.6	10.0	92.1	83.4	9.5	86.3
Other[b]	4.3	12.2	59.3	34.2	15.8	54.1	197.9	22.5	49.2
Total	35.2	100.1	76.5	217.0	100.0	59.9	878.8	99.9	55.4

Sources: U.S. Department of Health and Human Services, Health Care Financing Administration, Internet site http://www.hcfa.gov/stats/nhce96.htm, and unpublished data, 1996.

[a] The percentages do not add up to 100 because of rounding.

[b] "Other" includes: other professional services, home health care, vision products and other medical durables, nursing home care, and other personal health care.

TABLE 3.2 Amount and Percent Distribution of Personal Health Care Expenditures, by Source of Funds and Type of Expenditure, 1995

Type of Expenditure	Total	Out of Pocket	Third Party Payments							
			Total	Private Health Insurance	Other Private Funds[a]	Government Expenditures				
						Total	Medicare	Federal		State[c]
								Medicaid	Other[b]	
Amount (Billions)										
Total	878.8	182.6	696.2	276.8	27.3	392.1	184.0	83.1	36.5	88.5
Hospital care	350.1	11.4	338.7	113.1	11.3	214.3	112.6	37.2	25.5	39.0
Physician services	201.6	36.9	164.7	97.0	3.7	64.0	40.0	8.4	2.6	13.1
Dental services	45.8	21.8	24.0	22.0	0.2	1.8	—	0.9	0.1	0.8
Drug/drug sundries	83.4	49.8	33.6	22.1	—	11.4	—	5.6	0.3	5.6
Nursing home care	77.9	28.6	49.3	2.5	1.5	45.3	7.3	20.3	1.6	16.0
All other services[d]	120.0	34.0	86.0	20.0	10.6	55.3	24.0	10.8	6.3	14.1
Percent Distribution										
Total	100.0	20.8	79.2	31.5	3.1	44.6	20.9	9.5	4.2	10.1
Hospital care	100.0	3.3	96.7	32.3	3.2	61.2	32.2	10.6	7.3	11.1
Physician services	100.0	18.3	81.7	48.1	1.8	31.7	19.8	4.2	1.3	6.5
Dental services	100.0	47.6	52.4	48.0	0.4	3.9	—	2.0	0.2	1.7
Drug/drug sundries	100.0	59.7	40.3	26.5	—	13.7	—	6.7	0.4	6.7
Nursing home care	100.0	36.7	63.3	3.2	1.9	58.2	9.4	26.1	2.1	20.5
All other services[d]	100.0	28.3	71.7	16.7	8.8	46.1	50.0	9.0	5.3	11.8

Source: Katharine R. Levit et al., "National Health Expenditures, 1995," *Health Care Financing Review*, Fall 1996, 18(1), p. 211, Table 16.

Note: Numbers and percentages may not add to totals because of rounding.

[a] "Other Private Funds" includes: philanthropy, interest and dividend income, income from rental of office space, and other nonpatient income.

[b] Includes expenditures for maternal and child health programs, vocational rehabilitation programs, Public Health Service activities, Indian Health Service programs, workers' compensation programs, Veterans Administration Services, Alcohol, Drug Abuse and Mental Health Administration programs, and Defense Department programs.

[c] Includes state and local Medicaid payments.

[d] Includes other professional services, vision products and other medical durables, other personal care, and home health care.

government (61 percent) and private insurance (32 percent). Direct patient payments were smaller for hospital care than for any other medical service. On average, patients are responsible for 18 percent of expenditures for physician services and 60 percent of drug expenditures.

As the portion of the hospital bill paid for directly by the patient declined, so did the patient's and physician's incentive to question the prices charged by hospitals. The patient's use of the hospital is generally believed to be less responsive to the price charged than is the use of most other medical services. The declining portion of the hospital bill for which the patient is responsible, together with the small effect that price has on hospital use, removed patient and physician incentives to be concerned with how rapidly hospital prices increased or with the relative costs of hospitals. Under these circumstances, a more rapid increase in hospital expenditures would be expected. Conversely, a slower rate of increase in expenditures would be expected for those medical services for which patients paid a larger fraction of the bill and whose use is more affected by higher prices. These factors are important for understanding the changing composition of medical expenditures.

Hospital use and expenditures increased more rapidly than the other components of medical services, where consumers had to pay a larger portion of the bill. In recent years, because of Medicare limits on hospital expenditures, the introduction of utilization management, and growing competitive pressures, hospital expenditures have increased less rapidly than other components of medical care, thereby decreasing their share of personal medical expenditures. It is likely this trend will continue.

In 1965, before the introduction of Medicare and Medicaid, government expenditures represented 21 percent of personal medical expenditures. By 1995, the government share of personal medical expenditures climbed to 45 percent, with the greatest increases occurring in those sectors covered by Medicare and Medicaid, namely, hospital and physician services.

Over time, as shown in Table 3.3, direct patient payments for all medical services declined from 53 percent in 1965 to 21 percent in 1995. As more of the bill for medical services was paid by government and private insurance, the importance of price on the patient's use of the service and choice of a provider from whom to purchase that service diminished. The lessening of patients' price incentives enabled providers to more easily pass on higher prices and had important implications for the performance of the medical care market.

The government's financing of medical services has not been uniform for each of the components of medical care; it has been most concerned with cost containment in those areas to which it is financially committed. Higher prices for hospital services were of greater financial consequence and therefore of greater concern to the government than similar price increases for dental services, whose financing is predominantly private.

The sharp increase and change in composition of medical care expenditures indicate a need for a set of economic tools to predict equilibrium situations. To understand why ex-

TABLE 3.3 Percentage Distribution of Personal Health Expenditures by Source in the United States, 1965, 1975, 1985, and 1995

Source	1965	1975	1985	1995
		Amount (Billions)		
	$35.2	114.5	376.4	878.8
		Percent Distribution[a]		
Private[b]	79.3%	60.5	60.6	55.4
Out of pocket	52.6	33.3	26.7	20.8
Insurance benefits	24.7	24.8	30.2	31.5
All other	2.0	2.4	3.7	3.1
Public	20.7	39.6	39.3	44.6
Federal	8.5	27.0	29.6	34.5
State and Local	12.2	12.5	9.7	10.1

Source: U.S. Department of Health and Human Services, Health Care Financing Administration, Internet site http://www.hcfa.gov/stats/nhce96.htm, and unpublished data, 1996.
[a] The percentages may not add up to 100 because of rounding.
[b] After 1980 the category "All other" was expanded to include a greater percentage of what was formerly "Direct payments." "All other" now includes philanthropy, interest and dividend income, income from rental of office space, and so on, all considered nonpatient revenue.

penditures have increased so rapidly, it is necessary to determine why prices and quantities of medical care have been changing. Understanding the reasons for such changes is essential for forecasting and for anticipating the effects of public policy on prices, quantities, and expenditures in each of the medical markets.

The Interrelationship of the Different Medical Care Markets

Medical care, which is the output of the overall medical care market, is, in fact, the outcome of several interrelated markets. These include the markets for registered nurses, hospital services, physician services, and even health professional education. To be able to forecast the effects of a change in government policy on the medical care sector or to determine the effects of a natural change, such as an increase in the aged population, it is necessary to have a model of the medical care sector that describes the relationship of various submarkets and components of medical care to each other. The model that follows describes the various submarkets that comprise the medical care sector, demonstrates the way in which these different sectors are interrelated, and illustrates the usefulness of such a framework for forecasting and policy analysis (1). This overview of the medical care sector will also indicate the various subject areas to be covered in this book.

Three types of markets are present in the medical care sector, as shown in Figure 3.1. The patient's demand for a medical treatment (for a particular diagnostic category) is expressed by going to a physician whose determination of how to treat the patient is based

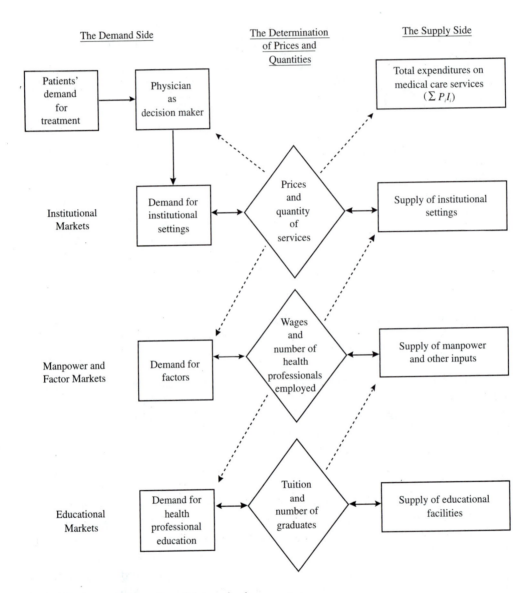

FIGURE 3.1 • An overview of the medical care sector.

on both economic and noneconomic factors. The physician's selection of one or more of several institutional settings—hospitals, outpatient facilities, nursing homes, the physician's office, or even home care—is based on the relative prices of each of those settings, the relative cost of each to the physician, and the efficacy of each in treatment. The demand for institutional care will depend on patient demand factors, physician considerations, and the relative price and efficacy of treatment in the different institutional settings. These institutional settings may thus be seen both as complements to and substitutes for one another.

(Under the traditional fee-for-service system, the physician is assumed to act as the patient's agent in determining which institutional settings will be used for providing care to the patient. Under traditional insurance coverage, each provider is paid separately. As managed care systems have developed, such as HMOs, the HMO receives an annual capitation fee and is responsible for providing all the medical services the patient might require. In both cases, the physician continues to determine the combination of institutional settings that will be used in patient treatment. The incentives facing the physician, patient, and the HMO, however, may differ. This issue will be discussed in greater depth; nevertheless, the model described is relevant for understanding and forecasting change under each of these different delivery systems.)

A change in the demand for different institutional settings that is the result of, for example, a change in the age of the population, will be reflected in institutional demands for manpower and other factor inputs (e.g., capital and supplies). These comprise the second set of markets to be analyzed. Such institutional demands for manpower and other inputs represent the demand side of the health manpower (and inputs) markets. The demand for a particular health manpower category, for example, will depend on factors relating to the patients' (and/or their physicians') demand for the institutional settings in which that manpower group is employed, the wages of the group, and the relationship of their wages to those of other health workers.

The demand for an education by prospective health professionals will depend on the demand for health professionals in the market just described. The demand for a health professional education, which is the amount that a person is willing to pay in terms of tuition and foregone income, is determined by the expected income and wages that might be earned (as determined in the manpower market) and by noneconomic motivating factors.

The supply side of each of these markets works as follows. The supply of health professional educational institutions (in terms, for example, of institutional capacity and faculty) and the demands for such education determine the number of graduates and the tuition rate to be charged. The number of graduates (the time required to educate each category of health manpower will, of course, vary) plus the existing stock of health manpower (less deaths and retirements) comprise the supply of health manpower at any given time. The supply of each category of health manpower in conjunction with the demands for such manpower will determine incomes and wages as well as employment (the participation rate). The outcomes of the health manpower (and other input) markets will affect the supply of services offered in different institutional settings. The cost of providing care in a given institutional setting will rise as the wages for a given manpower group rise and as more members of that manpower category are used to provide care. In each institutional setting, the costs of providing care together with the demands for care will determine how much care is provided; this is the outcome of the institutional markets. Total expenditures for personal medical care consist, then, of the prices of each institutional setting multiplied by the quantity of care provided in each setting.

To summarize the demand side of each of these separate markets, the demand for institutional care is derived from the initial demands for medical treatments. The demand for health manpower is similarly derived from the demand for institutional care, and the demand for a health professional education is derived from the demand for each health manpower profession. Similarly, the supply of medical services is based on the availability of the supplies in each of these other markets and on their costs.

To forecast the consequences of change in the demand or supply side of any part of this model, it is necessary to understand how the markets in each of the sectors operate. For example, legal restrictions on the tasks that health professionals are permitted to perform affect the demand for different health professionals, the wages they are paid, and consequently, the price and availability of medical service. Similarly, past subsidies to medical schools that have enabled them to set low tuition levels and fix the number of educational spaces irrespective of the demand for those spaces has affected the availability of physicians, their incomes, and the fees they charge. The performance of each of the separate markets in the medical care sector—the different institutional markets, manpower markets, and educational markets—will influence each of the other markets and the final price of and expenditures for medical care. A market in which price is higher and output is less than if it were functioning properly is subject to proposals for improving its performance.

APPLICATIONS OF A MODEL OF THE MEDICAL CARE SECTOR

The effects of alternative public policies on the final market—that is, on the price and availability of medical services—can be predicted, using the tools of supply and demand analysis, on the basis of an understanding of the different medical care markets and their interrelationships.

Our ability to forecast the likely consequences of changes in demand or supply conditions in medical care also requires an accurate overview of the medical care sector. Figure 3.2 describes the same markets discussed above by means of a different set of diagrams, showing each of the separate markets within the institutional, manpower, and educational markets in terms of a traditional supply and demand relationship.

A Demand Policy

As a result of an increase in health insurance in the population, we would expect to observe an increase in the demand for medical care (as would be shown by a shift in demand in Figure 3.2A). How much the demand for medical care will increase will depend, in part, on the importance of price to increased utilization (i.e., the price elasticity of demand for medical care). As a result of an increase in demand, depending on supply conditions in medical care, we would expect an increase in prices as well as an increase in medical care utilization. To forecast what will happen to prices and utilization for each component of medical care, we must examine how this increase in medical care demand

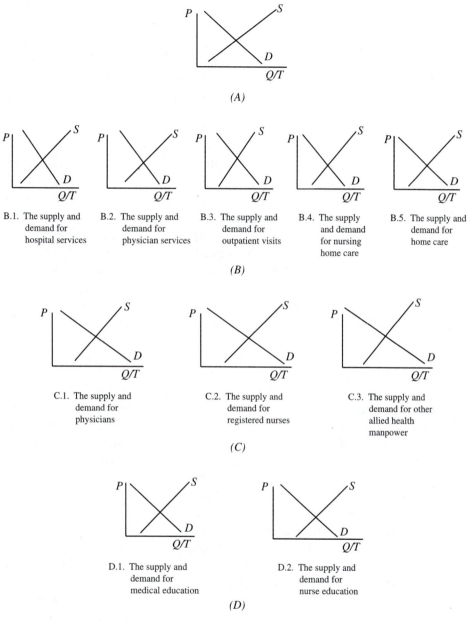

FIGURE 3.2 • An economic model of the medical care sector: (A) the market for medical care services; (B) the markets for institutional services; (C) the markets for health manpower; (D) the markets for health professional education.

is transmitted to each of the other markets. As a result of lower out-of-pocket prices to consumers for medical care, following greater insurance coverage, the demand for different institutional settings will increase; certain institutional settings will experience a larger increase in demand than others, depending, in part, on which population groups will increase their demand, what types of medical treatments will be demanded, and how important price is to utilization in each market. As a result of the increased institutional demand, prices in these settings will increase, as will the quantity of services provided. To increase their supply of services, the institutions affected will demand more inputs.

Various health professions will therefore experience an increase in demand for their services. Within each health manpower market, the employing institution's demand for a given health profession will be affected by the wages it would have to pay, the relative wages of other manpower groups that may be substituted for them, their relative productivity, the price of the output, and any legal restrictions that may prevent certain personnel from performing specified tasks. With the increase in demand for health manpower and given the existing stock (i.e., currently trained professionals) of that manpower group, wages and the employment rate in each of the health manpower markets will increase. Exactly how much each will increase will depend on the supply conditions (elasticity) and performance of each health manpower market. The resulting higher incomes will eventually increase the demand for an education leading to entrance into that profession. Thus, lowering an economic barrier to the use of medical care services by providing health insurance has increased demand for different institutional settings, manpower professions, and a health professional education.

The demand increase in each of the different markets will be followed by increases in prices as well as output. The size of the price and output increases in each market resulting from that initial increase in demand will depend on the size of the demand increase and the responsiveness of supply (supply elasticity) within each market. The less elastic supply is, the greater the price increase and the smaller the increase in output. It is precisely because of this effect on prices and output that an analysis of the efficiency of the supply side of each of the medical care markets becomes so important.

If the supply side of the market is relatively inelastic—that is, if it takes a relatively large price increase to bring about an increase in output—then demand programs will result in large price increases and small output increases; consequently, it will cost a great deal of money to achieve an increase in output. For example, according to Figure 3.3, an increase in demand will affect prices and quantity of services differently, depending on the elasticity of supply. If supply is relatively elastic (S_2), then an increase in demand, from D_1 to D_2, will be accompanied by a price increase, but it will be much less (P_2) than if supply were inelastic (S_1), in which case the new price would be P_1. Similarly, a much greater increase in services provided will occur under conditions of elastic supply (Q_2 versus Q_1). If the increase in demand were to occur as a result of a government subsidy program, and if supply were inelastic (S_1), the increased government expenditures for that

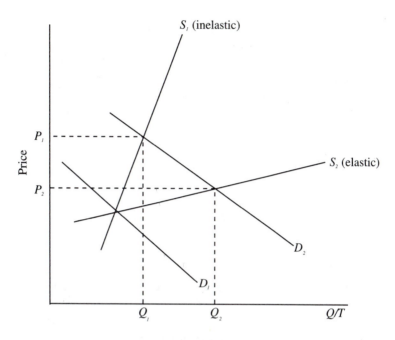

Quantity of medical services

FIGURE 3.3 • The effect on prices and medical services of an
increase in demand when there are different supply elasticities.

program would pay for higher prices (P_1) and less output (Q_1) than if supply were more
elastic (S_2).

It is thus important to understand what the supply elasticity is for each of the medical
care markets. If markets with relatively inelastic supply can be made more elastic, the potential benefits in terms of lower prices and increased output can be very great. Therefore,
we will examine each of the medical care markets in terms of economic efficiency to determine how well each performs. How do each of the markets respond to changes in demand? Could their prices be lower and outputs greater if changes were made in their
structure? By examining each of the medical care markets in terms of structure and performance, we can determine whether the efficiency of those markets can be improved
and what mechanisms will be most useful for improving economic performance.

Other demand policies will also be examined using the framework noted above. For
example, one way in which the government can reduce its expenditures on hospital services to the aged is to provide coverage for care in a less costly setting. Providing insurance coverage to the aged for services provided by a hospice would, assuming that the
hospice is a substitute for fewer hospital admissions, decrease the demand for hospital
care (a shift to the left in the demand for hospitals). As the demand for hospital services
decreases, the hospital's derived demand for its inputs and staff would similarly decrease.

As the out-of-pocket price to the aged for hospice services was reduced as a result of the government insurance coverage, there would be an increase in the quantity demanded of hospice services, with a consequent increase in the derived demand for inputs used by the hospice. Whether covering a lower-cost substitute to hospitals reduces the overall expenditure on services for that medical treatment depends on the relative cost and changes in use of each of those services. (Appendix 3 in Chapter 6 provides a detailed example of how to determine the savings of insuring a lower-cost substitute.)

A Supply Policy

A model of the medical care sector as described above is also useful for explaining how a supply subsidy might work. Typical governmental supply subsidies provide funds to educational institutions for increasing the number of health professionals. Such programs cause a shift to the right in the supply of the educational institutions and increase the schools' enrollment capacity. The effect is to increase the number of graduates in the educational market. As the number of graduates (e.g., physicians or nurses) increases and the supply of those particular health professionals in the health manpower market shifts to the right, the wages or incomes of the subsidized health professionals become lower than they might otherwise have been. The larger number of health professionals (those that were subsidized) and their relatively lower wages will result in an increase in demand for them in the institutional market (a movement down the institutions' demand for such personnel), since they will be substituted for other health professionals whose wages and numbers were not affected by supply subsidies. The effect on the institutional sector will be a shift to the right in their supply curve, since they can presumably produce the same quantity of services at a lower price (or a greater quantity of services at the same price). This is because the price of one of their inputs has been reduced as a result of the subsidy. Institutions will be affected differently by such a subsidy, since some institutions use relatively more of the subsidized input (e.g., hospitals use relatively more registered nurses) than others. The subsidy program's overall effect on the final price and quantity of medical care will vary, depending on how much of an increase in the input occurs as a result of that supply subsidy, how much of a decrease in the price of that input occurs, how much of that subsidized input is used in the production of medical care, and so on.

A completely specified model of the medical care sector should enable us to trace the effects of a supply subsidy program throughout each of the different medical care markets. We can then compare several supply subsidy programs on the basis of what it costs them to achieve a change in the final price and quantity of medical care services. Thus, such a model of the medical care sector allows us to compare alternative government supply subsidies, each of which is designed to increase the availability of medical care. Such subsidy programs need not be directed solely at a manpower category; they may be directed at any number of inputs, such as less-trained personnel who increase the productivity of more highly trained professionals, or they may provide subsidies for hospital construction. An overall model of medical care thus allows any number of supply subsidy programs to be evaluated on the basis of the cost of the subsidy and its final effect on the price and availability of medical care.

SUMMARY

The model of the medical care sector just described also serves to enumerate the different subject areas of this book. To understand the medical care sector it is necessary to learn about the theory of demand for medical care and the consequent derived demands within each of the other markets. In the demand section, as in all other sections, the theoretical discussion of demand will be followed by a review of studies that have attempted to estimate the theoretical variables discussed; the review will be followed by a summary of empirical estimates of the factors that affect demand.

After explaining the demand side of the medical care sector, we will examine the supply side of the different markets. In this way we hope to be able to judge the efficiency of each of the different medical care markets: hospital services, physician services, the market for physicians, the market for registered nurses, and the market for medical education. In addition to judging the efficiency of each of these markets, we will evaluate the relevant government policies that have an impact on these separate markets, such as health manpower legislation in the manpower markets. Finally, we will make public policy recommendations for improving efficiency within each of these markets, based on our analysis of their inadequate market performance.

This overview of medical care will also be used to discuss alternative approaches to its redistribution. Even though inefficiencies continue to exist in the medical care market, society may decide to increase the consumption of medical care to the population or to selected population groups. Such an overview suggests that it is possible to achieve an increase in consumption of medical care services either by shifting the demands for care or by increasing the quantity of a particular input on the supply side (i.e., shifting supply). Each of these policies will result in an increase in the quantity of medical care services consumed, as shown in Figure 3.4. For example, to increase the quantity of medical services consumed from Q_0 to Q_1 (based on a normative judgment that it is desirable to do so), either the demand for medical care can be increased from D_1 to D_2, or the supply can be increased from S_1 to S_2. Either of these policies will achieve the objective of increasing the use of medical care from Q_0 to Q_1. However, these alternative redistributive policies will differ in their costs and their effects on other population groups.

Demand and supply subsidies can be general, as when everyone in the population has access to that subsidy, or they can be targeted, such as providing the demand subsidy only to those with low incomes or subsidizing providers in low income areas. The cost of general versus targeted subsidies will differ as would the number of low-income persons receiving those subsidies.

The overview presented here illustrates why medical care is said to be the output of the

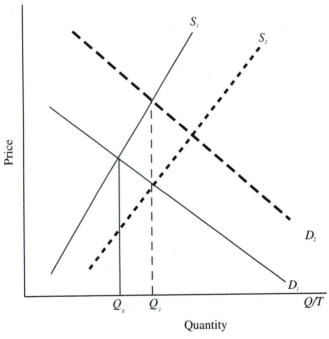

FIGURE 3.4 • Alternative demand and supply policies to achieve a redistribution of medical care.

medical care sector. The efficiency of the separate markets and their interrelationship affect the efficiency with which medical care is produced, the cost at which it is produced, and the growth of expenditures in this sector. The evaluation of the efficiency of each of these markets is, therefore, of prime concern for public policy.

The foregoing model of medical care also illustrates the alternative approaches that may be used to redistribute medical services and the means for evaluating them. These two concepts, efficiency and redistribution (equity), will be the basis on which both the separate markets and government policies will be analyzed throughout this book.

Key Terms and Concepts

- Health education markets
- Health manpower markets
- Institutional markets

- Demand subsidy effects
- Determinants of demand in each market
- Determinants of supply in each market

- Interrelationship of each type of market
- Outcomes of each market
- Supply subsidy effects

Review Questions

1. With an increase in demand for medical care, how will different supply elasticities affect total medical expenditures?
2. Assume that the price of a specific input (e.g., registered nurses) is subsidized. Trace through the effect of such a policy in all the medical markets and evaluate this policy in terms of its effect on the goal of increasing the level of the population's health. Second, evaluate this policy in terms of economic efficiency. Finally, evaluate this policy in terms of who benefits and who bears the cost.
3. Trace through the effects of increased use by insurance companies of preauthorization review of hospital admissions in each of the medical care markets.
4. Based on demographic projections, it is estimated that fewer female high school graduates will be available to pursue a nursing career. Trace through this demographic effect in each of the medical care markets.

REFERENCES

1. The description of the medical care sector in this section is based on an article by Paul J. Feldstein and Sander Kelman, "An Econometric Model of the Medical Care Sector," in H. Klarman, ed., *Empirical Studies in Health Economics* (Baltimore: Johns Hopkins University Press, 1970). Economists have developed other econometric models of the medical care sector. Perhaps the most ambitious of these is the one by D. E. Yett, L. Drabek, M. S. Intriligator, and L. J. Kimbell, *A Forecasting and Policy Simulation Model of the Health Care Sector* (Lexington, Mass.: Lexington Books, 1979).

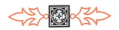

CHAPTER

Measuring Changes in the Price of Medical Care

THE USES OF A DEFINITION OF THE PRODUCT OF THE MEDICAL CARE INDUSTRY

How much has the price of medical care been increasing? Do rising Medicare expenditures indicate increased use of services, or are they the result of rising prices? Are physician fees falling as the result of the increased supply of physicians? Has competition in medical care reduced the rate of increase in medical prices? These are only some of the questions that are important to policymakers and define major areas of research in the economics of medical care. To answer these questions, accurate information on medical prices is essential.

Accurate price information consists of two parts: a definition of the output being measured and the actual price paid for that output.

What is the price of, for example, a hospital admission, and how has it changed over time? Is it the hospital's charges? Large insurers and HMOs do not pay charges; neither do Medicare and Medicaid. In fact, at any time a hospital may have negotiated over one hundred different prices for the same services with different organizations.

As difficult as it is to measure actual prices and their changes over time, measuring the output of the medical sector is even more difficult. A hospital admission in 1995 is not the same as one in 1985 and certainly not the same as one in 1965. The medical conditions treated in the hospital have changed as has the medical technology used to treat those diseases. Outcomes of hospital treatment have also changed.

More important, patients do not demand a hospital admission or a physician visit; they demand treatment for a particular disease. Hospital care, physician services, and home health care are actually inputs into a treatment. To determine whether medical prices are increasing it is necessary to determine how the costs of a treatment have changed over time. The treatment for heart disease involves drugs, hospital care, physician services, and so on, and the combination of these services or inputs has changed over time. Complicating the issue is that survival, the outcome of treatment for heart disease, has improved over time. Unless the cost of treatment is adjusted for survival and quality of life, the data will indicate that input costs (hospital care, etc.) and overall treatment costs have increased. But patients with heart disease are clearly better off today than patients thirty years ago.

Unless medical prices are adjusted for outcomes, they provide an inaccurate measure of price inflation.

From the patient's point of view, the demand for medical care is the demand for a treatment for some actual or perceived, current or potential, physical or mental disorder. After the patient consults a physician, a treatment is prescribed that often uses a combination of various inputs. Ideally, the costs and prices of medical care should be measured in terms of outputs, not just according to the inputs used in the treatment process. Using outputs rather than inputs would enable increases in input productivity and technological advances to be reflected both in the costs of providing a treatment and in its outcome.

Essential to any treatment measure of output is the need to adjust treatment costs for changes in treatment outcomes.

This chapter analyzes the measurement of prices, particularly in the field of medical care, beginning with a description of the functions and limitations of the CPI. This is followed by a detailed discussion of the medical care component of the CPI, which is still the most widely used index of medical care prices. The final section describes and evaluates another approach to measuring the price of medical care—one that is based on the use of medical treatment as the most appropriate unit of medical care output.

THE CONSUMER PRICE INDEX

What Should the CPI Measure?

The CPI is generally viewed as an index of the cost of living. The percentage change in the CPI from one year to the next is taken as a measure of the rate of inflation—the rate at which a family's income would have had to increase just to keep up with rising prices. Many union contracts contain provisions for automatically increasing wages in line with increases in the CPI. Social Security benefit levels are keyed to it as well, as are the pensions of retired federal employees. Private pension plans, however, are rarely affected by changes in the CPI. In all, the incomes of about half of the U.S. population are directly affected by changes in the CPI.

The CPI is viewed as an indicator of the nation's inflation rate and as such policymakers use it to determine monetary and fiscal policy. Further, the CPI, when it is used to deflate personal consumption expenditures in constructing national income accounts, affects estimates of real growth in the economy and productivity of the nation's labor force.

If the CPI were a true cost-of-living index, then it should measure the cost of maintaining a given level of welfare or utility, of remaining on a certain indifference curve. Accordingly, the cost of living is influenced by much more than the prices of goods and services that consumers buy. Tax rates influence the amount of gross income needed to maintain a certain level of welfare. Taxes that directly influence the prices of products, such as sales taxes, are reflected in the CPI; income taxes are not. On the other hand, governmental provision of more free-of-charge services, such as better highways or better fire departments, may increase the standard of living achievable at any level of income. One might argue that standards of living are also affected by changes in crime rates, environmental pollution, and other factors essentially beyond the individual's control.

Unless the above factors are considered in a cost-of-living index, it is not necessarily true that a household is better off when its gross income increases faster than the prices of the goods and services it buys (1).

Aware of the difficulty of measuring the cost of maintaining a level of welfare, the Bureau of Labor Statistics (BLS) has attempted a more modest task and designed the CPI to measure the change in the cost of purchasing a fixed market basket of goods and services representing average consumption patterns during some base period. A price index of this type, in which individual prices are weighted by base-year quantities, is called a Laspeyres index.[1] Thus, the CPI aims to measure how much the average household in its surveyed population will have to spend to buy the same market basket in the current year that it bought in the base year.

---

[1]It can be expressed by the following formula:

$$I_t = \frac{\sum_i Q_{bi} P_{ti}}{\sum_i Q_{bi} Pt_{bi}}$$

where
I_t = value of the index in year t
Q_{bi} = quantity of good i purchased in the base year
P_{bi} = price of good i in the base year
P_{ti} = price of good i in the year t
Such an index is often multiplied by some scaling factor so that it equals 100 in some particular year. Of course, if the index is multiplied by the same scaling factor in each year, percentage changes from year to year are not affected.

Even this limited view of the CPI, however, is not simple. The market basket purchased by the average household in the surveyed population is constantly changing, not only in response to price changes, but also in response to changes in incomes, tastes, and other factors as well. The quality of existing goods and services changes, and new products that had no counterparts in the past are introduced. It would be meaningless to go on pricing the same goods and services without making an allowance for these changes. In the following section, how the BLS resolves some of the major issues involved in constructing the CPI are discussed, together with the likely effects on the accuracy of the CPI.

Issues and Problems in Constructing the CPI

Population Coverage

The CPI was designed to measure price changes for urban wage earners and clerical workers; however, the definition of the covered population has changed over time (2). Until 1964, only families were included. At that time, single persons were added and the stipulation that household income should be less than $10,000 was dropped. After the 1964 revision of the CPI, its coverage included about 45 percent of the total U.S. population. In the 1987 revision of the CPI, a CPI was constructed for two population groups: all urban consumers (CPI-U) and wage earners and clerical workers (CPI-W) (3). The CPI-U is based on expenditures of all urban consumer units without regard to income or employment status. Excluded from the CPI-U are all rural and farm residents, military personnel, and those in institutions. Approximately 81 percent of all consumers and 80 percent of the noninstitutionalized population are included in the CPI-U.

The CPI-W is a more restricted sample that includes urban consumer units that receive more than half of their income from clerical or wage occupations and one or more of the household members had to be employed for at least thirty-seven weeks in an eligible occupation during the past twelve months. The CPI-W covers 38 percent of all consumer units and 42 percent of the noninstitutional population. Organized labor has supported the continued use of the traditional index (CPI-W) in contract escalation provisions because it believes that the more comprehensive index (CPI-U) will rise more slowly than the CPI-W.

Sampling Problems

The BLS updates the CPI market basket of goods and services about every ten years. The CPI (as of 1997), which was revised in 1987, is based on a survey of spending patterns for the 1982–84 period. Starting in 1998, the CPI will be based on a survey conducted in 1993–95. The survey consists of two components: (a) an interview survey to determine expenditures on those items (and quantity) that people purchase; (b) a diary, or record-keeping survey, in which individuals are asked to record a two-week diary of small, frequently purchased items. The BLS assigns weights to different items in the CPI based on data from these consumer expenditure surveys.[2]

Several aspects of the BLS sampling methodology may bias the CPI. The major criticism of these surveys has been that, at ten-year intervals, they are not conducted frequently enough. The BLS's weighting system was, until 1978, based on 1960–61 information. Until the 1987 revision, spending patterns were based on 1972–73 survey data. And until 1998, the CPI was based on buying patterns from a fifteen-year-old (1982–84) Consumer Expenditure Survey (CE). During any ten- to fifteen-year period, consumption patterns change and new products are introduced. These changes, however, are not picked up in the CPI until a new revision appears.

Table 4.1 indicates changes in the relative weights of major groups of items over the years. The years 1935–39, 1952, 1963, 1981, and 1996 were chosen because they correspond to major revisions in the CPI growing out of new consumer expenditure surveys. The 1981 weights are based on the 1972–73 survey and were first incorporated in the CPI in January 1978. December 1996 was chosen because it was the most recent data available.

The most striking trends in Table 4.1 are the declines in the importance of food and the increase in transportation costs in consumer budgets. The weight assigned to food has fallen considerably despite the fact that, as Table 4.2 shows, its price has risen as fast as the all-items index. The decline in the importance of food in consumer budgets probably reflects low-income elasticity rather than high-price elasticity. As per capita incomes have increased, a smaller fraction has been used to buy food. Food and housing remain, however, the most important elements in consumer budgets, together accounting for well over half of expenditures on the average.

The CPI is based on seven major product groups of items, such as food, medical care, and so on. These major groups are further divided into 69 expenditure classes, which in turn, are subdivided into 207 strata of items. The strata are the level at which the CPI is calculated. The strata subdivide into a total of 364 entry-level items; some strata may contain only one entry-level item, while others may contain several. The BLS samples these entry-level items in 44 geographical areas. The CPI is calculated and published for the 44 geographic areas and 207 strata of items which, when combined, result in 9,108 strata.

Probability sampling, which was introduced in the 1972–73 CPI revision, is used to determine how the price of an item changes over time. It is assumed that the other items in that expenditure class are changing in price, on the average, at the same rate as the item or items actually priced.

Within each geographic area sampled, a point-of-purchase survey is conducted in

---

[2]The national CPI is built up from indexes calculated for a sample of cities. Separate city indexes are published. Differences between city indexes, however, do not measure price differences between cities, but only indicate price changes for each city since the base period.

TABLE 4.1 Relative Importance of Major Components of the CPI, Selected Years (Percent)

Group	1935–39	December 1952	December 1963	December 1981[a]	December 1996[a]
All items	100.0	100.0	100.0	100.0	100.0
Food and beverages	35.4	32.2	25.2	17.5	17.5
Housing	33.7	33.5	34.0	46.0	41.2[b]
Apparel and upkeep	11.0	9.4	10.6	4.6	5.3
Transportation	8.1	11.3	14.0	19.3	17.1
Medical care	4.1	4.8	5.7	4.9	7.4
Entertainment[c]	2.8	4.0	3.9	3.6	4.4
Other goods and services[d]	4.9	4.8	5.7	4.0	7.2

Sources: U.S. Department of Labor, Bureau of Labor Statistics, *Handbook of Labor Statistics,* 1989, p. 485; data for December 1996 come from Internet site http://stats.bls.gov.

[a] CPI for All Urban Consumers.

[b] The rental equivalence approach to homeowner's costs: effective January 1985.

[c] Called "reading and recreation" before December 1977.

[d] "Other goods and services" now includes educational and "personal care" expenses, which were previously found under other categories. It also includes tobacco products; it no longer includes alcoholic beverages.

which consumers are asked how much they spend on each category of consumption and also where they make their purchases. Based on this survey, the BLS selects a sample of outlets (or, in the case of the medical care component of the CPI [MCPI], medical providers). Within each selected outlet one or more specific varieties of items are selected, the probability of the item selected is proportional to its sales based on the point-of-purchase survey.

Given this extensive sampling, there is still the problem, mentioned above, of outdated weights. Up until 1998, the weights for the CPI were based on the fifteen-year-old 1982–84 Consumer Expenditure Survey. Even the latest weights are not current at their time of introduction, but are based on a survey that was already five years old. These outdated weights, because of the substitution effect, may lead to an upward bias.

Substitution Bias

Because the CPI calculates price changes based on the Laspeyres index there is a substitution bias, which overstates inflation. The additional income required to purchase the base-year market basket in a later year will generally exceed the increase necessary to buy a market basket that is *equivalent in the eyes of the consumer* to that purchased in the base year. The CPI assumes that the consumer will purchase the same quantity of the item even though its price has risen. In fact, consumers will substitute away from those items for which price is rising more rapidly and this will lessen, to some extent, the impact of the general price increase.[3] For example, if videocassette recorders become relatively cheaper and movie theater tickets relatively more expensive, consumers may substitute home viewing for theater viewing with no loss of overall well-being. Studies have shown, however, that the substitution bias has had only a small upward effect on the CPI.

Quality Changes and New Products

Price changes that result from improvements in product quality should be omitted from a price index for measuring inflation. For example, if a color television set is substituted for a black-and-white set, the index should not reflect the full price difference between the two, since most of it will be due to product quality differences. If the CPI did not adjust for quality improvements in new cars, then between 1967 and 1994 the price of new cars would have risen 80 percent. For some products such as personal computers, consumer durables, apparel, and prescription drugs, quality change has been significant (4). Inadequate adjustment for quality change has led to an overstatement of inflation.

If the BLS considers the change in quality to be small, there is no adjustment for quality improvement; this causes an upward bias in the CPI. Otherwise, substitutions of new for old items are normally accomplished by linking. When the substitution is made, both the old and the new market baskets are priced. Percentage changes in the index prior to the link reflect percentage changes in the price of the old market basket; percentage changes after the link reflect percentage changes in the price of the new market basket. Thus, the price difference between the two market baskets at the time of the link is not reflected at all in the index.[4]

In many cases linking appears to be a good method of changing the CPI market basket. If the link is made at a time when one product is beginning to replace another in the market, but both are available and are purchased by some consumers, then the higher-

---

[3]An index that used current-year quantities as weights would understate cost-of-living increases because it would put too much weight on items whose prices had increased relatively slowly. Such an index is called a Paasche index. Clearly, some sort of average of a Laspeyres index and a Paasche index will yield a better measure of cost-of-living changes than either one individually. The Laspeyres formula is used primarily because of the high cost of continually collecting information on weights.

[4]The following is a simple hypothetical example of linking. Suppose that an EC has been represented by one item, black-and-white TV sets, and a decision has been made to price color sets instead. Let us say that the index for this EC was equal to 100 in year 1. The price of black-and-white sets rises from $150 to $165, from year 1 to year 2, which is an increase of 10 percent. The index, still based on black-and-white sets, rises to 110. At that point the link is made. Color sets go from $400 to $420, from year 2 to year 3, a 5 percent increase. The index, now based on the price of color sets, increases 5 percent to 115.5 in year 3. The $235 difference between the prices of color and black-and-white sets in year 2 never shows up in the index at all.

Year	B&W TV Sets	Index	Color TV Sets
1	$150	100	—
2	$165	110	$400
3	—	115.5	$420

priced one is worth the difference in price. However, when price changes are relatively small and quality improvements are large, linking understates the degree of quality improvement. For this reason, the BLS has explored other methods of making direct quality adjustments.[5]

The BLS has been criticized for introducing new items too slowly into the CPI. Initially, a new item tends to have a relatively high price. This price falls as production expands, and an increase in the number of producers leads to greater price competition. If consumers accept a new item while its price is relatively high, and if the item is absent from the index until after its price has fallen, the index will fail to register that fall in price of an item already important in consumer budgets. This problem occurs, for example, with the introduction of new drugs. The CPI will overstate inflation because it will miss the price declines of new goods.

In addition to the timeliness issue, new goods must be adjusted for price differences with the items they replace. It is difficult to estimate the extent of the CPI bias when a new good is substituted for another good because of price increases in the other good (substitution bias) and when a new good has quality improvements (quality bias). Some new goods provide the same services as the previous good but with a greater variety of services; some are of higher quality or lower price, and others provide entirely new services previously unavailable (e.g., cellular telephones).

Separating the many aspects of new goods, including timeliness, and adjusting for price differences between new and older goods is difficult and the extent of bias in the CPI for inadequately doing this is not easily determined.

It has been estimated that the overstatement of the CPI due to all of the various biases mentioned above is between 0.4 and 1.5 percent per year. The size of this bias is significant, given that the CPI is used to adjust federal revenues, such as Social Security payments and income tax brackets. In 1995, a 1 percent increase in the CPI raised federal outlays and reduced federal revenues enough to cause an increase of $6.5 billion in the federal deficit. Given these magnitudes, additional research to improve the accuracy of the CPI is being undertaken.

---

[5]The issue of adjusting for quality changes in a price index has received a great deal of attention from economists and statisticians. One proposed method for making such adjustments is the so-called hedonic technique. It can be applied to products for which many types are available at any one time, automobiles being perhaps the best example. Data are collected on the prices and characteristics of a number of different models at a point in time. Regression analysis is then used to estimate the contribution of different characteristics (in the case of the automobile, horsepower, fuel economy, interior room) to price. We can use this information to estimate what current models would have cost in the base year, based on their characteristics. The difference between these prices and the current-year prices would be estimates of the pure price change. To date, this method has not been used by the BLS. For a more complete discussion of this subject, see John Muelbauer, "Household Production Theory, Quality, and the Hedonic Technique," *American Economic Review,* 64, December 1974: 977–994, and Zvi Griliches, "Hedonic Price Indexes for Automobiles: An Econometric Analysis of Quality Change," in *The Price Statistics of the Federal Government* (Cambridge, Mass.: National Bureau of Economic Research, 1961), pp. 173–196.

Table 4.2 presents values for the CPI and its major component groups during the 1935–96 period. Since all the component indexes are scaled to equal 100 in 1982–84, those with the smallest values in 1935 increased the fastest in the 1982–84 period. The major component groups with the highest values in 1996 have increased the fastest since 1982–84. A one-point increase in an index is, of course, a smaller percentage increase today than it was in 1935. Table 4.2 shows that the indexes for the different major groups have had quite different patterns of increase over the years. Over the period as a whole, medical care has risen the most rapidly.

THE MEDICAL CARE COMPONENT OF THE CPI (MCPI)

Background of the MCPI

Rapidly rising medical prices have been the stimulus for proposals and legislation to reduce their rise. Much effort has been devoted to attempts to reduce the rise in hospital rates, physician fees, and prices of prescription drugs. Rising medical prices, which are a

TABLE 4.2 CPI and Major Groups, 1935–96 (1982–84 = 100)

Year	All Items	Food	Housing	Apparel and Upkeep	Transpor- tation	Medical Care	Entertain- ment[a]	Other[b]
1935	13.7	12.5	15.2	20.8	14.2	10.2	17.0	15.7
1945	18.0	17.3	18.2	31.4	15.9	11.9	25.4	20.0
1955	26.8	27.9	25.3	42.9	25.8	18.2	31.2	28.0
1965	31.5	32.2	29.2	47.8	31.9	25.2	39.1	33.0
1970	38.8	40.1	36.4	59.2	37.5	34.0	47.5	40.9
1975	53.8	60.2	50.7	72.5	50.1	47.5	62.0	53.9
1980[c]	82.4	86.7	81.1	90.9	83.1	74.9	83.6	75.2
1985[c]	107.6	105.6	107.7	105.0	106.4	113.5	107.9	114.5
1990[c]	130.7	132.4	128.5	124.1	120.5	162.8	132.4	159.0
1996[c]	156.9	153.3	152.8	131.7	143.0	228.2	159.1	215.4

Sources: U.S. Department of Labor, Bureau of Labor Statistics, *Handbook of Labor Statistics,* 1989; data for 1990 and 1996 come from Internet site http:\\stats.bls.gov

Note: The 1978 revision brought about several definitional changes, which have made it impossible to directly link pre- and post-1978 indexes for "entertainment" and "other."

[a] Entertainment includes most of what was called "reading and recreation"; entertainment excludes certain subcomponents found in "reading and recreation," such as TV and sound equipment, TV repair, and educational expenses.

[b] "Other" now includes educational and "personal care" expenses, which were previously found under other categories. It also includes tobacco products; it no longer includes alcoholic beverages.

[c] CPI for All Urban Consumers.

component of the CPI and have increased much more rapidly than the CPI, have caused the CPI to increase more rapidly than it would have otherwise. In 1996, medical care had a weight of 7.4 percent in the CPI-U, up from 4.9 percent in 1981, as shown in Table 4.1. An increase of about 13.5 percent in the MCPI would, in and of itself, increase the CPI by 1 percent. Through its effect on the overall CPI, the MCPI influences the CPI and has far-ranging effects on federal and private revenues and outlays as well as monetary policy to fight inflation. Determining the accuracy of the MCPI, therefore, is important for national policy as well as for evaluating the performance of the medical care sector.

The BLS views the MCPI, like the CPI, as an index of the price of a fixed bundle of goods and services. Four important issues are raised by this approach. First, is the weighting of the MCPI (and its individual components) an accurate reflection of its importance to the CPI? Second, are the prices recorded by the BLS accurate? Third, have the goods and services remained constant over time, or have new services been introduced and has quality changed? Fourth, how well do the goods and services priced by the BLS represent what consumers are purchasing? The remainder of this chapter discusses these four issues.

Table 4.3 presents an overview of movements in the MCPI and its component items since 1965. A glance at the table reveals that the medical services category has increased more rapidly than the medical care commodities category. The fastest-rising component of the MCPI has been the hospital room rate; a close second is prescription drugs.

Table 4.4 gives a breakdown of the relative weights of the items included in the MCPI as of December 1996. These weights are based on the 1982–84 Consumer Expenditure Survey data on quantities of medical goods and services consumed, updated to 1996 prices. Note that the weights for the CPI-U and the CPI-W are very similar.

The Weight of the MCPI in the CPI

The population covered by the MCPI and the overall CPI is, of course, the same. Since 1978, when the population coverage was extended to include the elderly, the population reflected in the MCPI has become more representative of the general population. Previously, when the aged, who are large consumers of medical services, were excluded, the weight assigned to medical care in the traditional CPI understated its importance in total consumption for the entire population; the relative weights of particular services within the MCPI were also different from the relative weights of those items in total U.S. medical care consumption. Hospital services, for example, are relatively more important for the elderly and unemployed than for urban wage earners and clerical workers. Dentists' fees are relatively less important. The MCPI has therefore become more representative of the general population.

Although the population has become more representative, an important factor affecting the weight of the MCPI is the exclusion of services that are paid for by the government on behalf of consumers. The CPI attempts to measure goods and services purchased by consumers. However, in expanding the population coverage of the CPI, the

TABLE 4.3 Trends in the MCPI, Selected Years, 1965–96 (1982–84 = 100 unless noted)

Item	1965	1970	1975	1980	1985	1990	1996
Medical care	25.2	34.0	47.5	74.9	113.5	162.8	228.2
Medical care commodities	45.0	46.5	53.3	75.4	115.2	163.4	210.4
Prescription drugs	47.8	47.4	51.2	72.5	120.1	181.7	242.9
Nonprescription drugs and medical supplies[a] (1986 = 100)						120.6	143.1
Medical care services	22.7	32.3	46.6	74.8	113.2	162.7	232.4
Professional services		37.0	50.8	77.9	113.5	156.1	208.3
Physicians' services	25.1	34.5	48.1	76.5	113.3	160.8	216.4
Dental services	30.3	39.2	53.2	78.9	114.2	155.8	216.5
Services by other medical professionals[b] (1986 = 100)						120.2	146.6
Hospital and related services					69.2	116.1	178.0	269.5
Hospital room	12.3	23.6	38.3	68.0	115.4	175.4	261.0
Other inpatient hospital services[c] (1986 = 100)						142.7	216.9
Outpatient services[d] (1986 = 100)						138.7	215.1

Sources: U.S. Department of Labor, Bureau of Labor Statistics, *Handbook of Labor Statistics,* 1975 and 1981 editions; Internet site http:\\stats.bls.gov.

Note: The only indexes available prior to 1978 are for urban wage earners and clerical workers. However, the table uses the more comprehensive All Urban Consumer indexes, which were introduced in 1978, for the year 1980. After the 1987 revision, all of the services include benefits paid by consumer-purchased insurance as well as consumer out-of-pocket expenditures.

[a] Excludes eyeglasses.

[b] Includes all consumer out-of-pocket expenses for eye care commodities.

[c] Consists of other hospital and inpatient services, including nursing and convalescent home service.

[d] Consists of emergency room services, laboratory fees, and x-rays.

BLS has added groups for whom the government, through Medicare and Medicaid, pays a large portion of their medical care services. In keeping with its general policy, the BLS does not attempt to reflect these governmental expenditures in the CPI weights. The MCPI is not designed as an index of the price of the bundle of medical care services *consumed* by its target population, but of those services *purchased* by it.

The importance of some of these points is illustrated in Tables 4.5, 4.6, and 4.7. Table 4.5 compares the weights of particular services in the MCPI with the weights of similar services from two additional data sources. They are the CE and total national expenditures from the National Health Accounts (NHA). The weights are compared for 1975, 1985, and 1995.

TABLE 4.4 Relative Weights of Items in the MCPI (December 1996)

	U (%)	W (%)
Medical care	100.0	100.0
Medical care commodities	17.3	16.7
Prescription drugs	12.1	11.4
Nonprescription drugs and medical supplies	5.2	5.3
Medical care services	82.7	83.3
Professional services	47.3	47.6
Physicians' services	25.7	25.8
Dental services	14.7	15.6
Eye care	4.6	4.5
Services by other medical professionals	2.3	1.7
Hospital and related services	31.0	32.0
Health insurance	4.4	3.7

Source: U.S. Department of Labor, Bureau of Labor Statistics, *Relative Importance of Components of the Consumer Price Index,* 1996, Table 1.

Note: Only health insurance premiums paid by the consumer are included in the CPI. The health insurance relative importance includes only that portion of the premium that is retained by the insurance carrier for administrative cost and profit, 9.7 percent of the total premiums for U and 10.6 percent for W. The portions that are paid as benefits have been assigned to the relevant medical care relative importances.

There are two major reasons why the weight of medical care services differs among the three data sets. The MCPI and the CE have a similar set of weights for the medical care expenditure categories. The major difference between the MCPI and the CE is that the CE covers the urban as well as rural populations, which the MCPI does not. Previously, the MCPI also excluded certain urban age groups, such as the aged. However, population differences between the MCPI and the CE have become smaller in recent years since the aged were included in the CPI in 1978. The population covered by the CE and the NHA are similar except for the elderly living in nursing homes; if this expense is paid by the elderly themselves or by third-party coverage, then it will be included in the NHA but not the CE.

The second reason for differences between the MCPI, CE, and NHA is the exclusion from the MCPI and the CE of payments made by third parties. Only out-of-pocket expenses and health insurance premiums paid by consumers are included in the MCPI and the CE. Previously, the MCPI did not allocate health insurance expenditures to their separate benefit areas. Currently, the MCPI weight for health insurance only shows that portion of the premium that is retained by insurance companies for administrative cost and profit; that portion of insurance spent on specific services is added to those services. The NHA includes all medical expenditures, including those by the government and employer-paid health insurance.

The exclusion of third-party payments from the MCPI and the CE is particularly im-

TABLE 4.5 Relative Weights of Items in MCPI, in Consumer Expenditures on Health Services and Supplies, and in Total National Expenditures on Health Services and Supplies, Calendar Years 1975, 1985, and 1995

	1975			1985			1995		
	MCPI[a] (Dec. 1975)	Consumer[b] Expenditures (1972–73)	Total Expenditures	MCPI[a] (Dec. 1985)	Consumer[b] Expenditures	Total Expenditures	MCPI[a] Dec. (1995)	Consumer[b] Expenditures	Total Expenditures
Medical services		80.1							
Hospital services	28.5	—[c]	40.2	26.4	26.6	39.3	30.7	31.2	35.4
Physicians' services	26.0	—[c]	18.3	27.0	27.2	19.5	25.7	24.8	20.4
Dental services	14.4	—[c]	6.1	15.1	15.7	5.1	14.5	14.1	4.6
Nursing home	—[c]	—[c]	6.6	—[c]	1.4	7.2	—[c]	1.4	7.9
All others[d]	15.5	0.0	13.1	8.8	8.7	13.2	6.9	7.0	17.0
Medical care commodities	12.0	16.5	11.9	18.9	16.9	10.2	17.4	16.4	9.8
Health insurance[e]	3.6	3.4	3.8	3.8	3.5	5.6	4.9	5.1	4.8
Total	100.0	100.0	100.0	100.0	100.0	100.1	100.1	100.0	99.9

Sources: U.S. Department of Labor, Bureau of Labor Statistics, *Relative Importance of Components of the Consumer Price Index,* various issues; U.S. Department of Labor, Bureau of Labor Statistics, *Consumer Expenditure Survey: Integrated Survey Data,* various issues, and unpublished data, 1996; U.S. Department of Health and Human Services, Health Care Financing Administration, Internet site http://www.hcfa.gov/stats/nhce96.htm, and unpublished data, 1996.

Note: Totals may not add up to 100.0 due to rounding.

[a] The index for all Urban Consumers is used.

[b] The amount of charges paid by consumer-paid health insurance has been allocated to specific services using the 1987 allocation rate provided to us by BLS.

[c] Data are not available. Prior to 1980, there is no breakdown of "medical services" in the Consumer Expenditure Survey. Also, there is no breakdown of "nursing home" from "other outpatient services" in MCPI; they are included in "hospital services."

[d] "All others" in MCPI includes "eye care" and "services by other medical professionals"; in consumer expenditures, it includes "eye care services," "services by other than physicians," "lab test, x-rays," "repair of medical equipment," and "other medical care services"; in National Health Accounts (NHA), it includes "other professional services," "home health care," "other personal health care," "public health activities," "research," and "construction."

[e] Health Insurance has been allocated to different services according to the allocation rate used by CPI in 1987. Health insurance includes only that portion of the premium that is retained by the insurance carrier for administrative cost and profit.

portant for certain services, such as hospital care, which are more likely to be covered by government (Medicare) and private insurance. Thus, the weight for hospital care is greater in total expenditures (NHA) than in the MCPI and the CE. Correspondingly, the weights of dentists' fees and drugs fall as we move across the three columns. Dental services and drugs are largely paid for by consumers, not the government or employers; thus, these components have a much larger weight with respect to what consumers spend but they represent a smaller portion of total medical expenditures, including government purchases.

Hospital expenditures have a weight that is almost 8 times greater than dental services in NHA but only twice as large in MCPI and CE. Since the price of hospital services has increased faster than the price of dental care, the MCPI understates the increase that has occurred in the MCPI over time. If the medical care price index was based on total medical expenditures (NHA), the MCPI would have increased faster than it did in the past decade, since total expenditures (NHA) give a heavier weight to the fastest-rising component, hospital care.

Nursing home services had no weight in the MCPI prior to the 1978 revision, since the CPI was limited to wage earners and clerical workers and excluded the elderly. Even though the aged are now included in the MCPI, there is a large difference between the CE and the NHA for nursing homes since the government is a large payer of nursing home services under Medicaid. The MCPI includes nursing homes in hospital services while the other two data sources separate nursing home expenditures.

Table 4.6 provides an indication of the importance of third-party payments. NHA expenditures in 1995 were more than 5 times greater than CE expenditures—$988 billion compared to $178 billion. For some services, such as dental care, there is almost a 100 percent difference, while for others, such as nursing homes, the difference is 30 times greater.

Table 4.7 shows how the weight of medical care within the CPI index would be different if the index covered the entire population and total medical expenditures rather than just consumer out-of-pocket payments. For 1975, 1985, and 1995, the CPI weight of medical care is compared with the weight of *consumer* expenditures on health services and supplies in personal consumption and with the weight of *total* expenditures on personal health care *plus* government purchases.

In the compared years, both of the former weights are smaller than the weight of medical care in personal consumption plus government expenditures; this reflects the large role government and employers play in financing medical services. It appears that the CPI weight of medical care will continue to understate the importance of medical care in total consumption, particularly if the role of government in this sector continues to expand and the CPI fails to include such expenditures in determining its weights.

Accuracy of Measured Prices in the MCPI

For the MCPI, as with the CPI, the BLS attempts to price items for which consumers have an out-of-pocket expenditure. For every such item, the BLS attempts to measure a

TABLE 4.6 Consumer Expenditures on Health Services and Supplies, and Total National Expenditures on Health Services and Supplies, 1995 (billions)

	1995	
	Consumer Expenditures	**Total Expenditures**
Medical services		
Hospital services	$55.8	$350.1
Physicians' services	44.2	201.6
Dental services	25.2	45.8
Nursing home	2.5	77.9
All others[a]	12.4	168.3
Medical care commodities[b]	29.3	97.2
Health Insurance	9.1	47.7
Total	178.5	988.5

Source: Katharine R. Levit et al., "National Health Expenditures, 1995," *Health Care Financing Review,* Fall 1996, 18(1): p. 201, Table 9 and p. 185, Table 5; U.S. Department of Labor, Bureau of Labor Statistics, Consumer Expenditure Survey, 1995, unpublished data.

Note: Totals may not add up exactly due to rounding.

[a] All others in Consumer Expenditures includes "eye care services," "services by other than physicians," "lab test, x-rays," "repair of medical equipment," and "other medical care services"; in National Health Accounts (NHA) it includes: "other professional care," "home health care," "other personal health care," "public health activities," "research," and "onstruction".

[b] The amount of charges paid by consumer-paid health insurance has been allocated to specific services using the 1987 allocation rate provided to us by BLS.

transaction price. A transaction price is the price a consumer actually pays for an item in the CPI market basket of goods and services. With regard to the MCPI, particularly for hospitals, transaction price data have not been used. Instead, the BLS relied on list prices.

The difference between hospital list prices (the charge to a full-paying patient) and the fees hospitals actually receive has been a major source of bias for the MCPI and, consequently, the CPI. There have been important changes in the percentage of patients that are full-paying and in how both private insurers and the government pays for hospital services.

Hospitals are paid different prices by different payers. Medicare changed from payment a per day to a payment per admission starting in 1983. Medicare's payment per admission also varies according to the patient's diagnosis. Medicaid also pays hospitals a different rate than does Medicare. In addition to government payers, hospitals also charge self-payers (those without insurance) a separate price, while those who are uninsured and unable to pay may not be charged anything. Lastly, private insurers and HMOs each negotiate separate prices with hospitals for their enrollees. And in the past decade there has been a large shift of the privately insured population into HMOs and preferred provider organizations (PPOs). Thus, a hospital may have upwards of one hundred different prices. List prices are not indicative of actual payments received.

TABLE 4.7 Weights of Medical Care in CPI, in Personal Consumption, and in Personal Consumption Plus Government Purchases, Calendar Years 1975, 1985, and 1995

	1975	1985	1995
Weight of medical care in CPI	6.4	6.5	6.3
Weight of consumer expenditure on health services and supplies in personal consumption	4.8[a]	4.7	5.4
Weight of total expenditures on health services and supplies in personal consumption plus government purchases[b]	10.3	12.2	15.7

Sources: U.S. Department of Labor, Bureau of Labor Statistics, *Relative Importance of Components of the Consumer Price Index,* various issues; U.S. Department of Labor, Bureau of Labor Statistics, *Consumer Expenditure Survey: Integrated Survey Data,* various issues; Katharine R. Levit et al., "National Health Expenditures, 1994," *Health Care Financing Review,* 17(3), Spring 1996: Table 10, p. 230; Katharine R. Levit et al.,"National Health Expenditures, 1995," *Health Care Financing Review,* 18(1), Fall 1996: Table 9, p. 201; U.S. Department of Commerce, Bureau of Economic Analysis, *Survey of Current Business,* various issues.

[a] 1972–73 figure

[b] Total expenditures on health services and supplies (total National Health Expenditures) as a percentage of consumer expenditures plus government purchases. The difference between consumer expenditures plus government purchases and GNP is that GNP includes private investments and net exports. Neither private investments nor net exports are relevant in determining the weight of health care expenditures on consumer and government budgets.

Over time, as competition among hospitals has increased, HMOs, PPOs, and private insurers have been able to negotiate larger discounts from hospitals' list prices. Thus the difference between list and transaction prices has become greater. As a result, the MCPI has been overstating the rise in hospital inflation—and this upward bias has become larger in more recent years.

While hospital services are given a lower weight in the MCPI than in total medical expenditures because government payments are excluded from the CPI calculation of weights, hospital services have risen faster than any other category in the MCPI. Thus, the bias in hospital prices has had a large impact on the rise in the MCPI as well as on the CPI.

From a policy perspective, the upward bias in the hospital services index has hidden the impact that hospital price competition has had in recent years.

Dranove et al. studied the magnitude of the upward bias in hospital prices when list prices rather than transaction prices are used (5). Using data from California hospitals for the 1983–88 period, they found that inflation in list prices exceeded the rise in actual prices by a factor of 2.

The BLS has recognized the discrepancy between hospital list prices and actual prices and is attempting to collect data on actual prices paid. In 1993, the BLS developed a producer price index (PPI) for hospitals based on actual prices. The PPI was used as a supplement to the CPI. Beginning in January 1997, the CPI pricing methodology for hospitals was similar to the PPI so as to more accurately reflect actual hospital prices.

The difference between list and actual prices has also been a problem for each of the other components of the MCPI. For example, with regard to physician services, the BLS previously gathered data from physicians on their usual or customary charges for particular services. However, the average fee received by the physician was a more relevant price. Customary charges differed from average prices *received* because customary charges were not the same as actual prices and not all charges were collected. Physicians participating in PPOs offer discounted fees to those patients. Previously, the physicians' fees component of the MCPI was based on customary charges, which could change at a different rate than the fees actually received by the physician. The BLS moved to correct this problem in the 1987 revision of the CPI by collecting physician fee data by payer type.

The measurement of prescription drug prices is a major area of concern with the MCPI. The rise in drug prices has been a source of concern for many, particularly the aged, since Medicare does not cover prescription drugs and a large part of the price is paid out of pocket. The rise in BLS's prescription drug price index has been used by the press and by legislators to propose limits on rising drug prices. Researchers believe that BLS's approach to measuring price increases results in a serious overstatement of the rise in drug prices.

When the patent protection of a drug expires and generic versions of the drug enter the market, consumers who act as though the branded and generic versions of the drug are equivalent benefit by paying less for the generic drug. The BLS, however, defines many products too narrowly; thus close substitutes are treated as though they were new goods. Consequently, the BLS does not pick up the price declines for those consumers who switch to the generic version. When a close substitute enters a market, such as with a generic drug, the BLS "links in" the generic drug to the index. Not all consumers of the branded drug, however, switch to the generic version, so for those consumers the linking process is appropriate since the generic version is not a good substitute. (When a generic version enters the market at a lower price than the branded drug, the branded drug often increases in price since those who continue to purchase the branded drug have a less price-elastic demand.)

There are three problems with the BLS approach of linking, which assumes the generic version is a completely separate good. First, the BLS does not include the generic version of the drug when it immediately comes on the market; instead, there is a lag period. Drugs, similar to other products, have a life cycle. When they are first introduced, their prices are relatively high; later in the cycle their prices decline. By linking the generic version after a lag time, the BLS misses the decline in price of that drug.

The same lag problem occurs with new branded drugs. New drugs frequently come down in price after their introduction, as production expands and competition among sellers increases. Because the price of the new branded drug is higher than existing, competing, drugs, the higher price purchasers are willing to pay reflects a difference in actual or perceived quality. It is thus appropriate for BLS to link these new drugs into its index and treat them as a new good. However, by the time the BLS links these new drugs into the drug price index, their price may have already declined, resulting in an overstatement of the index.

Second, the weight given to the generic drug by BLS in its index is too small. Even though BLS picks up the generic drug late, its market share continues to grow and thus its weight in the index should continue to increase.

Third, because the generic drug is treated as a separate good and linked in, the price decline experienced by those consumers who switch to the generic drug is not reflected in the BLS index.

Studying only a limited number of drugs to illustrate the problem of the prescription drug price index, researchers contrasted the BLS approach with alternative methods (6). The BLS approach assumes that the entry of generic drugs, once the patent protection of a branded good expired, was equivalent to a completely new product and was not to be compared to the branded product. The BLS approach would have resulted in a 14 percent price increase over a forty-five-month period. An alternative approach that assumes the generic and brand-name drugs are perfect substitutes results in a 53 percent decline in price. (An adjusted Paasche index, preferred by the researchers, declined by 48 percent.)

Thus, the potential bias in BLS's drug price index is quite substantial.

Quality Changes and New Products

A third major problem with regard to the MCPI is changes in quality. In the MCPI, as throughout the CPI, the BLS intends to trace movements in the price of a *constant-quality* market basket of goods and services. It is particularly difficult, however, to measure changes in the quality of most of the medical services priced. For example, the outcome of open heart surgery has improved over time; less invasive surgical techniques are being used; and improved drugs have lessened the need for surgical intervention and have prolonged life expectancy. Similarly, with regard to physician services, medical knowledge has improved, physicians are better trained than in the past, and together with improved technology, their diagnosis and treatment of illnesses have improved. A physician visit is not the same product or of similar quality as a visit ten or twenty years ago.

The intensity (inputs) of medical services has increased over time as have medical outcomes. The approach taken by the BLS, however, has been to ignore quality change and assume that any price increase is due solely to inflation.[6]

---

[6]Except, apparently, when an obvious method of adjustment is available. For example, in 1961 obstetricians' fees for obstetrical cases were substituted for general practitioners' fees for the same service. The obstetricians' fees were linked in—that is, the difference between their fees and those of general practitioners was attributed entirely to a quality difference. Similarly, if a service, such as a throat culture, was routinely given to all patients as part of a limited office visit, then that new service would be linked in to the price of that type of visit.

The problem of quality adjustment is particularly troublesome for hospital services, since it is the fastest-increasing component of the MCPI (7). Prior to 1972, hospital services were represented in the MCPI by daily room charges only. The index of semiprivate room charges was frequently cited as an index of the price of hospital care. This use of the semiprivate room charge not only ignored problems of quality change, but also presumed that the prices of other services not included in the basic room charge were changing at the same rate.[7] In 1972, an expanded hospital service charge index was introduced. It included the semiprivate room charge, the operating room charge, and the charges for eight specific ancillary services. The 1978 revision specified a much larger number of services for pricing.

Currently, the items that are priced in the hospital and related services index are individual components of a hospital admission. And the most important component in the hospital service charge index is the basic room charge, which is not a constant-quality item. Although the BLS recognizes that service quality might include levels of patient satisfaction, mortality rate from surgical procedures, frequency of postoperative infections, patient functional health status, and even intensity of resource utilization, it believes that no single measure can, by itself, offer a measure of the quality of a hospital service. Since increased hospital prices are not adjusted for quality improvements, BLS seriously overstates the rise in hospital and medical prices.

Health Insurance. The treatment of health insurance in the MCPI provides another example of the conceptual problems involved in adjusting for quality changes. Health insurance premiums may change in response to any of four types of changes: (a) changes in the price of medical services covered by the policy, (b) changes in the ratio of premiums collected to benefits paid out (the difference between the two is overhead expense), (c) changes in the comprehensiveness of the policy, and (d) changes in the average utilization of services by policyholders.

Types (a) and (b) are clearly price changes and should be reflected in an index of the price of health insurance. A change of type (c) represents a change in the nature or quality of the policy and thus ought not to be reflected in the index. It is less clear how to classify type (d). Changes in the average utilization of services by policyholders might occur in response to any number of things, such as changes in the incidence of illnesses (e.g., Aids), advances in medical knowledge or technology, and the introduction of cost-containment policies that place restrictions on his use of services. One might argue that premium changes of type (d) are pure price changes, since the policy itself is unchanged. For the uninsured, however, increases in medical expenses due to increased consumption of services would not be considered price increases. Also, a patient facing restrictions on their use of services is worse off than without such restrictions.

---

[7]The room charge index is also sensitive to changes in hospital pricing policies that may not affect the overall level of hospital charges. The extremely rapid increase in the semiprivate room charge index immediately after the introduction of Medicare was probably due in part to a movement away from the traditional policy of keeping room rates below actual costs and overcharging on ancillary services.

On balance, it is reasonable to make some adjustment for premium changes resulting from changes in average utilization of services, but how to make it is unclear. If premium increases due to utilization increases are not reflected at all in an index of health insurance prices, we are assuming that such increases are always worth their full price to policyholders. Conversely, if we treat all premium increases due to utilization changes as mere price increases, we are assuming that increased utilization is worth nothing.

From 1950 to 1964, the BLS included health insurance in the MCPI by pricing the most widely held Blue Cross-Blue Shield family plan in each sample area (note that the premiums of health insurance plans not priced were assumed to change at the same rate as those that were priced). All premium changes in the priced plans were reflected in the index, except those judged to be the result of changes in the comprehensiveness of policies, type (c) above. No attempt was made to adjust for premium changes of type (d), those due to changes in average utilization.

In the 1964 revision, the BLS discontinued a direct pricing of health insurance policies. Instead, it decided to price a bundle of services representing those covered by health insurance, and to make periodic adjustments for changes in the weight of the overhead component of health insurance premiums. These steps were designed to account for premium changes of types (a) and (b) and to eliminate the need to adjust for premium changes of types (c) and (d), since these are not reflected in the index in the first place.

Of the two methods that have been used, the former will show a more rapid increase during times of increasing health services utilization; the latter will show a more rapid increase when utilization is decreasing. Neither method is more obviously correct. The same method used in the 1964 revision was carried over to the 1978 revision with only slight modification.

In the 1987 revision, the BLS combined health insurance expenditures for specific medical services with other expenditures for those categories. Health insurance today only includes those expenditures not spent on medical services, such as administrative cost and profit, and this category is the result of a weighted average of the overhead of commercial insurers, Blue Cross and Blue Shield, HMOs, and supplementary policies for Medicare Part B. The health insurance component still represents premium payments made by consumers only. The BLS continues to experiment with direct pricing of health insurance premiums but considers it difficult to adjust premiums for changes in coverage (c) and utilization (d) (8).

An Input versus a Treatment Approach to Measuring the Rise in Medical Prices

The BLS constructs its MCPI by measuring how a fixed set of inputs, a day in the hospital, a physician office visit, drug prices, and so on, have increased over time. However, when some mental or physical disorder is perceived, a consumer is interested in purchasing a treatment, not a specific set of inputs. The specific goods and services—physician visits, hospital bed days, prescription drugs, and so forth—function as inputs that are combined to produce medical treatments. It is therefore reasonable to measure the cost of medical care by looking at specific illnesses and determining how the average cost per treatment episode has changed over time. Economists have found this cost-of-treatment approach to measuring medical care costs conceptually appealing.

A treatment approach for measuring changes in medical prices could reflect the effects on prices and quality of new medical technology, new drugs, and input substitution for providing a medical treatment. Treatment for a medical condition can be provided entirely in the hospital or it can be provided in part with hospital care, outpatient services, and home health care. With improvements in medical technology and the movement toward managed care, many surgical procedures previously performed in the hospital are now performed in outpatient surgery centers. The price of that treatment has been reduced. Similarly, suppose that hospital room charges increased, but that the increase was accompanied by shortened hospital stays without requiring increases in the use of other inputs. The MCPI would show an increase because of the increase in room charges. The cost-of-treatment index would increase less and perhaps even decline, depending on the net effect of the changes on costs of treatments.

Further, a treatment approach to measuring medical prices would facilitate adjustments for changes in treatment outcomes. The probability of recovery might be improved, and there may be a reduction in the amount of pain as well as improvements in the patient's well being and lifestyle.

In 1962, Anne Scitovsky detailed a proposal for a treatment index that would combine separate indexes of the treatment costs for specific illnesses into a composite index, weighting each component by the percentage of total medical expenditures spent on that illness in a base year (9). This procedure is analogous to the method by which the various component indexes are aggregated into the all-items CPI.

Recognizing that her proposed index would not adjust automatically for such changes in the quality of treatments, Scitovsky suggested that for each illness included in the calculation of the index, a single objective indicator of quality be chosen. The average number of disability days might be appropriate for some infectious diseases or conditions requiring surgery; the number of live births per one hundred pregnancies might be the quality measure for maternity cases. Using these quality indicators to adjust the individual cost-of-treatment indexes would have "the great merit of making possible more complete and systematic correction for quality changes." (The issue of how to deal with changes in the quality of treatments is a major point of contention in the debate over the merits of this approach to measuring the cost of medical care.)

A modification of the original Scitovsky idea arose out of a comment by Yoram Barzel. Using the example of polio, he argued that although the costs of treating individual cases of polio may have remained constant or possibly increased, the introduction of the polio vaccine has led to a drop in the total cost of polio because its incidence has been curtailed. Barzel contended that it is more appropriate to look at the *expected* treatment costs of an illness than at the treatment costs of cases that actually occur (10).

The prevention of a case of illness clearly represents an output that is superior to the successful treatment of a similar case. Concentrating on the costs per case of treating specific illnesses ignores the influence of preventive medical care. An index that measures the costs of medical treatments should reflect the role of preventive care, otherwise it gives a misleading view of changes in the price of care and the productivity of the industry.

An actual cost-of-treatment index has not been constructed. However, in several studies Scitovsky examined the treatment costs of a selected group of illnesses covering the 1951–64, 1964–71, and 1971–81 periods. These studies made no adjustments for changes in treatment quality (11). The study was limited to cases treated by physicians at the Palo Alto Medical Clinic (PAMC), a multispecialty, largely fee-for-service group practice of about 140 physicians in Palo Alto, California. Data on treatment costs were obtained from the records of PAMC and Stanford University Hospital, where nearly all patients requiring hospitalization were treated. Data on costs of treatment rendered outside PAMC or Stanford Hospital were obtained from the patients directly.

Table 4.8 presents a summary of the findings on the changes in treatment costs for the conditions studied. It is striking that in so many cases the percentage increases in treatment costs exceeded the percentage increases in the MCPI. These results are surprising because unless it can be shown that the quality of treatments for these illnesses improved substantially over the period, these results seemed to belie the allegation that the MCPI overstates increases in the price of medical care by failing to account for productivity improvements.

A number of possible explanations were offered for the differences between the rates of increase in the estimates of treatment costs and the MCPI. Scitovsky found that the prices of ancillary hospital services were rising particularly rapidly. These services were not even priced by the BLS at that time, and the MCPI may have been biased downward by their omission. It is also possible that for the sample of illnesses chosen, treatment costs rose faster than the cost of medical care in general. Further, medical care prices tend to be higher in larger cities, and since Palo Alto doubled in size and became part of the San Francisco metropolitan area during the 1951–64 period, part of the higher costs for the treatment approach may be the result of more rapid medical price increases in Palo Alto. The MCPI for San Francisco also increased faster than the national MCPI during this period.

The greater increase shown in the cost-of-treatment approach can also be attributed to a closing of the gap between customary and average charges for physicians' services. Scitovsky used data on actual charges for services rather than customary charges, which was BLS practice. Since average actual charges were increasing faster than customary charges—the practice of cutting fees for low-income patients was becoming less prevalent—this accounted for part of the differences in results. For example, for pediatricians in PAMC from 1951 to 1964, the average charge increased 54 percent more than the customary charge for an office visit and 31 percent more for a home visit.

A final reason why the cost-of-treatment approach rose more rapidly than the BLS index for medical care is that the latter measures only the price of an input, while the

TABLE 4.8 Percentage Increase in the Costs of Treatment of Selected Illnesses, 1951–81

	1951–64	1964–71	1971–81
Otitis media	69	31	113
Appendicitis			
Simple	73	79	254
Perforated	86	115	235
Maternity care	73	56	257
Cancer of the breast	103	70	254
Forearm fractures (children)			
Cast only	52	17	183
Closed reduction, no general anesthetic	85	102	173
Closed reduction, general or regional anesthetic	355	62	253
Myocardial infarction	NA	126	294
Pneumonia (nonhospitalized)	NA	31	114
Duodenal ulcer (nonhospitalized)	NA	12	184
MCPI	55	47	129

Sources: Anne A. Scitovsky and Nelda McCall, "Changes in the Cost of Treatment of Selected Illnesses, 1951-1964-1971," *Health Policy Program, Palo Alto Medical Research Program,* August 1975: 10, 17; Anne A. Scitovsky, "Changes in the Costs of Treatment of Selected Illnesses, 1971–1981," *Medical Care,* 23(12), December 1985: 1347.

cost-of-treatment approach also includes the quantities of inputs used. Those diseases for which the treatments remained basically the same increased less than the MCPI. For example, treatment for an ulcer during the 1964–71 period did not change very much; however, during the 1971–81 period, there were important diagnostic and treatment changes. During the earlier period ulcer treatment costs rose less rapidly than the MCPI, while in the latter period it rose more rapidly. There were important quality changes as a result of these diagnostic and treatment changes with regard to healing and prevention of a recurrence.

More Recent Cost-of-Treatment Studies

Several researchers recently completed a study using the cost-of-treatment approach to indicate the extent of bias in the MCPI. The researchers constructed two new indexes of medical care prices, which they then applied to a particular disease: acute myocardial infarction (MI) or heart attack. The two indexes were a service price index and a cost-of-living index (12).

The service price index focuses on the services actually used in treatment and conceptually is a price index of particular medical treatments over time; it is similar to the current MCPI, which also measures how the price of services has changed over time. Neither the service price index nor the MCPI adjusts rising prices for quality improvements or for changes in inputs.

The cost-of-living index is an attempt to incorporate quality change. The index measures how much "consumers would be willing to pay (or would have to be compensated) to have today's medical care and today's prices, when the alternative is base period medical care and base period prices" (p. 11).

Treatment of heart attack victims was chosen as the treatment to be studied because heart disease (which is more inclusive than heart attacks) accounts for almost one-seventh of medical spending and treatment costs for heart attacks have risen rapidly in recent years. A heart attack is also a readily definable episode with a beginning and a measurable outcome, survival. Given the outcome measure it becomes easier to establish a value for such a treatment than for other types of treatment with different types of outcomes.

Two sources of data were used for the study: (a) detailed data on services, prices, the discharge abstract, and demographic information for all heart attack patients admitted to a single major teaching hospital for the 1983–94 period and (b) data on Medicare patients who had a heart attack during the 1984–91 period.

Neither the service price index nor the cost-of-living index was adjusted for factors affecting the incidence of illness, such as changes in lifestyle, which would affect the expected cost of heart disease. Further, the authors recognize that if their study were to be extended to examine the price of all medical services, then multiple treatment indexes would have to be calculated and adjustments made for their changing weights over time.

The authors found that the service price index rose less rapidly than a method based on the MCPI. The study results are summarized in Table 4.9. All of the annual percent increases are adjusted for inflation. Over the time period studied (1983–94), the MCPI rose 3.4 percent per year. The hospital services component of the MCPI rose even more rapidly, 6.2 percent annually. The BLS approach, as previously discussed, uses list prices for a constant set of services over time. As a comparison, the authors constructed a "synthetic" MCPI, which was based on list prices for hospital services used in treatment of a heart attack. This synthetic MCPI increased by 3.3 percent annually, more slowly than the BLS's hospital services index of 6.2 percent. In an attempt to reflect actual rather than list prices, a second synthetic MCPI was created, which was based on the hospital's accounting costs. This index rose by 2.4 percent annually.

A second problem with BLS's MCPI, in addition to using list rather than transaction prices, is that it continues to price a specific item, such as a day in the hospital, even though the number of days may have decreased; the MCPI does not adjust for changes in inputs used. The mix of treatments provided to heart attack patients has changed over time. In 1984, 65 percent of heart attack patients at the hospital studied received Medical Management; by 1994, only 23 percent of patients were treated with this approach. Similarly, the comparable percentages for the earlier and the more current period were: catherization only, 20 percent and 21 percent; angioplasty, 3 percent and 30 percent; and bypass surgery, 11 percent and 27 percent. There has been a dramatic shift over time to more expensive treatment methods.

Even within each of these treatment methods, there have been shifts in the inputs used

TABLE 4.9 Annual Rates of Change in Various Medical Price Indices, Adjusted for Inflation, 1983–94

Index	Real Annual Change
Service Price Indices	
Basic Components Price Indices	
MCPI	3.4%
Hospital Component	6.2
Room	6.0
Other Inpatient Services	5.7
Synthetic MCPI for MTH—Charges	3.3
Synthetic MCPI for MTH—Costs	2.4
Patient Weighted Price Index—Laspeyres	2.8
Patient Weighted Price Index—Five-Year Chain Index	2.1
Patient Weighted Price Index—Annual Chain Index	0.7
Cost of Living Index (1984–91)	−1.1%

Source: This table is based on David M. Cutler et al., "Are Medical Prices Declining?," NBER Working Paper #5750 (Cambridge, Mass.: National Bureau of Economic Research, September 1996).

for treatment. For example, the use of operating room time increased by 38 percent for bypass surgery patients, while their length of stay declined by 22 percent.

To account for this shift to more expensive treatment methods and shifts in the use of inputs within each treatment type, the authors developed a set of additional patient weighted price indexes (PWPIs) that could be reweighted or "chain weighted" at different intervals. One chain-weighted PWPI reweights the mix of treatments every five years; the other recalculates the weights every year. These chain weighted indexes are compared to a price index, similar to the MCPI (referred to as the Laspeyres PWPI), which does not reweight the change in mix of treatments. Over the time period studied, the Laspeyres index increased by 2.8 percent per year. The five-year chain-weighted index rose 2.1 per cent per year and the chain-weighted index that was reweighted annually increased by only 0.7 percent per year.

The main reason for the lower rate of increase in the latter index is the weight placed on room charges. The length of stay in the hospital decreased sharply over that time period (36 percent), while the hospital room charge increased by 60 percent. Unless these changes in inputs are recognized (for example, by more frequent reweighting, which would have captured the decrease in length of stay), the MCPI is likely to have a serious upward bias.

The above treatment indexes did not attempt to adjust prices for changes in the outcome of treatment. To remedy this, the authors constructed a cost-of-living index to adjust treatment costs for changes in life expectancy. To calculate this, it was necessary to estimate the value of an additional year of life less the costs of producing that additional year. (To place a value on the additional years remaining after a heart attack, several different values of an additional life year were used.)

When the BLS approach was contrasted with the cost-of-living index, the authors found that the latter index actually decreased (adjusted for inflation) by about 1 percent per year—a difference of 4 percent per year between the two indexes. The authors conclude that the MCPI approach substantially overstates the amount of price inflation. Further, rather than the rapid price increases that have been indicated by the MCPI, the inflation-adjusted price of medical care may have been falling over this time period. The authors caution that the estimate of the cost-of-living index is dependent on the assumed value of life.

The authors conclude that by adjusting for both differences between list and actual prices paid and by including changes in the mix of treatments actually used (annual chain-weighted PWPI) the result is a much slower rate of increase in medical prices, about 0.5 percent per year as compared to 3.3 percent per year (synthetic MCPI charges), adjusted for inflation. Further, if the MCPI were actually a cost-of-living index, then medical prices would be falling rather than increasing.

Assuming that the results of the above study can be generalized to other medical services, the MCPI seriously overstates the rise in medical price inflation.

While this study provides some indication how much the MCPI is upward-biased, it should be kept in mind that the study is based on data from one teaching hospital, using one disease type (heart attack patients), where the services are provided within the hospital, and uses one outcome measure, additional life years. Constructing a new MCPI price index based on this approach would be highly useful, but also quite difficult.

Evaluating the Cost-of-Treatment Approach

The results of the above studies clearly show that in the absence of adjustments for changes in actual prices paid, changes in the mix of treatments, and improvements in treatment outcomes, the MCPI has a serious upward bias. In evaluating the merits of the cost-of-treatment approach to measuring the costs of medical care, it is important to consider whether a practical method exists for making adjustments for changes in treatment quality.

Three serious problems hinder the implementation of a cost-of-treatment approach. The first is that the quality of a medical treatment is truly multidimensional; a single quality indicator for each illness might be too simplistic. The probability of recovery, the expected number of disability days, the probable extent of physical impairments once recovery is complete, the painfulness of the treatment, and the amenities provided along with it are only some of the relevant aspects of the quality of a treatment. Determining how different treatment methods affect these different aspects of quality might be very costly, although such information would obviously be useful for other purposes besides the construction of a medical care price index.

The second problem, which would still be troublesome even if complete information existed on the technical aspects of the outcomes of different treatment methods, arises when placing values on differences in treatment quality. What value, for example, should be placed on a slightly lower probability of death from a particular disease, or on a little less pain? The problem of determining such values is as much conceptual as technical; its solution is not clear. A reduction in the frequency of miscarriages certainly represents an improvement in the quality of maternity care. However, is it appropriate to assume that an obstetrician who is 99.9 percent successful in delivering babies is exactly twice as good as one who delivers only one live birth for every two cases handled? A doubling of the success rate in delivering babies or in treating an illness might imply more than a twofold increase in quality. But exactly how much more? This is the kind of question that must be answered if a cost-of-treatment index is to be adjusted correctly for changes in quality of treatments.

Third, should the *expected* treatment cost of an illness be used rather than the average costs of cases actually treated? Since the expected cost is the probability of contracting an illness times the average cost of treatment, it can be influenced by preventive medical care. The movement to capitation payment provides HMOs and their providers with a financial incentive to substitute preventive services for more costly acute care. In principle, an expected-cost-of-treatment index could be calculated in the manner described earlier. For each illness, the total cost of treatment would be averaged over the number of cases treated plus the number of cases prevented. However, it is not simple to distinguish the number of cases eliminated by preventive medical care alone. Incidence rates of illnesses are influenced by many factors, including nutrition, personal health habits, lifestyle, and environmental factors such as pollution levels. The simple method of comparing the incidence of an illness in a base year with that in a later year and taking the difference as a measure of the effects of preventive care is not satisfactory. Other factors may be responsible for the difference. If birthrates go down and less is spent on maternity care, for example, does this mean that the medical care industry is more productive? Is it more productive if the nation decreases its consumption of cigarettes and the incidence of lung cancer goes down? Surely the answer is no in both cases. Ideally, then, the effects of preventive care on incidence rates should be computed separately from those of other factors when preparing an index of expected treatment costs. Multivariate statistical techniques might be used for this task, but it is questionable whether precise estimates could be obtained.

Despite its limitations, the cost-of-treatment approach retains a theoretical appeal; it would enable more meaningful comparisons to be made of the cost of medical care, both cross-sectionally and over time. The fixed-bundle-of-goods-and-services method of pricing medical care used by the BLS yields results that are difficult to interpret meaningfully. The treatment of an illness seems a more appropriate notion of medical care output than the physician's visit, the hospital patient day, or the other, more conventional units used by the BLS. Still, enormous practical difficulties and perhaps considerable cost would be involved in actually constructing a cost-of-treatment index as a substitute for the MCPI. In addition, some conceptual problems involved in this approach have not been solved adequately, most notably the issues of how to deal with changes in the quality of medical treatments and how to take account of the preventive aspects of medical care.

SUMMARY

In summarizing our discussion of the MCPI, we might emphasize four points. First, the MCPI is not designed as a comprehensive price index for all medical care utilized in the United States. Although it was originally targeted to a population that was not representative of the entire United States in terms of medical care consumption, its representativeness has improved since 1978. However, the MCPI still neglects the increasingly important share of medical care purchased by government. Second, the sampling procedures used have become more sophisticated, so that the MCPI is likely to resemble more closely the index that would have been calculated if all the relevant data (rather than samples) had been used. In the most recent revision, the price data collected from providers are becoming more representative of what patients, insurance companies, and other organizations actually pay the provider. Third, the difficulty in accounting for quality change and the introduction of new products raises questions about what the MCPI does and what it ought to measure. And, lastly, there is serious concern that the MCPI greatly overstates the amount of medical price inflation.

APPENDIX: HEALTH INSURANCE PREMIUMS AS A MEASURE OF THE PRICE OF MEDICAL CARE

Still another approach to assessing the price of medical care is to measure it in terms of health insurance premiums. Melvin Reder reasons that "if medical care is that which can be purchased by means of medical insurance, then its 'price' varies proportionately with the price of such insurance" (13). The apparent advantages of this price-of-insurance approach are its simplicity and the fact that productivity changes that influence the cost of providing care would automatically be reflected in the index. For example, technical changes that lower the cost of providing treatments would lead to downward pressure on insurance premiums and thus hold down the index of the price of medical care. Improvements in preventive care, which we have seen would be difficult to assess in a cost-of-treatment index, would also show up automatically in a price-of-insurance index. Preventive measures, to the extent that they lowered the expected cost of medical care, would also lower the costs of providing health insurance and would thus be reflected in this kind of index.

However, users of this approach will encounter the familiar conceptual problems involving the issue of quality change. A health insurance policy need not remain a constant-quality good over time, even if the language of the policy remains unchanged. Changes in the incidence of illnesses may occur, for example, for reasons beyond the control of the medical care industry. Such changes may affect the utilization of medical services and thereby raise or lower health insurance premiums. Alternatively, physicians may develop more input-intensive treatment methods over time, improving the quality of care but also raising insurance premiums. In neither case would it be correct to price the insurance policy as though it were a constant-quality item.

Consider a third example: Suppose that there were increases in both hospital capacity and physicians in a previously underserved area. It is likely that the amount of illness left untreated would drop, that treatments would generally be more complete, and that travel time and waiting time would decrease. Health insurance premiums would have to increase, but surely such premium increases would not be pure price changes. The improvement in care may more than compensate the population for the increase in premiums. And, lastly, the increasing restrictiveness of health plans in limiting choice of provider has resulted in lower premiums, but this change should not be treated as a pure price decrease, since the enrollee is not as well off as previously.

It appears, then, that the price-of-insurance approach is subject to the same basic problem that plagues the other methods of pricing medical care that we have examined: How can we quantify that component of price change that represents the value consumers place on increased quality (or loss they attach to lower quality)? Adjusting a price-of-insurance index for quality change would be at least as conceptually and practically difficult as adjusting a cost-of-treatment index.

Key Terms and Concepts

- Consumer expenditures
- Consumer price index
- Market basket of goods and services
- Quality change
- Weighting of goods and services

- Actual versus list prices
- Cost-of-treatment price index
- Input-based price index
- Linking
- Medical care price index

Review Questions

1. Evaluate the present medical care price index. What should the MCPI conceptually measure? What are its limitations?
2. Contrast the Scitovsky and MCPI approaches for measuring changes in the price of medical care.
3. Why do you think, as Scitovsky found, that the costs of episodes of illnesses have increased faster than the prices of the medical care goods and services used in treating the illnesses?
4. It has been proposed that the change in insurance premiums for a given package of

benefits be used as an alternative to the current medical care price index. Evaluate this proposal.

REFERENCES

1. For a further discussion of the appropriateness of the CPI as a cost-of-living index, see Janet L. Norwood, "Indexing Federal Programs: The CPI and Other Indexes," *Monthly Labor Review,* 104, March 1981: 60–65.

2. See U.S. Department of Labor, *The Consumer Price Index: History and Techniques,* Bulletin 1517, 1966, especially p. 84. Also see Ina K. Ford and Philip Sturm, "CPI Revision Provides More Accuracy in the Medical Care Services Component," *Monthly Labor Review,* 111, April 1988: 17–26.

3. For a general discussion of the 1987 revision of the CPI, see Ford and Sturm, *ibid.,* and Charles Mason and Clifford Butler, "New Basket of Goods and Services Being Priced in Revised CPI," *Monthly Labor Review,* 110, January 1987: 3–22.

4. Brent R. Moulton, "Bias in the Consumer Price Index: What Is the Evidence?", *Journal of Economic Perspectives,* 10(4), Fall 1996: 159–177.

5. David Dranove, Mark Shanley, and William D. White, "How Fast Are Hospital Prices Really Rising?," *Medical Care,* 29(8), August 1991: 690–696.

6. Zvi Griliches and Ian Cockburn, "Generics and New Goods in Pharmaceutical Price Indexes," *American Economic Review,* 84(5), December 1994: 1213–1232.

7. Elaine Cardenas, "The CPI for Hospital Services: Concepts and Procedures," *Monthly Labor Review,* July 1996: 32–42. Also see Brian Catron and Bonnie Murphy, "Hospital Price Inflation: What Does the New PPI Tell Us?," *Monthly Labor Review,* July 1996: 24–31.

8. See "Appendix: Test of Direct Pricing of Health Insurance Premiums," in Ford and Sturm, *op. cit.*

9. Anne Scitovsky, "An Index of the Cost of Medical Care—A Proposed New Approach," in Solomon J. Axelrod, ed., *The Economics of Health and Medical Care* (Ann Arbor, Mich.: Bureau of Public Health Economics, University of Michigan, 1964), pp. 128–147.

10. Yoram Barzel, "Cost of Medical Treatment: Comment," *American Economic Review,* 58, September 1968: 937–938.

11. Anne Scitovsky, "Changes in the Costs of Treatment of Selected Illnesses, 1951–65," *American Economic Review,* 57, December 1967: 1182–1195; Anne Scitovsky and Nelda McCall, "Changes in the Costs of Treatment of Selected Illnesses, 1951–1971," Health Policy Discussion Paper, University of California School of Medicine, San Francisco, September 1975; and Anne Scitovsky, "Changes in the Costs of Treatment of Selected Illness, 1971–1981," *Medical Care,* 23(12), December 1985: 1345–1357.

12. David M. Cutler, Mark McClellan, Joseph P. Newhouse, and Dahlia Remler, "Are Medical Prices Declining?," Working Paper Series (Cambridge: National Bureau of Economic Research), Working Paper 5750, September 1996.

13. Melvin Reder, "Some Problems in the Measurement of Productivity in the Medical Care Industry," in V. Fuchs, ed., *Production and Productivity in the Service Industries* (New York: Columbia University Press, 1969), p. 98.

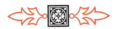

CHAPTER

The Demand for Medical Care

THE PURPOSE OF DEMAND ANALYSIS

One of the purposes of an analysis of the demand for medical care is to determine those factors which, on the average, most affect a person's utilization of medical services. At any point in time many factors influence the consumer's choice to seek medical treatment of a given intensity. It would be virtually impossible to explain completely every individual's utilization of medical services, but certain factors are important for most persons. Demand analysis seeks to identify which factors are most influential in determining how much care people are willing to purchase. The better our understanding of those factors, the better we will be able to explain variations in utilization among population groups and among areas.

Such an understanding will also enable us to forecast future utilization more accurately; to do so, each of the factors affecting demand is forecasted separately. If, for reasons of social policy, it was desirable to increase a certain population group's use of medical care, then by our understanding of which factors affect demand, such a change could be achieved. Thus an understanding of which factors affect demand, and to what extent, will enable us to explain variations in use of medical services. That knowledge can be used to forecast demand more accurately and to bring about changes in utilization if so desired.

DEMAND VERSUS NEED AS A BASIS FOR POLICY AND PLANNING

At various times it has been proposed that the planning of health facilities and health manpower be based solely on estimates of need for medical care in the population. Need has generally been defined as the amount of medical care that medical experts believe a person should have to remain or become as healthy as possible, based on current medical knowledge.[1] The Lee and Jones research of the 1930s was one of the classic studies using medical need as the basis for determining physician requirements in the country (1). The Hill–Burton formula for planning hospital facilities (initiated in the late 1940s) also used need as the criterion for the number of beds required in an area. Four and one-half beds per thousand population was the standard for determining whether additional beds should be added. (If population density was fewer than six persons per square mile, then the standard became 5.5 beds per thousand.)

The assumption underlying the use of need as a basis for public policy in medical care is that need itself is, or should be, the main determinant of hospital and physician use. Need, however, is only one factor affecting demand for care; basing resource allocation decisions solely on medical need will result in a misallocation. If the estimated quantity of services required to meet medical need exceeds the quantity that people will actually use, then there will be an underutilization of hospitals and physicians—resources that could have been used elsewhere or in another manner. If, on the other hand, people demand more medical care than would be provided based solely on a need criterion, then there will be excess demand and increased waiting times. Shortages of facilities and manpower are costly because they waste a patient's time—time that could have been spent in a more productive manner.

Thus, planning based solely on medical need is likely to result in the use of either too few or too many resources. These consequences are shown in Figure 5.1. Planning according to medical need is shown by a vertical line, since need is independent of price. (Need is also independent of the prices of other services, of income, and of insurance coverage. Changes in these other factors would not change need, as medically defined.) The number of medical facilities determined by need is shown along the horizontal axis (e.g., Q_0 equals four beds per one thousand population). If utilization is less than need (Q_1) or

---

[1]J. Jeffers et al. state: "An accurate specification of a population's 'needs' for medical services requires perfect knowledge of the state of its members' health, the existence of a well-defined standard of what constitutes 'good health,' and perfect knowledge of what modern medicine can do to improve ill (or below standard) health. It must be acknowledged that existing diagnostic procedures are not capable of providing perfect knowledge of the state of any population's, or even an individual's health. It also must be acknowledged that a clear-cut consensus as to what constitutes 'good health' does not exist among health professionals." James R. Jeffers, Mario F. Bognanno, and John C. Bartlett, "On the Demand Versus Need for Medical Services and the Concept of 'Shortage,'" *American Journal of Public Health,* 61(1), January 1971: p. 47.

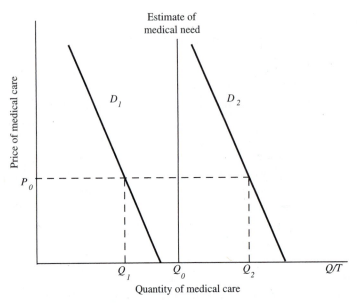

FIGURE 5.1 • Need versus demand as the basis for planning in medical care.

greater than need (Q_2) at a given price (P_0), then either too many (Q_0–Q_1) or too few (Q_2–Q_0) resources will be allocated to medical facilities.

When need is viewed as one factor affecting demand, then greater or lesser needs for care would be represented by different demand curves; for example, D_2 may include a greater amount of need than D_1. Changes in medical need cause a shift in the demand for care. If preventive care reduces the future need for acute medical services, this may be shown by a shift to the left in the demand for acute care (e.g., from D_2 to D_1).

Planning according to demand would reduce the waste of resources and patients' time. If utilization is less than medical need (e.g., utilization equals Q_1), then by understanding which factors affect demand and by knowing how much demand can be changed when one of these factors is changed, demand can be increased so that quantity demanded at the market price equals medical need. Conversely, if a decrease in utilization is desired where it exceeds need (e.g., utilization equals Q_2), utilization can also be decreased by influencing one of the factors affecting demand.

Using demand analysis does not mean that medical need is disregarded. Instead, additional demand factors, as well as need, are used to estimate utilization. The emphasis, then, is on accurately forecasting demand. Once demand has been forecast, we can decide, based on value judgments, whether demand should be increased or decreased. Planning according to medical need alone is based on the assumption that medical need should be the only criterion for determining utilization, which is a value judgment that not everyone shares. Everyone may not place the same value on fulfilling all or even a certain percentage of their medical needs. Some may not be willing to pay the necessary price or to spend the necessary time to receive all the medical care that medical experts believe they should receive. Disregarding demand factors is likely to result in a waste of resources as well as a failure to ensure that those persons with the greatest need receive care.

Underlying demand analysis is the assumption that people allocate their scarce resources among different goods and services in a way that maximizes their utility. Some persons might say, however, that medical care does not provide any utility, since the patient does not desire to purchase it. Many goods fall into this category: auto repair services, legal services, and home repairs. The desirability of the service is not relevant to the applicability of demand analysis. "Undesirable" services could simply be redefined, as in the case of medical care, to mean those services that provide benefits by alleviating or eliminating illness.

As the price of medical services is reduced, there will be, on average, an increase in the quantity demanded. At some point, the marginal benefits derived from additional units of medical care declines. For example, diagnostic uncertainty decreases as more specialists' services and tests are used. In addition, the probability of recovery from particular illnesses varies, depending on the quantity of medical care used. Some medical services provide reassurance to patients; others provide amenities. Some medical services are a substitute for services performed by the family in the home. Patients and their families differ in their perception of the value of these different aspects of medical care, which reflects differences in the amounts they are willing to pay for these perceived benefits.

There is great variability in the use of medical care due to the unpredictability of the individual incidence of illness. Variability in medical care use and in incidence of illness, however, averages out over large groups of individuals. It is therefore possible to forecast the average demand for care, as opposed to the demand by any particular individual. The estimated demand curve represents the average of many individuals' perceived benefits from additional units of medical care in relation to the price they are willing to pay for those additional benefits.

Since patients differ in both their perception of medical benefits and in their willingness to pay for additional medical services, who is to judge how much medical care should be used? If the patient makes this determination, then, as is the case in a market-oriented system, he would use medical services to the point where the marginal benefit of the last unit equals the price paid for that unit. If, however, medical need is the criterion for rationing medical care, then regardless of the patient's willingness to pay, he would not be allowed to receive more medical care than others believe is needed.

In most markets in the United States, output quantity and quality are based on the concept of consumer sovereignty. Consumers are assumed to be the best judges of how to use their resources to increase their own utility; how they choose to spend their money, together with the cost of producing those goods, determines the variety and quality of the goods and services being produced.[2] The concept of consumer sovereignty in medical care is not uniformly accepted by health professionals, whose task it then becomes to develop an alternative set of criteria sufficiently specific to determine not only the quantity of resources to be spent on medical care but also the method by which these limited resources are to be allocated among different patients and institutional settings. These alternative criteria must substitute for all those allocative functions that would, in a system of consumer sovereignty, be performed by prices and differing consumer demands. In addition, an alternative system should make explicit the values underlying its distribution of medical care.

The determination of optimal output in a market, whether it is made with respect to medical care demand, the manpower markets, or the health education markets, is based on the concept of marginal benefits and marginal costs. When the marginal benefits of a service are equal to the marginal costs of producing that service, the output of that service is considered to be optimal. If the marginal benefits are either greater or less than the marginal costs of producing a service, consumption in that market is considered to be economically inefficient (i.e., resources are misallocated in that they are not placed in their highest-valued uses). Efficiency in consumption, therefore, is one criterion by which the output of different medical care markets will be evaluated. The other criterion is efficiency in production: whether the output is produced at minimum cost. Economic efficiency in consumption and in production are criteria that economists use to evaluate the performance of different markets. In medical care, the criterion of efficiency in production is more widely accepted than the criterion of efficiency in consumption, for which some persons would prefer to substitute a need criterion. Applying the criterion of efficiency in consumption to each medical care market, however, should sharpen the debate on the underlying values and criteria for defining optimal output in each market: Should consumers' or health professionals' perception of marginal benefits prevail?

Whether or not people accept the criterion of efficiency in consumption, demand for medical services must still be analyzed if we are to be able to forecast use of services more accurately.

A MODEL OF THE DEMAND FOR MEDICAL CARE

The Demand for Medical Care Derived from the Demand for Health

The traditional theory of consumer demand assumes that consumers purchase goods and services for the utility provided by those specific purchases. A reformulation of consumer

---

[2]Deciding whether incomes should be redistributed is independent of deciding who should determine the goods and services to be produced in society. If society determines that certain population groups do not have sufficient incomes, their incomes can be supplemented.

demand, however, draws a distinction between goods and services purchased in the market and more fundamental objects of choice, referred to as commodities (2). If the commodity demanded by consumers is good health, then health can be produced by goods and services purchased in the market as well as by the time devoted to preventive measures. Within this framework, the demand for medical care is derived from the more basic demand for health.

According to Michael Grossman (3), consumers have a demand for health for two reasons: (a) it is a consumption commodity—it makes the consumer feel better; and (b) it is an investment commodity—a state of health will determine the amount of time available to the consumer. A decrease in the number of sick days will increase the time available for work and leisure activities; the return to an investment in health is the monetary value of the decrease in sick days.

A view of medical care demand as being derived from the demand for health implies the following. First, increases in age result in an increase in the rate at which a person's stock of health depreciates. Over the life cycle, people will attempt to offset part of the increased rate of depreciation in their stock of health by increasing their expenditures on, and use of, medical care. Second, the demand for medical care will increase with increases in a person's wage. The higher the wage, the greater the value of an increase in the number of healthy days. A consumer who is paid a high wage will also substitute purchases of medical care services for his own time when producing the commodity health. We would thus expect to observe a positive relationship between increased wages and greater expenditures on the demand for medical care. Third, it is hypothesized that education has a negative effect on the demand for medical care. More highly educated people are presumed to be more efficient in producing health. They are, therefore, likely to purchase fewer medical care services.

This view of medical care demand provides a rationale for including in the demand model certain factors believed to affect demand, traditionally known as taste variables, because they influence the individual's demand for health. The importance of the patient's time in relation to the demand for medical care will also be included in the demand model. Analyzing the demand for medical care as being derived from the individual's demand for health provides a better basis for determining which factors should be included in a model of demand for medical care, and for hypothesizing their effects.

Determinants of the Demand for Medical Care

A discussion of the demand for medical care requires an economic framework not only for surveying the literature on factors affecting demand, but also for evaluating empirical research on demand. If a demand study excludes relevant factors affecting demand, perhaps because they are not easily measured or because the investigator is unaware of their importance, then its results are likely to be inaccurate.

Variations in the demand for medical care are determined by a set of patient and physician factors. The patient's demand for medical care is essentially the demand for a treatment, and variations in demand are a result of variations in the number, type, or quality of treatments demanded. This demand is typically initiated by the patient. The physician then combines various inputs to provide a treatment of a given quality. The patient's determinants of demand are her incidence of illness or need for care, a set of cultural-demographic factors, and economic factors. The roles of the physician as advisor to the patient and as a supplier of a service are discussed separately below.

Empirical studies on the demand for medical care should thus describe, first, how different factors affect the patient's demand for medical care, and, second, what determines how the physician will provide care for a given treatment. For purposes of clarity, the patient and physician phases will be described sequentially, although they occur simultaneously. The aim of empirical research, then, is to derive an estimate of the relationship between patient and physician factors and use of medical care.

The assumption of choice is implicit in studies of demand. Choices are made with respect to the amounts of medical care purchased and of the combinations of components of care that produce a treatment. If choice in these areas were not possible, much less variation in medical care use would be observed when nonmedical factors, such as cultural and economic background, are analyzed. Less variation would also exist in the manner in which a treatment is provided. The patient's and physician's degree of choice depends on two factors: knowledge and the availability of substitutes. It is often assumed that no close substitutes within the field of medical care exist. Even if this were true (which it is not), families might still differ in their demand for medical services because they attach different values to the expected benefits of increased use or because their knowledge of these benefits varies. Within the field of medical care itself, the substitutability of components in providing a treatment appears to be increasing. Not only are ambulatory services and home health care partial substitutes for hospitalization, but the increased use of outpatient surgery provides an additional substitute for hospital care. These, then, are the reasons underlying the assumption that the patient exercises choice in his demand for medical care and the physician exercises it in the treatment provided.

Factors Affecting the Patient's Demand for Medical Care

As we have noted, the factors affecting a patient's demand for medical care are incidence of illness, cultural-demographic characteristics, and economic factors. The first two, stemming from the family's perception of a medical problem and their belief in the efficacy of medical treatment, shape the consumer's desire for medical care. When translating this desire into an expenditure, the family is limited by the extent of its available resources. Determining the amount to be spent on medical care becomes a part of the problem of allocating scarce resources among alternative desires. Each of these general factors affecting a patient's demand for care is discussed below.

Actual or perceived illness or desire for preventive medicine will determine whether an individual is in the market for medical care at any point in time. The onset of illness and the use of a hospital is for many people an unexpected occurrence. Thus, for individuals, illness may be considered a random event, but with respect to the age and sex of the population as a whole, illness has a fair degree of predictability. As individuals age, the incidence of illness increases and morbidity patterns change; chronic diseases become a more important determinant of the need for medical care. Although medical expenditures are approximately the same for both sexes in the early years, there is a difference in the need for medical care among men and women, holding constant marital status and age.

Later in life, expenditures incurred by women exceed those incurred by men, primarily because of obstetrical charges, although the difference persists beyond the childbearing ages. The relationship between age and use of medical services, however, is not simply linear nor is it the same for each type of medical service. For example, the relationship between age and use of hospital services is different from that which exists between age and the use of dental services. Even for hospital care, there are differences in admissions and in length of stay by age group. Although these population characteristics may not affect each of the components of medical care in the same manner, they are important in explaining variations in the use of these services.

Marital status and number of persons in the family also affect the demand for medical care. Single persons generally use more hospital care than do married persons. The availability of people at home to care for an individual may substitute for additional days in the hospital. Family size also affects demand; a larger family has less income per capita (although not necessarily proportionately less) than does a small family with the same income.

Higher levels of education may lead to increased efficiency in a family's purchase and use of medical services. A greater amount of education in the household may enable a family to recognize the early symptoms of illness, resulting in a greater willingness to seek early treatment. Such families are likely to spend more for preventive services and less for more acute illnesses later. Years of education in a household may be a proxy measure for a greater awareness of the need for medical care, for different attitudes toward seeking care, and for greater efficiency in its purchase and production. Differences in education among families are expected to result in differences in use and expenditures for medical services.

Although it is important to determine the effect that cultural-demographic factors have on the demand for medical services, such factors are not subject to sudden changes, nor are they generally the instrument of public policy. The age structure changes gradually, as do attitudes. The effect that economic factors have on the demand for medical services is of more immediate value for purposes of forecasting and policy.

The economic factors contributing to medical services demand are income, prices, and the value of the patient's time. They affect not only whether a patient will seek medical care, but also the extent of the care once treatment is undertaken. Economic factors may not have much of an effect on whether a maternity patient goes to a hospital (although they may influence the choice of hospital), but once she has been admitted, they affect her length of stay. Each of these economic factors is briefly discussed.

A number of studies have examined the relationship between family income and expenditures on medical care and also the effect of income on use of medical care. When these studies are based on survey data, it is often found that families with higher incomes have greater expenditures for medical care, although the percentages of income spent on medical care decline as income increases. In other words, the income elasticity of medical care expenditures is less than 1; that is, the percentage increase in medical care expenditures is less than the percentage increase in income (4).

The manner in which family income is measured must be understood if the effect of income, as it is derived from medical care surveys, is to be interpreted correctly. A family's income in any given year may be abnormally low or high because of the temporary loss of employment, windfall gains, or other unexpected events. Empirical evidence suggests that total consumption is not raised or lowered to correspond with temporary changes in income. Rather, a family's level of consumption is determined primarily by its expected normal or permanent income (5). If transitory income has little or no effect on total expenditures, and families that are sick are likely to be below their normal incomes, then survey data that merely show the relationship between income and expenditures include both permanent and transitory income. Since transitory income is included in the income reported by the survey, although it presumably has little effect on expenditures, the reported survey relationship between income and expenditure is likely to be understated. If the effects of transitory income can be removed, the income elasticity of medical expenditures will be increased. Thus one reason why estimates of the effect of income on medical care expenditures are low is that it is difficult to determine the relationship between permanent income and medical care expenditures from survey data.

Another reason estimates of income elasticity derived from survey data are biased downward is that employer contributions to health insurance premiums are not normally included in survey data. Such employer contributions do not constitute taxable income for employee recipients. The higher the income tax bracket, the larger the potential tax saving to the employee and the greater the incentive to have the employer pay for health insurance. If, for persons with higher incomes, a greater proportion of medical expenditures is reimbursed by third-party payers, then survey data showing the relationship between family income and out-of-pocket expenditures will understate the true income elasticity.

Once survey data are corrected for transitory income and employer-paid health insurance premiums, it appears that the income elasticity of medical care expenditures is approximately 1; that is, a 10 percent increase in income will lead to a 10 percent increase in expenditures on medical care.

The price of a service and the use of that service are, according to economic theory, inversely related: as the price is reduced, purchase or use of the service will increase. Knowledge of price elasticity of demand for medical services is therefore of great importance for public policy. Many persons have generally assumed, however, that prices have very little effect on use of medical services. If national health insurance is to result in greater use of medical services, its proponents must assume that the use of medical services is responsive to changes in price; if not, national health insurance will not result in any changes in use but merely in a redistribution of income.

It is useful to clarify why market demand curves are negatively sloped. People often think of medical services as acute, such as medical care following an auto accident or the need for heart surgery, in which case price is unimportant. In such life or death situations, people will not buy more or less medical care if the price is changed. Medical services, however, consist of more than emergency cases. There are many situations where a person might stay an extra day in the hospital, depending on the price she may have to pay for that extra day, or based on the relative price of inpatient versus outpatient surgery a person might choose the least expensive setting. Many medical services are postponable, can be performed in different institutional settings, or simply provide the patient with reassurance. The use of these services is more responsive to prices.

The market demand for medical services or for any of its components, such as the demand for physician services, is the horizontal summation of thousands (within a community) or millions (large urban areas) of individual demands for that service. Even though many individuals may not change their use of medical services when the price of that service changes, some persons might. Those who go to the hospital or physician for emergency reasons are added together with those who use services for other reasons. Further, even though many persons may not be aware of the price that is being charged, others are. Thus, when the demands for medical services are added up—namely, how much each person will demand at different prices—the slope of the demand curve is based on those individuals who are responsive to price as well as those who enter the market at a lower price.

Obviously the market demand for specific services whose use is more emergent will have price inelastic demands compared to those services that are less emergent. And when the market demands for all of these services are added together, the slope of the demand curve will reflect the use of the less emergent services.

Thus, as in any market it is not average persons but marginal purchasers—those who are responsive to price—who provide the demand curve with its negative slope.

Figure 5.2 illustrates how individual demands are summed to obtain the market demand. Individual demand curves are represented by d_A, d_B, d_C, and d_D. The first two demand curves are completely price inelastic; those individuals will purchase the same quantity regardless of the price. Individuals d_C and d_D, however, will change the quantity demanded based on price. To derive the market demand curve, the quantities each person will buy at each price are summed up. When these four demand curves are horizontally summed to derive the market demand curve, the market demand curve's negative slope is based on individuals represented by d_C and d_D.

Before discussing estimates of price elasticity of demand for medical services, it would

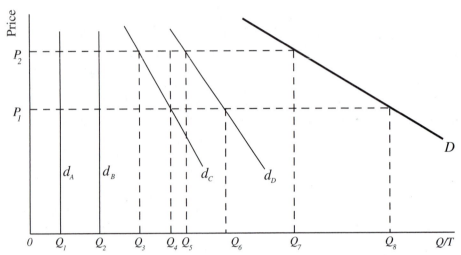

FIGURE 5.2 • Summing individual demands to obtain market demand.

be useful to discuss what the relevant price variable should represent. Patients do not usually pay the medical provider's stated price or charges. Part or all of the price (as in the case of Medicaid patients) is paid by a third-party payer or by the government on the patient's behalf. Any estimate of price elasticity of demand should be based on the net or the out-of-pocket price paid by the patient. Health insurance is one of the most important factors reducing the patient's price. Insurance coverage represents a movement down the individual patient's demand curve, which increases the quantity of services demanded. For all individuals, the existence of insurance coverage represents a *shift* in the overall demand for medical care.

The effect of insurance on the individual's demand for care and on the aggregate demand for care is explained graphically and more completely in the appendix to this chapter. Although, as will be discussed, estimates of price and insurance elasticities have generally been found to be inelastic with respect to demand for medical services, these estimates vary by type of medical service and by seriousness of illness.

Certain institutional settings can substitute for others in treatment of an illness. An analysis of the demand for any one component may be inaccurate if it omits the substitutability and demand for other components. Because a patient can be treated for an illness with different combinations of hospital care, outpatient services, and home health care, different lengths of stay in the hospital may reflect differences in the use of other institutional settings. Therefore, a demand analysis of any one component of care should include net prices to the patient of substitutes and complements. Again, the relevant price to the patient of these substitutes and complements is the out-of-pocket, not the stated, price.

One important reason why estimated price elasticities of demand for medical care are expected to be low is that time costs may represent a relatively large portion of the total price of ambulatory medical care. In addition to prices and income, the consumer's time is a constraint that affects the type of goods and services purchased. Consumer time may be considered an input into the production of a good or service. Cooking a meal and consuming it at home, for example, requires more consumer time than does eating in a restaurant.

When time costs are high, people will substitute purchased services for their own time. Since time has an opportunity cost, it is also scarce and should be viewed as one of the resource constraints facing the consumer. The importance of including time costs, as well as the money costs of consuming a good or service, is that it enables us to explain and predict consumer demand more accurately. If either time or money costs of a service decrease, the quantity demanded would be expected to increase. For example, people with higher earned incomes, such as businesspeople, typically have a higher cost of time; consequently, they have a higher demand for air travel than do those with low time costs, such as students.

In medical care, time is used in traveling to a provider and in waiting to be treated. The following example illustrates how differences in time costs affect the price elasticity of demand for a service. Assume that the patient's out-of-pocket price for visiting a medical provider is $10 and that the time costs are $20; the total price of the visit is therefore $30. If the elasticity of the medical service with respect to the total price were −1.0, meaning that a 10 percent change in the total price results in a 10 percent change in use, and if the out-of-pocket price dropped 50 percent (from $10 to $5), the result would be only a 20 percent decrease in the total price of care (from $30 to $25). This 20 percent change in the total price would lead to a 20 percent change in use because the price elasticity is −1.0. Thus, when an out-of-pocket price is reduced by 50 percent and use increases only 20 percent, the calculated price elasticity is −0.4. The demand for that service is thereby estimated to be price inelastic. Thus, as time costs contribute a larger proportion of the total price, the calculated price elasticity of demand becomes smaller, while the time price elasticity increases (6).

In the past, as third-party coverage and government reimbursement covered a greater portion of the bill, time costs began to represent a greater proportion of the patient's total cost. Changes in money and time costs have important implications for the consumption of medical services. Analyses of the impact on the demand for physician services of a change in insurance coverage, from no out-of-pocket price to the introduction of a 25 percent co-insurance provision, found that the use of such services substantially decreased, primarily among those enrollees with the lowest time costs. This increase in the money price of the service, to a 25 percent co-pay, represented a much larger increase in total price to persons with low time costs than it did for those with higher time costs. For example, home visits, which involve the lowest time costs, experienced twice as large a decline as other types of visits. Further, enrollees decreased their demand for care of minor illnesses considerably more than their demand for medical care of other conditions (7). Nonprofessionals (i.e., those with lower time costs) had a much greater reduction in the number of annual examinations as their out-of-pocket price increased. Female dependents, who have lower time costs than female subscribers, had a larger reduction in visits when the money price of a visit was increased.

Three policy implications follow from the findings that time costs have an important effect on the demand for medical services. First, as out-of-pocket prices to patients decrease, demand for medical care becomes more responsive to the cost of time. If the quantity of medical care supplied does not increase sufficiently to meet increased demands, as is the case under a system similar to the Canadian health care system, then the likely method of rationing is to allocate care to those who can afford to wait. Those with a low time cost are more likely to receive care than are those with a high opportunity cost of time.

Second, society has determined that certain population groups should receive an increase in their use of medical services. Although the money prices to these groups have been reduced, it may be desirable to reduce their time costs to increase further their use of services. Locating clinics closer to these population groups will lower their travel costs and increase utilization.

Third, when planners determine the number and size of hospitals, the patients' time costs should be considered, together with institutional costs, as the relevant costs for planners to minimize. Consumers are willing to pay higher money prices to decrease their time costs. Unless time and money costs are both included in the planning of medical facilities, planners might attempt to lower the costs of hospital or other facility costs by building fewer though larger units, thereby increasing travel time costs to patients.

The Role of the Physician in the Demand for Medical Care

In nonmedical markets the consumer, with varying degrees of knowledge, selects the goods and services that she desires. In medical care, however, the patient does not decide, for example, which hospital to enter or the form of treatment she is to receive; instead, the patient selects a physician who makes these choices. When acting on the patient's behalf, the physician, as the patient's agent, uses her awareness of the patient's financial resources and medical needs to act as the patient would if she had the knowledge and medical authority to make the decision (8). When choosing the components of care to be used in treatment, the physician is guided not only by their efficacy but also by their relative prices to the patient. For example, previously, if a patient had Blue Cross insurance and could be treated either as an outpatient or as an inpatient, but Blue Cross only covered inpatient hospitalization, it was less costly *to the patient* to be hospitalized. This choice of treatment settings by the physician on the patient's behalf, however, resulted in higher total health care costs.

Evidence that physicians made such choices on the patient's behalf is documented in many studies relating hospital utilization to patients' insurance coverage. Although physicians' behavior is also affected by other factors discussed below, the fact that they often act in the patient's financial and medical interest can be used to predict medical and hospital use according to the patient's financial, sociodemographic, and medical characteristics. The more a physician is aware of and acts in accordance with the patient's needs, desires, and financial interests, the stronger is the empirical relationship between such patient characteristics and use of medical services.

With the growth of more comprehensive (fee-for-service) health insurance, financial constraints became less important and physicians prescribed the highest quality of medical care for their patients. This was rational behavior on the part of the physician and the patient, since the marginal benefit of additional tests and other services, no matter how small, was probably greater than the out-of-pocket price the patient had to pay. The physician was able to practice what Victor Fuchs has referred to as the "technologic imperative" (9). In other words, medicine was able to prescribe the best technically possible care. No consideration was given as to whether the marginal benefits of that additional care exceeded the marginal costs of producing it.

Utilization review mechanisms, however, may prevent the physician from acting solely in the patient's interest. For example, insurance companies and HMOs increasingly review the appropriateness of admissions and length of stay. A physician will find it difficult to prescribe hospital care and/or a length of stay that satisfies the patient's preferences when it conflicts with these review mechanisms. To the extent that such institutional arrangements and sanctions exist, the relationship between utilization and patient characteristics (both economic and noneconomic) will be less clear.

There is a more important reason why the physician may not act solely in the patient's interest. As one of the inputs into the patient's medical treatment, the physician has an economic interest in the manner in which a treatment is provided. The physician has a dual role. A physician is both the patient's advisor and a supplier of medical services. As a supplier of a service, the physician has a financial stake in the services used in treatment. In prescribing care to a patient, the physician is acting not only in the patient's interest as an advisor, but also in his own interest as a supplier of services. One of the more obvious examples of the effect of this dual role is when physicians prescribe additional tests for the purpose of protecting themselves against a possible malpractice suit. The physician is able to shift certain costs from himself to the patient and the patient's third-party payer.

According to traditional economic theory, an increase in the supply of physicians would lead to a movement down the market demand curve for physician services with a consequent decrease in price and an increase in quantity demanded of physician services. With a price inelastic demand for physician services, a decrease in price would decrease physicians' incomes.

Contrary to economic predictions, when the supply of physicians (the physician to population ratio) increased, researchers observed an increase in both price and quantity, with no decrease in physician incomes. Traditional economic theory would have predicted falling prices, an increase in quantity demanded, and a decline in physician incomes. This empirical observation of higher physician to population ratios and higher physician prices gave rise to the belief that physicians could increase their own demand.

(This subject is discussed more extensively, together with appropriate diagrams, in Chapter 10.)

According to the demand creation hypothesis, when the supply of physicians increases and the demand facing each physician decreases, physicians will prescribe additional treatments so as to maintain their incomes. When faced with a relatively high demand, a physician will have little incentive to prescribe additional treatments that may or may not be needed. When demand falls, however, physicians are hypothesized to increase both their output and price to maintain their incomes. Given the lack of patient information regarding treatment needs and extensive insurance coverage, the physician is able to take advantage of her advisory role and recommend additional services.

(Many similar advisor-supplier relationships exist with purveyors of other goods and services that consumers purchase—for example, real estate agents and auto mechanics.)

Findings that physicians have been able to induce demand for their services have several policy implications. First, increased patient knowledge would lessen the physician's ability to create additional demand. The patient (or the insurer acting on the patient's behalf) can obtain additional information by requiring prior approval from the insurer and/or receiving a second opinion from another physician whenever surgery is recommended. An alternative approach was to rely on tissue review committees within hospitals to reduce unnecessary surgery. The problem with such institutional arrangements, which were not very successful, is that as long as other physicians in the hospital were financially unaffected by the medical practice of their colleagues, they had little incentive to be concerned with their colleagues' behavior. A third approach is to provide the physician with a financial incentive to avoid unnecessary surgery. One such approach is to encourage methods of physician reimbursement that are unrelated to the quantity of services provided, for example, capitation, which is discussed more completely in subsequent chapters.

In summary, there is a potential conflict in the physician's role as both an advisor to the patient and as a supplier of a medical service. To the extent that the physician acts as the patient's agent, considering the patient's needs and financial resources, we would expect to find a strong relationship between the patient's characteristics and her demand for medical care. On the other hand, to the extent that the physician is also concerned with maintaining his income as the physician to population ratio increases, changes in the supply of physicians would be included in a demand analysis. Under fee-for-service payment, the physician's role as the patient's agent has been affected by the lack of patient information and extensive insurance coverage. With improvements in computer technology, purchasers of physicians' services, such as insurers and large employers, are finding it easier to monitor physicians' behavior and penalize demand inducement.

A Review of Selected Empirical Demand Studies

A number of studies have attempted to estimate price and income elasticities of demand for medical services. These studies have been based on the fee-for-service system and have differed with regard to the theoretical variables included in the demand model, the measurement of the theoretical variables, data, statistical techniques, and methods used for analysis. Most of the demand studies have attempted to estimate the relationship between economic factors and total medical care expenditures as well as separately for expenditures on hospital and physician services, while holding constant the effect of other, noneconomic, factors. Very few studies have been able to measure the effect of economic factors by type of medical diagnosis or by seriousness of illness. Ideally, it would be desirable to know price elasticities at different deductible, co-insurance levels, and incomes, holding constant such factors as health status, time prices, and noneconomic factors. It would then be possible to forecast more accurately changes in utilization if prices were increased or decreased, as under proposed national health insurance plans.

When expenditures, rather than visits or hospital utilization, are used as the dependent variable, estimated price and income elasticities are generally higher, presumably because expenditures include some measures of quality. Physician visits, hospital admissions, and patient days do not enable the investigator to differentiate between visits that include a greater intensity of services, use of specialists, or changes in the length of the visit. Expenditure data reflect quality as well as quantity of services; therefore, price and income elasticity estimates based on expenditure data partly measure the demand for quality as well as the demand for quantity of services. When expenditure data are used, however, it is particularly important that prices be accurately measured. If, for example, a physician charged a higher price to higher-income persons, part of the difference in expenditures between high- and low-income persons was a result of price differences and not of differences in quantity or quality.

The importance of time costs on demand has not often been included in statistical demand studies. Only a few studies have estimated time price elasticities. Failure to include time explicitly as a factor affecting demand for services may result in incorrectly attributing its effect to other factors.

Demand studies have also differed with respect to the inclusion of substitutes and complements in the demand model. The demand for hospital care depends, in part, on the price of home health care. The availability of data on substitutes and complements has generally been limited. Excluding such factors from the statistical estimation of demand may affect the price elasticities of demand for hospital services or other services whose demand is being analyzed.

The measurement of income has also distorted the results of demand studies. Ideally, it is desirable to measure the effect of usual or permanent income, but when surveys collect income data, the incomes of those surveyed may be temporarily high or low. If, for example, a person is sick and his income is temporarily low, but expenditures are related to his usual income, the person will show up in the survey as having a low income but a high expenditure. Thus, if demands for medical services are related to usual and not temporary income, the estimate of income elasticity will be too low when it is measured using temporary incomes.

Data used in demand studies have also differed by level of aggregation. Some studies have been based on state averages; others have used individuals as the unit of observation. In those studies where the level of aggregation encompasses a state, certain factors known to affect demand, such as age, may turn out to be statistically insignificant because there is insufficient variation between states according to age. Use of individual data, however, has generally resulted in lower elasticity estimates. When individual data are used, many individuals in the sample may not have had any utilization during the period covered and it is often difficult to separate the effect of economic factors from all other variables.

The databases from which elasticity estimates were derived have changed over time. Initially, researchers used state data, which included only gross measures of prices and the degree of availability of insurance coverage. There were then a number of studies that used claims and premium data from specific insurance companies. Comparisons have also been made among individuals having different insurance policies. Occasionally, there were instances of a natural experiment, as when a co-payment was introduced in the insurance plan for a particular group of people. The RAND Health Insurance Study was designed as an experiment and has resulted in many studies on the effect of prices on use of services. As the data have improved, it has become possible to develop better measures of prices, as well as to show the effect of income-related co-payments and health status.

The foregoing discussion of empirical demand studies provides some indication of the great variety of variables used, how economic factors are measured, and the sources of data. Such studies have also used different methods of statistical estimation. Most studies have used a single-equation approach, although some have used simultaneous equations. Differences in statistical estimation methods could also result in different elasticity estimates. Given these differences in approach, data, and methods, it is not surprising that large variations exist in the statistical estimates of price and income elasticities.

The following is a brief summary of the results of statistical demand studies. Table 5.1 describes elasticity estimates for the overall market demand for hospital, physician, and other providers' services rather than for individual providers; as such, the price elasticity estimates are lower, since individual providers have better substitutes than hospital or physicians' services in general.

The market demand curves for hospital and physician services are price inelastic. The price elasticity for hospital admissions and physician visits is roughly −0.2.

Insurance coverage for hospital services (and physician in-hospital services) is currently quite high—approximately 90 percent of the hospital bill is paid for by private or public insurance. It is therefore unlikely that hospital use will increase rapidly if the remaining out-of-pocket prices were to be paid for under any form of comprehensive national health insurance plan. Also, utilization review methods would serve to limit increases in hospital use if the remaining financial barriers were removed. Physician office visits, however, have less complete coverage. Any policy that lowers the price of physician office visits could result in a substantial increase in demand for physician services.

The demand for nursing home care among private-pay patients appears to be price elastic, between −1 and −2. Thus policies to include nursing home care under Medicare

TABLE 5.1 Selected Results on Price Elasticities of Demand for Medical Care

Study	Dependent Variable	Elasticity
W. G. Manning et al. (1987)	Hospital admissions	−0.14 to −0.17 (depending on co-insurance)
M. S. Feldstein (1977)		−0.20
J. Newhouse and C. Phelps (1976)		−0.17
G. J. Wedig (1988)	Physician visits	−0.11 to −0.35
W. G. Manning et al. (1987)		−0.17 to −0.31 (depending on co-ins)
Newhouse, Phelps, and Marquis (1980)		−0.09 to −0.13
F. Goldman and M. Grossman (1978)		−0.03 to −0.06 (pediatric visits)
J. Newhouse and C. Phelps (1976)		−0.16
Lamberton, Ellingson, and Spear (1986)	Nursing home services	−0.76
B. R. Chiswick (1976)		−0.73 to −2.40 (different proxies for price)
M. S. Marquis and S. H. Long (1995)	Insurance enrollment	−0.30 to −0.40
J. Gruber and J. Poterba (1993)		−1.80
W. G. Manning and M. S. Marquis (1989)		−0.54
P. F. Short and A. K. Taylor (1989)		−0.32
R. Feldman et al. (1989)		−0.31

Sources: B. Chiswick, "The Demand for Nursing Home Care: An Analysis of the Substitution Between Institutional and Noninstitutional Care," *Journal of Human Resources,* 11(3), Summer 1976: 295–316; R. Feldman et al., "The Demand for Employment-Based Health Insurance Plans," *Journal of Human Resources,* 24(1), Winter 1989: 115–142; M. Feldstein, "Quality Change and the Demand for Hospital Care," *Econometrica,* 45(7), October 1977: 1681–1702; F. Goldman and M. Grossman, "The Demand for Pediatric Care: An Hedonic Approach," *Journal of Political Economy,* 86(2), April 1978: 259–280; J. Gruber and J. Poterba, "Tax Incentives and the Decision to Purchase Health Insurance: Evidence from the Self-Employed," NBER Working Paper #4435 (National Bureau of Economic Research, Washington, D.C., August 1993); C. E. Lamberton, W. D. Ellingson, and K. R. Spear, "Factors Determining the Demand for Nursing Home Services," *Quarterly Review of Economics and Business,* 26(4), Winter 1986: 74–90; W. G. Manning et al., "Health Insurance and the Demand for Medical Care: Evidence from a Randomized Experiment," *American Economic Review,* 77(3), June 1987: 251–277; W. G. Manning and M. S. Marquis, *Health Insurance: The Trade-off Between Risk Pooling and Moral Hazard* (Santa Monica: R-3729-NCHSR, RAND, 1989); M. S. Marquis and S. H. Long, "Worker Demand for Health Insurance in the Non-Group Market," *Journal of Health Economics,* 14(1), May 1995: 47–63; J. Newhouse and C. Phelps, "New Estimates of Price and Income Elasticities for Medical Services," in R. Rosett, ed., *The Role of Health Insurance in the Health Services Sector* (New York: National Bureau of Economic Research, 1976); J. P. Newhouse, C. E. Phelps, and S. Marquis, "On Having Your Cake and Eating It Too: Econometric Problems in Estimating Demand for Health Services," *Journal of Econometrics,* 13(3), August 1980: 365–390; P. F. Short and A. K. Taylor, "Premiums, Benefits, and Employee Choice of Health Insurance Options," *Journal of Health Economics,* 8(3), December 1989: 293–311; G. J. Wedig, "Health Status and the Demand for Health: Results on Price Elasticities," *Journal of Health Economics,* 7(2), June 1988: 151–163.

or a new long-term care program would result in large increases in use and expenditures on such care.

The estimates of price elasticity of demand for health insurance vary widely, from −0.3 to a price elastic −1.8. The price elasticity refers to the loading or administrative charge, that is, the amount above the pure premium. (This subject is discussed in great detail in Chapter 6 on the demand for health insurance.) Reductions in the administrative costs of insurance will, the more price elastic is the demand for insurance, result in a greater number of persons purchasing health insurance.

Table 5.2 shows firm-specific price elasticities (cross-price elasticities), namely, what the effect would be on a specific hospital or physician if they changed their price and their competitors did not. Since any one hospital, physician, or health insurance plan has relatively good substitutes, namely, competing hospitals, physicians, and health plans, firm-specific price elasticities are expected to be price elastic. Hospital specific price elasticities are about −1.12, that is, if a hospital lowered its price by 10 percent it would increase its admissions by 11 percent. Physicians have higher cross-price elasticities, between −1.75 and −5. Given the larger number of physicians, their greater similarity

TABLE 5.2 Firm-Specific Price Elasticities

Study	Dependent Variable	Elasticity
T. R. McCarthy (1984)	Physician services	−3.07 to −3.32
R. H. Lee and J. Hadley (1981)		−2.80 to −5.07
R. A. McLean (1980)		−1.75 to −2.16
R. Feldman and B. Dowd (1986)	Hospital services	−1.12
D. M. Cutler and S. Reber (1996)	Health insurance plans	−2.00
B. Dowd and R. Feldman (1994/95)		−7.90
P. F. Short and A. K. Taylor (1989)		−2.60 to −5.30
W. P. Welch (1986)		−2.00 to −6.20

Sources: D. M. Cutler and S. Reber, "Paying for Health Insurance: The Tradeoff Between Competition and Adverse Selection," unpublished paper, Harvard University and National Bureau of Economic Research, 1996; B. Dowd and R. Feldman, "Premium Elasticities of Health Plan Choice," *Inquiry,* 31(4), Winter 94/95: 438–444; R. Feldman and B. Dowd, "Is There a Competitive Market for Hospital Services?" *Journal of Health Economics,* 5(3), September 1986: 277–292; R. H. Lee and J. Hadley, "Physicians' Fees and Public Medical Care Programs," *Health Services Research,* 16(2), Summer 1981: 185–203; T. R. McCarthy, The Competitive Nature of the Primary-Care Physician Services Market, *Journal of Health Economics,* 4(2), June 1985: 93–117; R. A. McLean, "The Structure of the Market for Physicians' Services," *Health Services Research,* 15(3), Fall 1980: 271–280; P. F. Short and A. K. Taylor, "Premiums, Benefits, and Employee Choice of Health Insurance Options," *Journal of Health Economics,* 8(3), December 1989: 293–312; W. P. Welch, "The Elasticity of Demand for Health Maintenance Organizations," *Journal of Human Resources,* 21(2), Spring 1986: 252–266.

and closer location to each other, any one physician is a closer substitute than is one hospital to another.

Different health plans, such as competing HMOs, and even different types of health plans, such as HMOs, indemnity plans, and PPOs, are also substitutes for one another. Similar health plans are obviously closer substitutes than are different types of health plans. As shown in Table 5.2, if any one health plan increased its premium by 10 percent relative to that of a competing health plan, the health plan could lose more than 20 percent of its enrollment to its competitors.

The estimates of elasticity of demand with respect to time, shown in Table 5.3, are surprisingly high: −1 on the number of sick child visits (using the parent's wage as the opportunity cost of time); −0.6 to −1 with respect to travel time to a public outpatient department; and −0.2 to −0.3 to a private physician's office. Waiting time elasticities of demand are lower, between −0.05 and −0.12.

When income elasticities of demand for medical expenditures are estimated based on aggregations of individuals or through cross-national comparisons, medical services are found to be income elastic; greater than +1.0, that is, as income increases by 10 percent,

TABLE 5.3 Time-Price Elasticities for Physician Services

Study	Dependent Variable	Elasticity	
J. P. Vistnes and V. Hamilton (1995)	Physician visits	−1.05	
R. M. Coffey (1983)		−0.09	
F. Goldman and M. Grossman (1978)	Physician visits	−0.06 to −0.07	
J. Acton (1976)	(travel time)	−0.60 to −1.00	(to public outpatient dept.)
		−0..25 to −0..37	(to private physician's office)
J. Acton (1976)	Physician visits	−0..12	(to public outpatient dept.)
	(waiting time)	−0.05	(to private physician's office)

Sources: J. Acton, "Demand for Health Care Among the Urban Poor with Special Emphasis on the Role of Time," in R. Rosett, ed., *The Role of Health Insurance in the Health Services Sector* (New York: National Bureau of Economic Research, 1976); R. M. Coffey, "The Effect of Time Price on the Demand for Medical-Care Services," *Journal of Human Resources*, 18(3), Summer 1983: 407–424; F. Goldman and M. Grossman, "The Demand for Pediatric Care: An Hedonic Approach," *Journal of Political Economy*, 86(2), April 1978: 259–280; J. P. Vistnes and V. Hamilton, "The Time and Monetary Costs of Outpatient Care for Children," *AEA Papers and Proceedings*, 85(2), May 1995: 117–121.

expenditures on medical care will increase by more than 10 percent. These results are shown in Table 5.4.

There is a difference in estimated income elasticities when aggregated data as compared to individual data are used. As discussed earlier, persons with higher income are more likely to have employer-paid health insurance; the growth in insurance coverage, both as a percentage of the bill paid and in terms of the type of medical services covered, is income-related. Thus at any point in time, the relationship between out-of-pocket expenditures

TABLE 5.4 Estimated Income Elasticities of Demand for Medical Services

Study	Dependent Variable	Elasticity
U-G Gerdtham et al. (1992)	Medical care expenditures	1.33
R. E. Leu (1986)		1.18 to 1.36
J. P. Newhouse (1977)		1.31
E. Kleiman (1974)		1.22
P. Feldstein and J. Carr (1964)		1.00
F. Goldman and M. Grossman (1978)	Physician services	1.32 (pediatric visits)
V. Fuchs and M. Kramer (1973)		0.57
R. Anderson and L. Benham (1970)		0.63
M. Silver (1970)		0.85
C. E. Lamberton, W.D. Ellingson and K.R. Spear (1986)	Nursing home care	1.07
W. J. Scanlon (1980)		2.27
B. R. Chiswick (1976)		0.55 to 0.89

Sources: R. Anderson and L. Benham, "Factors Affecting the Relationship Between Family Income and Medical Care Consumption," in H. Klarman, ed., *Empirical Studies in Health Economics* (Baltimore: John Hopkins University Press, 1970); B. Chiswick, "The Demand for Nursing Home Care: An Analysis of the Substitution Between Institutional and Noninstitutional Care," *Journal of Human Resources,* 11(3), Summer 1976: 295–316; P. Feldstein and J. Carr, "The Effects of Income on Medical Care Spending," *Proceedings of the Social Statistics Section of the American Statistical Association* (1964); V. Fuchs and M. Kramer, *Determinants of Expenditures for Physicians Services in the United States, 1948–1968* (New York: National Bureau of Economics Research, Occasional Paper 117, 1973); Ulf-G Gerdtham et al., "An Econometric Analysis of Health Care Expenditure: A Cross-Section Study of the OECD Countries," *Journal of Health Economics,* 11(1), May 1992: 63–84; F. Goldman and M. Grossman, "The Demand for Pediatric Care: An Hedonic Approach," *Journal of Political Economy,* 86(3), April 1978: 259–280; E. Kleiman, "The Determinants of National Outlay on Health," in M. Perlman, ed., *The Economics of Health and Medical Care* (London: Macmillan, 1974); C. E. Lamberton, W. D. Ellingson, and K. R. Spear, "Factors Determining the Demand for Nursing Home Services," *Quarterly Review of Economics and Business,* 26(4), Winter 1986: 74–90; R. E. Leu, "The Public–Private Mix and International Health Care Costs," in A. J. Culyer, and B. Jonsson, eds., *Public and Private Health Services* (Oxford: Basil Blackwell, 1986): 41–63; J. P. Newhouse, "Medical-Care Expenditures: A Cross-National Survey," *Journal of Human Resources,* 12(1), Winter 1977: 115–125; W. J. Scanlon, "A Theory of the Nursing Home Market," *Inquiry,* 17(1), Spring 1980: 25–41; M. Silver, "An Economic Analysis of Variations in Medical Expenses and Work Loss Rates," in H. Klarman, ed., *Empirical Studies in Health Economics* (Baltimore: John Hopkins University Press, 1970).

and income is positive but not income elastic. Over time, however, the income effect, which includes the amount paid by insurance, is more pronounced. Similarly, cross-national studies examine total medical expenditures and income, regardless of whether these expenditures are paid directly by the consumer or through government.

The finding that medical expenditures are income elastic means that medical expenditures will continue to increase at the same or higher rate as income. Medical care is, therefore, likely to continue to absorb an increasing share of this country's resources.

Physician services, except for pediatric visits, appear to be inelastic with respect to income.

In more recent studies, the income elasticity of demand for nursing home care by private-pay patients was estimated to be highly income elastic, between 2.3 and 2.8.

The RAND Health Insurance Experiment (RAND) was a controlled experiment to determine the effect of different insurance co-payments on use of medical services. As such, it has greatly increased our knowledge of the effect of deductibles and income-related cost sharing on the demand for medical services (10). Under the experiment, participants were randomly assigned to one of fourteen insurance plans for three to five years. One of the insurance plans provided free care (no deductibles or cost sharing), while the others involved different cost-sharing percentages. The cost-sharing plans differed according to the family's co-insurance rate, which was either 25, 50, or 95 percent. The 95 percent plan was the same as an income-related catastrophic plan. The maximum annual dollar expenditure of the family under these plans was income-related; it was either 5, 10, or 15 percent of income, up to a maximum of $1,000.

The RAND study concluded, consistent with traditional economic theory, that as the co-insurance rate rose, overall use and expenditure fell, for adults and children combined. These results are presented in Table 5.5. Compared to the free care plan, a co-insurance rate of 25 percent resulted in a 19 percent decline in expenditures; higher co-insurance rates, 50 and 95 percent (subject to a maximum out-of-pocket amount), resulted in over 30 percent declines in expenditures. In other words, per person expenditures in the free care plan were 23 percent higher than in the 25 percent plan and 50 percent higher than in the 50 percent co-insurance plan. The probability of a physician visit in a year was 7 to 18 percent lower in the cost-sharing plans than in the free care plan, while hospital admissions were 21 to 29 percent lower. For the Individual Deductible Plan, which had co-insurance for ambulatory services (95 percent) and free inpatient services, the respective probabilities were 13 and 11 percent lower than the free plan.

Price elasticities for the 0–25 and 25–95 percent ranges of co-insurance were calculated according to the type of care received by the patient (e.g., outpatient, hospital, and all care). As shown in Table 5.6, for the 0–25 percent plan, the price elasticity was −0.17 for each of the above types of care. Under the 25–95 percent plan, the elasticity estimates were −0.31, −0.14, and −0.22 for outpatient, hospital, and all care, respectively. For outpatient care under the 25–95 percent plan, these estimates varied according to whether the treatment was for well care (−0.43) or for chronic care (−0.23).

TABLE 5.5 Differences Between Plans in Predicted Total Expenditures per Person and in the Probability of One or More Physician Visits or Hospital Admissions (All Participants)

	Expenditures	Physician Visits (Probability as a Percent of Free Plan)	Hospital Admissions (Probability as a Percent of Free Plan
Free care	$430	100	100
25 percent co-insurance	81%	93	79
50 percent co-insurance	67%	89	71
95 percent co-insurance	69%	82	75
Individual deductible plan, 95 percent co-insurance	77%	87	88

Source: Adapted from Joseph P. Newhouse et al., *Some Interim Results from a Controlled Trial of Cost Sharing in Health Insurance* (Santa Monica: R-2847-HHS, RAND Corporation, January 1982).

A concern with increased cost sharing is that it causes people to delay seeking needed medical care. Further, lower use rates associated with increased cost sharing may have adverse health effects on individuals. To examine these effects on health, the RAND study included measures on self-reported health status indicators, measures of physiologic health, and health practices, such as smoking, weight, and use of preventive services (11). Since participants were randomly assigned to health insurance plans, differences in use rates were due to cost-sharing provisions of the plan and not to the health of the participants. Individuals with the free care plan improved on three of the eleven health status indicators—vision, blood pressure, and dental health. Free care members scored better on three of the twenty-three physiologic measures (two vision measures and blood pressure). The effect of the free care had small effects on health practices; blood pressure control and early detection of cancer improved although they were offset by decreases in other health practices. The authors state that "the average appraised mortality risk for

TABLE 5.6 Price Elasticities for Various Types of Care

Range of Nominal Co-insurance Variation	Type of Care					
	Outpatient				Hospital	All Care
	Acute	Chronic	Well	All		
0–25 Percent	0.16	0.20	0.14	0.17	0.17	0.17
25–95 Percent	0.32	0.23	0.43	0.31	0.14	0.22

Source: W. G. Manning et al., "Health Insurance and the Demand for Medical Care: Evidence from a Randomized Experiment," *American Economic Review,* 77(3), June 1987: 251–277.

people on the free plan was very close to the risk for those with cost sharing." Even when those at elevated risk were compared, the effect "rarely differed between insurance plans" (p. 303).

The authors concluded by saying that "despite the limited gains in health, free care leads to large differences in utilization for the healthy. Because most people are healthy, it is expensive and inefficient to use free care for all as the method to assure the health needs of the few."

The impact of cost sharing, however, was found to have a larger effect on lower-income persons, particularly children (12). A panel of experts divided episodes of care into those in which medical care produces usually effective treatments and usually less effective treatments. It was determined that for those conditions in which medical care is highly effective, the probability of poor children in the cost-sharing plan having an episode of treatment was 44 percent less than children in the free plan; for nonpoor children the probability was only 15 percent less. Poor adults in the cost-sharing plan had a 41 percent lower probability of seeking treatment than adults in the free plan, while for nonpoor adults it was 29 percent lower.

The poor are at greater risk of not receiving treatment when such treatment would be effective than are the nonpoor, particularly poor children. This finding should be kept in mind with regard to any government proposals for national health insurance in which cost sharing is not income-related.

AN APPLICATION OF DEMAND ANALYSIS: EXPLAINING ANNUAL CHANGES IN PERSONAL MEDICAL EXPENDITURES

Personal health care expenditures increased from $23.7 billion in 1960 to almost $1 trillion by 1995. The average annual rates of increase have, however, varied over time. Before the introduction of Medicare and Medicaid in 1966, personal health care expenditures increased at an annual rate of 8.3 percent. Afterward, the annual percentage increases were more rapid. Between 1965 and 1975 and between 1975 and 1985, it was 12.5 and 12.7 percent per year, respectively. Between 1985 and 1995, the rate of increase slowed to 8.9 percent per year.

These rapid increases in medical expenditures in the post–Medicare period have been the result of increased demands for medical care, the increasingly large involvement of government in the financing of medical care, and increases in the costs of providing such services. Together, these changes in demand and supply have resulted in increased prices and quantities for medical services, each of which constitute part of the increase in medical expenditures.

Although many of the factors affecting demand and supply have changed gradually, the price of medical services has sharply increased. In addition, the population has increased, there have been changes in its age distribution, and personal incomes have increased—all of which have led to increased demands for medical care. A more detailed analysis of changes in medical care expenditures would examine additional demand factors, but the changes in prices, incomes, and population and its changing composition can be used to provide a rough approximation of the importance of these demand factors in contributing to increases in medical care expenditures during these periods (13).

As shown in Table 5.7, the rise in the price of medical care as measured by the medical care price index contributed substantially to each period's increase in medical care expenditures. Before 1965, medical prices contributed less than 30 percent of the annual percentage increase in expenditures. However, after the introduction of Medicare and Medicaid in 1966, the increase in medical prices contributed between 50 and 75 percent of the annual percentage increase in medical expenditures. When the rate of increase in medical prices is subtracted from the rate of increase in medical expenditures, the result is the average annual percentage increase in the *real* quantity of medical care purchased.

To explain changes in the quantity of medical care purchased during this period, we must first adjust for changes in the population, which will give us the annual percentage increase in the quantity of medical care per person. Subtracting the rate of increase in population from the rate of increase in real medical output yields the annual percentage increase in quantity of medical care per person during this period. As shown in Table 5.7, population changes explain only a small percentage of the overall rate of increase in medical expenditures, particularly in the post-1965 period. During the latter period, population was increasing at approximately 1 percent per year, while medical expenditures were increasing more rapidly than in the past.

Per capita incomes were rising (although at different annual rates of increase) during the different periods examined. If an income elasticity of 1.0 is assumed—that is, demand for medical care will increase at the same rate as the increase in income—then part of the annual percentage increase in medical care can be accounted for by increased per capita incomes. In the post-1965 period, real (adjusted for inflation) per capita incomes were rising less rapidly than previously.

In addition, because medical care prices have been increasing at a faster rate than prices in the rest of the economy, the rate of increase in medical prices relative to the prices of other consumer goods and services can be used to represent an increase in the price of real medical care services. With an increase in the price of a service we would expect a decrease in demand for that service; the size of the decrease in demand for medical care depends on its price elasticity of demand. Assuming that the price elasticity of demand for medical services is −0.2, which means that the demand for medical care is relatively price inelastic, a 1 percent increase in price would lead to a 0.2 percent decrease in quantity demanded. With reference to Table 5.7, the rate of increase in the quantity of medical care will decline by 0.2 multiplied by the relative rate of increase in the price of medical care.

TABLE 5.7 Factors Affecting Changes in Personal Health Care Expenditures

Factor	Average Annual Rate of Change (%)			
	1960–65	1965–75	1975–85	1985–95
Personal health care expenditures	8.3	12.5	12.7	8.9
Accounted for by:				
Rise in price of medical care (CPI Medical Care)	2.5	6.6	9.1	6.9
Population increase (resident population)	1.5	1.1	1.0	1.0
Rise in real personal income per capita, increasing medical expenditures by an equal percentage (income elasticity = 1.0)	3.5	2.7	2.2	1.2
Decline in quantity demanded because of rise in relative price of medical care (price elasticity = −0.2)[a]	−0.2	−0.2	−0.4	−0.7
Changes in population distribution (aging population)[b]	0.1	0.5	0.6	0.2
Total accounted for	7.4	10.7	12.5	8.6
Unexplained residual	0.9	1.8	0.2	0.3

Sources: U.S. Department of Health and Human Services, Health Care Financing Administration, Internet site http://www.hcfa.gov/stats/nhce96.htm, and unpublished data, 1996; Bureau of the Census, *Statistical Abstract of the United States, 1996,* 116th ed.: Table 2, p. 8; Table 692, p.448; Table 746, p. 484; *Economic Report of the President, Transmitted to the Congress, February, 1996* (Washington, D.C.: U.S. Government Printing Office: 1996), Table B-30, p. 315; Daniel R. Waldo et al., "Health Expenditures by Age Group, 1977 and 1987," *Health Care Financing Review,* 10(4), Summer 1989: Table 3, pp. 116–117 with corrections supplied by Daniel Waldo.

[a] Annual change in relative price of medical care has been calculated by substracting the annual rate of change in CPI from the annual rate of change in MCPI.

[b] The impact of aging population on personal health care expenditures has been calculated using the following method: for each year, three population age groups are used (under 19, 20–64, and 65+) and for each age group constant age-specific health care expenditure per capita equal to the 1987 value is assumed throughout. The impact of aging population during a given time period is calculated as a ratio of total health care expenditure (sum of the products of health care expenditure per capita in the age group [HEPC$_{i87}$] and percentage of total population in the same age group [POPi]) from two time periods (jk).

$$IMPACTkj = \Sigma \, (POPij * HEPC_{i87}) \, / \, \Sigma \, (POP_{ik} * HEPC_{i87})$$

Over time the composition of the population has changed. In 1965, 9.2 percent were over 65 years of age. By 1995, 12.7 percent were 65 and over. Since those over 65 have greater demands for care than the rest of the population, an adjustment was made for the aging of the population.

When these factors affecting demand are summed up for the different periods, most of the annual percentage increase in medical expenditures can be accounted for. The amount of the unexplained residual was greatest (1.8 percent per year) in the period right after the introduction of Medicare and Medicaid, 1965 to 1975, than in the two subsequent ten-year periods (0.2 and 0.3 percent annually).

It is likely that the large unexplained residual in the post–Medicare period, which is the percentage increase in real medical care output that cannot be explained by the demand factors we have described, represents changes in the *type* of medical services produced. When medical prices were used to adjust expenditures to determine real output increases, it was assumed that the price increases were pure price increases and that the output produced was similar over time. Innovations in medical technology have, however, changed the medical product over time. Further, after Medicare was introduced, the age distribution of hospital patients changed; the aged constituted a larger proportion of patients. The aged require more costly types of service than do the nonaged. Also, after Medicare, hospitals increased their service quality by adding more facilities and services and increasing ratios of personnel per patient, both of which contribute to an increase in real expenditures per person in the post–Medicare period. It is likely that if the foregoing analysis included these additional factors, the price increase would have been smaller (since it also reflects changes in product and quality over time) and that the size of the unexplained residual would be much lower.

THE DEMAND FOR MEDICAL CARE FACED BY THE FIRM

Up to this point, the determinants of demand for medical services have been discussed. The demands for hospital care, physician services, nursing, and home care are derived from the demand for treatment. Based on empirical estimates, the market demand for hospital and physician services was determined to be relatively price inelastic. However, it is important to distinguish between the overall market demand for a service such as hospital care, which does not have very good substitutes, and the demand facing an individual provider. While the overall demand for hospital care may be relatively inelastic with respect to price, the demand facing an individual hospital, especially in a community with several hospitals, will be much more price elastic, since any one hospital is a possible substitute for another. (The strategic implications and anti-trust concerns of this difference in price elasticity between firm and market demand are discussed in subsequent chapters.)

To determine the demand facing an individual firm, a two-step approach is needed. First, the provider (e.g., a hospital) must estimate the overall market demand for hospital care. To do so, it is necessary to estimate demand by type of service, such as obstetrics, and by market area. For each service, the factors affecting demand must be specified and an estimate derived of the relative importance of each factor (i.e., the elasticity of each factor with respect to hospital care). Factors that should be included in an overall demand forecast include, as discussed in the demand model, measures of need, sociodemographic variables, and economic measures. Since the first two sets of variables change gradually, short-range forecasts must place greater emphasis on the economic variables. Substitutes for hospital care, particularly certain procedures that may be performed in outpatient surgery centers, can result in dramatic decreases in use of the hospital.

A forecast of hospital demand must include some estimate of how each of the factors affecting demand will change over time. For example, the likely growth of HMOs in a market area must be estimated. Once an estimate of the population enrolled in an HMO is determined, then the effect of HMOs on hospital use is required, again by type of service. For each of the factors affecting demand, an estimate of how such factors will change over time, together with their likely effect on demand, is required. This approach should provide an overall estimate of demand by type of service.

The second step in a demand forecast for an individual provider is to determine what proportion of the overall market demand will be received by the individual provider, that is, the hospital's market share. The market share, by type of service and by geographic area, will depend on the individual hospital's characteristics relative to its competitors, such as the hospital's price relative to other hospitals' prices; the relative reputation of the hospital; its distance from various zip codes compared to other hospitals in the market area; and the number and location of its primary care physicians relative to other hospitals. It is important for the provider to be able to relate its characteristics (relative to other health providers) to its market share. For example, knowing the importance of prices relative to those of their competitors will provide an indication as to the effect on their market share of a change in relative prices. (The importance of relative prices or other provider characteristics will vary by payer group; prices or reputation will be more important to some purchasers than others.)

By forecasting demand in this two-step process, namely, overall market demand and then relative market shares, a provider can determine whether a decrease in its demand was the result of a decrease in overall market demand or a decrease in its market share. It is possible that a hospital's admissions have fallen because of a decline in overall demand for hospital care but that its market share has increased. Similarly, the decline in a hospital's admissions may have been the result of a decline in its market share in a market where the overall number of admissions has remained constant. The hospital's competitive performance is clearly different under these two scenarios.

Having some understanding of the factors that affect a hospital's market share can suggest how that hospital should allocate resources to increase its market share. By making rough calculations as to the effect of each of the factors affecting market share, the hospital can conduct cost/benefit analyses; the hospital can allocate resources to recruitment of primary care physicians, advertising to enhance its reputation, and so on, so that the effect on market share *per dollar spent* on each of these activities is equal. Although it is difficult to derive precise estimates of such allocations, merely thinking in terms of marginal costs and marginal benefits of alternative allocations should improve the decision-making process.

Forecasting demand has become more important to providers in an increasingly competitive environment. Not only must providers forecast their demands so as to establish their staffing patterns, but providers must be able to determine how to increase their market shares relative to their competitors. Demand and market share forecasts are important not only to hospitals, medical groups, and other medical providers, but also to health insurance companies and health maintenance organizations. An understanding of demand analysis should improve the ability to forecast demand in the foregoing situations.

SUMMARY

An understanding of the factors affecting demand for medical services is essential if one is to be able to explain differences in demand among different population groups. In addition to need, there are economic factors, such as out-of-pocket price, time costs, and income, as well as cultural and demographic factors. Although all these factors are important in a demand analysis, economists are particularly concerned with the economic factors since they change more quickly. It is also through changes in the economic factors, such as out-of-pocket prices and time costs, that public policy is able to change demands for care.

Estimates of price and income elasticities (the percent change in quantity of medical services resulting from a 1 percent change in price or income) are important for quantifying differences in demand and for forecasting demands for medical services.

It is important to distinguish between market and firm (individual physician or hospital) demand curves. Firm demand curves are more price elastic because there are better substitutes to an individual firm than there are to hospital or physician services. If all the individual firms were able to collude by acting as one firm, thereby facing the less price elastic industry demand for their services, they would be able to increase their prices. It is this type of collusive behavior that is anticompetitive according to the anti-trust laws.

The role of the physician as the patient's agent has been subject to a great deal of discussion and research. A physician can be hypothesized to act as either a perfect or imperfect agent on behalf of the patient. When the physician is a perfect agent, the physician is expected to act solely in the patient's interest, prescribing treatment according to both the patient's medical needs and economic resources. As an imperfect agent, the physician manipulates information so as to benefit herself as well as her patient. In a fee-for-service setting, imperfect physician agents induce additional demand for their services so as to maintain or increase their income.

To counteract fee-for-service physicians who act as imperfect agents, insurance companies have introduced cost containment approaches, such as utilization management, which attempt to correct the imbalance of information between the physician and the patient. When physicians are capitated, it becomes necessary to monitor physician behavior to prevent imperfect physician agents from decreasing patient access to care.

APPENDIX: THE EFFECT OF CO-INSURANCE ON THE DEMAND FOR MEDICAL CARE

A diagram may clarify the effect of co-insurance on the demand for medical care. Figure 5.3 shows the relationship between the price of medical care and the quantity demanded, with all other determinants of demand held constant. When the price is P_1, the quantity demanded will be Q_1. When insurance has a co-insurance feature, the person using medical services would have to pay the amount of the co-insurance, which is the difference between the proportion that the insurance pays and the price charged. The price paid by the patient would be P_2, which is, for example, 20 percent of P_1; the third-party payer would pay the remainder of the price, $P_1 - P_2$. As a result of the 80 percent price reduction, the patient will now demand Q_2 of medical services. (The actual increase in quantity demanded as a result of the decrease in price due to co-insurance will depend on the size of the co-insurance and the price elasticity of demand.) As long as there is some responsiveness of price to quantity demanded, co-insurance will increase demand by lowering the price the patient will pay for medical care.

Although insurance coverage represents a *movement* down an individual's demand curve, the aggregate effect of an increase in coverage is to cause a *shift* in the demand for medical care. For example, according to the demand curve represented by D_1 in Figure 5.4, an individual would demand Q_1 units of medical care if the out-of-pocket price was $10 per unit. If the individual were now provided with insurance requiring that only 20 percent of the total price be paid, then at a price of $10 per unit the individual need only pay $2. Therefore, the individual would move down the demand curve and consume Q_2 units at a price of $2 per unit. The actual price of Q_2 units is not $2 per unit but $10 per unit; the third-party payer pays 80 percent, or $8 per unit. Thus, the actual demand curve for medical care has shifted to the right. Similarly, if the initial price were $15, the patient with demand curve D_1 would consume Q_3 units of medical care. With the introduction of an 20 percent co-insurance program, the patient would move down his demand curve and consume Q_4 units at a price of $3 per unit. The total price per unit at Q_4 is, however, $15 per unit. Each of the points on the original demand curve (D_1) now represents only 20 percent of the total price. The new demand curve (D_2) represents the relationship between the total price per unit (20 percent of which is paid for by the patient and 80 percent by the third-party payer) and the quantities demanded at these different prices. (As the patient co-payment becomes less, the demand curve will rotate to

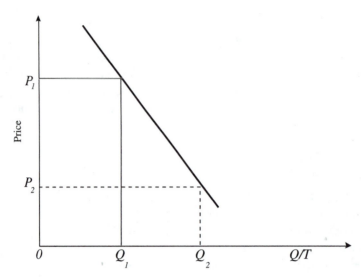

FIGURE 5.3 • The effect of co-insurance on the demand for medical care.

the right; it will become completely vertical when the patient is not required to make any out-of-pocket payments for medical care.)

The analysis of the effect of insurance becomes more complicated when there is a co-insurance provision *and* a rising supply curve for medical care. For example, according to Figure 5.5, the patient's original demand curve is D_1. The provision of health insurance with a co-insurance feature (for simplicity, it is assumed to be 50 percent with the re-

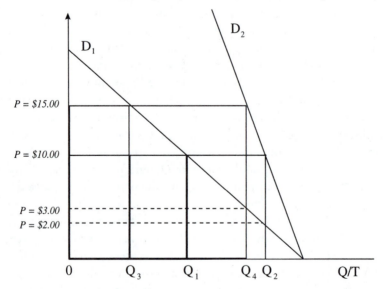

FIGURE 5.4 • Insurance as a shift in the aggregate demand for medical care.

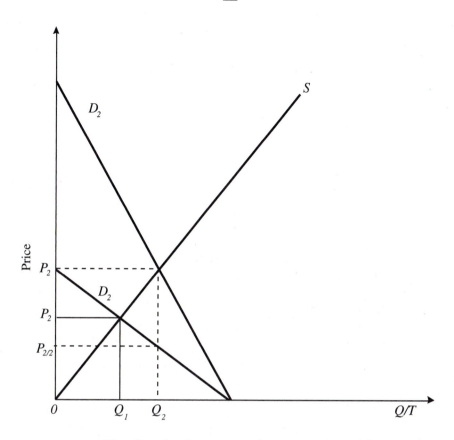

FIGURE 5.5 • The effect of co-insurance on the aggregate demand for medical care with a rising supply curve.

mainder being paid by the government) will result in a shift in demand to D_2, which represents the amount that both the patient and the government will pay for medical care. Every point on demand curve D_2 represents a doubling of the price for a given quantity over D_1, since it is a 50 percent co-insurance program. So far the analysis is similar to the previous example. However, since the new demand curve (D_2) intersects the supply curve at a higher price than previously, a new equilibrium price and quantity of medical care, P_2 and Q_2, will be established. Q_2 is thus the only quantity at which the public pays one-half the price of the medical care ($P_2/2$) that is also an equilibrium position. Thus the price the consumer will pay with a 50 percent co-insurance is greater than 50 percent of the original market price ($P_1/2$). The introduction of a percentage co-payment feature does not mean that the consumer's price will be a similar percentage of the original market price. Nor does it mean that the amount of care used will increase by that same proportion. The greater the co-insurance paid for by the government (or other third party), the greater the consumer's use of medical services will be, but the actual price the consumer must pay and the amount actually consumed will depend on the elasticity of both demand and supply. The more elastic demand and supply are, the greater will be the increase in quantity and the less the rise in price.

Key Terms and Concepts

- Demand creation
- Demand versus need
- Efficiency in consumption
- Efficiency in production
- Optimal rate of output
- Time costs

- Cross-price elasticities
- Determinants of demand
- Firm-specific price elasticities
- Market demand and relative market shares
- Physician as the patient's agent
- Price and income elasticities

Review Questions

1. If the price of medical care were set to zero for everyone, would individual demands for medical care still differ? Under what conditions would you favor a "negative" price for medical care?
2. Why do economists tend to reject the concept of need as the sole determinant of use in favor of the concept of the demand for medical care?
3. What are the various consequences if hospital planning in the United States is done according to need (or the use of bed to population ratios) rather than demand?
4. What variables should be included in a comprehensive measure of the price a person pays to consume medical care?
5. Define cross-price elasticity of demand. What is the meaning (in words) of a cross-price elasticity of demand of +6.5? Would you expect the goods to be substitutes or complements?
6. Discuss the determinants of the demand for medical care.
7. Why might the estimate of the income elasticity of demand for medical care be higher if one adjusts for health status than if one does not?
8. Price and nonprice methods (such as professional judgment or age of patient) have been used to ration medical services. Discuss the welfare implications of using each approach.

9. Evaluate the statement, "Medical care is never free, although the individual recipient may pay nothing."

10. How can a model of demand for hospital care be used to explain changes in hospital utilization over time?

11. How can a model of demand for medical care be used to explain the rise in medical expenditures over time?

12. How could you use a model of demand for medical care for purposes of policy (e.g., improving equity)? For example, as a national health policy analyst, you desire to increase the utilization of ambulatory medical care of low-income people. How would you use the results for demand analysis to suggest recommendations?

13. What are the differences between forecasting the demand for hospital services and forecasting the demand for a particular hospital's services? How would you determine the demand for your hospital's services? Be explicit regarding the factors that would be included in the analyses, including the reasons for their inclusion.

14. The physician has a dual role in medical care, as the patient's agent and as a supplier of a service. Under what circumstances would these roles be in conflict? What empirical evidence supports each of these different roles?

15. What factors might cause physicians to experience an increase in the number of requests for annual physical examinations even though they do not change their fees for this service?

16. It has been said that there is economic inefficiency on the demand side of the medical care market. What are both the reasons for and effects of this economic inefficiency?

17. It has been said that extensive (both public and private) insurance coverage resulted in an "erosion of the medical marketplace." Explain this statement.

REFERENCES

1. Roger Lee and Lewis Jones, *The Fundamentals of Good Medical Care* (Chicago: University of Chicago Press, 1933).

2. Kevin J. Lancaster, "A New Approach to Consumer Theory," *Journal of Political Economy,* 74(2), April 1966: 132–157.

3. Michael Grossman, "On the Concept of Health Capital and the Demand for Health," *Journal of Political Economy,* 80(2), March–April 1972: 223–255.

4. A number of surveys have collected data on family income and expenditures on medical care. A few of the better-known surveys are those conducted by the National Center for Health Statistics as part of the Health Interview Survey and published in Series 10, *Vital and Health Statistics* (Washington, D.C.: U.S. Department of Health, Education, and Welfare, various years). The National Opinion Research Center, University of Chicago, has also conducted national surveys on medical expenditures. These surveys, which have been conducted at five-year intervals beginning in 1953, have been presented in various publications, such as Odin W. Anderson, Patricia Collette, and Jacob Feldman, *Changes in Family Medical Care Expenditures: A Five*

Year Resurvey (Cambridge, Mass.: Harvard University Press, 1963). More recently, the Deppartment of Health and Human Services has undertaken national surveys of medical care expenditures (1977, 1982, and 1987), which are referred to as the National Medical Care Expenditure Survey.

5. The distinction between permanent and transitory components of income and their relationship to consumption are discussed by Friedman in terms of his permanent income theory of consumption in Milton Friedman, *A Theory of the Consumption Function* (Princeton, N.J.: Princeton University Press, 1957).

6. For a more complete discussion of the role of time in the demand for medical care, see Charles E. Phelps and Joseph P. Newhouse, "Co-insurance, the Price of Time, and the Demand for Medical Services," *Review of Economics and Statistics,* 56(3), August 1974: 334–342. See also Jan P. Acton, "Demand for Health Care Among the Urban Poor, with Special Emphasis on the Role of Time," in Richard Rosett, ed., *The Role of Health Insurance in the Health Services Sector* (New York: National Bureau of Economic Research, 1976).

7. Anne A. Scitovsky and Nelda M. Snyder, "Effect of Co-insurance on Use of Physician Services," *Social Security Bulletin,* 35(6), June 1972: 3–19.

8. For a discussion on agency theory, see David Dranove and William White, "Agency and the Organization of Health Care Delivery," *Inquiry,* 24(4), Winter 1987: 405–415.

9. Victor Fuchs, "The Growing Demand for Medical Care," *New England Journal of Medicine,* 279(4), July 25, 1968: 190–195.

10. A shorter version of the study results without appendixes is contained in Joseph Newhouse et al., "Some Interim Results from a Controlled Trial of Cost Sharing in Health Insurance," *New England Journal of Medicine,* 305(25), December 17, 1981: 1501–1507. See also Emmett B. Keeler and John E. Rolph, "How Cost Sharing Reduced Medical Spending of Participants in the Health Insurance Experiment," *Journal of the American Medical Association,* 249(16), April 29, 1983: 2220–2222.

11. Emmett B. Keeler et al., "Effects of Cost Sharing on Physiological Health, Health Practices, and Worry," *Health Services Research,* 22(3), August 1987: 279–306.

12. Kathleen N. Lohr et al., "Use of Medical Care in the RAND Health Insurance Experiment, Diagnosis and Service-Specific Analyses in a Randomized Controlled Trial," *Medical Care,* 24(9), Supplement, September 1986: S1–S87.

13. The discussion in this section is based on an earlier article by Victor Fuchs, "The Growing Demand for Medical Care," *New England Journal of Medicine,* 279(4), July 25, 1968: 190–195.

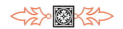

CHAPTER

The Demand for Health Insurance

APPROPRIATENESS OF HEALTH INSURANCE COVERAGE

Although the number of services covered and the percentage of the bill paid by health insurance have increased over time, insurance coverage still varies greatly by population group, by services covered, and by percentage of the medical bill covered. In pointing to the percentage of the medical bill covered by insurance as a measure of its "adequacy," anything less than 100 percent coverage (or at least a "high" percentage) is deemed by some to be "inadequate." The policy recommendations that follow from such a normative judgment are based either on the assumption that inadequacy is the result of insufficient financial means on the part of consumers for purchasing the appropriate amount of insurance, or that the inadequacy is a result of the health insurance industry's failure to provide more appropriate coverage. The recommendations based on this normative judgment of inadequate health insurance are that the government should either provide comprehensive coverage under its own auspices or subsidize the purchase of health insurance.

To determine the "appropriateness" (or optimal amount) of health insurance coverage in the United States, appropriateness in an economic sense must be defined. It is also important to determine whether there are market conditions that distort the consumer's ability to select the economically appropriate quantity of health insurance coverage. In this chapter, therefore, we examine the determinants of the demand for health insurance. In Chapter 8 we examine the economic efficiency of the health insurance market to determine whether there are (or have been) distortions on the demand or supply side of that market that result in either "too much" or "too little" (or insufficient varieties) of health insurance offered. The conclusions with respect to the supply side of that market should indicate the appropriate role of government, if any, as a regulator or provider of health insurance.

HEALTH INSURANCE TERMINOLOGY

As a preface to the analysis of the demand for health insurance, a brief discussion of a number of concepts used in health insurance is in order.

Deductibles

When consumers pay a flat dollar amount for medical services before their insurance picks up all or part of the remainder of the price of that service, this is referred to as a deductible. Deductibles may be set in a number of ways: they may apply to each unit of service, or they may be cumulative—for example, once $250 has been paid by the consumer for medical services within a year, the third-party payer will contribute to the cost of additional services. Deductibles may also be established either on a family basis or for each individual. Deductibles may also be related to family income, with higher deductibles being required of persons with higher family incomes, as has been proposed under certain national health insurance schemes.

An important reason for using a deductible is that it lowers the administrative costs of claims processing in a situation where there are many small claims and the cost of handling these claims is high. These transaction costs are likely to exceed the amount people are willing to pay for insurance against small claims. Typically, people are more willing to pay the transaction costs of handling large, unexpected claims. Thus, by lowering the transaction costs for small claims, the consumer is more likely to be able to buy insurance (at a lower premium) for protection against large medical expenditures. A large percentage of families incur small medical expenditures within a year, while a small percentage of families incur very large expenditures. This phenomenon is illustrated in Figure 6.1A. The insurance costs of covering medical expenditures would obviously be lowered if a deductible were placed at the low end of the expenditure spectrum, as indicated by line A in Figure 6.1A. Further, the deductible provides the consumer with an incentive to shop around for the best price when the deductible is greater than the price of the service.

The case against deductibles is generally made on the grounds that the deductible, no matter how small, may be a deterrent to needed care. Further, a flat deductible, irrespective of family income, is a greater burden on low-income families than on high-income families.

The effect of the deductible on use of services is complex. If there is a deductible, once the deductible is exceeded and additional services are free, the deductible will have no effect on decreasing the use of services. Once the deductible has been paid, the patient will use the services as though their price were "zero." If the deductible has not been exceeded, the price of the services will determine (other things being held constant) how much they will be used. A deductible by itself, therefore, will either tend to result in greater use of services (similar to a zero price) when a low deductible is used, or if the deductible is high,

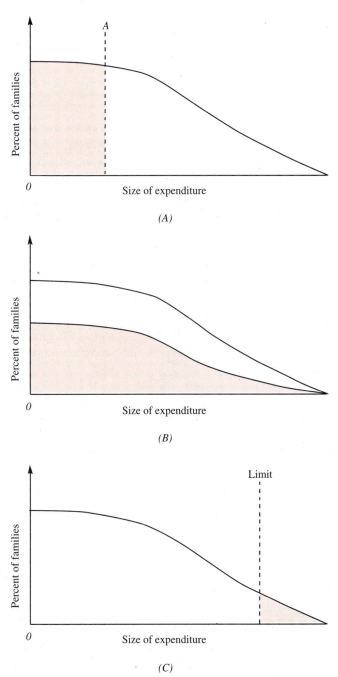

FIGURE 6.1 • The expected distribution of family medical expenses with different types of co-payments; (A) the imposition of a deductible; (B) a co-insurance provision; (C) a maximum or limit to coverage.

it will tend to make insurance coverage irrelevant to many users of care. The effectiveness of a deductible depends on the size of the deductible, the expected medical expenditures of the family (if on a family basis), and family income.

Co-insurance

When the third-party payer reimburses the patient for a certain fraction of the price of the service, the arrangement is termed co-insurance. A co-insurance level of 80 percent in effect lowers the price to the patient of those covered services by 80 percent. The patient pays the remaining 20 percent herself. If the price of the services should rise, the insurance would pay 80 percent of the new, higher price. Co-insurance levels can also vary by service covered and by family income. The advantage of co-insurance is that it reduces the price of the service and still provides the patient with an incentive to seek out less costly providers. The effectiveness of a co-insurance feature will depend on how responsive utilization is to lower prices, which is the price elasticity of demand. If use is not responsive to price, co-insurance will merely be a way of reducing the cost of the insurance package to the consumer. Depending on the level of co-insurance and the price elasticity of demand, co-insurance can change the distribution of medical expenditures, as shown in Figure 6.1B. Co-insurance would result in the consumer's paying for the shaded portion of Figure 6.1B, while the third-party payer would pay for the remainder of the medical expenses.

Stop Loss Levels, Limits, and Maximums

Deductibles and co-insurance can add up to a large financial loss to a person who has a serious illness. Insurance therefore includes a "stop loss." Once the patient's out-of-pocket medical expenses (deductible and co-insurance) reach a certain dollar amount, typically $2,500, then the patient is no longer responsible for additional out-of-pocket payments.

While stop loss levels are meant to protect the patient from a large financial loss, limits and maximums are similarly used to protect the insurance company from large losses. Insurance companies often include $1 or $2 million lifetime limits on how much they are willing to reimburse for a patient's medical expenses. Expenditures above that limit become the responsibility of the patient. This approach shifts the cost of very large expenditures, generally considered to be catastrophic, to the patient incurring him instead of distributing them among all insured persons. Limits have been used in the past by Blue Cross, such as when it covered hospital services up to a maximum of thirty days in the hospital. Mental health benefits have had low maximums, typically $50,000. (Legislation enacted in 1996 requires mental health benefits to be the same as medical benefits.) The part of medical expenditures that is excluded by limits and maximums is generally the tail of the distribution, as shown in Figure 6.1C. Large expenditures, incurred by a small percentage of families, are generally not responsive to prices; to exclude this part of the distribution from coverage appears to be particularly unwise, since large, unexpected losses to a small percentage of the population meet the criteria defining insurance risks. If the objective of using limits is to enable the insurance company to lower its insurance premium to consumers, an alternative approach would be to use a small deductible for the many families that have small expenditures. This front-end deductible, when applied to many families, would be less of a financial hardship than would a catastrophic expense befalling a small percentage of the population.

Insurance coverage for the tail of the distribution (i.e., the large expenditures incurred by a small percentage of the population) is generally referred to as major medical or catastrophic insurance. Major medical coverage was an innovation introduced by the commercial insurance companies in the late 1940s to compete with Blue Cross, which until that time was the dominant third-party insurer selling hospitalization insurance up to a maximum limit.

Other Forms of Coverage

Insurance contracts may include any or all of the above in various combinations of deductibles, co-insurance, and limits. Other aspects of insurance coverage should also be briefly mentioned. Some coverage may specifically exclude certain diseases for which the potential insurance purchaser was treated in the previous year; this is referred to as a preexisting condition. Allowing immediate coverage for preexisting conditions would be like allowing a person whose house was on fire to buy insurance to cover his loss; a person would have no incentive to buy insurance while healthy. Other kinds of insurance coverage may include continuation of salary if a person becomes ill, or disability benefits if a person is unable to be fully rehabilitated once an illness has been incurred.

Indemnity versus Service Benefits

When Blue Cross was started in the 1930s, it provided a "service" benefit for hospital care, which meant that the price to the patient for the stay in the hospital (up to a maximum period) was reimbursed in full to the hospital. There were no cost-sharing provisions, deductibles, or co-insurance features for the patient. An indemnity benefit, which was offered by commercial insurance carriers, differed from a service benefit in that it reimbursed the patient, not the hospital, a predetermined amount for the patient's medical costs. The amount of reimbursement was often a fixed dollar amount per hospital day or admission or a percentage of the bill. The patient had an incentive to minimize the cost of the illness. Naturally, the hospitals that had founded Blue Cross preferred the service-benefit approach, since it meant that they would be reimbursed for all their services and the patient would have no incentive to shop around for the least expensive hospital or a less costly nonhospital provider. By providing coverage only for hospital care, Blue Cross made nonhospital services more costly to the patient; therefore, hospital use was encouraged when other, less costly settings could have been used to treat the patient. Further, hospitals would incur lower collection costs if they could bill Blue Cross for all their patients instead of having to collect from each patient. A more detailed discussion of the Blue Cross service benefit policy and a comparison between it and an indemnity policy is provided in Appendix 1 of this chapter.

THE THEORY OF DEMAND FOR HEALTH INSURANCE

The consumer's demand for health insurance represents the amount of insurance coverage that he is willing to buy at different prices (premiums) for health insurance. Additional insurance coverage will be purchased if the insurance premium (actually, the loading charge) declines. Once the consumer has some insurance, the marginal benefit of increasing the comprehensiveness of insurance declines the more comprehensive the coverage. *When the marginal benefit of additional coverage equals the marginal cost (to the consumer) of buying that additional coverage, then the "appropriate" amount of insurance will have been purchased.*

According to this definition, 100 percent coverage of all medical expenses would be demanded by the consumer only when insurance is sold at its pure premium; that is, no administrative cost is added. At positive administrative prices for insurance, the consumer would demand less than 100 percent coverage. This is because the marginal benefit of the last unit of insurance coverage would be purchased only if the price of that additional coverage to the consumer were very small. Adding an administrative price to the pure premium would cause the total price of those last units to be greater than their marginal benefits. The consumer would purchase additional coverage only to the point where the benefit of additional coverage equaled the total price of additional coverage.

Keeping in mind that the appropriateness of the amount of insurance coverage consumers will buy will be related to their perception of the value of additional coverage compared with the additional cost of that coverage, the demand for health insurance will be examined under two conditions. In the first situation it is assumed that there is no "moral hazard." The demand for medical care is assumed to be completely price inelastic; that is, patients cannot affect the size of their loss once they are ill (1). The second situation considers the demand for insurance coverage when moral hazard exists.

To understand the factors that affect the demand for health insurance, it is necessary to be familiar with the economic theory underlying the purchase of insurance. This discussion should clarify why people buy insurance for some risks and not for others. The economic theory of insurance is then used to predict the type of insurance expected to be most prevalent in the health field.[1]

Underlying the demand for insurance is the assumption that an individual wishes to

---

[1]Throughout this analysis, for the sake of simplicity, it is assumed that utility functions are independent, that is, the degree to which others have insurance to cover their medical loss does not affect an individual's desire to subsidize another person's purchase of insurance.

maximize her utility, which is the usual assumption made in demand analysis. Since a person does not know whether she will have an illness, consequently, a loss of wealth to pay for it, the individual who seeks to maximize her utility when subject to uncertain events seeks to maximize her *expected* utility. That is, the person can choose between two alternative courses of action:

1. She can purchase insurance and thereby incur a small loss in the form of the insurance premium, or
2. She can self-insure, which means facing the small possibility of a large loss in the event that the illness occurs, or the large possibility that the medical loss will not occur.

To determine whether consumers will purchase insurance for an unexpected medical event or self-insure and bear the risk themselves, it is necessary to compare courses 1 and 2 to determine which choice provides them with a higher level of utility.

The use of expected utility, as discussed by M. Friedman and L. Savage in their classic article (2), assumes that the consumer selects among alternative choices according to whether one choice is preferred to the others, and ranks these choices according to how much one choice is preferred over another (i.e., cardinal rankings). Although one can think of the utility function as having no unique origin or unit of measure, once some unit of measure and a point of origin are accepted, the utility function of an individual can be described for all levels of wealth. Further, for an individual to purchase insurance, she must believe that the marginal utility of wealth is decreasing; although the preference is for more wealth rather than less wealth, additional wealth has a lower marginal utility. The relationship between total utility and wealth is shown in Figure 6.2A; as will be shown, unless the utility function exhibits this relationship to wealth, the "rational" individual will not purchase insurance.

To illustrate the choices an individual has who is trying to decide whether to purchase health insurance, we will assume that if an illness occurs, it will cost \$8,000. If the individual is currently at W_3, meaning that his wealth is \$10,000, then if the event occurs, \$8,000 must be paid out, thereby moving the individual to wealth position W_1. (The corresponding utility levels at W_3 and W_1 are U_3 and U_1, respectively.) Let us assume that the probability of the individual's requiring medical services costing \$8,000 is 0.025— 2.5 percent. The "pure premium" of the insurance that would cover the actuarial value of the expected loss would therefore be $0.025 \times \$8,000 = \$200$.

The pure premium is a function of *both* the size of the expected loss (\$8,000) and the probability of it occurring (0.025) *for a large group of people* (the law of large numbers). If the person were to buy insurance priced at the actuarial value of the expected loss, he would pay \$200, thereby reducing his wealth, with certainty, to point W_2 on Figure 6.2A, which represents \$9,800. Let us further assume that as a result of purchasing insurance and decreasing wealth to \$9,800, the individual is now at U_2, which is equivalent to

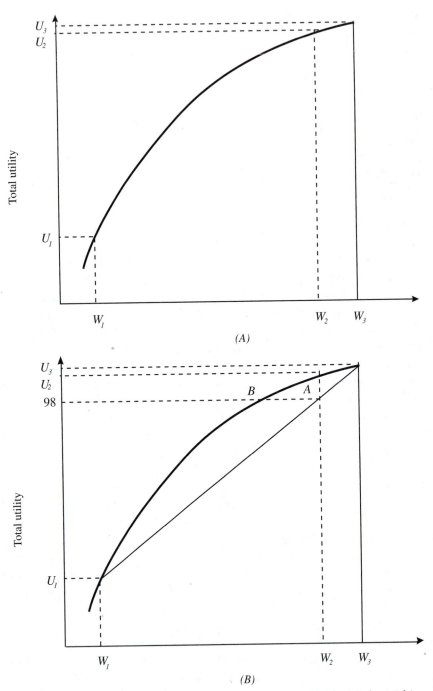

FIGURE 6.2 • The relationship between total utility and wealth; (A) diminishing marginal utility with increased wealth; (B) expected utility.

being at a total utility level of 99, U_3 being 100 and U_1 being 20. The choices facing the individual therefore are:

a. To purchase insurance for $200 and move to a lower level of utility, 99, or
b. Not to purchase insurance and have a 2.5 percent chance that he will incur an $8,000 loss and thereby move to a utility level of 20 ($U_{1)}$, which is associated with a wealth position of $2,000, or face a high probability of 97.5 (100 − 2.5 percent) that a loss will not be incurred and thereby remain at a wealth position of $10,000 with an associated utility level of 100.

To compare choices *a* and *b*, we must use expected utility. The expected utility of choice *b* is the weighted sum of the utilities of each outcome, with the weights being the probabilities of each outcome. Therefore, the expected utility of choice *b* is

$$P(U_1) + (1 - P)(U_3) = 0.025(20) + 0.975(100) = 98$$

To determine whether a person would buy health insurance, we compare the utility level of choice *a,* which represents purchasing insurance and thereby leaves the person at utility level $U = 99$, with the expected utility level of choice *b,* which represents not purchasing insurance and thereby results in an expected utility level $U = 98$. Since the utility level of choice *a* is greater than that of choice *b,* we predict that the person would purchase insurance. In this example it is assumed that the insurance is sold at the actuarially fair premium and that the utility function with respect to wealth is similar to the one described in Figure 6.2A—namely, diminishing marginal utility with respect to increased wealth.

The expected utility of choice *b,* $U = 98$, is shown in Figure 6.2B, by the straight line drawn on the utility curve extending from U_3, W_3, to U_1, W_1. The straight line represents expected utility for different probabilities that the illness will occur. The *lower* the probability that the event will occur, the closer the expected utility will be to the point farthest to the right on the utility curve. As the probability that the loss will occur increases, the expected utility value moves down to the left on the straight line, closer to the point represented by U_1 on the curve. In other words, if the loss is certain to occur, the individual will be at W_1 ($2,000) with a corresponding utility level of U_1 (= 20). Since the calculation of expected utility is based on the weighted sum of the probabilities of being at the different utility levels, as the probability of being at U_1 increases, the expected utility estimate declines in a linear fashion.

To show that expected utility declines linearly, the probability of the event occurring can be assumed to increase from 0.05, to 0.10, to 0.15, to 0.20. The expected utility of each of these events would then be as follows:

$$P(U_1) + (1 - P) (U_3) = 0.05(20) + 0.95(100) = 96$$
$$= 0.10(20) + 0.90(100) = 92$$

$$= 0.15(20) + 0.85(100) = 88$$
$$= 0.20(20) + .80(100) = 84$$

Because the individual's actual utility curve (decreasing marginal utility with respect to wealth) is always above the expected utility line (constant marginal utility with respect to wealth), the individual will always buy insurance if it is sold at its actuarially fair value (its pure premium). Thus, a risk-averse person will prefer to take a certain loss (the premium) rather than accept the uncertainty of a loss, even though the expected value of the loss is equal.

Insurance, however, is never sold at its pure premium because there are administrative, claims-processing, and marketing costs. These costs are referred to as the loading charge and are, in effect, the price of insurance. To determine whether an individual, as represented in Figure 6.2B, will buy insurance when there are these additional costs, the maximum amount above the pure premium he would be willing to pay for insurance must be calculated.

Referring back to Figure 6.2B, W_3–W_2 represents the dollar amount of the pure premium for an $8,000 loss that has a 2.5 percent probability of occurring. Since the utility level with insurance is greater than the expected utility level (99 versus 98), the person purchasing insurance will be willing to pay an amount above the pure premium that makes the actual utility level *after* the additional payment equal to the expected utility level. When the actual utility level is equal to the expected utility level (at $U = 98$), the person will be indifferent as to whether she purchases insurance or self-insures. If an additional payment places the individual's actual utility level below her expected utility level, the person would be better off self-insuring; that is, the person would be willing to pay an amount above the pure premium as long as his expected utility is not greater than his actual utility.

This discussion is illustrated in Figure 6.2B. Point A is the expected utility without insurance. If one draws a straight line from point A to where it crosses the actual utility curve, then at this point, B, a person's actual utility level and expected utility level are the same, $U = 98$. The distance from A to B on the wealth axis is the additional amount above the pure premium that a person would be willing to pay for that insurance. At every point along the expected utility line, which represents a different probability of the event occurring, there is an additional amount above the pure premium that a person would be willing to pay for insurance. At points close to W_1, which represent a high probability that a person will incur a large enough loss to leave her at wealth position W_1, a person would be willing to pay a smaller amount above the pure premium; the distance between the expected utility line and the actual utility curve, which would leave her at the same level of utility, is closer at that point.

As shown in Figure 6.3A, with an expected utility level at point E, the pure premium would be $W_3 - W_4$, which is a large amount, since the probability of the loss's occurring is quite high. A person would be willing to pay an additional amount above the pure pre-

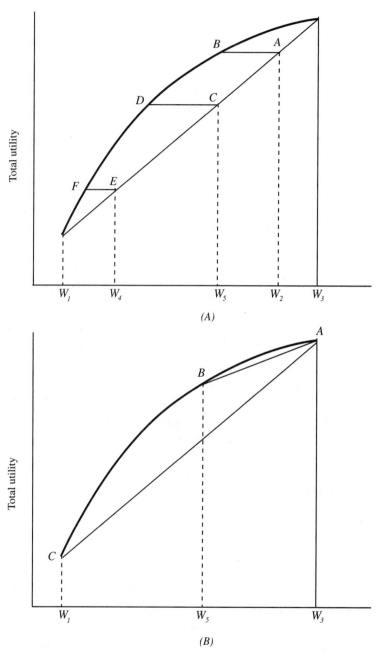

FIGURE 6.3 • The amount above the pure premium an individual is willing to pay for health insurance; (A) according to different probabilities of the event occurring; (B) according to different magnitudes of the expected loss.

mium equal to the distance *EF,* since at point *F* expected utility is equal to actual utility. Any amount greater than *EF* would place the person at a lower point on her actual utility curve. Actual utility would then be less than the expected utility of not buying insurance. The amount above the pure premium, which is equal to the distance *EF,* is smaller than at another part of the graph, for example, *CD.* At point *C* a person is willing to pay an additional amount equal to *CD,* which would make the actual utility level indicated by *D* equal to the expected level indicated by *C. CD* is greater than *EF* because the probability of the loss's occurring is larger at point *E.* As the loss becomes almost certain to occur, the person can save for the event instead of paying the same amount (equal to the pure premium) to an insurance company *plus* an additional amount to cover other insurance company costs. In the case of near-certain events, such as annual medical or dental checkups (probabilities approximately 1.0), it would be cheaper to self-insure. At large probabilities and at very small probabilities (very rare events) a person is willing to pay less over the pure premium than at other, more intermediate probabilities.

Another factor that influences how much over the pure premium the person is willing to pay for insurance is the magnitude of the expected loss. When the expected loss is relatively large, as shown in Figure 6.3B, a person can lose W_3-W_1 ($8,000) if the illness occurs and they do not have insurance. If, on the other hand, the loss is relatively small, as for a visit to the dentist for a filling, this loss will be represented by a smaller possible loss in wealth if it occurs, W_3-W_5. The expected utility line for the large loss is *AC;* for the small loss it is *AB.* The distances W_3-W_1 (expected utility line *AC*) and W_3-W_5 (expected utility line *AB*) represent different-size losses with the same probabilities of occurrence. The area between the actual utility curve and the expected utility line is much greater for the large loss than for the small one. Given the same probability that either the large or the small loss will occur, a person is willing to pay a larger amount above the pure premium for the large loss than for the small one.

To determine the demand for health insurance, we must now combine the preceding discussion of risk aversion (the total utility curve of the individual that increases but at a decreasing rate), the probability that a loss will occur, the magnitude of that loss if it should occur, and information on the price of insurance—that is, the amount charged above the pure premium. To illustrate the price–quantity relationship of the demand for health insurance, reference is made to Figure 6.4.

The price of insurance along the vertical axis in Figure 6.4 is the amount *above* the pure premium (the loading charge) that the person must pay for insurance; along the horizontal axis is the probability that the event will occur. The curved line starting at 0 probability of the event's occurring and ending at a probability of 1.0 (certainty) is the amount above the pure premium that the person is willing to pay for insurance. This area is taken from the previous figures and is merely the distance between the actual utility curve and the expected utility line. Since insurance is never sold at a price just equaling the pure premium (included are costs for marketing, administration, and claims processing), the price of insurance is represented by line *AA* in Figure 6.4. The reason it increases

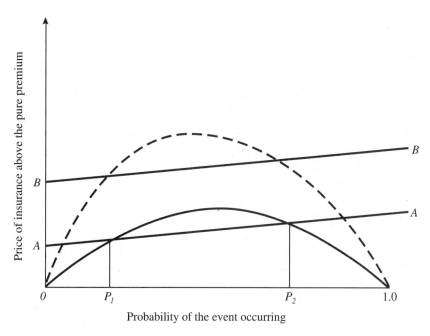

FIGURE 6.4 • The relationship between price of insurance and quantity demanded.

as the probability of the event's occurring increases is that there are greater administrative costs, such as record keeping and verification, when claims are more frequent (have a higher probability of occurring). Since line *AA* intersects the solid curved line representing the amount above the pure premium the person is willing to pay for insurance, the person will buy insurance for events that fall between P_1 and P_2. Between those two points the price the person has to pay for insurance is *less* than the amount he would be willing to pay, meaning that he would be better off (at a higher level of utility) if the insurance were purchased.

The price of insurance is *greater* than the amount she is willing to pay for events that have either a very small probability of occurring (the area $0–P_1$) or a very high probability of occurring (to the right of P_2). Based on Figure 6.4, we would predict that illnesses having both a very small probability of occurrence as well as those that have a high probability of occurrence (i.e., routine care) would be unlikely to be insured against by individuals. If required to purchase insurance for these two events, an individual would be worse off, since the marginal benefits to be derived from that coverage would be smaller than the marginal costs (price) of insurance!

If the price of insurance were to rise to line *BB,* we would expect the individual represented by the solid curved line to self-insure—that is, to demand *less* insurance coverage. With a higher price of insurance, the new price will now *exceed* the additional amount above the pure premium the individual is willing to pay. Regardless of the probability of the event's occurrence, the individual would be worse off if more had to be paid for insurance than he was willing to pay. Only if the magnitude of the loss, as shown by the dashed curved line, were greater than price line *BB* would the individual purchase insurance for that probable loss. Thus, as the price of insurance rises, the individual will be less likely to insure for certain events. This inverse relationship between the price of insurance and the quantity of insurance demanded is the demand schedule for insurance.

A person is also more likely to insure against events that have a greater magnitude of loss than against events with smaller possible losses. This aspect of the demand for health insurance can be seen with reference to the price of insurance (*BB*) in Figure 6.4 and the two curved lines representing different possible losses. Referring back to Figure 6.3, we saw that the amount above the pure premium that a person was willing to pay was less for small losses than for large losses, given the same probability of the event's occurring. One interesting implication of this relationship between the price of insurance and the size of the loss is that as the cost of medical care has risen, so has the size of the probable loss, and this by itself has resulted in an increase (a shift) in the demand for health insurance.

In summarizing this theory of the demand for health insurance, attention should be drawn to two areas: (a) the factors that affect the demand for health insurance, and (b) the welfare implications (is the person better or worse off?) of requiring an individual to purchase health insurance against all types of medical illness, the routine as well as the low-cost services. The following factors would affect the demand for health insurance:

1. *How risk-averse is the individual.* If she has a utility curve that is increasing but at a decreasing rate (i.e., diminishing marginal utility with respect to increased income), the individual is willing to pay an amount above the pure premium for insurance coverage. (Risk-averse people have a greater demand for insurance.)

2. *The probability of the event occurring.* As shown in Figure 6.3, for those events that have a very low or a very high probability of occurring, a person is willing to pay less above the pure premium than for events that have a more intermediate probability of occurring. (The demand for health insurance is lower when the probabilities of the event occurring are either very high or very low.)

3. *The magnitude of the loss.* The larger the magnitude of the loss, as in Figure 6.3, the greater will be the amount above the pure premium that the individual is willing to pay for insurance. (The demand for insurance will be greater, the greater the size of the loss.)

4. *The price of insurance.* (Also known as the loading charge). The higher the price of insurance (the amount above the pure premium), the individual will insure against fewer events. (The higher the price the lower will be the quantity of insurance demanded.)

5. *The income of the individual.* The size of a person's income and wealth will affect the amount above the pure premium she is willing to pay for health insurance. At both low and high incomes the marginal utility of income is either relatively high or low,

so that such persons might prefer to self-insure (3); the distance between the expected and actual utility curve is less at both high and low incomes than for intermediate income levels.

Low-income persons, in addition to being unwilling to spend much above the pure premium for insurance, also have available a low-price substitute if they become ill— Medicaid. However, those with high incomes have an incentive to purchase employer-paid health insurance because it is a fringe benefit and is not considered to be taxable income. The tax treatment of health insurance is discussed below.

The demand for health insurance is affected by the tax treatment of health insurance premiums. This tax subsidy for the purchase of health insurance lowers the price of insurance to those with high income. As incomes increase and people move into higher tax brackets, there is greater incentive for them to demand fringe benefits from their employers rather than increases in their cash incomes. Health insurance premiums paid by the employer are excluded from the taxable income of the employee (not just federal taxes, but state and Social Security taxes as well).

The favorable tax treatment of health insurance as an employer-paid fringe benefit lowers its price and has led to a much greater demand for insurance than would have otherwise occurred. (See Appendix 2 for a graphical illustration of this issue.) It has been estimated that in 1994 this tax incentive for the purchase of health insurance resulted in a loss in federal government revenues (excluding lost state income taxes) of approximately $74 billion a year. The tax treatment of health insurance coverage is, in effect, a subsidy for the purchase of health insurance and is greater for persons in higher income tax brackets.

For example, a person in a 33 percent marginal tax bracket can purchase insurance, as an employee fringe benefit, at less than its pure premium. If the insurance policy's loading charge is approximately 10 percent, a person in a 33 percent tax bracket would be willing to purchase insurance with before-tax dollars since the tax subsidy exceeds the price (loading charge) of the insurance. (The price elasticity of demand for health insurance has been estimated to be between −0.2 and −1.0 [4].) Thus an important reason for the increasing comprehensiveness of health insurance coverage for small claims ("first-dollar coverage") is that the premium for such losses is *less* than the actuarial value of such losses as the individual moves into higher and higher tax brackets. This government tax policy has stimulated the demand for health insurance and has increased its comprehensiveness.

Marginal tax brackets have been declining over time. The highest tax bracket has decreased from 87 percent in 1963 to 70 percent in 1980 to 39 percent currently. This decline in marginal tax brackets has increased the effective price of health insurance and is likely to lead to a decline in its comprehensiveness.

Previously, cost-based reimbursement and the use of service benefit policies removed any incentives that may have existed either for the patient to shop around or for the provider to provide care more efficiently. These policies increased the magnitude of a medical loss and thereby increased the demand for health insurance. If the provider's costs are reimbursed in full, regardless of what other hospitals may charge, and if the patient is not required to pay any portion of the hospital's bill, as is the case under a service benefit policy, then any incentives for cost constraint on either the demander or the supplier have been removed. This method of provider reimbursement, preferred by hospitals and accepted by Blue Cross, increased hospital costs, increased the magnitude of the probable loss due to a hospital episode, and thereby resulted in a further *increase* in the demand for protection against such large losses.

An important factor that affects the price of insurance (loading charge) is whether the individual is part of a large employee group. Group policies are sold at substantially lower prices. In part, the reduced price reflects lower administrative costs per individual; some of the administrative and claims processing costs are handled by the group itself and there are lower marketing costs. (Another reason for lower prices to group members, discussed below, is that there is less likelihood of adverse selection. Individuals seeking to purchase health insurance may be doing so because they expect to use such coverage in the near future. To guard against such self-selection and the possibly higher risks associated with it, the price of the policy will be higher to an individual than to a person who is a member of a group, which he joined so as to have a job rather than because he was ill and wanted insurance.) The higher price of insurance (the loading charge) to persons who are not part of a group leads to a smaller demand for health insurance.

Whether a group is self-insured or purchases insurance from an insurance company will affect the expected loss, hence the insurance premium, and consequently, the demand for insurance. In the past ten to fifteen years, states have enacted many state mandates. All insurance companies are required to include in their insurance policies their respective state mandates. There are more than 750 state mandates in all the states. These mandates are generally of three types: coverage for specific medical conditions, such as substance abuse, in vitro fertilization, and hair transplants (Minnesota); the services of specific health providers, such as chiropractors; and inclusion of certain population groups, such as newborns and the handicapped.

Any employer that becomes self-insured is exempt from state regulation, including state mandates and state health insurance premium taxes, according to the 1974 federal Employee Retirement and Security Act (ERISA). These cost savings are significant and are an important reason why many large firms have decided to become self-insured (5). It is believed that many small businesses would offer health benefits to their employees if state mandates were eliminated.

One additional factor affecting the price and demand for health insurance is technology (6). The growth in medical technology over the past several decades has made it possible to treat certain diseases that were previously untreatable. These treatment costs, however, are quite large; for example, organ replacements and medical care of low birthweight babies cost hundreds of thousands of dollars. Once a treatment for a previously untreatable condition becomes available, there is an increased probability that an individual may require such a treatment. Further, the magnitude of the loss is increased. Both of these factors, the probability of a loss and its magnitude, should cause an increase in the demand for health insurance.

It has been said that there are three stages of technology development. The first is "nontechnology," in which hospital and medical care offers little hope of recovery or improvement from the disease; thus treatment costs are low. The second is "halfway technology," which treats the disease once it has been incurred, for example, organ transplants or surgery for cancer patients. Halfway technology is typically very expensive. The third stage is "high technology." This stage is characterized by an understanding of the disease process, thereby making it possible to prevent the onset of the disease. An example of technology in this stage is immunizations. Technology is relatively inexpensive in this stage.

In the past three decades the medical sector has been characterized by the development of halfway technologies for many diseases. These technological developments, by raising the probable loss of a medical event, have increased the demand for health insurance.

As health insurance has covered new technology, it has stimulated the demand for insurance while at the same time raising the price of insurance, thereby decreasing the quantity of insurance demanded. Health insurance provides for treatment of an illness with whatever technology is currently available as contrasted with providing only the state of technology available at the time the contract was written. The demand for health insurance is increased when the latest (nonexperimental) technology is covered, since the probable loss is increased if halfway technology becomes available to cover a previously untreatable illness. The insurance premium, however, is also increased since the new technology is costly. "In the long run, the price of private health insurance depends upon the state of technology" (7). As the premium increases, the quantity demanded decreases, leading to a larger number of uninsured.

In addition to which state of technology is covered, the method used by the insurer to pay for the new technologies has further increased the price of insurance. Previous retrospective cost-based payment to hospitals (and no out-of-pocket payment by patients) eliminated provider efficiency incentives while providing an incentive to the patient and physician to perform the service as long as there was some positive marginal benefit, even though the marginal benefit was less than the resource costs of providing the treatment. Thus the insurance system encouraged the development of halfway technologies while increasing the cost of insurance.

There is a circular process to the demand for health insurance and the development of technology. While technology has increased the demand for insurance, insurance has stimulated the growth of technology. The investment in technology depends on its profitability, which is related to the potential size of its market, whether insurance (either private or government) will pay for it, and the cost of developing the technology. Since the demand for technology is derived from the demand for hospital and physician services, the method of provider payment affects the demand for technologies. The change in hospital payment to fixed prices per admission, selective contracting among hospitals, and the development of capitation-based systems (whereby medical providers receive a fixed payment per enrollee regardless of the quantity of medical services delivered), is changing the demand for new technologies. The emphasis is on cost reducing rather than just quality-enhancing technology. A substitution in the type of halfway technology being demanded is also occurring, from caring for the patient in a hospital to being able to provide the treatment in an outpatient setting and in the patient's home.

The circular relationship between technology and insurance ultimately affects investment in technology, the type of technology developed, the demand for insurance, the cost of that insurance, and the rise in medical expenditures.

The demand for health insurance is thus affected by economic variables, price and income, the tastes of the individual for risk aversion, and the size of the probable loss.

It is interesting to speculate on the welfare implications of this theory of demand for insurance. In attempting to maximize their utility, consumers will allocate their income so that the marginal benefit from each of the goods and services they consume equals the prices they must pay for those goods and services. If the price (which represents the marginal cost of producing those goods and services) exceeds the marginal benefits to them, they will be worse off by purchasing those goods and services. They can increase their utility by cutting back on those goods and services for which the marginal benefit is less than the price that must be paid and using the funds saved to purchase other goods and services whose marginal benefits (per dollar) are greater. In this manner they will achieve a higher level of utility than by any other allocation process. If, however, consumers are *forced* to purchase a good whose price is greater than its marginal benefit, they clearly end up worse off than before. Forcing consumers to pay a price for a good that is higher than its marginal benefit is a situation that can occur in the health field if all consumers are required to have complete comprehensive insurance coverage against all of their medical expenses.

As shown in Figure 6.4, there are two situations in which the price of insurance will exceed the amount above the pure premium that the consumer is willing to pay. The first is for medical losses that have either a very high or a very low probability of occurring. In Figure 6.4, the area to the right of P_2 represents medical losses that have a high probability of occurring; these routine medical expenses are for such purchases as physician office visits, a dental visit, and over-the-counter drugs. Comprehensive insurance coverage to include such routine medical expenses would necessitate a price, perhaps in the form of a tax on consumers, that would have to exceed what they would be willing to pay above the actuarial value of those losses; requiring consumers to pay that price by law clearly leaves them worse off than if they could self-insure for those losses.

A second situation in which a consumer is made worse off by being required to purchase complete insurance coverage is where there are small medical losses. The price of insurance for that coverage (line *BB*) is greater than the amount above the pure premium (the solid curved line) the consumer would be willing to pay.

It might be argued that since the price of insurance is less than the aggregate amount consumers would be willing to pay in all situations, requiring insurance coverage for even those medical expenses that they would prefer not to insure against would, on an aggregate basis, still leave them better off with insurance than without. However, as long as the different forms of coverage are divisible and do not have to be sold together, consumers would be better off with *some* coverage than with either complete coverage or none at all.

The welfare implication of mandatory insurance coverage that covers all medical losses, no matter how small or routine and expected they may be, is that some consumers will be worse off than if they had a choice and could self-insure in those situations.

AN APPLICATION OF THE THEORY OF THE DEMAND FOR HEALTH INSURANCE

The theory of the demand for health insurance can now be used to explain why we observe some people insuring against certain types of medical loss (e.g., hospital care) and not others (e.g., dental care). (When we later introduce the concept of moral hazard, we will see that although people may buy insurance for hospital services, they still may not insure against all hospital expenses, preferring to bear some of the costs themselves.) Also, since not everyone is a "risk averter" (their expected utility curve may be equal to or greater than their actual utility curve with respect to wealth), we would expect some people not to buy *any* health insurance. They would do so, not out of ignorance or irrationality, but because they are not risk averters (i.e., for the same reason that some people gamble).

Before the price of health insurance was greatly reduced as a result of being widely available as a fringe benefit, a sizable percentage of the uninsured, 37 percent, according to a survey conducted in the mid-1950s, indicated that they felt they were just as well off without health insurance (8). The potential market for health insurance at that time was less than 100 percent of the population. As the price of medical care increased over time (i.e., the size of the potential medical loss became larger), and as personal income also increased, the demand for health insurance also grew. More recently, only about 10 percent of the uninsured believe they are just as well off without health insurance.

To determine how well the foregoing model of demand for health insurance predicts the type of health insurance found in the population, we examine the purchase of insurance coverage by type of medical expense. Costs for hospitalization and for surgery would seem far more likely to qualify as high expected losses, with a relatively low probability of occurrence, than would medical losses such as physician office visits, optometric services, drugs, and dental care, all of which involve relatively smaller medical expenses and are considered by families to be more routine and budgetable.

In examining older rather than more recent data (before the sizable effect on demand of the tax subsidy for health insurance), we find that the economic theory of demand for health insurance is able to explain the type of health insurance observed in the population quite well. Using data from a 1957–58 household survey of the U.S. population, medical expenses by type of service were classified according to whether they had a high or a low probability of occurring and whether they had a high or a low potential loss if they did occur. Low probability of occurrence was arbitrarily defined by whether 20 percent of the population incurred an expense for that medical service during the past year; high potential loss was also arbitrarily defined by whether the average cost incurred by persons using that medical service was greater than $40. These data are shown in Table 6.1, together with the actual percentage of expenditures covered by insurance for each of the medical services examined.

According to the data, the prevalence of insurance was generally consistent with what the economic theory of demand for health insurance would lead us to expect. Those medical services that have a low probability of occurrence and a high expected loss are more likely to be covered by insurance than are those expenses with either a high or a low probability of occurrence and low expected loss.

The costs of a medical event have greatly increased over time, leading to an increase in the demand for insurance. Also contributing to an increase in demand was the growth in incomes and the rise in inflation throughout the 1960s and 1970s. As incomes and inflation increased, more employees preferred to receive additional income in the form of health insurance, which was not subject to personal income taxes. Thus, although the

TABLE 6.1 Classification of Medical Services by Probability of Occurrence, Potential Loss, and Insurance Benefits, 1957–58

Type of Medical Service	Probability of Occurrence	Magnitude of Expense	Percent of Expenditures Covered by Insurance	Expenditures on This Type of Service as a Percent of Total Medical Expenditures
Hospital care	Low	High	58	23
Physician charges for:				
Surgery	Low	High	48	7
In-hospital visits	Low	High		
Office visits	High	Low	7	24
House calls	High	Low		
Drugs and medicines	High	Low	1	20
Other medical services	Low	Low	1	8
Dental care	High	Low	—[a]	15

Sources: R. G. Rice, "Some Health Insurance Implications of the Economics of Uncertainty," unpublished paper presented before The American Public Health Association, October 6, 1964. Columns 1 and 2 based on data published in O. W. Anderson, P. Collete, and J. J. Feldman, *Changes in Family Medical Care Expenditures and Voluntary Health Insurance: A Five Year Resurvey* (Cambridge, Mass.: Harvard University Press, 1963).
[a]Less than one-half of 1 percent.

percentage of medical expenditures covered by insurance has greatly increased since the period covered by the data cited above, we would still expect to observe a difference in the distribution of medical expenses covered by health insurance. Those medical services having a lower probability of occurrence and a high potential loss are still more likely to have more of their expenses covered by insurance than are those services considered to be routine and/or with a relatively lower potential loss. The same relationship holds for more recent data as well.

Aggregate data for 1994 support the finding that where the probability of use is low and the expected cost is high, the percent of the bill paid for by insurance is highest. Consumer out-of-pocket expenditures for short-term hospital care are approximately 3 percent of total hospital expenditures, with the remainder being paid for by private insurance and government programs. For physician services, approximately 19 percent of total expenditures are out-of-pocket; the out-of-pocket percentage is 49 percent for dental care, 59 percent for eyeglasses (and other medical durables), and 62 percent for drugs (9).

In summary, the model of demand for health insurance suggests that a measure of the adequacy of health insurance should *not* be the percentage of aggregate medical expenses covered by health insurance, with anything less than 100 percent being considered inadequate. Instead, the adequacy of health coverage should be examined separately for each type of medical service. Even if everyone were a risk averter, we would not expect people to buy insurance for all of their medical expenses. The price of insurance (i.e., the amount above the pure premium) for some medical expenses would exceed the amount some people would be willing to pay. Requiring everyone under such circumstances to purchase health insurance for *all* of their medical expenses would make people *worse off,* since the costs of the coverage for some expenses would exceed the benefits.

BIASED SELECTION IN HEALTH CARE MARKETS

Adverse Selection

The earlier discussion of demand for health insurance assumed that the insured population belonged to the same risk group, that is, that they all had the same probability of incurring an illness. The pure premium was based on the average expected loss of that group. An individual, however, is more knowledgeable about her own health status than is the insurance company. High-risk individuals therefore have an incentive to purchase insurance at a premium that is based on a lower-risk group. The insurance company's concern that this difference in information will lead to high-risk individuals purchasing insurance based on a lower-risk group's premium is referred to as "adverse selection."

Insurance companies realize that population groups have differing levels of risk. However, if the insurance company is unable to distinguish between high and low risks, the insurance premium will reflect the average risk of the two groups. In this situation, the high-risk group will purchase insurance since a premium based on the average risk of the two groups is still lower than a premium based solely on their own risk group. Low-risk individuals may not purchase insurance since a premium based on the average of the two risk groups would be greater than their own risk-based premium. Adverse selection would result in a biased sample of those who purchase health insurance; predominately more higher-risk individuals would purchase insurance at a premium that is based on a lower-risk group. (Insurers' concern with adverse selection would also occur if they were unable, because of legal prohibitions, to use certain risk factors for determining a premium.)

When adverse selection occurs, the insurance company loses money. To remain in business, the insurance company must raise its premium to reflect the proportionately greater number of high-risk individuals. As the premium is increased, more low-risk individuals drop out. To prevent their losing the less risky subscribers, insurance companies are reluctant to raise their premiums without also imposing restrictions on use at the higher premium (10).

The above discussion is illustrated in Figure 6.5. Assume the following: both high- and low-risk individuals have the same relationship between total utility and wealth; they each have $10,000; and if an illness occurs, the loss is $8,000. Low-risk individuals have only a 0.2 probability of incurring an illness, while high-risk individuals have a 0.8 probability. It is further assumed that there are an equal number of low- and high-risk individuals.

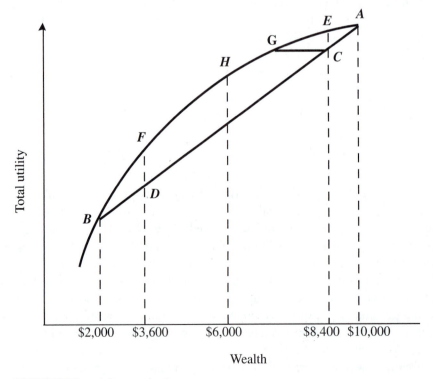

FIGURE 6.5 • Adverse selection.

The pure premium for the low-risk group is $1,600 ($8,000 multiplied by 0.2) and a resulting wealth position of $8,400. For high-risk individuals the pure premium would be $6,400 ($8,000 multiplied by 0.8) and a resulting wealth position of $3,600.

The straight line *AB* shows the expected utility of an $8,000 loss occurring at different probabilities. If health insurance were sold at the pure premium to each risk group, both risk groups would be willing to purchase insurance. The low-risk individual would be at a higher utility level, *E,* which is greater than the expected utility, *C.* The low-risk individual would also be willing to pay distance *CG* in excess of the pure premium. (High-risk individuals would also be willing to purchase insurance sold at the pure premium since their actual utility, *F,* is above their expected utility, *D.*)

If the insurance company cannot distinguish between high- and low-risk individuals, the pure premium will be based on the average risk of the two populations. The pure premium for everyone would then be $4,000 ($8,000 multiplied by 0.5). High-risk individuals would purchase the insurance because they would be at a higher utility level, *H* instead of *F.* Low-risk individuals, however, would not buy insurance since their utility level with insurance, *H,* would be lower than *G,* which is the maximum amount above the pure premium they would be willing to pay.

The approaches used by insurance companies to protect themselves against adverse selection attempt to redress the information imbalance. Excluding from insurance coverage (up to one year) for preexisting conditions, which the individual may be aware of but not the insurance company is one such approach. Similarly, the insurance company may require the individual to have tests performed so as to have the same information as the individual. Insurers may require a minimum period before certain services are covered (e.g., ten months for obstetrics care). Low-risk individuals may "signal" (i.e., provide information on their risk status) by their willingness to accept insurance policies that contain high deductibles and co-insurance.

Preferred Risk Selection

"Preferred risk selection" occurs when insurers receive the same premium for everyone within a group but the risks within that group vary. The insurer then tries to select the low-risk individuals while receiving a premium that is based on the average risk of the group. Preferred risk selection is caused by a difference in the premium and the risk level of the individual. As shown in Figure 6.5, the average premium received by an insurer would be $4,000, which would cover both low- and high-risk members of that group. The insurer, however, would be able to increase their profits if they could receive that average premium and attract just the low-risk members of that group.

Approaches used by insurers to attract low-risk individuals include offering benefits, such as well baby services and sports medicine clinics, that low-risk individuals would find appealing, while deemphasizing services, such as having a cancer center, cardiac care specialists, and transplant services, which would be attractive to high-risk individuals.

Those aged eligible to participate in Medicare are able to voluntarily join an HMO.

The HMO receives a premium for the aged based on their age and sex, within a geographic area. That premium is based on 95 percent of what those aged would have cost the government had they remained in the traditional Medicare program. Since the premium is based on the average medical expenditures of the aged within that risk group, the HMO has an incentive to select the healthier aged within each risk group. In recruiting aged to join their HMO, the HMOs do not enroll the aged by mail, for fear that the bedridden might join up. Instead the aged are invited to meetings. Also the aged are permitted to leave the HMO with thirty days' notification. Thus it has been alleged that some HMO physicians will inform enrollees who require expensive surgery that the HMO can perform it, but if they were to disenroll, they could be cared for at the university hospital, which has better specialists and facilities.

Studies have been conducted to determine whether the government saves money when they pay HMOs 95 percent of the average cost for the aged enrolling in an HMO. These studies indicate that the government still loses 6 percent; in other words, if the aged who enrolled in HMOs remained in the traditional Medicare program, the government would have spent 11 percent less on those aged (11). Thus the HMOs enrolling the aged are, on average, receiving a preferred risk group. The risk adjustment factors used by the government account for only about half of the risk selection of new Medicare HMO enrollees. Over time their medical costs rise the longer they remain enrolled in the HMO.

The importance of preferred risk selection to an insurer can be seen by the data presented in Table 6.2. One percent of the population incurs 30 percent of total medical expenditures (as of 1987). The top 5 percent of the population incurs 58 percent of total medical expenditures and 10 percent of the population incurs 72 percent of total expenditures. If an insurer were able to enroll the remaining 90 percent, while receiving a premium based on the average, it would make a great deal of money. The problem of preferred risk selection is important for Medicare because 48 percent of those in the top 1 percent of those with the highest expenditures are over age 65 (12). (The increase over time in medical expenditures for those in the highest expenditure categories are likely due to the development and availability of new medical technologies.)

Concluding Comments on Risk Selection

Adverse selection would be limited if all individuals were required to have health insurance. Individuals would then have no need to join a health plan only when they became ill. Adverse selection could still be a problem at open enrollment time when an individual who becomes ill and who is in a less comprehensive, more restrictive health plan decides to switch to a more comprehensive, less restrictive plan. The more comprehensive plan would receive an adverse risk group. This problem is somewhat mitigated by the fact that the individual who wants to switch can only do so once a year and then must wait several months before enrollment in the new plan.

TABLE 6.2 Distribution of Health Expenditures for the U.S. Population, by Magnitude of Expenditures, Selected Years, 1928–87

Percent of U.S. Population Ranked by Expenditures	1928	1963	1970	1977	1980	1987
Top 1 percent	—	17%	26%	27%	29%	30%
Top 2 percent	—	—	35	38	39	41
Top 5 percent	52%	43	50	55	55	58
Top 10 percent	—	59	66	70	70	72
Top 30 percent	93	—	88	90	90	91
Top 50 percent	—	95	96	97	96	97
Bottom 50 percent	—	5	4	3	4	3

Sources: Data for 1928 are from I. S. Falk, M. C. Klem, and N. Sinai, *The Incidence of Illness and Receipt of Medical Care among Representative Families* (Chicago: University of Chicago Press, 1933); data for 1963 are from R. Andersen, J. Lion, and O. W. Anderson, *Two Decades of Health Service: Social Survey Trends in Use and Expenditures* (Cambridge, Mass.: Ballinger, 1976). Data for 1970 are from National Center for Health Services Research tabulations of the 1970 CHAS/NORC survey; for 1977, from the 1977 National Medical Care Expenditure Survey (NMCES); for 1980, from the 1980 National Medical Care Utilization and Expenditures Survey (NMCUES); and for 1987, from the 1987 National Medical Expenditure Survey (NMES).
Adapted from: M. L. Berk and A. C. Monheit, "The Concentration of Health Expenditures: An Update," *Health Affairs*, 11(4), Winter 1992: 145–149.

Health insurers have competed on their ability to select low-risk groups. An insurer may therefore be more profitable, not because it is more efficient, but because it is better at attracting a preferred risk group. To limit preferred risk selection, each group should have a risk-adjusted premium. In this way, insurers would no longer have an incentive to select low-risk groups; each risk group would have a premium that reflects their risk. Instead, insurers would have to compete on price (premium) for each risk group. The more efficient insurers would then be those who are better able to manage risk. Accurate, risk-adjusted premiums would change the nature of insurance competition from risk selection to risk management. Unfortunately, developing risk-adjusted premiums under the Medicare program has not yet met with much success. A great deal of research is devoted to developing better risk adjusters for the aged besides age and sex. (Biased selection is further discussed in Chapters 8 and 12.)

THE DEMAND FOR HEALTH INSURANCE UNDER CONDITIONS OF MORAL HAZARD

The previous discussion demonstrated that even when the demand for medical care is assumed to be completely price inelastic, people would still not demand completely comprehensive health insurance because of selling and transaction costs (loading charge). In this section the concept of moral hazard is introduced to show that its existence also results in a demand for health insurance coverage that is less than 100 percent of a person's medical expenses (13).

If demand for medical care were inelastic with respect to price, the individual's demand curve in the event of illness would look like D_1 in Figure 6.6; that is, the individual would demand Q_1 units of medical care. In the case of moral hazard, it is possible for the patient to affect the size of his loss; therefore, there is some price elasticity to the individual's demand curve. Thus, if an individual became ill, the quantity of medical care that he would demand would depend, in part, on the price that had to be paid for that care. If insurance covered the entire cost of the illness episode, the individual represented by demand curve D_2 would demand Q_2 units of medical care. The presence of some elasticity in the individual's demand curve indicates that the individual will demand different quantities of medical care depending on how much must be paid for that care. Since insurance lowers the price of medical care to individuals, they will consume more care than if they had to pay the entire price themselves. It is this behavior of individuals that is termed "moral hazard."

To the individual consuming medical care under these circumstances, it is perfectly rational behavior—he is equating the marginal cost of purchasing that care with the marginal benefit of additional units. Since the marginal benefit of additional units of medical care decreases as the quantity of medical care consumed increases, the individual will continue to consume additional units as long as the marginal benefit of those additional units exceeds their additional cost. Insurance coverage that reduces the price of care to zero under these circumstances results in an inefficient use of medical resources. Since the individual with insurance consumes medical care until the marginal benefits and marginal costs of the last units are equal, this will be at a point where the "true" marginal costs (the costs of *producing* those units) are greater than the marginal benefits. "Too much" medical care will be consumed, and the value of those additional units will be less than the costs of their production. This is illustrated in Figure 6.6 at the point where Q_2 units of medical care are consumed by an individual with 100 percent insurance coverage, with the costs of producing each unit indicated by the supply curve (S).

Another implication of the existence of moral hazard is that although individuals with insurance will consume Q_2 units of medical care if they become ill, they may be unwilling to purchase an insurance policy that provides such extensive coverage. As both consumers of medical care and purchasers of insurance, individuals are expected to consider the price involved in both cases: as consumers of medical services, greater utilization resulting from having insurance will result in their having to pay a higher premium for it. Instead of paying that higher premium, an individual may well prefer to self-insure or to purchase a less comprehensive insurance policy. For example, with reference to Figure 6.6, assume that an individual has both a 0.5 probability of not incurring any medical illness during the year, in which case her demand for medical care would be zero units, and a 0.5 probability of requiring medical care for an illness during that year. If the individ-

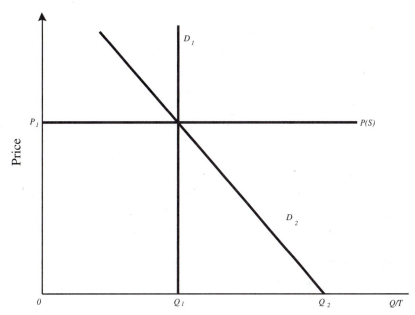

FIGURE 6.6 • The demand for medical care under conditions of moral hazard.

ual required medical care, with a corresponding demand curve of D_1, the individual would consume Q_1 units (which represents 100 units) at a cost of $10 per unit. The pure premium in this situation would be 0.5(0) + 0.5($1,000) = $500 per year. If, however, the individual's demand curve were D_2 (where Q_2 represents 200 units of medical care), the pure premium under these circumstances would be 0.5(0) + 0.5($2,000) = $1,000 per year.

These differences in premiums resulting from the price elasticity of the demand curve may be great enough for some individuals to prefer self-insurance, in which case the expected loss to them would be $500 per year [0.5(0) + 0.5($1,000)]. They would consume Q_1 units of medical care if they became ill because, even though their demand curve may be represented by D_2, they would have to pay P_1 dollars per unit (which is the intersection of D_2 and S) and would consequently consume Q_1 units of care.

Individuals differ in their demands for medical care. If Figure 6.6 represents different demands for medical care, and one individual's demand is D_1 while the average demand among the rest of the population is D_2, then a premium for comprehensive insurance to the individual represented by demand curve D_1 would be based on a utilization level indicated by Q_2, multiplied by a price of P_1. Under these circumstances an individual may well prefer self-insurance, which would mean a 0.5 probability (as in the previous case) of being ill and, if so, paying a price P_1 multiplied by Q_1 units of medical care. In both examples, *requiring* the individual to purchase comprehensive insurance that is the same as that which is purchased by the rest of the population will make the individual worse off (the marginal costs of the premium for the comprehensive coverage will exceed the marginal benefits of that insurance).

As a result of the effect of moral hazard on the use of medical care, several approaches have been used to limit utilization. One approach, which was not successful, was to rely on internal hospital utilization review committees. As long as hospitals were reimbursed for their costs, physicians were paid separately by Blue Shield, and the patient was not responsible for any part of the bill (under a service benefit policy), none of the participants had an incentive to use the utilization review committee to impose a cost on any of the other participants.

Two other approaches which have been more successful are to introduce incentives on the part of either the physician or the patient. Under managed care systems, such as health maintenance organizations, the physician is likely to have an incentive (e.g., bonuses at the end of the year) if the organization's expenditures are less than their premium income. Other managed care systems use utilization review; the utilization review organization is separate from the providers being reviewed and failure to follow the utilization review guidelines results in financial penalties to either the patients or their physicians.

Another incentive approach for reducing utilization occurs when deductibles and co-insurance are included as part of the health insurance package. Some persons, when purchasing insurance, might prefer intermediate choices between the extremes of comprehensive coverage or self-insurance. Deductibles and co-insurance enable consumers to bear some of the risk themselves and pay a smaller premium than if all their medical costs were covered by insurance.

In Figure 6.7A, the pure premium for comprehensive insurance would be represented by utilization level Q_2, multiplied by price P_1 (multiplied by the probability of 0.5). The cost of self-insurance would be P_1 multiplied by Q_1 (0.5). The cost of an insurance policy with a co-insurance feature that lowered the price to the patient from P_1 to P_2 would cost $P_1 - P_2$ multiplied by a utilization level of Q_3 (0.5). The pure premium for a policy with a co-insurance feature would be in between the premiums of the two other alternatives. The availability of co-insurance would make insurance more attractive to some people who would prefer no insurance if their only other choice were comprehensive insurance.

In his article on the economics of moral hazard, Pauly also discusses the use of deductibles to reduce the costs of insurance premiums. Using only deductibles results either in the consumption of the same amount of care as in the case of no insurance, or conversely, in consumption of the same amount of care as in the situation of complete insurance coverage. This effect of deductibles on utilization is illustrated in Figure 6.7B. Without insurance, the individual represented by demand curve D_1 would, in the event of illness, consume Q_1 units of medical care; with complete insurance coverage the same individual would consume Q_2 units of medical care. If a deductible were instituted for the individual with complete coverage, then before the insurance would pay the medical costs, the individual would have to use and pay for Q_3 units of medical care at a cost of

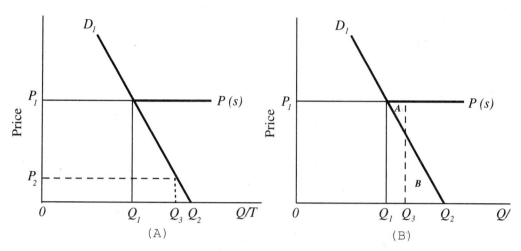

FIGURE 6.7 • The effect of (A) co-insurance and (B) deductibles on the demand for medical care.

P_1 times Q_3. After that amount had been paid, the price of additional care (assuming no co-insurance feature) would be zero and he would consume Q_2 units of care.

If the individual decides not to consume up to the deductible, which is P_1 times Q_3 units of medical care, she will merely act as though she has no insurance and use Q_1 units of care. Whether or not the individual will pay the deductible ($P_1 \times Q_3$) and then consume up to Q_2 units of medical care depends on whether the excess amount that must be paid for the deductible, area A in Figure 6.7, which is above the individual's demand curve, is less than the "consumer surplus," represented by area B. The consumer surplus is the area under the demand curve that consumers would be willing to spend, but do not have to, since it would be at no cost if they first bought Q_3 units of care. If area B exceeds area A, consumers will then pay the deductible and consume Q_2 units of medical care.

Just as the effect on utilization of the co-insurance feature will depend on the price elasticity of demand and the amount of the co-insurance, the effect the deductible has will also depend on its size and the price elasticity of demand. In our discussion of deductibles and co-insurance, differences in income have been ignored; it is obvious that any co-payment feature that is unrelated to income levels will have a more important effect on lower-income persons than on higher-income persons.

The existence of moral hazard thus has two effects. The price (premium) of health insurance is increased because utilization is increased when the consumer does not have to pay anything out of pocket (the moral hazard issue). Second, there is a decrease in the demand for health insurance when the insurance premium is increased, because of the previous increase in utilization. Although the existence of moral hazard results in "overuse" and a consequent increase in the premium while at renewal time the higher premium results in a lower quantity demanded of insurance, both of these behaviors are rational, given the consumer's demand curve for medical services and for insurance and the prices of each.

The conclusion to be drawn from the discussion of the demand for health insurance, whether moral hazard is assumed to exist or not, is that even if all individuals were risk averters, insurance coverage for 100 percent of all of their medical expenses should not be required for all persons. When there are transaction costs for administering claims, and when people have different demands for medical care, no single insurance policy is best for everyone. Some persons will prefer to have only some type of medical expense covered; because of the existence of moral hazard, others will prefer to have some cost-sharing features.

SUMMARY

The preceding discussion on the demand for health insurance offers an approach to answering the following questions: How much health insurance should the population have (i.e., what percent of total health expenditures should be covered by insurance), and what components of medical services should health insurance cover? The answers would indicate the degree to which the provision of health insurance in the population is economically efficient. Government intervention to increase or to change the type of health insurance in the population can then be evaluated in terms of whether such action moves the population closer to or further from what would be an optimal quantity and type of health insurance.[2]

To discuss the efficient amount and type of health insurance in the population, it is necessary to have criteria to evaluate what is efficient and what is inefficient in the purchase of health insurance. Assuming competition in the provision (supply) of health insurance, the price at which health insurance is sold will equal the marginal costs of providing it. In a competitive market, the suppliers will also respond to demands for different types of health insurance coverage and provide such coverage at a price that reflects the cost of producing it (these two assumptions are discussed in Chapter 8).

The condition for economic efficiency on the demand side is that consumers purchase the type of and quantity of health insurance coverage to the point where its price equals the marginal benefit to them from additional insurance coverage. Since the demand curve indicates the marginal benefit to be derived from the purchase of health insurance, if the cost of additional insurance exceeds its marginal benefit, consumers will be better off purchasing less coverage. When the quantity of health insurance demanded is equal to the cost of providing that insurance, the individual will purchase the appropriate quantity; that is, the conditions of economic efficiency are met. At that point, the marginal cost of producing health insurance equals the marginal benefit to the consumer of that additional coverage.

---

[2]This discussion assumes no redistribution of medical services; when national health insurance proposals are discussed later, this assumption will be changed. Another assumption, which will subsequently be discussed, is that there are no externalities in the provision of personal medical services. Since redistribution of medical care to low-income persons may in fact have external effects, the efficient distribution of health insurance coverage may necessitate a different amount and type of insurance to low-income groups.

The demand for health insurance was analyzed under two assumptions: first, that no moral hazard existed, in that the price of medical care did not affect its utilization or the quality of care demanded; and second, that moral hazard did exist, meaning that there is some price elasticity with respect to the demand for quantity and quality of medical care. In the first situation it was shown that individuals would *not* want to insure against all events. Insurance would be more likely for those medical services where the expected loss is greater and where the probability of the event's occurring is neither extremely high nor rare. Requiring insurance for all losses and all probabilities of their occurring, as well as for all individuals, would be economically inefficient; the cost of the insurance would exceed the marginal benefits to the consumer of additional coverage.

Based on this discussion, what percentage of the distribution of health expenditures should be covered by health insurance? The distribution of health expenditures is skewed, as shown in Figure 6.1: many people have relatively small expenditures; a smaller percentage of the population have larger expenditures. We would expect the large expenses with a low probability of occurrence to be covered by insurance, which suggests that the curve shown in Figure 6.1 should be modified. At a *minimum,* the tail of the distribution (relatively large expenditures for a small percentage of the families) should be covered by insurance, through major medical or catastrophic insurance, as shown in Figure 6.8. Further, since the administrative costs of handling small claims are likely to exceed the amount above the pure premium that people that are willing to pay for relatively routine, smaller expenses, a deductible might be included for such expenses, as represented by the shaded portion of the curve in Figure 6.8.[3]

When the demand for health insurance under conditions of moral hazard was discussed, it was shown that given the differences in preferences among people in their demands for medical care, it would be preferable to offer people more than an all-or-nothing choice. People might prefer some co-payment that would reduce the size of the medical expenses in the middle area of Figure 6.8. Insurance, in this instance, would cover less than 100 percent of medical expenditures (different components of the distribution of medical expenses would be covered at different percentages), and the premium for such insurance would be much lower than if it covered the entire distribution of medical expenses.

In discussing other factors affecting the demand for health insurance, the tax de-

---

[3]It has been claimed that deductibles and co-insurance provisions in health insurance will result in a decline in the demand for preventive services, which are lower-cost, more predictable medical services. Evidence of this alleged adverse effect is difficult to find. One can make the case that if preventive services have an effect on future medical demand, presumably insurance companies should be willing to subsidize the purchase of such services. Most, if not all, health insurance actually precludes such services from coverage. Similarly, HMOs and prepaid health plans have cut back on their use of preventive services, again presumably indicating that the costs of such services are greater than their potential savings. Thus, if co-payments actually reduce the demand for preventive care, it is not clear that increased demand for such services would have favorable cost/benefit ratios.

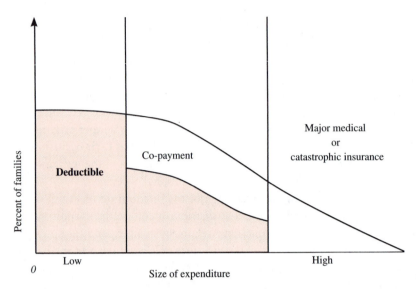

FIGURE 6.8 • The effect of health insurance on the expected distribution of medical expenses among families.

ductibility of premiums was mentioned; as incomes increase and people move into higher tax brackets, they have a greater incentive to purchase insurance against more, though smaller, medical expenses. The effect of the tax deductibility of health insurance premiums is a movement *away* from economic efficiency in the demand for health insurance. The "true" cost of health insurance has not been lowered, but its price to higher-income consumers has been. They will, therefore, be purchasing "too much" health insurance. The tax treatment of health insurance premiums has reduced the price of insurance against smaller, more predictable medical expenses to higher-income people to a point that may be *below* the actuarial value of those expenses. If the tax deductibility of health insurance premiums were no longer allowed, there would be less distortion in the purchase of health insurance, because the decision to purchase would more closely correspond to the cost of the insurance and the perceived marginal benefits to the consumer of that additional coverage. (The tax subsidy for the purchase of health insurance is discussed more technically in Appendix 2.)

An important question raised by the discussion of the demand for health insurance is which components of medical care should be covered by health insurance. When only one component of medical care, such as hospital services, is covered by insurance, the price of hospital care to the consumer relative to the prices of other forms of care has been distorted. The decision to use the different forms of care is based, in part, on the relative prices the patient must pay for such care. Inasmuch as these relative prices will not reflect the relative costs of care, moving toward greater economic efficiency in the use of medical care will require the patient to face prices proportional to the costs of such care. An example of insurance coverage that distorted the use of medical components by distorting the relative prices of medical care faced by the consumer was the Blue Cross service benefit policy. A service benefit policy provided very complete coverage for just hospital care, while it excluded nonhospital care; this led to an inefficient (more costly) form of treatment when services that could be performed on an outpatient basis were instead performed in a hospital. Competitive pressures have forced Blue Cross to provide coverage for nonhospital services.

Certain types of health insurance do not distort the relative prices faced by the patient when seeking care. One example is indemnity insurance, which reimburses the patient a fixed dollar amount or the same percentage co-insurance on all services. Patients and/or their physicians therefore have an incentive to minimize the cost of a medical treatment, and the relative prices of the different components of medical services are not artificially distorted.

A second approach is the use of capitation payments (by or on behalf of patients) to an organization to cover the cost of medical services. Under these arrangements, a decision maker, generally a physician, prescribes that combination of services so that the relative costs of different medical services used by the patient equals their relative marginal benefits. HMOs are organizational arrangements whereby the patient is covered by a capitation payment system.

Finally, the method of provider reimbursement affected economic efficiency in the demand for health insurance. The previous method of cost-based hospital reimbursement resulted in higher health care costs. These higher costs increased the size of the probable loss, thereby resulting in a greater demand for health insurance than if other, more efficiency-oriented payment mechanisms had been used.

An important reason for understanding the demand for medical care, as well as the demand for health insurance, is to be able to determine whether the quantity (and quality) of medical care consumed is optimal. The optimal rate of output of medical care will be achieved when the price of that care (which is presumed to equal the costs of producing that care under a competitive system) is equal to the marginal benefit of that care. As has been shown, the type of insurance coverage that existed (service benefit coverage) and the tax treatment of health insurance premiums are two reasons why prices in medical care to consumers have been (and still are) distorted, thereby resulting in consumption of a nonoptimal amount of medical care.

To determine whether the price of medical care to the patient reflects the minimum cost of producing that care, it is necessary to turn to an analysis of the supply side of the medical care market.

APPENDIX 1: THE ALLOCATIVE INEFFICIENCY OF BLUE CROSS' SERVICE BENEFIT POLICY

Blue Cross' service benefit policy provided complete coverage against hospital expenses, in a semiprivate room accommodation. A person with Blue Cross did not have to pay any of the charges for hospital care (up to a maximum number of days), but had to pay the full price for any other forms of medical services, such as outpatient services or nursing home care, used in the treatment of that illness. Blue Cross' service benefit policy caused an "overuse" of hospital care relative to other medical components used in treatment. The consequence was a cost of treatment that was higher than if other, less costly, but equally efficacious forms of care were used.

The foregoing conclusion is illustrated in Figure 6.9. Assume that treatment for a medical illness can be achieved with varying amounts of hospital and/or physician services. This substitutability in the use of components for treatment is shown by the indifference curves in Figure 6.9. The shape of the indifference curve indicates the degree of substitutability among components, and it depends on the particular illness and its seriousness. The budget constraint *AB* indicates the quantity of physician and hospital services that patients can purchase without insurance; if they spent all their funds on physician services, they could purchase *OA* units of physician services; if they spent all their funds on hospital care, they could purchase *OB* units of hospital care; or they could purchase some combination of the two. The slope of the budget constraint indicates the relative prices of physician and hospital services. With no insurance, a patient with a particular illness and with budget constraint *AB* will consume *OC* units of physician services and *OD* units of hospital care. If the patient had indemnity insurance that reimbursed a

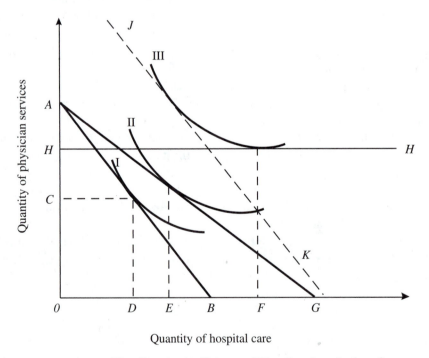

FIGURE 6.9 • The allocative inefficiency of Blue Cross' service benefit policy.

given amount of money for medical care, then if the patient became ill, the budget constraint would shift out parallel and become *JK*. With indemnity insurance the patient could purchase more medical care than previously. The slope of the new budget constraint would remain the same; the relative prices of the components used in treatment would not change but the patient could buy more of each, thereby moving to a higher indifference curve (III). The effect of indemnity insurance is similar to an increase in income when the patient is ill.

However, if the patient merely had hospitalization coverage with a co-insurance feature, the price of hospital care to the patient would be reduced, and the budget constraint would rotate to the right and become *AG*. The patient could now purchase more hospital care. The effect on the mix and quantity of components used when there is just insurance for hospital care and not for any of the other components is similar to the income and substitution effects of a price change. The patient will use relatively more hospital care, since the price of hospital care relative to out-of-hospital care has been reduced. This is the substitution effect. The income effect will be an increase in the use of both components, as long as they are normal goods.

If the patient were now to receive a service benefit policy, hospital care becomes essentially free, since there is no out-of-pocket cost to the patient. The substitution effect of this price reduction to the patient becomes even greater than in the previous case. Line *HH* is horizontal, to indicate that there is no price constraint on the purchase of additional units of hospital care. (It is lower than point *A* because, presumably, it would require more of the consumer's income to purchase the policy; hence less would be available to purchase physician services.) The individual, when ill, will use relatively more hospital care than in any of the previous cases. Because there is some disutility to being in the hospital, use of the hospital will not increase infinitely. Patients, through their physicians, will substitute hospital care for nonhospital services when these nonhospital services would be equally efficacious. In the case above, diagnostic testing would be free to the patient if performed in the hospital, whereas the full price would have to be paid if it were performed outside the hospital. We would therefore predict that such testing would be performed in a hospital.

The misallocation of resources resulting from a service benefit policy is shown as follows. The budget constraint *JK,* since it is tangent to indifference curve III, would make the patient as well off as would the service benefit policy; however, the combination of services used in the treatment represents the use of fewer resources. The slope of line *JK* represents the relative prices of hospital and physician services if the patient had an indemnity type of insurance or had to pay the full price of these services in the event that he did not have insurance. The relative prices of physician and hospital services are assumed to represent their relative marginal costs. The quantity of hospital care used in treatment with a service benefit policy is given by the point where indifference curve III is tangent to line *HH*. Since the patient is equally well off at any point along the same indifference curve, the least costly combination of services would be achieved by using the medical components according to their relative prices (as well as their relative benefits in treatment). The magnitude of misallocation is the difference between line *JK* and a line with the same slope intersecting the point of tangency between the indifference curve and line *HH*.

Although quality of hospital care is not shown in these diagrams, part of the increase in quantity of hospital care may be viewed as an increase in quality. Since the price of hospital care to the patient has been reduced to zero with a service benefit policy, the patient will also demand higher-quality hospital services, such as requesting the removal of an appendix in a teaching hospital when a smaller, less care-intensive community hospital would be equally satisfactory. This demand for increased quality of hospital services will result in an even greater misallocation of resources.

In this discussion, the allocative inefficiency resulting from insurance that provides coverage just for hospital care depends on how much the price of hospital care is subsidized relative to the prices of other medical components (the most severe case being the Blue Cross service benefit policy), the degree of substitutability of hospital care for other forms of care, and the price elasticity of demand both for hospital utilization and for increased hospital quality.

The effects of a hospital service benefit policy were threefold. First, the hospital was used when other less expensive but equally effective forms of treatment could have been used, thereby raising the cost of producing medical care. Second, hospital use increased to a point where the additional benefits to the patient of time spent in the hospital were very low. The real cost of resources to produce the additional care was greater than the price faced by the patient, thereby resulting in a situation where the marginal cost of producing the additional care *exceeded* the marginal value to the patient of increased use. Third, there was a much greater demand for quality of hospital services on the part of patients and their physicians because the price of higher-quality services to the patients was zero and quality may be considered a normal good; therefore, they demanded increased quality to the point where the additional benefits derived from it equalled the price they faced. Since the price of higher-quality hospital services was zero, the amount of quality demanded was greater than it would otherwise have been; the cost of resources used in producing higher-quality care, at the margin, exceeded their additional benefits. These, then, were the three misallocative effects of different types of hospital insurance policies, with the greatest misallocation occurring in the case of a service benefit policy.

One approach for remedying these inefficiencies was to use utilization review (UR) procedures. These review mechanisms attempt to reduce excess utilization by making patients liable if they do not follow the utilization guidelines. Alternatively, the distortion in the relative prices of care to the patient, which has brought about these inefficiencies, could be changed. Another approach for correcting such inefficiencies, without placing the financial incentive on the patient, is to provide incentives to the *physician* to use the least costly mix of components. Capitation payment of medical services, such as used by HMOs, is an example of such an incentive system.

APPENDIX 2: THE TAX ADVANTAGE OF HEALTH INSURANCE AS A FRINGE BENEFIT

Employees may receive increased income from their employer in either cash or as a fringe benefit in the form of health insurance. The cost to the employer of either choice is the same. To an employee in a high tax bracket, however, employer-purchased health insurance may be worth more than an equivalent payment in cash.

If an employee receives an income of $1,000 a week, then, as shown in Figure 6.10, the employee's budget line is I_1M_1. If the employee spent her entire income on other goods and services, the employee could purchase quantity OI_1 of other goods and services each week. If she chose instead to purchase just health insurance with her weekly income, the employee could purchase a maximum of OM_1 quantity of health insurance each week. The slope of I_1M_1 represents the relative prices of health insurance and all other goods and services. The combination of health insurance and other goods and services that the employee will actually purchase depends on the employee's tastes and preferences.

Assume that the employee receives a raise of $200 a week. If the employer gave the raise to the employee in cash, the employee's budget line would increase to I_2M_2. In

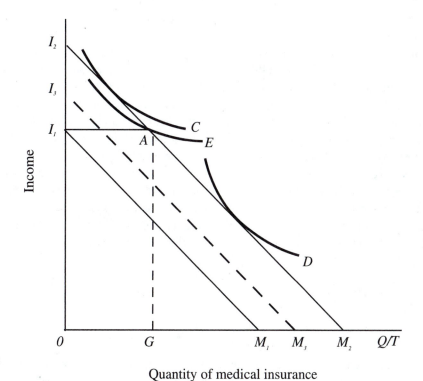

FIGURE 6.10 • Fringe benefits versus money income.

addition to being able to purchase more health insurance, the increased cash would enable the employee to purchase more of other goods and services.

If the employee has to pay income taxes (and Social Security taxes) on a cash raise, then the after-tax value of that cash raise is reduced and is shown by the budget line I_3M_3. The after-tax budget line would depend on the employee's marginal tax bracket. The higher the marginal tax rate of the employee, the lower will be the new budget line.

If, instead of cash, the employer uses the money to purchase health insurance for the employee, which is not considered as taxable income, the employee's budget line changes to I_1AM_2. The budget line becomes horizontal from I_1 to A. The employee receives OG quantity of health insurance while retaining her current income. (The cash amount of the raise divided by the price of health insurance equals quantity OG.) Thus the employee receives OG quantity of health insurance and still has a budget line of I_1M_1. The employee can still purchase OI_1 of other goods and services (if she spent her entire income) or can purchase GM_2 of additional health insurance (for a total quantity of OM_2 if she spent her entire income on health insurance).

An employee who prefers more of other goods and services rather than additional health insurance would, with a cash raise, be on indifference curve C. An employee who prefers additional health insurance would move to indifference curve D after a cash raise. If the cash raise is then taxed so that the new after-tax income is budget line I_3M_3, those employees could no longer be on indifference curves C and D; they could only be on an indifference curve that is tangent to the budget line I_3M_3. With a fringe benefit, however, both employees could move to higher indifference curves. The employee preferring additional insurance can attain indifference curve D. Indifference curve C is still unattainable under fringe benefits; the highest indifference curve achievable by that employee is indifference curve E. However, E is still preferable to any indifference curve on budget line I_3M_3.

Employer-purchased health insurance is in the interest of the employees. As long as employees pay taxes on their cash income but not on employer-purchased health insurance, they have an incentive to receive additional income in the form of fringe benefits. The higher the employees' marginal tax bracket, the greater is their incentive for more comprehensive insurance, such as first-dollar coverage, as well as new types of coverage, such as vision and dental benefits. If health insurance fringes were taxed at the same rate as cash income, employees would demand less health insurance (14).

APPENDIX 3: THE EFFECT ON THE INSURANCE PREMIUM OF EXTENDING COVERAGE TO INCLUDE ADDITIONAL BENEFITS

As insurance companies compete with one another, it becomes important for them to be able to provide a given set of benefits at the lowest possible cost. Benefit design is important in a price-competitive market. Since a treatment for an illness can be provided using a combination of settings (e.g., hospital, physician's office, and home care), insurance companies are adding less costly substitutes to their policies. Similarly, as a consequence of its hospital service benefit policy, Blue Cross has broadened its coverage to include out-of-hospital care. The hoped-for effect of adding additional coverage is that substitution away from the hospital toward lower-cost substitutes will occur and the insurance premium can be reduced.

To determine whether adding coverage for a nonhospital benefit will reduce the total costs of care (i.e., the premium), the following information is needed:

1. the price elasticity of demand for the newly covered benefit;
2. the co-payment factor for the new benefit;
3. the cross-elasticity of demand between hospitalization and the new benefits;
4. the cross-elasticity of demand between the new benefit and any complementary components of care; and
5. the relative prices of hospital care, the new benefit, and any other complementary components affected.

This information would be used in the following manner to determine whether adding a new insurance benefit would lower the insurance premium. Assuming that the demand for hospital care is as it appears in Figure 6.11A, then without any insurance, the patient would have to pay the full cost of a hospital episode if he became ill; the patient would have to pay P_{H1}, and according to his expected demand, would use Q_{H1} days of hospital care. The consumer's total expenditures for hospital care would be $(P_{H1} \times Q_{H1})$. With an insurance policy that provided complete coverage for hospital care but not for substitutes to the hospital, such as the Blue Cross service benefit policy, the price of hospital care to the patient would become "zero," and the expected utilization in the event of illness would be Q_{H2}. The total expenditure for hospital care in this case would be $(P_{H1} \times Q_{H2})$.

Including in the insurance contract home health visits with a co-insurance feature will now result in a lower price to the patient, from P_{M1} to P_{M2}, and an increase in utilization of home health visits, from Q_{M1} to Q_{M2}, as shown in Figure 6.11B. The amount of the increase in home health visits will depend on the price elasticity of demand for home health visits and the size of the co-insurance payment. The cost to the insurance company of covering home health visits is that part of the actual price that the insurance company will have to pay $(P_{M1} \times P_{M2})$, multiplied by the number of home health visits, $Q_{M2.}$ (The patient would pay the remainder, $PM_2 \times Q_{M2}$.)

If the new benefit acts as a partial substitute for hospital care, then with the reduction in the price of home health visits, patients (through their physicians) will demand less hospital care. How much less hospital care will be demanded will depend on the cross-elasticity of demand between hospital utilization and the price of home health visits, which is equal to the percent change in hospital utilization divided by the percent change in the price of home health visits. This is shown in Figure 6.11A by a shift in the demand

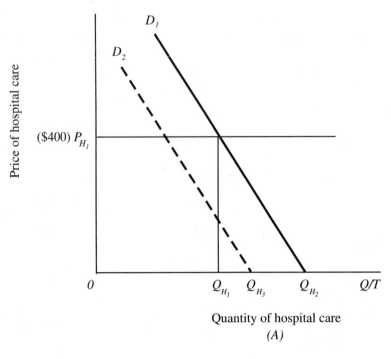

Quantity of hospital care

(A)

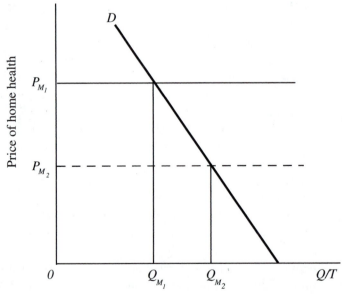

Quantity of home health visits

(B)

FIGURE 6.11 • The effect on hospital utilization of insuring out-of-hospital services: (A) hospital utilization, (B) home health visits.

for hospital care to the left, indicated by demand curve D_2. Since the price of hospital care to the patient with his initial insurance policy has been assumed to be "zero," the new quantity demanded will be Q_{H3}. The size of the shift in demand for hospital care will depend on the magnitude of the cross-elasticity of demand and the size of the reduction in the price to the patient of the new benefit.

The savings in hospital expenditures to the insurance company of including coverage for a nonhospital service would be the difference in hospital utilization ($Q_{H2} - Q_{H3}$), multiplied by the price of hospital care, P_{H1}. If the savings in hospital expenditures were greater than the cost to the insurance company of adding the new benefit, the total cost (the premium) would be reduced.

In actuality, other services might be affected by the provision of a new benefit (i.e., subsidizing home health visits). If there are medical services that are complementary to the use of home health visits, there will be an increase in use of these complementary services (a shift to the right in their demand curve). These additional costs may be borne by the patient rather than by the insurance company if the complementary service is not insured.

Following is a numerical example of a change in benefit design illustrating whether insuring a nonhospital service will reduce the total cost of an insurance premium. Let us assume the following values for each of the data required in our example:

1. Hospital utilization (Q_{H2}) when home health visits are not covered by insurance is 800 patient days per 1,000 population.
2. The price of hospital care is $400 per day.
3. The price of a home health visit is $40.
4. Home health visits are 600 per 1,000 population.
5. The price elasticity of demand for home health visits is −1.0 (a 10 percent decrease in price leads to a 10 percent increase in home health visits).
6. The cross-elasticity of demand between hospital patient days and the price of home health visits is + 0.2 (a 10 percent decrease in the price of a home health visit leads to a 2 percent decrease in hospital patient days).
7. After home health visits are included in the insurance coverage, the co-insurance rate is 20 percent; that is, the patient has to pay only 20 percent of the price of home health visits. (It is also assumed that the price of home health visits remains at its previous level.)

With this information we can now calculate the change in the cost of the premium as a result of including home health visits with a 20 percent co-insurance feature.

The total cost of the premium per 1,000 population before the new benefit is added to the coverage is

$$\frac{TC}{1,000} = P_{H1} \times \frac{Q_{H2}}{1,000}$$

$$\frac{\$320,000}{1,000} = \$400 \times \frac{800}{1,000}$$

or $320 per person. The total cost of the premium *after* home health visits are covered at a 20 percent co-insurance rate is

$$\frac{TC}{1,000} = P_{H1}\left(\frac{Q_{H3}}{1,000}\right) + 0.8P_{M1}\left(\frac{Q_{M2}}{1,000}\right)$$

which is

$$\frac{\$303,360}{1,000} = \$400\left(\frac{672}{1,000}\right) + 0.8(\$40)\left(\frac{1,080}{1,000}\right)$$

or $303.36 per person.

The difference is computed as follows:

1. The increased expenditure on home health visits is

$$0.8(\$40)\left(\frac{600}{1,000}\right)(1.8) = \frac{\$34,560}{1,000}$$

This is the percentage of the home health price paid by the insurance company (0.8), multiplied by the price of home health visits ($40), multiplied by the number of home health visits per 1,000 population (600/1,000), multiplied by the percent increase in home health visits as a result of the 80 percent reduction in home health prices to the patient (a −1.0 price elasticity multiplied by a 80 percent reduction in price) leads to an 80 percent increase in utilization, hence, 1.8.

2. Subtract the saving on decreased hospital utilization, which is

$$\$400\left(\frac{128}{1,000}\right) = \frac{\$51,200}{1,000}$$

This is the price of hospital care, multiplied by reduction in patient days as a result of a lower price of home health visits. (The cross-elasticity of +0.2 when multiplied by a 80 percent reduction in the price of home health visits is equal to a 16 percent reduction in hospital utilization; this is then multiplied by 800/1,000.)

3. The net effect of the savings on hospital expenditures less the increased home health expenditures is

$$\frac{\$51,200}{1,000} - \frac{\$34,560}{1,000} = \frac{\$16,640}{1,000} \text{ or } \$16.64 \text{ per person}$$

Given the data and assumptions used in this example, the effect of insuring home health visits would be a net decrease of $16.64 per person in the total cost of the premium ($303.36 versus $320 per person).

In the preceding example, insuring an out-of-hospital service would further reduce the insurance premium if the price of hospital care increased faster than the nonhospital service, the substitutability between the two services (cross-elasticity) increased, and the price elasticity of demand for the nonhospital service were reduced.

Adding insurance coverage for an out-of-hospital service is more likely to reduce hospital utilization when this service is used *in conjunction with* hospital care in treatment of an illness episode. An example of this is case management for catastrophic care. If, however, home health visits are covered by insurance and used separately, not as part of the treatment for an illness, there may be a large increase in home health utilization without any consequent lowering of hospital utilization (15). A major medical policy, which covers all the medical services used in treatment (after a sizable deductible has been paid), is more likely to result in substitution away from the more costly components.

Key Terms and Concepts

- Adverse selection
- Deductibles and co-insurance
- Loading charge
- Moral hazard
- Pure premium
- Risk aversion

- Decreasing marginal utility of wealth
- Expected and actual utility
- Indemnity versus service benefits
- Optimal amount of health insurance
- Preferred risk selection
- Probability of loss occurring
- Tax-exempt employer-paid health insurance
- The size of the expected loss

Review Questions

1. How would you use utility analysis to analyze the following statement?
   Consumers should purchase health insurance policies that cover 100 percent of all medical care expenses. Anything less than 100 percent coverage reflects either irrational consumer behavior or market failure in the insurance industry. (Organize your discussion around diagrams.)

2. Explain why health insurance is more common for hospital expenses than for ambulatory care expenses.

3. How will a change in the price of medical care affect the demand for health insurance?

4. Discuss each of the factors affecting the demand for health insurance. Indicate the effect that each has on demand.

5. What are the welfare implications of having everyone purchase the same (very comprehensive) health insurance coverage?

6. What is "moral hazard"? How does its existence affect the demand for health insurance? What approaches have been used by insurance companies to control its existence?

7. What is adverse selection? How does its existence affect the market for health insurance? What are some ways in which insurance companies try to protect themselves from adverse selection?

8. What information would you need to know (and how would you use it) to determine whether expanding benefit coverage (e.g., covering hospice services) would lower the cost of an insurance premium?

9. In what way do technological innovations, such as an inexpensive new drug that would replace the need for cardiac surgery or the development of organ transplants, affect the demand for health insurance?

10. Trace through each of the medical markets the effects of making employer-paid health insurance premiums taxable to the employee.

11. It has been proposed that employer-paid health insurance be taxed as part of an employee's income. Evaluate this proposal in terms of economic efficiency, equity (be sure to define efficiency and equity in your answer), and who you think would be likely to favor and oppose this proposal.

12. Evaluate Blue Cross's hospital service benefit policy in terms of economic efficiency. If the service benefit policy was inefficient, how could Blue Cross survive in a competitive insurance market? Why were hospitals in favor of it?

REFERENCES

1. The discussion in this section borrows heavily from an unpublished article by J. J. German, "A Note on the Economic Theory of Insurance with Implications for Health Insurance," mimeographed, January 1967; and the article by Dennis Lees and Robert Rice, "Uncertainty and the Welfare Economics of Medical Care: Comment," *American Economic Review,* 55(1), March 1965: 140–154. The comment by Lees and Rice (as well as the comment by M. Pauly in the next section of this chapter) were written in response to Kenneth J. Arrow, "Uncertainty and the Welfare Economics of Medical Care," *American Economic Review,* 53(5), December 1963: 941–973. Arrow claimed that the market for health insurance requires government intervention because there are gaps in consumers' health insurance coverage, and that this is evidence that the market is not producing certain services that consumers are willing to purchase. Lees

and Rice argued that Arrow's claims are not evidence of market imperfections but rather are the result of transaction costs. For example, "the transaction cost to the individual of completing and filing applications and forms, paying premiums, keeping records, etc., as well as possible costs of obtaining information, may be of sufficient magnitude to make insurance policies against certain losses not worthwhile." Arrow replied that individuals who cannot take advantage of the economies of group health insurance will face too high a transaction cost (i.e., the price of insurance is greatly in excess of its pure premium) and thus may not purchase health insurance.

2. M. Friedman and L. Savage, "The Utility Analysis of Choices Involving Risk," *Journal of Political Economy,* 56(4), 1948: 279–304.

3. On this last point, see the discussion by Jan Mossin, "Aspects of Rational Insurance Purchasing," *Journal of Political Economy,* 73(4), July/August 1968: 553–568.

4. Susan M. Marquis and Stephen H. Long, "Worker Demand for Health Insurance in the Non-group Market," *Journal of Health Economics,* 14(1), May 1995: 47–63; and Jonathan Gruber and James Poterba, "Tax Incentives and the Decision to Purchase Health Insurance: Evidence from the Self-Employed," *Quarterly Journal of Economics,* 109(3), August 1994: 701–733. In a review article Pauly concludes, "The results generally support the view that the impact of loading ... on insurance purchases is significantly negative. The actual numerical estimates of the elasticity of insurance with respect to the loading 'price,' however, vary considerably, ranging from about –0.2 . . . to numbers greater than unity" (p. 644). Mark V. Pauly, "Taxation, Health Insurance, and Market Failure in the Medical Economy," *Journal of Economic Literature,* 24(2), June 1986: 629–675.

5. Jon R. Gabel and Gail A. Jensen, "The Price of State Mandated Benefits," *Inquiry,* 26(4), Winter 1989: 419–431. This article includes results from studies also conducted by Gail A. Jensen and Michael Morrisey. A more recent study finds that state mandates have very little effect on the rate of insurance coverage of small firms; see Jonathan Gruber, "State-Mandated Benefits and Employer-Provided Health Insurance," *Journal of Public Economics,* 55(3), November 1994: 433–464.

6. The discussion in this section is based on Burton A. Weisbrod, "The Health Care Quadrilemma: An Essay on Technological Change, Insurance, Quality of Care, and Cost Containment," *Journal of Economic Literature,* 29(2), June 1991: 523–552.

7. *Ibid.,* p. 540.

8. E. Friedson and J. Feldman, *Public Attitudes Toward Health Insurance,* Research Series 5 (New York: Health Information Foundation, 1958).

9. Katherine R. Levit et al., "DataView: National Health Expenditures, 1994," *Health Care Financing Review,* 17(3), Spring 1996: Table 17, p. 240.

10. M. Rothschild and J. Stiglitz, "Equilibrium in Competitive Insurance Markets: An Essay on the Economics of Imperfect Information," *Quarterly Journal of Economics,* 90(4), 1976: 629–649.

11. Randall S. Brown and Jerrold W. Hill, "The Effects of Medicare Risk HMOs on Medicare Costs and Service Utilization," in Harold S. Luft, ed., *HMOs and the Elderly* (Ann Arbor, Mich.: Health Administration Press, 1994).

12. Marc L. Berk and Alan C. Monheit, "The Concentration of Health Expenditures: An Update," *Health Affairs,* 11(4), Winter 1992: Exhibit 2, p. 148.

13. The discussion in this section is based on the article by Mark Pauly, "The Economics of Moral Hazard: Comment," *American Economic Review,* 58(3), June 1968: 531–537. In Pauly's comment to Arrow's reply to Lees and Rice, he argues that even if there are certain economies in government provision of health insurance that would lower transaction costs, other costs may more than offset such possible savings. In addition to a loss of consumer choice, the existence of "moral hazard" would cause consumers to demand less insurance "at the premium its behavior as a purchaser of insurance and as a demander of medical care under insurance makes necessary." In other words, the existence of moral hazard would result in higher prices for insurance and, consequently, a decreased demand. The lack of complete health insurance coverage in the private market can also be explained by moral hazard, which would not be lessened even if government were somehow able to reduce the transaction costs of insurance to individuals.

14. The reader is referred to the following articles for a more complete discussion of the welfare loss of excess health insurance coverage: Mark V. Pauly, "A Measure of the Welfare Costs of Health Insurance," *Health Services Research,* 4(4), Winter 1969: 281–292; Martin S. Feldstein, "The Welfare Loss of Excess Health Insurance," *Journal of Political Economy,* 81(2), March–April 1973: 251–280; Roger Feldman and Bryan Dowd, "A New Estimate of the Welfare Loss of Excess Health Insurance," *American Economic Review,* 81(1), March 1991: 297–301; and Joseph P. Newhouse, "Medical Care Costs: How Much Welfare Loss?" *Journal of Economic Perspectives,* 6(3), Summer 1992: 3–21.

15. A recent study of Medicare's home health care program found that such visits did not substitute for inpatient admissions and were used primarily to provide long-term care. H. Gilbert Welch, David E. Wennberg, and W. Pete Welch, "The Use of Home Health Care Services," *The New England Journal of Medicine,* 335(5), August 1, 1996: 324–329.

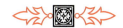

CHAPTER

7

The Supply of Medical Care: An Overview

DETERMINANTS OF SUPPLY

The concept of economic efficiency is relevant to both the demand and the supply side of an industry. When evaluating economic efficiency, we are concerned that the rate (and type) of output be "optimal." Economic efficiency in demand is related to economic efficiency in supply through prices. The optimal rate of output occurs when the marginal benefit of the last unit equals the price of that unit, which in turn equals the marginal cost of producing that last unit. Several reasons were given why economic efficiency does not occur on the demand side. For example, since employer-purchased health insurance is not included as part of employees' taxable income, the price of insurance is lowered, resulting in more comprehensive coverage than if employees had to pay the full price (with after-tax dollars). Also, the limited information available to patients on prices, physician quality, their diagnosis, and treatment needs has made it possible for some physicians to manipulate patient demands for medical services.

In our examination of the supply side of the medical care sector, the criterion of economic efficiency is also important. If the various markets within the medical care sector are not economically efficient, the cost of medical care will be higher than it should be. By examining the reasons for deviations from economic efficiency, we can make policy recommendations to improve the efficiency of the market and reduce the rise in the cost of medical care.

The economic efficiency of the supply side of the medical care sector also has important implications for redistributive policies. If the supply side of medical care is relatively

163

inelastic, requiring relatively large price increases to produce an increase in medical care output, this will influence the type of redistribution programs proposed on the demand side, specifically, redistributive programs to disadvantaged population groups. The cost of a national health insurance program would be greater and the availability of services diminished when supply is more inelastic. Because of greater total expenditures, higher prices, and less output, the political feasibility of instituting such a program, as well as its comprehensiveness, will be reduced.

Greater price inelasticity will benefit providers by resulting in higher prices, wages, and incomes for providers of medical services. These price increases will be financed by the rest of the population, which will result in their having lower incomes.

As shown in Figure 7.1, a relatively inelastic supply curve, represented by S_1, would, with an increase in demand from D_1 to D_2, result in a greater price rise and a smaller increase in services provided than if the supply of medical services were more elastic. A more elastic supply schedule could produce the same level of output (Q_1), but at a lower cost. Or for the same increase in demand, provide $Q_2 - Q_1$ more services at a smaller increase in price: P_2 rather than P_1. Total cost after the increase in demand would be $P_1 \times Q_1$ in the inelastic case versus $P_2 \times Q_2$ in the situation where supply is more elastic. In the latter case more of the increase in total expenditures would go for increased medical services, whereas in the former there would be more rapid price increases with a smaller increase in services.

The elasticity of an industry's supply is affected by that industry's market structure and

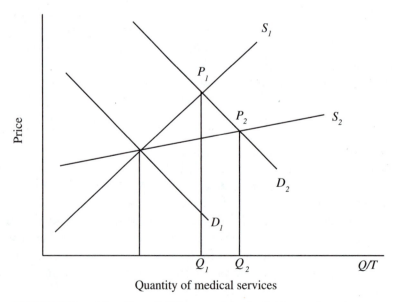

FIGURE 7.1 • The effect of different supply elasticities on the price, quality, and cost of national health insurance.

by the nature of the production function for producing that service. Each of these topics is examined with regard to their effect on supply elasticity and appropriate public policy, if indicated.

Market Structure

Markets can be characterized by their "structure"; that is, by the number of purchasers and suppliers within that market. Markets that have a large number of buyers and suppliers are considered to be competitive; no individual buyer or seller has influence over the market price. Monopoly occurs when there is only one supplier of a service. Input markets can also be characterized by whether they are competitive or monopolistic. (While firms are suppliers in the services market, these same firms are demanders in the input market.) Again, monopoly can occur in either the services market and/or the input (health manpower) market. (A single purchaser in a market that may have few or many sellers is a monopsonist [discussed in Chapter 15].)

Many economists believe that there is a relationship between the structure of a market and its conduct or behavior and ultimately to how well that market performs. Markets that are characterized by many buyers and suppliers are believed to result in greater economic efficiency (lower prices relative to costs and greater output) than markets characterized by fewer suppliers. Such generalizations, however, must be tested against each particular market, its conduct, and hence its performance, since some markets with few firms can be very competitive and achieve economically efficient outcomes.

There are two important determinants of the number of firms in an industry: the extent of economies of scale in relation to the size of the market and barriers to entry. There are several types of entry barriers, the most permanent being those that are legally granted, such as licensing (e.g., health manpower and certificate of need for facilities) and patents to promote technological innovation. An entry barrier can also occur when industry suppliers or their inputs are either directly or indirectly subsidized (through tax laws), thereby providing existing firms with a cost advantage over other firms.

Most industries are characterized by a market structure that is intermediate between competition and monopoly. Oligopoly markets are dominated by a few firms; each is aware that their actions, such as the price they set, will be matched by their competitors. Because firms in oligopoly markets recognize their interdependence with competitors, collusion is more prevalent in these types of markets.

Monopolistic competition is characterized by a large number of firms (similar to a competitive industry) that produce an output that is slightly differentiated from the other firms. These output differences may be a result of real or perceived differences in the types of services offered, patient location, quality, or reputation. Since the products or services are somewhat different, monopolistically competitive firms face a slightly downward sloping demand curve and therefore have some influence over the pricing of their services (similar to the monopoly model). The prices set by such firms, however, cannot differ too greatly from those of their competitors, or they will suffer large losses in their market share. Monopolistically competitive markets are similar to competitive markets in terms of economic efficiency.

An analysis of the determinants of market structure will be undertaken for each of the medical care markets examined. Based on that analysis it should be possible to determine whether there are sufficient numbers of purchasers and suppliers for that market to be competitive. The relative market shares of competitors will be examined as well as firm concentration ratios to characterize the structure of each market. (An important part of calculating market shares and concentration ratios is correctly defining the relevant product market, namely, how close a substitute certain services are, and the geographic market, that is, how close another hospital has to be for it to be considered a good substitute to a particular hospital.)

Market shares and concentration ratios, however, are inadequate, by themselves, for determining market competitiveness; they do not indicate *potential entry* into that industry by other firms. Although a market may be highly concentrated, entry by other firms may not be very costly, thereby leading the firms in the market to act competitively.

Competitive Behavior

Market structure influences how firms in an industry compete. In purely competitive markets firms do not engage in collusive pricing strategies because of the difficulty of coordinating such behavior among a large number of firms and the incentive for each firm to cheat. Instead, prices approximate the costs of providing the service. In highly concentrated markets the costs of negotiating collusive prices among competitors are lower and therefore more likely to occur. (Competitive industries with a large number of suppliers often seek legislation to enable them to achieve what a competitive market does not permit, namely, regulated prices and limits on entry.) More highly concentrated markets (and markets where consumer information is limited) are also characterized by a pricing strategy that results in price discrimination, whereby different prices (unrelated to cost) are charged to different purchasers.

Product strategies also differ by market structure. The products and services produced in markets where there are a large number of suppliers are often relatively similar. More highly concentrated markets often invest in research and development to develop new services. Such firms also spend more on advertising, with the purpose of differentiating their services from those of their competitors, enabling them to raise their price and increase profits. While the likelihood of collusive arrangements are greater in more concentrated industries (and therefore must be monitored) so is the likelihood of innovation and change.

Thus the competitive behavior of firms in the different medical markets will also be analyzed.

Market Performance

Each medical market's performance will be evaluated in terms of whether it approximates economic efficiency. In highly competitive markets, each firm is both technically (maximum output for given inputs) and economically (least-cost combination of inputs used) efficient. As shown in Figure 7.2, the industry price is determined by the intersection of demand and supply (industry supply in the short run is the summation of each firm's marginal cost curve). And, in equilibrium, since each firm sells at the industry-determined price, price approximates marginal cost and average total cost, and each firm is producing at the minimum point on the long-run average cost curve, thereby taking advantage of economies of scale. Consequently each firm is efficient—otherwise they could not survive—and the right number of firms exist in the industry. The long-run industry supply curve (not shown) is determined by entry of new firms, which in a constant cost industry (input prices and productivity unchanged) will be horizontal.

The rate of output in a competitive industry is considered to be optimal, since price, which reflects marginal benefit, is equal to marginal cost (assuming no externalities). Profits are normal in that price equals average total cost, and included in cost is a normal rate of return on capital and the opportunity cost of the owner's efforts.

Price/cost ratios are used to indicate the extent to which prices are competitively determined in an industry. The higher price is relative to cost, the greater is the firm's market power. Firms with market power have less price elastic demand curves for their services. If the competitive industry characterized in Figure 7.2 were to become monopolized, for example, by all the firms merging into one (or by all the firms acting as a cartel), then the remaining firm would have as its demand curve the industry demand curve. The new firm's demand curve would be less price elastic than the (horizontal) demand

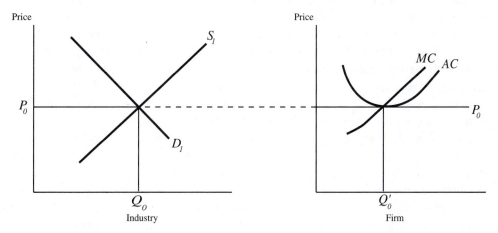

FIGURE 7.2 • The industry and the firm under long-run competitive equilibrium.

curves faced by the earlier competitive firms. Previously, each competitive firm faced a highly elastic demand curve because the services provided by the other firms were good substitutes. With only one firm in the industry, the price elasticity of the firm's demand curve would be determined by how good a substitute other industries' services are to its own.

A firm with market power has greater discretion in setting prices, its output, level of quality, and the type of service it provides. (Market power is defined as the ability of a firm to profitably increase its price [and/or decrease quality and access to services] and sustain that increased price for a period of time without an offsetting loss of volume.) Market power therefore distorts efficient outcomes; prices are higher, output is lower, profits are greater, and responsiveness of the firm to purchasers is less than would occur in a highly price-competitive market.

Competitive markets should not be evaluated on whether those who are uninsured or who have low incomes receive access to medical services. It is not the function of competitive firms to subsidize the poor and sick. To ensure that the poor and sick do receive care, government must provide them with subsidies. Competitive markets can then be evaluated in terms of how efficiently they provide those subsidized services.

Public Policies

Although few industries approximate the competitive ideal and long-run equilibrium may never be attained because underlying conditions are constantly changing, the tendency of the industry is to move in the indicated direction. The competitive model, more than any other model, is better able to predict the outcome. The usefulness of the competitive model, therefore, is with regard to its predictions and the effect of its assumptions on performance. For example, each market will be examined to determine whether there are any barriers that limit entry of new firms, a crucial assumption underlying competitive market structures that will affect the industry's performance. Further, how well certain assumptions, such as availability of information and purchaser and provider incentives, are fulfilled will affect competitive behavior, and, consequently, performance.

Market performance can presumably be improved through alternative approaches. First, the actual market can be restructured to more closely approximate a competitive industry and greater reliance placed on competitive pressures to achieve the goal of economic efficiency. An example of this approach is the applicability and enforcement of the anti-trust laws that seek to prevent monopolization of an industry. Alternatively, greater emphasis can be placed on regulation and centralized decision making to achieve the desirable outcomes of a competitive market. Under either of these public policy approaches there needs to be a comparable set of measures by which to evaluate the performance of each market. Unless there is agreement on the desired outcome measures, regulatory and market competitive approaches cannot be compared. The two approaches suggested for improving market performance—increased regulation and greater reliance on market pressures—will be analyzed according to the economic criteria of economic efficiency.

A competitive market will result in a more elastic industry supply curve than if, for example, that industry were subject to entry barriers. With increased demand, a competitive industry will produce a greater output at a lower price. However, even in a competitive industry, the industry supply curve may be less elastic than is economically feasible because of the nature of the production function and possible restrictions on the use of various inputs. These issues are now discussed.

EVALUATION OF ECONOMIC EFFICIENCY IN SUPPLY

Characteristics of Production Functions

Underlying the supply of any good or service is the production function, which describes the technical relationship between the output of that service and the resources (inputs) used to produce it. If the output were nursing care per patient, then included in the inputs would be the number of and type of nurses on the nursing unit. This technical relationship between nursing care per patient and the types of nurses may be expressed in the following general form:

$$Q_{npc} = f(\text{RNs, LPNs, NAs, UN})$$

where Q_{npc}, which represents quantity of nursing patient care, is functionally related to the number of registered nurses (RNs), licensed practical nurses (LPNs), nursing aides (NAs), and the type of nursing unit (UN).

Certain characteristics of medical production functions are important to understand since they affect the cost and quantity of care provided. First, the various inputs (e.g., types of nurses) are, to some extent, substitutable for one another in the production of nursing care. The substitutability is not one-to-one (i.e., one LPN cannot substitute for one RN). RNs presumably have more skills as a result of their additional education, and therefore LPNs can substitute for some but not all of the tasks RNs perform.

The second characteristic of production functions is the concept of marginal productivity of each input, which is the additional output achieved by increasing each input by a small amount (holding the other inputs constant). The marginal productivity of each input, together with information on the relative prices (wages) of different inputs, determine which combination of inputs is less costly (since they are substitutable) for producing a given level of output or for meeting an increase in output.

The relative marginal productivities of any two inputs should be equal to their relative prices or wages. For example, if an RN costs twice as much as an LPN, then, at the margin, the RN should be twice as productive as the LPN. Similarly, if an RN contributed one and a half times more than an LPN to patient care, increases in patient care should not necessarily be achieved through increases in the number of RNs. If RNs' wages were twice as great as those of LPNs, it would be less expensive to achieve an increase in nursing care by increasing LPNs rather than RNs, assuming no change in quality.

A third characteristic of production functions is the distinction between the "short" and "long" run. Not all the inputs can be varied simultaneously at each point in time. At any time, the decision maker can vary the combination of nurses and their numbers on the nursing unit. To change the type of nursing unit itself, by enlarging it or improving it through greater use of monitoring mechanisms, would take longer. The "long run" is that period of time in which the administrator can vary not only the number and type of nurses but also the size and character of the nursing unit. The "short run" is that period of time in which the administrator can vary the other inputs but not make changes in the nursing unit itself. Another example of the short versus the long run is with regard to physician services. In the short run, an increase in physician services can be achieved by having the physician work longer hours or by hiring additional personnel. In the long run, medical schools may increase the number of physicians, which are the fixed input in the short run.

When one input is fixed in the short run, this gives rise to the "law of variable proportions" (commonly known as the law of diminishing returns), which states that after some point, continued increases in the variable input (RNs) will result in the marginal productivity of that input declining.

The law of variable proportions is the reason why the industry supply schedule in the short run (the sum of each firm's marginal cost curve) is rising. To increase output the firm increases its variable inputs, whose marginal productivity eventually declines; consequently the marginal cost of additional output rises. (Marginal cost is equal to the wage divided by marginal productivity.) If there is an increased demand for the industry's output, more resources must be drawn into production, and it will be necessary to pay higher wages to bid these resources away from their current use. Thus, in addition to the rising marginal cost curve (because of the law of variable proportions), the marginal cost curve will shift up as the price of inputs rises. In the long run, when all the inputs in the production function can be varied, the supply schedule will become more elastic (i.e., it will require less of an increase in cost to increase supply).

These distinctions between the short and long run are important for determining the extent of economies of scale in producing nursing and other types of medical care. The concept of "returns to scale" is another characteristic of production functions. With an increase in the demand for nursing care (derived from an increased demand for medical and hospital care), all the inputs, including the nursing unit, can be increased in the long run. When the nursing unit is expanded by increasing all of its inputs, and the output increases by a larger percent, then economies of scale are said to exist; the cost per unit of output will decline (the long-run average cost curve is falling). Constant (and decreasing) returns occur when output expands by a similar (lesser) percent. Returns to scale (consequently the long-run average cost curve) determine which size of unit or facility is less costly, that is, lower cost per unit of output.

One further aspect of the production function is worth mentioning. Technical change typically results in a greater output being produced with the same or fewer inputs. One such example of technical change that has led to a decrease in inputs for treatment of a patient is the use of new drugs, which has decreased the use of more expensive institutional care. However, in medical care, technical change has usually meant that illnesses that formerly could not be treated can now be cared for and current illnesses will have a higher probability of a successful outcome or a shorter recovery period. Such technical change often expresses itself through a change in medical care *output* (i.e., an increased probability of recovery) and may result in increased rather than decreased use of inputs, such as improved diagnostic imaging equipment. Thus, both types of technical change have occurred in medical care. It is important to hold the effects of technical change constant when analyzing the production function for medical care.

These characteristics of production functions, input substitutability, marginal productivity of each input, the law of variable proportions, and returns to scale determine the nature of costs and, consequently, supply of medical services, in the short and long run.

Assumptions Underlying Medical Services Production and Cost Functions

Several important assumptions underlying production functions and cost minimization must be examined to determine whether they are fulfilled in certain medical markets. The first is the assumption of substitutability in the use of inputs to produce a given output. In the health field there are a number of legal restrictions on the tasks that various health professionals are permitted to perform. Even if a nurse is capable of performing certain tasks that are reserved solely for the physician, the nurse may not be permitted to perform them because she would be violating the state practice acts. Similarly, attempts by nursing organizations to require the use of fixed ratios, such as the number of RNs per inpatient day, result in a more costly production process since a change in relative wages between RNs and other personnel will change the least-cost combination of inputs, hence the ratio of RNs per inpatient day.

The effect of these legal restrictions is to limit the extent to which inputs may be substituted in producing a given level of output. When legal restrictions prevent substitution from occurring when it would not result in a diminution of the quality of care, the legal restrictions have increased the cost of producing that care. The "costs" of restrictive practices, therefore, are the additional resources required to produce a given level of care for a given level of quality.

A second assumption used in determining the least-cost combination of inputs is that the relative prices of the inputs used in production are not distorted. For example, if the government subsidizes certain inputs, such as hospital capital or educational programs for health manpower, then the relative price of the subsidized input has been lowered and relatively more of it will be used in production. From a societal perspective, subsidizing just one input results in economic inefficiency in producing that output. If it is desired to increase production of that output, it would be less costly to subsidize the output itself, rather than any one input used in producing that output.

And, lastly, there is the assumption that decision makers are desirous of minimizing the cost of producing their output. This last assumption is particularly important when nonprofit hospitals (not previously subject to price competition) and medical schools are examined.

Economic efficiency in production requires decision makers to use information on the marginal productivity and the relative prices of their inputs to produce the output at minimum cost. Decision makers of nonprofit organizations, however, may have goals other than cost minimization. To the extent that the decision makers' goals differ from cost minimization, and they do not compete in a price-competitive market and/or that the provider payment mechanisms enable them to pursue these other goals, the supply curve of medical care will be less elastic. In other words, it will take larger price increases to produce an increase in services than it would if the objectives and constraints were similar to those of a competitive industry. The objectives of nonprofit hospitals and medical schools will be examined to determine the effects of such objectives on industry performance.

Production Functions at All Levels of the Medical Sector

The example of the production function used earlier (nursing care), the information required to be able to minimize costs (marginal productivity and relative prices), and the assumptions underlying the behavior of the decision makers (a desire to minimize costs), can be applied equally well to other levels of the medical sector. For example, with regard to medical services, the physician faces a production function in providing an office visit that includes such inputs as the physician's own time, the time of one or more types of assistants, diagnostic tests and equipment, and the size and layout of the physician's office.

How the delivery of medical services should be organized—namely, the combinations of institutional settings that are least expensive for producing patient care—is essentially a discussion of a production function and cost minimization at a very aggregate level. For example, traditional fee-for-service practice, health maintenance organizations, and managed care are different delivery systems, each offering differing incentives to the various decision makers. In each delivery system, the decision maker faces a production function in providing treatment for an illness of a particular diagnosis and of a given level of severity. The inputs are the different institutional settings, such as a hospital, a physician's office, or the patient's home.

To determine which delivery systems (combinations of inputs or institutional settings) are least expensive, information is needed on the marginal productivities and the relative costs of the different institutional settings, as well as an understanding of the objectives of the decision makers and the incentives they face. As will be discussed, changes in financial incentives and removal of certain legal restrictions have had important effects on changes in the organization of medical care.

SUMMARY

In evaluating the performance of each of the medical markets in the remaining chapters of this book, the first step will be to examine the market structure for each of the separate markets, beginning with the insurance market, then the institutional settings in which care is provided, proceeding to the manpower markets, and ending with the education markets. Each market will be compared to a hypothetically competitive medical market. The competitive market is used as the yardstick for comparison, since it is inclusive of the conditions necessary for economic efficiency. The performance that might be expected under a competitive market will then be compared with what is observed in the particular medical market. Any divergence in performance between what is expected theoretically and what is observed will be analyzed in terms of differences in the structure and assumptions underlying the hypothetically competitive and actual markets.

To the extent that there are indications of inadequate performance in any particular market, the assumptions that underlie a competitive industry will be examined: Is entry by other firms permitted? What are the payment and incentive mechanisms in that industry? And what are the goals and objectives of the suppliers? Major segments of the medical sector, such as hospitals and medical schools, are dominated by nonprofit firms. Do their objectives, which differ from those of for-profit firms, lead to either desirable or undesirable differences in performance? Finally, what have been the effects on performance of barriers to entry into various medical markets that have been advanced on the grounds of consumer protection?

Key Terms and Concepts

- Barriers to entry
- Competitive markets
- Market performance
- Market power
- Monopolistic markets
- Monopoly markets
- Oligopoly

- Determinants of market structure
- Economies of scale in relation to market size

- Geographic market definition
- Optimal rate of output
- Product market definition

Review Questions

1. The following affect the supply of medical care, price of medical care, the prices of inputs, and technological or scientific knowledge. Explain how an increase in each of the above, while the effect of the other two are held constant, will cause changes in supply.
2. Economists claim that there have been and are several causes of economic inefficiency in medical care. List three basic causes, and for each describe why it results in economic inefficiency and poor performance in medical markets.
3. How has the lack of information affected the structure of the medical care market?
4. Contrast the differences in technical versus economic efficiency with respect to the provision of medical services.
5. What information does a decision maker need to minimize her costs of production?
6. Would a decision maker use an input if it is subject to diminishing returns?
7. Apply the concept of a production function and the idea of "marginal rate of substitution" to an HMO. Show how this knowledge may be used for deciding on the settings to be used in providing a medical treatment.
8. Assuming a price-competitive medical market, what is the likely effect on the relative proportion of hospital and physician services used in providing a treatment of the large increase in the supply of physicians?
9. How has the elasticity of supply of medical services affected the government's cost of expanding health care to the poor and uninsured?
10. Why should a competitive market be used as a yardstick for evaluating the performance of the different medical care markets?

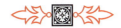

CHAPTER

The Market for Health Insurance: Its Performance and Structure

ECONOMIC EFFICIENCY

It is important to determine how efficiently each sector of the medical care market performs. If these separate submarkets do not perform efficiently, then there may be a legitimate role for public intervention to increase the efficiency of the marketplace. Government intervention to increase efficiency is different from, and should be kept separate from, government intervention to redistribute the output of the medical care market. A government policy that attempts to do both simultaneously, either through a government agency or comprehensive regulation, may do neither as well as separate policies directed toward either efficiency or equity.

Economic efficiency with regard to the supply of health insurance usually means that there are no entry barriers; that the number of firms in the market is the "right" number—that is, each firm operates at a minimum point on the long-run average cost curve; that each firm attempts to minimize its cost of production—that is, achieve internal efficiency; and that the firms are price-competitive. However, even if the health insurance industry is economically efficient in the supply of health insurance, imperfections may exist in the input market in which insurance companies are demanders or purchasers of physician and hospital services. Physicians and hospitals are suppliers of these inputs. To the extent imperfections exist in these "input" markets, the price of health insurance will be higher and there will be less variety in the types of health insurance products sold.

The performance of the health insurance market will therefore be evaluated not only on how competitive it is but also on whether suppliers of medical services have placed restrictions on an insurer's ability to purchase medical services and on the sale by insurers of certain types of insurance products. Hypotheses will be offered to explain possible divergence from economic efficiency, since any intervention to improve economic efficiency in this market should be consistent with the reasons for inadequate performance.

THE DEMAND SIDE OF THE HEALTH INSURANCE MARKET

The Market Demand for Health Insurance

The factors affecting the aggregate demand for health insurance, as discussed previously, are the price of insurance, the probability of loss, the magnitude of the loss if it occurs, the income of the consumer, and how risk-averse the individual is. With increases in the price of medical care, the size of the potential loss increases, which in turn causes an increase (shift to the right) in the demand for health insurance. Increased incomes lead to a greater demand for fringe benefits, which also results in an increase in the demand for health insurance. (An increase in the aggregate demand for health insurance represents an increase in the percentage of the population with some insurance, an increase in the portion of the bill covered by insurance, as well as coverage for new benefits.) The price elasticity of the overall market demand for health insurance is considered to be approximately −1; for each 1 percent increase in the price of insurance there will be a 1 percent decrease in the demand for insurance (1).

The Demand for Health Insurance Faced by the Individual Insurance Firm

Health insurance was traditionally provided by Blue Cross and Blue Shield (BCBS) plans, which were nonprofit (although several are converting to for-profit), and commercial insurers, which are for-profit. As new health insurance products have developed, the most notable being HMOs, commercial insurers and BCBS plans, which previously offered only indemnity and service benefit policies, now also offer HMO options to their subscribers. Similarly, independent HMOs offer their group enrollees an indemnity option in addition to an HMO. Another option offered by HMOs is a point-of-service (POS) plan, which allows an HMO's enrollee to seek care from a non-HMO provider but at a high co-payment, usually 40 percent.

The variety of health insurance products has grown rapidly since the early 1980s, as have the methods of provider reimbursement. Whereas the insurance industry was once dominated by indemnity and service benefit policies with providers paid fee-for-service, managed care and HMOs are currently the fastest-growing forms of health insurance. Managed care broadly defined refers to both HMOs and health insurance (both indemnity and service benefit policies) that use utilization management. Appropriate use of medical services, such as prior authorization for a hospital admission or for outpatient surgery, review of the patient's length of hospital stay, case management of catastrophic care, and monitoring physicians' utilization patterns are examples of utilization management.

Health insurers also include a PPO as an option to their enrollees. PPOs are a closed panel of providers who are willing to discount their prices and/or who have lower use rates than other providers. (PPOs are a means of price competition between providers who are part of a PPO and those who are not.) Enrollees who use a PPO provider pay a lower co-payment, usually 10 percent, while they may pay 30 percent of the provider's fee if they use a non-PPO provider. PPO providers hope to receive a greater number of a firm's employees in return for discounting their prices and/or being more appropriate users of services. PPOs have developed rapidly since the mid-1980s.

Finally, a number of larger companies have decided on self-insurance (whereby they, rather than the insurance company, bear the financial risk of their employees' medical expenses) as an alternative means of providing their employees with health insurance. The employer may then contract with an insurer or a third-party administrator (TPA) to provide administrative services only (ASO), including processing of claims. Smaller companies are also considering this option, together with a reinsurance component, to protect themselves against an employee's catastrophic medical expenses. The advantage of self-insurance is that companies are able to lower their health insurance costs since they are exempt from all state health insurance mandates, such as mandated benefits that the insurance must include, and inclusion of certain providers, such as chiropractors and faith healers.

(Because there are economies of scale in administering health insurance and larger employer groups are more likely than smaller firms to self-insure [a substitute available to them], larger groups receive lower insurance prices [loading charges] than smaller firms.)

Thus the health insurance market consists of the commercial insurers' indemnity plan, based on fee-for-service payment, service benefit plans (BCBS), HMOs, PPOs, and self-insured companies. Fee-for-service plans are predominately managed care, since they include utilization review mechanisms. In addition to their own plans, commercial insurers and BCBS also market HMOs, PPOs, and ASO contracts to employers who are self-insured. There are also independent TPAs, HMOs, and PPOs who market their services directly to employers.

The "product," health insurance, differs both according to "real" characteristics, such as type of coverage, patient cost-sharing arrangements, methods of claims payment, and the provider panel, as well as according to perceived differences in product, such as reputation for payment of claims. We would therefore expect to observe premium differences between insurance firms in accordance with these product differences. If the price of insurance differs between firms by a greater amount than what is justified by product differences, we would expect groups of insured persons to switch their insurance coverage.

Insurance companies will therefore compete among themselves for the insured population on the basis of price as well as in terms of product differences. If insured groups move between insurance firms according to differences in prices and products, the market will perform in an efficient manner. The "product" will be expected to change over time and also to conform more closely to the preferences of the insured group.[1] If additional firms selling insurance enter the industry, we would expect the resulting price competition to bring the price of insurance (the loading charge) relatively close to the pure premium; that is, the cost of administration, claims processing, and marketing functions would be produced efficiently and there would be no excess profits in the industry. (The more price elastic the demand curve facing the individual insurance firm, the closer the price will be to average costs; there will also be less likelihood of excess profits in the long run.)

The efficient performance of this industry is not contingent on each consumer's having perfect information regarding all the price and product differences among firms. The costs of acquiring such information are clearly too great for an individual; however, large groups, such as those with employee benefit managers, would be expected to develop such expertise. Also, since approximately 85 percent of private insurance is purchased by groups, it is the information acquired by these groups that brings about competition among insurance firms. The behavior of these informed groups will be sufficient to produce a more competitive rate structure for all groups. However, because such information is costly to acquire, we might also expect the product and price differences to be more favorable to large groups that acquire it.

Given the wide varieties of health insurance available to purchasers of health insurance, namely, individuals (representing about 15 percent of the private health insurance market) and groups (85 percent), both large and small, each type of health insurance has relatively good substitutes. As will be discussed below, how good a substitute one type of insurance is for another depends on how large a price increase by one insurer causes enrollees to shift, either to competitors offering the same type of insurance or to a different type of health insurance.

Regardless of how responsive the overall market demand for health insurance may be to the price of insurance, the demand curve facing each firm is more price elastic than the aggregate demand for insurance. The simple reason is that while there are fewer substitutes for health insurance, there are good substitutes available for any one firm selling insurance. To the extent that there are good substitutes for each insurer's plan and the different types of health plans are considered by purchasers to be good substitutes for one

---

[1]Since there are such large differences in the costs of handling a group and an individual, we would expect that most individuals in a group would prefer to forgo the benefits of individually tailored policies to take advantage of the lower cost of a single group policy.

another, then the demand curve facing each health insurer is very price elastic. With a highly price elastic demand curve, a firm will be unable to increase its premiums, relative to other firms, without losing sufficiently large market share to make the price increase unprofitable.

Important to determining the number of competing firms as well as the different types of health insurance marketed is the industry's market structure.

THE SUPPLY SIDE
OF THE HEALTH INSURANCE MARKET

The market structure of the health insurance market is determined by economies of scale, any barriers to entry into the market, whether any firms have cost advantages over other firms, and whether there are regulations inhibiting competition among firms.

Economies of Scale

Economies of scale, given the size of the market for health insurance, determine how many firms can compete in the sale of insurance. Economies of scale will also indicate whether the insurance business is a "natural" monopoly; that is, can the functions performed by insurance companies be performed less expensively by just one firm? (Another aspect of efficiency in production concerns whether each firm is itself operating in the most efficient manner.)

It has been difficult to separately estimate the extent of economies of scale in supplying health insurance from differences in the firm's efficiency and the functions it performs. Many companies differ in the administrative functions they perform, and they do not perform them equally well. The range of administrative functions includes marketing and selling policies, processing applications and policies, maintaining the policy file, processing claims, reviewing claims, and paying claims. The variety of contracts offered, each entailing a different cost, and the extent to which the company has group or individual policies (it is more costly to handle individual policies) also differ among firms.

Several studies have attempted to empirically estimate the extent of economies of scale among different health insurance carriers. Using data from the early 1970s, Vogel and Blair examined economies of scale for commercial health insurance companies only, since their output mix (e.g., variety of contracts, percentage of nongroup policies, etc.) was so different from that of Blue Cross. The authors determined that economies of scale do exist and that the administrative cost ratio declines with increased size of operation. When economies of scale were investigated separately for Blue Cross and for Blue Shield (in their non-Medicare business), no economies of scale were found. The authors then included in their analysis BCBS plans that had merged. They observed lower administrative costs for these merged, larger firms. Based on these studies, the authors concluded that economies of scale do exist in the nonprofit sector, although the gains from such economies are offset by internal inefficiency ("x-inefficiency") because they are nonprofit firms (2).

In a follow-up study, Blair and Vogel undertook a "survivors" analysis to test for economies of scale among health insurers (3). In this type of analysis, firms are assigned to different categories according to their size. The growth of firms in each size category is studied over time. If substantial economies of scale exist, then firms in the largest classes will grow rapidly at the expense of firms in the smaller size categories. Smaller firms will either have to expand their scale of operation (and/or merge) or they will be forced to leave the industry. The authors found that all but the smallest size categories expanded over the 1958–73 period. They concluded that economies of scale existed but that they were not as large as originally believed, since other size categories also grew.

The authors also attempted to determine whether economies of scale exist in the administration of Medicare Part A (hospital claims payment). They found results opposite of what they expected. Administrative costs per claim increased with the size of the firm. The interpretation of this finding was that the cost-based method used by Medicare to pay intermediaries encouraged higher administrative costs (4). An experiment in which the government awarded Medicare Part B contracts on the basis of a competitive bid found that submitted bids were quite low relative to their historical cost and lower than carriers reimbursed on a cost basis (5). Sizable savings to the government are possible if Medicare intermediaries were chosen and paid according to a competitive bid rather than the current cost-based payment system. Intermediaries would have a greater incentive to be internally efficient as well as to take advantage of economies of scale.

Even though economies of scale exist in the insurance industry, as indicated by the above studies, and there are financial requirements for becoming a supplier of health insurance, such as minimum reserve requirements, given the very large size of the market, there can be a sufficient number of firms for the industry to be competitive. A firm selling health insurance in one city can easily market its product in another city while centralizing all other administrative functions. There are over one thousand for-profit commercial health insurers and more than sixty Blue Cross and Blue Shield plans.

Blue Cross and Blue Shield Cost Advantages

Differences in costs between firms, unrelated to their efficiency, have, however, given some types of firms a competitive advantage over other firms, thereby affecting the industry's structure. Blue Cross and Blue Shield plans received two important cost advantages over commercial insurers that enabled them to increase their market shares at the expense of their competitors.

Favorable Tax Treatment

Because Blue Cross plans were nonprofit, they were exempt from both federal and state premium taxes. On average, commercial insurers pay a 2 percent state tax on their total premiums. However, since administrative expenses are typically 10 percent of premiums, 2 percent of total premiums is equal to 20 percent of administrative expenses. Thus the Blues' tax exemption was a significant portion of administrative expenses. Studies have found that the competitive advantage of the Blues' exemption from state premium taxes enabled Blue Cross to increase its market share between 1 and 6.7 percent (6).

In return for such favorable tax treatment, however, the Blues have been subject to greater regulation by state insurance commissioners, who must approve their premium increases. Several states have limited premium increases that the Blues wanted to charge their nongroup (individual) enrollees, which the Blues claim have caused them to lose money on this line of business. To escape such regulation, a number of Blue Cross plans have converted to mutual insurance companies.

The Blues lost their federal (but not state) tax-exempt status under the 1986 tax reform legislation. A Government Accounting Office (GAO) report found that the pricing practices of the Blues were similar to those of the commercials, namely, experience rating of large groups; there were few subsidies for high-risk individuals enrolling in the Blues; the Blues had profit-making subsidiaries; and "all these activities tend to reinforce the perception that the plans are similar to commercial companies" (7).

The Blue Cross Hospital Discount

The second, and perhaps more important, competitive advantage that Blue Cross had over commercial insurers is that Blue Cross received a discount from hospital charges that was not available to commercial companies for the same care in the same institution. The size of the hospital discount to Blue Cross was as high as 27 percent in some states. According to one study, this greater discount for the Blues resulted in an average increase in their market share of 7 percent (8).

The competitive consequences of Blue Cross' cost advantages were as follows. A firm in a competitive market with a cost advantage could undercut the prices of other firms and drive them from the market. If this were to occur, the public would benefit from that cost reduction in terms of lower prices. However, researchers found that BCBS plans having a cost advantage were able to increase their market shares, but not to the extent thought possible. The researchers developed several hypotheses as to how Blue Cross plans used their competitive advantage.

Because the Blues were controlled by the hospitals, it was in the hospitals' interest to provide the Blues with a competitive cost advantage, namely, a discount (9). In this way the price of Blue Cross coverage was lowered relative to commercial insurance. Hospitals benefited by assisting the growth of a more expensive type of hospital coverage. Hospitals were consequently able to increase their costs and charges faster than they would have otherwise.

Weller distinguishes between discounts that are procompetitive (i.e., a firm is a tough bargainer and tries to get the lowest price possible from its suppliers) and discounts that are anticompetitive (i.e., a supplier gives a favored purchaser a preferential price). Based on the findings that Blue Cross plans were started and controlled by hospitals and that those Blue Cross plans with relatively high market shares were also in areas where hospital costs were relatively high, Weller concluded that the hospital discount could be explained more adequately in terms of anticompetitive behavior on the part of hospitals (10).

Another study concluded that in addition to benefiting hospitals, the Blue plans were less efficient. Thus their cost advantage was also used to benefit their management and employees, in terms of higher salaries and internal "slack" within the organization (11).

Blue Cross plans are no longer controlled by hospitals. As Blue Cross competes with other insurers, hospitals and Blue Cross have developed an adversarial relationship. However, even if the cost advantages that led to such a large share were removed, the large market share of the Blues still provide those Blue plans with increased market power, hence a competitive advantage (12). A Blue Cross plan that is the dominant insurer in an area is able to extract a discount from hospitals because of its purchasing power than is an insurer with a small market share. The hospital must continue to give a discount to a dominant insurer if it is not to suffer large losses of patients to competitive hospitals.

A recent study finds that the Blues are using their large market share (monopsony power) to extract greater price concessions from hospitals and that in the current price competitive health insurance market, these reduced input costs are being passed on to employer groups as reduced premiums (13).

Blue Cross is a loose federation of independently operating plans joined together by an interplan system for handling claims incurred in other areas. The national Blue Cross organization provides certain important functions, such as representing all Blue Cross plans in their relations with the federal government and testifying on legislation affecting the health insurance industry. Each Blue Cross and Blue Shield plan had a monopoly within its market over its type of service.[2] Blue Cross plans did not compete with one another as did commercial insurers. If one Blue Cross firm was more efficient and wished to expand its market, it could not enter another Blue Cross plan's area. Each Blue Cross plan benefited by being the designated representative of Blue Cross's reputation and by being the only one to offer the Blue Cross insurance package to subscribers. Commercial companies, on the other hand, competed with one another as well as with Blue Cross.

Current competitive pressures in the insurance market and the consequent separation of hospitals' and Blue Cross' interests have resulted in Blue plans competing with one another and entering each other's markets, such as in Ohio. Such competitive behavior was initially opposed by the national Blue Cross organization, which owns the Blue Cross trademark and licenses other plans to use it. However, given the applicability of the anti-

---

[2]Each Blue Cross plan was required to sign up 75 percent of the hospitals and beds in its area. M. Olson claims that "this requirement ensured that no Blue Cross plan could select only the most efficient hospitals in its area. Its effect was to reduce competitive pressures on less efficient hospitals." Mancur Olson, "Introduction," in Mancur Olson, ed., *A New Approach to the Economics of Health Care* (Washington, D.C.: American Enterprise Institute, 1981), p. 10.

trust laws to the health field, Blue Cross plans can no longer divide up markets among themselves. Competition among Blue Cross plans is increasing and making the insurance industry still more competitive.

The structural aspects of the insurance market have affected competition among insurers. While there are economies of scale in the production of health insurance, given the size of the insurance market, there are a sufficient number of insurers to make the health insurance market quite competitive. Blue Cross, however, has received preferential tax exemptions and hospital discounts, two artificial cost advantages over commercial insurers that have provided them with competitive advantages. These cost advantages have provided the Blues with greater market shares than they might otherwise have had, their hospitals with more advantageous benefits, as well as benefiting Blue Cross management. Had it not been for their relatively greater administrative inefficiency and their more costly hospital benefit package, the commercial insurers would have suffered an even greater loss of market share.

Table 8.1 shows the population covered and relative market shares both over time and by type of carrier. While the overall market share of commercial insurers is greater than Blue Cross and Blue Shield, in any one market these data may be misleading. Within any one market there are usually several commercial insurers, but generally only one Blue Cross and Blue Shield plan. Thus, particularly in the Northeast and Midwest, the Blue plans have a much larger market share than any one commercial insurer; in a number of states their market share exceeds those of all the commercial insurers. (It was not possible to separate out duplicate coverage among commercials, BCBS, and independent plans. An employer that self-insures, for example, may use an insurance company to administer their claims processing [ASO contract]; this would show up as an increase in independent plans as well as insurer's market share.)

Of interest in Table 8.1 is the dramatic changes in market shares by type of insurance company. Independent plans, which include HMOs, company self-insurance plans, and administrative service contracts only, increased their share of the market from 5 percent in 1970 to 65 percent in 1995; this increased growth came at the expense of traditional indemnity plans and Blue Cross, which have lost market share. The decline in market shares of BCBS plans has been dramatic.

INDUSTRY CONDUCT AND COMPETITIVE BEHAVIOR

When HMOs began to enter the group health insurance market in the early to mid-1980s, they set their premiums just below the premiums charged by traditional insurers. This practice was referred to as "shadow pricing." At the time, most (if not all) of the premium was paid by the employer on behalf of the employee. When the employee did pay part of the premium, it was not related to cost differences between different health plans. The employees' choice of health plan was therefore unaffected by differences in prices between health plans. To compete against the traditional plan, which offered unlimited

TABLE 8.1 Enrollment of Persons with Hospital Expense Protection, 1950–95

	Net Number of Persons Insured			Gross Number of Persons Insured		
Year	Civilian Population (Thousands)	Total Number (Thousands)[a]	Percent of Population	Commercial Insurance Percent of Total[a]	Blue Cross-Blue Shield Percent of Total	Independent Plans Percent of Total[b]
1950	150,790	76,600	50.8	48.3	50.7	5.7
1955	162,967	101,400	62.2	52.8	50.0	6.4
1960	178,140	122,500	68.8	56.5	47.4	4.9
1965	191,605	138,700	72.4	55.9	45.6	5.0
1970	201,895	158,800	78.7	56.5	47.3	5.1
1975	213,789	178,200	83.4	55.8	48.5	7.4
1980	225,621	187,400	83.0	56.3	46.3	17.7
1985	236,219	181,300	76.8	55.4	43.4	30.4[c]
1990	247,763	181,700	73.3	45.7	39.0	47.4[c]
1995	251,538	185,300	70.9	41.3	35.4	64.8[c,d]

Sources: *Book of Health Insurance Data—1997–98* (Washington, D.C.: Health Insurance Association of America, 1997), p. 39, Table 2.10; U.S. Bureau of the Census, Statistical Abstract of the United States, 1997, 117th ed. (Washington, D.C.: U.S. Department of Commerce, 1997–98), p. 8, Table 2.

[a] The data in this column refer to the net total of persons protected, that is, duplication among persons protected by more than one kind of insuring organization or more than one insurance company policy providing the same type of coverage has been eliminated. Included in the BCBS and commercial percentages are administrative services only (ASO) agreements and their sponsorship of HMOs and PPOs, which are also counted as independent plans.

[b] "Independent plans" includes self-insured plans, plans employing third-party administrators, and HMOs.

[c] For 1984 and later, estimates of persons covered by "independent plans" have been developed by HIAA in the absence of other available data.

[d] In 1995, within independent plans, the 64.8 percent is comprised of HMOs, 32 percent, and self-insured, 33 percent. This is an increase from 1990 when the 47.4 percent was comprised of HMOs, 20 percent, and self-insured, 27.4 percent.

choice of provider, HMOs, with their restricted provider panels, offered more benefits. Although the HMO had a lower cost of providing care, it still charged premiums that were only slightly below those of the non-HMO health plans. The difference between their premiums and costs of care were used to provide the employee with greater benefits and increase the HMOs' profits.

Employers initially believed that offering an HMO option to their employees would reduce insurance premiums because the HMO's lower cost would be passed on to the employer. However, this did not occur because the HMOs used shadow pricing. To receive the cost savings resulting from managed care and the employees' use of a restricted provider panel, employers turned to PPOs. PPO providers were paid fee-for-service; thus employers believed that the price discounts and lower use rates of their employees would result in lower claims expense, hence lower insurance premiums.

The rapid growth in HMOs did not occur until employers received some of the savings in the form of lower premiums and/or employees became responsible for paying the difference between the lowest-cost plan and the plan they chose.

Another form of competitive behavior engaged in by insurers as well as by HMOs was preferred risk selection. When an HMO was offered along with a traditional health plan to an employer group, at similar premiums, the traditional plan received an adverse risk group. HMOs were able to attract a lower-risk group of employees through design of their benefit package (e.g., emphasizing well baby care). Also, those who were at higher risk or who were ill wanted to continue with their own physicians, rather than switch to the HMOs' restricted provider panel. It was for this reason that traditional health plans, when offered along with HMOs, wanted to be assured that they would receive a minimum percent of the employees in a group (e.g., 50 percent of the employees). Alternatively, the insurer would offer the employer a choice of different plans, managed fee-for-service and an HMO, at the same premium for each age-sex risk group, and the insurer would then make the monetary transfers between its own plans. Similarly, to internalize the cost of adverse selection to the non-HMO plan, when a single HMO is offered to an employee group, the HMO also offers a non-HMO product along with their HMO, for the same premium, so as to provide an employee group with more choices.

There are subtle methods by which a health insurer can achieve a preferred (low) risk group when the premiums of the different risk groups are not risk-adjusted. The plan can contract with new specialists compared to specialists who have been in practice longer (and whose chronically ill patients would follow them into the health plan). The health plan can advertise in newspapers rather than keeping brochures in physicians' offices, where the population reading them are, on average, sicker than those who read the newspaper. And waiting rooms for pediatric patients can be attractive and waiting times short, compared to waiting times and access to referrals for chronically ill patients.

Various methods have been proposed to reduce risk selection through the use of risk-adjusted premiums. Risk adjustments can be up-front, in that the premium is adjusted to reflect the characteristics of the group insured, or it can be retrospective, whereby monetary transfers are made among health plans based on their claims experience.

To date, risk-adjusted premiums have not been widely used by employers. (Nor have they been used by medical groups accepting subcapitation payments from HMOs.) Medicare pays HMOs a risk-adjusted premium for those aged who join an HMO. However, the risk factors used by Medicare have been insufficient to fully account for the preferred risk group received by HMOs. Risk adjustment is an area that is receiving a great deal of attention and research funding.

Risk-adjusted premiums would reduce competition among insurers to select preferred risks. Risk-adjusted premiums would incentivize insurers to compete on their administrative expense (loading charge) and on how well they manage risk. Risk-adjusted premiums provide efficient insurers with an incentive to accept high-risk patients. A risk-adjusted premium that fairly reflects the expected expense of high-risk patients provides insurers with an incentive to innovate and to manage the care of high-risk patients.

THE PERFORMANCE
OF THE HEALTH INSURANCE MARKET

The health insurance industry is a supplier of insurance and a demander of medical services; it thus operates in two different markets. (An HMO that has its own hospitals and physicians can be similarly analyzed as a competitor against other insurers and as a delivery system competing against other providers.) As a supplier of health insurance, insurers can be a price-competitive industry even though the markets in which they purchase medical services may be monopolistic. To the extent that the medical services market is not price-competitive, then that part of the insurance premium that goes for claims expenses will be higher. Subsequent chapters examine the competitiveness of different provider and manpower markets. The competitiveness of provider markets, however, does affect the cost of medical services and the types of products that health insurers can market.

Figure 8.1 illustrates the separate components of the health insurance premium. The loading charge, which includes administrative and claims-processing costs, marketing expense, reserves against losses, and profits, represents approximately 8 percent of the premium when insurance is sold to groups. (When sold to the individual market, the loading charge is much higher, reflecting higher marketing costs and higher reserves.) The claims expense is affected by risk factors of the group, such as age and sex of the employees, the type of industry (e.g., construction workers or accountants), location (to reflect medical costs in that region), the benefit package desired by the employees, the medical inflation rate in the coming year, and which cost containment policies, such as the size of the deductible, are included in the benefit package.

The size of the loading charge is related to the various cost containment options. Cost containment policies increase administrative expense while reducing claims expenses. Unless the additional cost of cost containment is less than the savings from reduced claims expense, these policies would not be undertaken. Thus higher administrative expenses of managed care companies are not necessarily an indication of inefficiency.

Price competition among traditional insurers reflected competition over the size of the loading charge. Actuaries estimated the expected claims expense, given the above risk factors of the group, the group's location, benefits, and so on. Insurers had an incentive to minimize their loading charge and to also compete on risk selection—selecting lower-risk enrollees to lower their claims expense. If insurer risk selection were minimized (through use of risk-adjusted premiums), then price competition among insurers would be based on how well they are able to reduce the loading charge and on how well they can manage risk, that is, use those institutional settings and medical practices that are most appropriate, thereby reducing the costs of caring for sick patients.

Competition among health insurers until the early to mid-1980s was based on their premiums, the most important component being the size of the loading charge, and risk selection. Cost containment measures such as utilization review and PPOs were viewed as an intrusion into the practice of medicine by the medical profession.

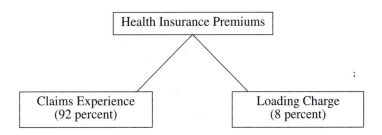

FIGURE 8.1 • The determinants of health insurance premiums.

The introduction of utilization management and the use of provider panels dramatically changed the role of health insurers with regard to the practice of medicine. Insurers no longer passively accepted physicians' treatment decisions. Instead they established practice guidelines and reviewed physicians' medical decisions. Provider panels affected the patient's choice of provider. This change in the insurers' role did not (and was not able to) occur until the anti-trust laws became applicable to the medical services industry in 1982.

Thus, two important aspects of market performance to be discussed are price and product competition among insurers. Price competition among insurers reduces the loading charge and eliminates any excess profits; premiums reflect the cost of producing health insurance. Product competition forces insurers to respond to the insured population's preferences for different types of insurance. Included in the discussion of product competition is a discussion of insurers' previous inability to offer certain products, such as cost containment and risk management.

Insurer Price Competition

To provide some indication of the competitiveness of the health insurance industry, it is important to examine the pricing of health insurance policies.

The price of insurance is the benefit/premium ratio, which is the percent of the total premium paid out in benefits to each insured group. If, for example, the premium for each member in a group were $1,000 per year and the utilization experience of that group resulted in an average payout of benefits equal to $900 per member per year, the benefit/premium ratio would be 0.9. The difference between benefits and total premiums (the "loading charge") goes for administration, claims processing, marketing, and insurer profit. In a price-competitive market, each of the components of the loading charge would be efficiently produced and a competitive rate of profit would be included.

When the benefit/premium ratio is close to 1.0, the group is "experience rated," that is, the premium reflects the expected experience of the group (and the loading charge is competitively produced). The more the health insurance industry approximates a competitive industry, the closer the benefit/premium ratio would be to 1.0. In a competitive industry we would expect groups to change insurance companies when their benefit/premium ratio surpasses the amount they are willing to pay for real or perceived product differences between firms.

When information is inadequate or when monopolies exist in the sale of health insurance, there will be greater divergence from 1.0 in the benefit/premium ratio.

One indication of the performance of the industry is the variation in benefit/premium ratios when size of group is held constant; the smaller the variation, the more efficient the market. (Because of economies of scale in administering different-size groups, the larger the size of group, the closer the benefit/premium ratio would be to 1.0.)

Table 8.2 shows the ratios of expenditures (benefits) to premiums by different types of insurance plans for the 1955–95 period. Two points are of interest in this table. First, differences in the benefit/premium ratio between group and individual policies indicate the large savings to an individual from participating in a group plan. Second, the benefit/premium ratios for the Blues, commercials, and independent plans appear to follow the same underwriting cycle; these ratios rose through the 1970s and then declined throughout the 1980s (14).

The use of the benefit/premium ratio as a measure of industry performance has diminished in more recent years. Previously, when almost all health insurance consisted of indemnity plans and insurers performed only administrative tasks, the benefit/premium ratio was an indication of how much was spent on administration and how much on the delivery of medical services. With the growth of managed care and multiple types of health plans, however, the benefit/premium ratio no longer simply measures the division of medical and administrative expense (15).

Currently, a low benefit/premium ratio can indicate increased responsibility by the insurer for medical management functions, such as utilization review, quality assurance, and provider profiling, functions that have as their purpose lower medical costs. Further, health plans today offer a variety of products, from indemnity, to closed panels of providers, an HMO option, an open-ended HMO (where the patient can use non-HMO providers and pay a percent of the charge), as well as a variety of pharmacy benefits for the different health plans, life and disability insurance, dental plans, and mental

TABLE 8.2 Ratio of Benefit Expenditures to Premium Income, According to Type of Plan, 1955–95

Year	All Plans	Blue Cross-Blue Shield	Commercial Insurance Companies			
			Total	Group Policies	Individual Policies	Independent Plans[a]
1955	0.721	0.933	0.725	0.839	0.530	0.912
1960	0.760	0.929	0.789	0.904	0.529	0.965
1965	0.793	0.938	0.819	0.936	0.547	0.906
1970	0.860	0.964	0.872	0.958	0.581	0.962
1975	0.868	0.960	0.886	0.984	0.511	0.867
1980	0.901	0.970	0.847	0.897	0.580	0.936
1985	0.843	0.904	0.798	0.834	0.583	0.886
1990	0.886	0.893	0.819	0.842	0.646	0.899
1995	0.877	0.887	0.822	0.843	0.686	0.929

Sources: Numbers for commercial insurance companies and independent plans, 1955–75, were developed from data provided in Marjorie Smith Carroll and Ross H. Arnett, "Private Health Insurance Plans in 1978 and 1979: A Review of Coverage, Enrollment and Financial Experience," *Health Care Financing Review,* 3(1), September 1981: 55–88. The remainder of the data (All Plans, Blue Cross and Blue Shield, and the data for 1980–95) comes from *Source Book of Health Insurance Data—1997–98* (Washington, D.C.: Health Insurance Association of America, 1997), pp. 42–48, Tables 2.13, 2.18.

[a] "Independent plans" include plans that offer health services on a prepaid basis and self-insured health plans.

benefits. This greater range of products and benefits has increased the administrative and marketing cost to the insurer. (These are not wasteful expenditures since they are in response to purchaser demands.) Similarly, insurers differ in their percentage of individual, small group, and large employer enrollees, which affect their marketing and enrollment costs.

The relative closeness of these ratios between the different insurers and to a benefit/premium ratio of 1, suggests that this has been a relatively price-competitive industry. More recently, however, measures other than the benefit/premium ratio, discussed below, are more indicative of the price competitiveness of this industry.

Price Sensitivity among Health Plans

A second indication (in addition to the benefit/premium ratio) of the price competitiveness of the health insurance industry is consumers' willingness to switch health plans in response to changes in their out-of-pocket premiums.

In a typical large employer setting, employees have a choice of several health plans and are able to change health plans during open enrollment periods. Once enrolled in a health plan, there are switching "costs" of changing plans. The employee has to learn more about the other health plans and their provider networks, and possibly establish a relationship with a new provider. If switching costs are sufficiently high, employees may remain in a plan even if their monthly out-of-pocket premium (co-premium) has increased relative to the co-premiums of alternative plans. High switching costs would therefore limit price competition among health plans.

The importance of a change in relative co-premiums on employee switching behavior was recently studied (16). In 1994, the University of California, a large employer, changed the method by which it contributed to its employees' health plan premiums. At each of the university's nine campuses, there were two fee-for-service plans (a "high option" indemnity plan and a PPO) and several HMOs. Prior to 1994, the university had paid the full premium for most plans and subsidized the cost of the most expensive plans. In 1994, the university limited its contribution to the cost of the least expensive plan; employees had to pay the additional cost (co-premium) of more expensive plans.

The change in employee contributions for their health plans between 1993 and 1994 provided a natural experiment to measure the impact of price on switching of health plans. Table 8.3 shows that 50 percent of those who had to pay for a fee-for-service plan switched plans. One-half of those switching joined a free HMO while the remainder joined a free fee-for-service plan. With regard to the HMOs, 30 percent of those in HMOs that required a co-premium switched, predominately to a free HMO.

To determine the relationship between the size of the co-premium and the likelihood

TABLE 8.3 Plan Switching by Type of Plan

	FFS Plans		HMO Plans	
	Free	Pay	Free	Pay
Number of employees (1993)	7,139	9,928	4,4854	12,573
Percent not switching plans	94.21	49.88	95.40	69.70
Percent switching into . . .				
a free FFS plan	—	25.30	2.49	1.30
		[50.48]	[54.19]	[4.30]
a pay FFS plan	0.15	—	0.07	0.11
	[2.66]	—	[1.55]	[0.37]
a free HMO	5.00	22.93	1.69	28.42
	[86.44]	[45.74]	[36.69]	[93.57]
a pay HMO	0.63	1.79	0.35	0.35
	[10.90]	[3.58]	[7.56]	[1.76]

Source: T. C. Buchmueller and P. J. Feldstein, "The Effect of Price Switching among Health Plans," *Journal of Health Economics,* 16(2), 1997: 231–247.

Note: Figures in brackets represent the percentage of switchers in each column choosing each type of plan. Pay and free plans are defined respectively as plans requiring and not requiring a monthly employee premium in 1994. Monthly premiums increased between 1993 and 1994 for all pay plans, and were constant (at zero) for all free plans.

that employees would switch plans, a multivariate analysis was undertaken that held constant the employee's age, income, length of time in the plan, and so on. Based on those results, Table 8.4 was constructed, which shows the probability of switching at higher co-premiums. Thus, with no change in relative premiums, for various reasons 5 percent of enrollees switch each year. With a co-premium up to $10 a month (and a free plan available), 26 percent of the enrollees would be expected to switch health plans. With a co-premium up to $20 a month, 30 percent would switch (34 percent of those in HMOs would switch). With a co-premium up to $30 a month, 42.5 percent of those in an HMO would switch to a free HMO.

This study shows that relatively small co-premiums have a large effect on the probability of switching health plans. The high price sensitivity of health plan choice found in the above study is supported by other studies, one of which found the cross-price elasticity of a health plan's demand curve to be −7.9 (17).

These findings indicate that the demand curve facing the individual health plan is very price elastic; small relative price increases will cause much greater percentage decreases in their enrollment, making such price increases unprofitable.

A further indication of the insurance industry's price competitiveness was the approach used by Blue Cross for many years to price its insurance coverage (community rating) and how market forces caused a change in that approach.

The Efficiency and Equity Aspects of Community Rating

Proposals have been made at both the federal and state levels to require health insurers to use "community rating" as a basis for establishing health insurance premiums. Community rating, as contrasted to experience rating, charges subscribers the same premium, regardless of the experience or risk factors, that is, age and sex, of the group.

An early example of the use (and consequences) of community rating was by Blue Cross. Aged persons, who had much higher hospital use rates than younger persons, were

TABLE 8.4 Simulated Probability of Switching Plans in Response to Various Premium Increases

	All Plans, All Coverage	HMOs Only, All Coverage
Probability of switching if . . .		
ΔPREM = 0	0.052	0.052
ΔPREM = 10	0.264	0.251
ΔPREM = 20	0.296	0.341
ΔPREM = 30	0.329	0.425

Source: T. C. Buchmueller and P. J. Feldstein, 1997, "The Effect of Price Switching among Health Plans," *Journal of Health Economics,* 16(2), 1997: 231–247.

charged the *same premium.*[3] The benefit/premium ratio for aged persons was, therefore, greater than 1.0; the benefits paid on their behalf exceeded the premiums they paid for insurance. Since the average benefit/premium ratio for all groups in a community rating system had to be close to 1.0, this meant that low users of hospital services had benefit/premium ratios much less than 1.0.

The effect of community rating, when the expected costs of groups differ, is that a subsidy is provided to high-use groups, financed by a (regressive) "tax" on lower-use groups. A large intergenerational transfer would be expected to occur, wherein younger age groups subsidize older age groups, who have higher use rates (18). Any such "subsidy-tax" system can be evaluated on the basis of two economic criteria: (a) its effect on efficiency—namely, does it affect the quantity of health insurance purchased? and (b) its equity—does such a redistribution scheme cause higher-income subscribers to subsidize lower-income subscribers?

With regard to the efficiency aspects of community rating, low-user groups are typically low-risk groups. There is a certain amount above the pure premium that an individual is willing to pay for health insurance. Charging low-risk groups a much greater amount above their pure premium than if they were experience-rated results in fewer low-user groups purchasing insurance. Low-user groups might decide that they would be better off if they self-insured (no insurance) rather than pay the community rate. Depending on the price elasticity of demand for insurance, low-user groups would demand less insurance under community rating.

Similar to an excise tax that is placed on some goods and services and hence distorts their relative prices, a community rate is a tax on the insurance premium of a low-risk person. The result of such a "tax" is a decreased demand for health insurance coverage. Changing from a community rating system to one based on experience rating should result in the low-risk group's purchasing more health insurance. It is for this reason that community rating is considered economically inefficient. (A similar inefficiency occurs when a monopolist charges a price for a service that exceeds its cost of production.)

Community rating does not permit low-risk groups to purchase insurance at its costs of production, which is its actuarial value plus administrative cost.

Community rating is also inefficient because it subsidizes and therefore increases unhealthy lifestyle behavior. As long as there is some price elasticity to unhealthy lifestyles, community rating removes the financial incentive to reduce such activities, such as smoking, being overweight, having high blood pressure, and so on. Further, community rating decreases an employer's incentive to undertake risk-reducing behavior among its employees for the purpose of reducing both the employer's and employees' medical expenses.

Perhaps the main reason for community rating, according to its advocates, is that it

---

[3]Even under community rating, however, premiums differed according to whether the individual was married or single and whether he belonged to a group.

enables those who would otherwise not be able to afford health insurance to pay the premium. Without relying on government subsidies, community rating subsidized high-risk (presumably low-income) persons by taxing low-risk (presumably higher-income persons).[4] However, community rating not only is an inefficient mechanism for redistributing medical care but it has contrary redistributive effects.

Using risk factors such as age and sex as a basis for determining a medical insurance subsidy assumes that all high-risk people have lower incomes than low-risk people. However, many older people have higher incomes than those who are younger. The direction of the subsidy, however, goes from the younger (low-risk) to the older (high-risk) person, regardless of their relative incomes. Further, the actual subsidy goes to the group that *uses* more medical services, not necessarily to the group that has the highest risk of hospitalization.

Empirical studies document the unintended redistributive effects of community rating (19). A study of Michigan Blue Cross revealed that under community rating the most heavily subsidized group were auto workers. The next most heavily subsidized group was comprised of health care professionals—physicians, nurses, and other hospital employees. These subsidized groups had higher than average incomes. What occurred under community rating was that the subsidy-tax concept operated in reverse: higher-income persons were subsidized by lower-income persons. Similarly, if community rating were to be geographically based, then there would be unintended wealth transfers from poorer, rural communities to wealthier, urban communities that have higher health care expenditures.

If everyone agreed on the value judgment that subsidies should be provided to lower-income families to purchase health insurance, these values could be realized more efficiently through a system of direct subsidies to those families instead of attempting such redistribution indirectly through community rating.[5]

The community rating concept was inefficient because it raised the price of health insurance to low-user groups, thereby decreasing their demand for health insurance. Their demand for health insurance was less than if they had been experience-rated. Community

---

[4]An additional reason suggested for community rating is that it is insurance with a longer time horizon. Since everyone grows old, the young (low-risk) who subsidize the aged eventually receive such a subsidy themselves. However, when the premium (based on average risk) exceeds what a low-risk premium would cost, low-risk individuals would buy less insurance. Subsidized high-risk individuals would buy more insurance. This is inefficient (one cannot purchase insurance at the cost of producing it) as well as being an unstable situation; it therefore could not exist in a price-competitive insurance market. Instead, it would be more equitable to vary the insurance premium over time according to age, since age (a proxy for risk) is highly correlated with income and assets. Thus an age-adjusted premium would be more equitable over time than community rating.

[5]Blue Cross' goals did not include being the most efficient welfare agent. Instead, Blue Cross may have attempted to increase its enrollment, and in so doing, allocated its taxes and subsidies according to a policy that facilitated the greatest increase in its growth. This policy would result in charging lower premiums to groups whose demands are more elastic, such as large unions, and higher premiums to groups with less elastic demands, instead of matching the subsidy to income level.

rating was also an inefficient method of distributing subsidies for the purchase of health insurance.

Community rating, as a pricing system for health insurance, could not survive in a price-competitive market. For community rating to have survived as long as it did was an indication of Blue Cross' market power. Competitive forces would cause insurance premiums to become experience-rated. Competitors would sell health insurance to lower-user groups at a price that approximated their expected experience rate. As low-user groups switched their insurance coverage, the community-rated premium to the remaining subscribers would increase, in turn causing additional groups that were subsidizing others to change their insurance coverage. As expected, Blue Cross abandoned community rating as competition from commercial insurance companies increased.

Since community rating cannot be instituted by a single insurer in a competitive market, its advocates have attempted to legally mandate community rating. President Clinton's 1993 plan for health reform, which was rejected by Congress, included such a proposal. However, additional empirical evidence of its consequences is provided by the experience of New York State, which enacted community rating that took effect April 1993.

New York health insurers were required to offer a community rate regardless of age or medical condition. The effect was predictable. Large numbers of young healthy people dropped their coverage as their rates increased; some insurers increased their rates as high as 79 percent (20). The insurance pool began to consist of a greater number of older, sicker persons. The average age of policyholders increased as did the average claim expense, which, for some insurers, doubled. (The cost of an average claim increased 46 percent for the individual market.) As a result, the community-rated premium was expected to further rise, continuing the process. An important consequence of this legislation was that the total number of insured persons *decreased,* increasing the number of uninsured by four hundred thousand.

Legally mandating community rating eventually results in insurers engaging in preferred risk selection. If the benefits coverage is not mandated along with community rating, then insurers would compete for low-risk groups by structuring their benefits accordingly (e.g., including higher deductibles, emphasizing wellness programs, and deemphasizing chronic care specialists). It is more likely that along with community rating a standard benefit package would also be mandated. However, insurers could still attempt to enroll low-risk groups according to where they locate their providers, the services they emphasize, and access to referrals for specialists. An additional problem with mandating a standard benefits package is that subscribers have different preferences regarding the benefits they are willing to purchase and the size of the deductible and co-payment desired (both of which determine their premium).

Maintaining a community rate with a single set of benefits, when subscribers differ in their utilization experience and in their preference for benefits and cost sharing, is highly inefficient. Diversity in consumer preferences can be dealt with most efficiently by a health insurance system that offers a variety of benefits, cost-sharing arrangements, and rate structures. If it is determined that the members of certain groups have incomes that are inadequate to purchase a "minimum" level of health insurance, and if society desires that they should have at least a minimum level of health insurance, subsidies can be provided directly to those groups instead of mandating a community-rated insurance scheme for all persons that would subsidize higher-income persons by imposing a regressive tax on those with lower incomes.

Product Competition in the Health Insurance Market

An important factor affecting competition and performance in the health insurance market is whether insurance carriers are able to respond to consumer demands, that is, whether there are any restrictions on the products health insurers can market. In this regard, the (previous) unavailability of cost containment products is discussed.

The Previous Unavailability of Cost Containment Products

An important development that has occurred over the past decade has been the introduction of cost containment programs by the health insurance industry. Cost containment methods include utilization review, such as preauthorization prior to being admitted to a hospital, concurrent review (review of length of stay while in the hospital), second opinions for surgery, as well as HMOs, and PPOs. These cost containment approaches differ from the use of deductibles and cost sharing, which have long existed, in that these newer approaches place a third party between the traditional patient–physician relationship. The physician's decision-making authority is subject to review.

The rapid increases in medical expenditures and health insurance premiums are not a recent phenomenon. Why therefore weren't insurance companies previously more aggressive in adopting such measures in their attempts to control rising costs? One study examining the potential savings to an employer from adopting utilization review found that it was very effective in reducing hospital use and medical expenditures; the savings to cost ratio was found to be 8 to 1 (21).

One possible reason for the unavailability of such restrictive cost control insurance products was insufficient demand by the purchasers of health insurance, employers and employees. Employer-purchased health insurance is exempt from federal, state, and Social Security taxes; thus the employee does not bear the full cost of rising medical expenditures. The after-tax value of the savings to employees from more restrictive cost containment methods was too low given the high marginal income tax rates during the 1960s and 1970s. Many employees also believed that health benefits were a hard-won benefit and that restrictions on those benefits would be a "give back." Further, firms engaged in overseas competition were provided with import protection; for example, the auto companies benefited from "voluntary" quotas being placed on Japanese imports, which made it possible to pass on higher employee costs (in the form of medical care) to consumers in the form of higher auto prices. (With a less price elastic demand curve as a result of decreased availability of foreign substitutes, increased employee health costs resulted in higher auto prices; in the 1980s, with more import competition and a more elastic demand curve, increased employee medical costs caused greater decreases in production and employment, thereby increasing employer and employee concern with rising medical costs.)

While it is possible that there might not have been much demand for such restrictive approaches among firms, it is unlikely that all firms and purchasers would have been opposed to such measures. It is therefore necessary to examine supply side reasons why cost control measures were not offered.

A second explanation for the previous lack of cost control programs is that any insurer who innovated in developing such programs would be copied by other insurers. The innovator would not gain any competitive advantage and would incur costs if the innovation did not work. Similarly, if an insurance company is successful in changing the practice style of physicians, then the physicians would treat their patients from other insurers in a similar manner; the innovating insurer would incur the costs of inducing physicians to change and not receive any competitive advantage (22).

The third, and most likely, explanation for the lack of cost control methods is based on anticompetitive behavior by providers.

Health insurance consists of three components: the pooling of risks, the administration of claims, and the expense of physician and hospital services. In a competitive market, an insurance company will be able to lower its costs (hence increase its profits or lower its premiums), if, in performing the risk function, it selects preferred risks (individuals who are less costly) and if it is efficient in the administration of claims. Insurance companies would be able to reduce their costs for medical services if they are able to purchase hospital and physician services at lower prices or have their subscribers use fewer such services. Health providers have always been more concerned with the prices they received and whether controls were placed on the use of their services than on how insurance companies pool their risks and administer their claims.

Competition among insurance companies on the basis of how well they are able to reduce provider prices or utilization is contrary to the economic interests of physicians and hospitals. Blue Cross and Blue Shield plans were developed and controlled by hospitals and physicians and therefore would not be expected to engage in such cost control activities. When insurance companies did initiate such activities, physicians (and other health providers) engaged in anticompetitive behavior to prevent the insurer from continuing such actions.

During the early 1930s, insurance companies in Oregon placed restraints on physician utilization. Preauthorization of services and monitoring of claims were used. When faced with competition, the insurance companies acted to lower their costs. Physicians accepted such constraints on their behavior since it was during the Depression; physicians did not have as many patients and were unsure of their ability to collect from those they did have. Consumers benefited from these cost containment measures through lower insurance premiums. The response to this situation by the Oregon medical society was twofold: first, the society threatened physicians who participated in such insurance plans with expulsion from the medical society; and, second, the medical society started its own insurance plan. The medical society–sponsored plan did not use aggressive utilization review procedures. With the growth of their own insurance plan, physicians were encouraged to boycott other insurance plans. The effect of these policies was to increase the growth of the insurance plan sponsored by organized medicine and to cause a decline in the other insurance plans. To have physicians participate in their plans, these other plans then had to become less aggressive in their cost containment efforts (23).

Additional examples of such anticompetitive behavior were organized medicine's actions against capitated plans, such as HMOs; the Michigan State Medical Society's threat to boycott Blue Shield; and the organized refusal by the Indiana Federation of Dentists to submit radiographs to insurance companies, resulting in their losing an anti-trust case (24).

Anticompetitive actions by medical organizations made it difficult for insurers to compete by offering certain types of products that reduced medical expenses through the use of cost control methods. (Co-pays and deductibles did not interfere with physician pricing or decision making and were, therefore, acceptable to providers.) Through their anticompetitive behavior providers precluded certain types of coverage from being offered in the insurance market.

The Supreme Court's ruling in 1982 that upheld the applicability of the anti-trust laws to the health professions made such anticompetitive behavior illegal.

Throughout the 1980s, the demand for cost control methods increased among employers and employees. The reduction of federal tax rates in 1981 also served to stimulate demand for such cost containment products by decreasing the tax subsidy for more comprehensive insurance. Free of anticompetitive restraints on the types of insurance products they were able to offer, insurance companies are better able to match their insurance products to the preferences of each employer group.

Federal and State Health Insurance Regulation

Federal Legislation

In 1996, health insurance regulatory reforms were enacted at the federal level. The first (the Kassenbaum–Kennedy bill) removed certain health insurance market imperfections. Included in the legislation were *guaranteed issue,* whereby health insurers have to offer group health insurance to groups willing to purchase it. Thus insurers would not be able to deny coverage to groups they believe would be high-risk. *Guaranteed renewal* requires health insurers to renew all health insurance policies, precluding them from dropping individuals or groups who incur high medical costs. Consistent with the concept of insurance, persons who purchase insurance should not lose it once they incur a serious illness. *Portability* is important because employees are often reluctant to leave their jobs because they cannot take their health insurance with them. Under the new legislation employees are able to continue their insurance coverage if they move to another employee group or if they become self employed. *Limitations on preexisting exclusions* means that once an individual has met the (usual twelve-month) preexisting exclusion limit for any illness, an insurer cannot reimpose another twelve-month waiting period if the employee changes jobs. Employees are thus more likely to be able to change jobs without fear of being without health insurance if they or a family member have an illness.

In addition to the above, the new law expands the tax deductibility of health insurance premiums (up to 80 percent from the current 30 percent) for the self-employed by the year 2006. This will begin to eliminate an inequity that exists between the self-employed and those employed by groups, who currently receive 100 percent tax deductibility of their premiums. In 1996, Congress also enacted legislation that required insurance benefits for mental health to be equal to an employer's medical benefits. Opponents are concerned that mandating such benefit increases will raise the price and consequently decrease demand for health insurance.

State Health Insurance Regulation

States have also enacted health insurance laws. Some have improved the functioning of the insurance market, such as the establishment of high-risk pools. Others, such as mandated community rating, reduced limits on preexisting exclusion waiting periods, mandated benefits and providers, rate regulation of insurance premiums, and "any willing provider" laws, have had an adverse impact on economic efficiency.

Washington State provides an example of the equity and efficiency consequences in the individual health insurance market from eliminating the preexisting waiting period (25). In 1995, the insurance commissioner decreed that for a given period of time the twelve-month waiting period for preexisting conditions be eliminated and after that, the preexisting waiting period should only be three months. Adverse selection began. Those who were sick purchased insurance, some from their hospital beds. Those with chronic conditions left the state's high-risk pool to purchase less expensive private coverage. The insurance companies immediately filed for large rate increases for those with individual coverage as claims increased. Individuals who had insurance began to drop their coverage as their premiums increased. The demand for insurance declined further because low-risk individuals believed that they could buy insurance once they became ill, given the short waiting period. The insurance commissioner attempted to limit insurers' rate increases and lawsuits were filed by the insurers against the insurance commissioner. Health insurers who did not sell individual coverage opposed government subsidies to offset these higher claims costs since the subsidies would help their competitors who did sell individual coverage. Given the losses incurred by the insurers and the uncertainty over future rate increases, the number of insurers participating in the individual market decreased.

SUMMARY

The market structure of the health insurance industry was examined with respect to the extent of economies of scale, whether barriers to entry existed, and whether any insurers had any cost advantages over other insurers.

It appears that economies of scale do exist in the administrative function. However, large

Blue Cross and Blue Shield companies, which were less subject to competitive pressures, appear to have had internal "slack," which more than offset gains resulting from economies of scale. Therefore, if monopolies were created to administer any national health insurance scheme, either at a national or regional level, to take advantage of economies of scale, the lack of competitive pressures as a result of having a monopoly might cause administrative costs to be higher than if more firms competed against one another.

Blue Cross has benefited from several cost advantages over their commercial competitors. Many Blue plans are exempt from state premium taxes and they received a discount from hospital charges. These cost advantages, particularly the hospital discount, provided the Blues with greater market power, which enabled them to sell more comprehensive health insurance. This benefited hospitals and led to higher health care costs. The Blues themselves also benefited from these cost advantages. A firm's efficiency is affected by its objectives and the extent to which it is subject to competitive pressures. As a result of these cost advantages, the Blues' increased market power enabled them to have greater organizational slack than would have been possible in a more competitive market.

The Blues' higher market share, based on their previous preferential treatment by hospitals, has also provided them with an advantage over other insurers in today's competitive market, since their greater volume enables them to demand a greater discount from hospitals. These higher discounts also make it difficult for a new insurer to enter the market. Thus in a number of markets the Blues continue to maintain short-run competitive advantages over the commercials.

The applicability of the anti-trust laws to the health field has removed an important market imperfection affecting the type of health insurance products that insurers were permitted to sell. Previously, medical societies had been able to act anticompetitively to restrict an insurer's sale of cost control programs that interfered with physicians' decision-making authority. The previous role of providers in limiting the sale of cost control products by insurers illustrates the importance of competition in provider markets on the price and quantity of medical care. The demand for medical services and the supply of those services are linked together by the health insurance market. Thus, even if the health insurance market were competitive, restrictions in provider markets (either anticompetitive or legal) can have adverse effects on consumers.

Important to understanding the previously limited and generally ineffective approach used by Blue Cross to limit hospital expenditure increases, namely, to favor controls on increases in the number of beds, was the fact that Blue Cross was started, supported, and controlled by hospitals. Hospitals used Blue Cross as a means of increasing the demand for hospital care and of ensuring payment to hospitals for their services. As such, it was not in hospitals' interest to have Blue Cross provide any coverage to patients other than for hospitalization. Out-of-hospital coverage could serve only to decrease hospital utilization. Similarly, it was not in the interests of hospitals to have Blue Cross include any co-payments such as co-insurance, because this would provide patients with an incentive to shop around for the least costly hospital.

To compete with Blue Cross, commercial companies offered lower-priced coverage by including patient cost sharing and coverage for out-of-hospital care. Blue Cross, whose benefits were entirely for hospital care, could have kept its premiums from rising rapidly by more aggressive monitoring of hospital utilization and strict limits on how much they paid hospitals. This, would, however, have placed Blue Cross in an adversary position with the hospitals that controlled Blue Cross. Therefore, the only other cost containment approach was to control hospital utilization and costs indirectly by decreasing the availability of hospital beds in an area. Blue Cross was already committed to reimbursing hospitals for all of their beds, whether or not they were filled. If Blue Cross could prevent new hospitals from being built, Blue Cross would not be in conflict with existing hospital administrators and in that way limit hospital utilization. (Existing hospitals would further benefit since entry by new hospitals would be eliminated). Blue Cross' premium consisted of a greater portion of hospital costs than did the premiums of commercial companies; therefore, Blue Cross's premium would be reduced by a proportionately greater amount if utilization were reduced.

Increased competitive pressures among insurance companies forced Blue Cross to undertake more direct and effective cost control approaches, such as preauthorization for hospital admission, utilization review, out-of-hospital coverage, and forming hospital PPOs. These intensified competitive pressures changed Blue Cross' traditional relationship to hospitals. To survive in this new competitive environment, Blue Cross had to develop a more adversarial relationship with hospitals.

Competitive markets force insurers to minimize their administrative costs and to respond to insured groups' demands for different types of insurance coverage. The incentives inherent in such competition are more effective for achieving economic efficiency in the demand and supply of health insurance than having one large firm administer a standard insurance policy for everyone. Innovations in benefit packages and in cost minimization are more likely to occur when there are strong competitive pressures than when firms, whether they are for-profit or nonprofit, are protected from such competition.

Blue Cross was established by hospitals and grew at a rapid rate because it was able to see the vast potential demand for coverage of health care costs. The commercial insurance companies, entering the market after Blue Cross, also grew, because of their product and pricing innovations. They offered a benefit coverage (major medical insurance) that was different from that offered by Blue Cross, they offered indemnity payments rather than a service benefit policy to subscribers and providers, and they priced their premiums according to the experience of the group. The newest entrants, HMOs and PPOs, were a response to market demand for lower premiums that was not being met by the traditional insurers. Unless competition were possible, it is unlikely that consumers would have been offered a greater choice in benefits, cost-sharing arrangements, premiums to match their own experience, and types of insurance products.

The benefits of health insurance competition appear to be passed on to the purchasers of insurance. As shown in Table 8.2, the benefit/premium ratio appears to average at approximately 0.9 over time. As insurance companies attempt to reduce the two components of their premium, the loading charge and benefit expenditures, and as these cost savings are passed on to the purchasers, the premium will rise less rapidly and the difference between benefits paid and premiums will become smaller. (As insurance companies perform more administrative functions, such as utilization review and case management, the costs of these functions will increase the loading charge.)

The performance of the health insurance market has been improving over time. Prices are relatively close to costs (as indicated by the benefit/premium ratio), employees have become more price sensitive in their choice of health plan (as their co-premium reflects higher cost plans), and there is greater variety in the types of health insurance products offered.

A growing concern with regard to efficiency and equity, however, are regulations enacted by some states and those being considered by other states. These regulations, such as shorter waiting periods for preexisting conditions, community rating, and state mandates, decrease the demand for insurance by allowing people to wait until they are ill before they buy insurance (shorter waiting periods), impose a regressive "tax" on low-income groups to subsidize the care of those who are older and at higher risk (community rating), and increase the cost of health insurance (state mandates), thereby decreasing the demand for insurance.

Key Terms and Concepts

- Health maintenance organizations (HMOs)
- Point-of-service plan (POS)
- Portability
- Preferred provider organizations (PPOs)
- Third-party administrator (TPA)
- Shadow pricing

- Benefit/premium ratio
- Community rating
- Experience-rated
- Guaranteed issue and renewal
- Preexisting exclusion
- Risk-adjusted premiums

Review Questions

1. Outline the structure of the insurance industry. Does its structure deviate from the purely competitive model? What changes, if any, would you suggest to alter the performance of this industry?

2. How is a "pure" premium calculated?

3. What does the loading charge consist of?

4. Is a benefit/premium ratio close to 1 necessarily a sign that the industry is being efficient and minimizing the cost of medical services?

5. What are the possible consequences of community rating on economic efficiency and equity?

6. What factors affect the price elasticity of demand for an individual insurance company? Is there a difference in the price elasticity of demand facing the individual insurance company as compared to the overall market demand for health insurance?

7. Explain why multiple-option plans, such as PPOs, HMOs, preauthorization for admission, and cost containment programs, such as preauthorization for admission, did not emerge sooner in the health insurance market.

8. What evidence would enable you to evaluate whether the health insurance market is price-competitive?

9. What is the difference between "experience" rating and "community" rating?

10. Why do insurers and HMOs have an incentive to engage in preferred risk selection?

11. What are some methods by which insurers and HMOs try to achieve preferred risk selection?

12. What would be the effect on risk selection of using "risk-adjusted" premiums?

13. Blue Cross had several cost advantages over commercial insurance companies. Blue Cross received a discount from hospitals, did not have to pay taxes, and did not have to earn and distribute profits to shareholders. What effect should these cost advantages have had on Blue Cross's market share? What hypotheses have been suggested to explain the lack of such an expected effect on market share?

14. What would be the hypothesized effect on the types of insurance plans purchased if a limit were placed on the amount of employer-purchased health insurance that is tax-free income?

15. Do all-payer systems, whereby the state regulates hospital charges so that every purchaser pays the same price for hospital care, enhance competition among insurers? Who do you believe would be for and against all-payer systems?

16. Indemnity insurance, whereby the insurance company pays a specified dollar amount when an episode of illness occurs, and HMOs are two different approaches for handling moral hazard in medical care. Do you agree?

17. Would you expect the price of insurance (the loading charge) to be the same for small employers as for very large employers? (*Hint:* consider both demand and cost factors in your explanation.)

18. What factors affect the price elasticity of demand for an individual insurance company?

19. How have anticompetitive restrictions by medical societies affected the prices and types of products offered in the health insurance market?

20. In the 1970s, prior to price competition, why was Blue Cross more interested than

the commercial insurers in placing limits on the growth in hospital beds (Certificate of need legislation)?

REFERENCES

1. See footnote 4, Chapter 6.
2. Ronald J. Vogel and Roger D. Blair, *Health Insurance Administrative Costs,* Social Security Administration, Office of Research and Statistics Paper 21, October 1975.
3. Roger D. Blair and Ronald J. Vogel, "A Survivor Analysis of Commercial Insurers," *Journal of Business,* 51(3), July 1978: 521–529.
4. Roger D. Blair, Jerry R. Jackson, and Ronald J. Vogel, "Economies of Scale in the Administration of Health Insurance," *Review of Economics and Statistics,* 57(2), May 1975: 185–189. Also, in another study of the performance of Medicare (Part A) processing costs, H. E. Frech found lower cost per dollar processed, lower average processing time (in days), and fewer errors per $1,000 processed in for-profit as compared to not-for-profit firms. H. E. Frech III, "The Property Rights Theory of the Firm: Empirical Results from a Natural Experiment," *Journal of Political Economy,* 84(1), February 1976: 143–152.
5. Stephen T. Mennemeyer, "Effects of Competition on Medicare Administrative Costs," *Journal of Health Economics,* 3(2), August 1984: 137–154.
6. H. E. Frech, "Blue Cross, Blue Shield, and Health Care Costs: A Review of the Economic Evidence," in Mark V. Pauly, ed., *National Insurance: What Now, What Later, What Never?* (Washington, D.C.: American Enterprise Institute, 1980), pp. 251–252; and Killard Adamache and Frank Sloan, "Competition Between Non-Profit and For-Profit Health Insurers," *Journal of Health Economics,* 2(3), December 1983: 225–243. The importance of the state tax exemption as a Blue Cross competitive cost advantage has diminished as more firms have become self-insured and because of ERISA thereby are no longer subject to such premium taxes.
7. *Health Insurance: Comparing Blue Cross and Blue Shield Plans with Commercial Insurers,* Report to the Chairman, Subcommittee on Health, Committee on Ways and Means, House of Representatives (Washington, D.C.: U.S. General Accounting Office, July 1986), p. 20.
8. Adamache and Sloan, *op. cit.*
9. Frech, "Blue Cross, Blue Shield, and Health Care Costs," *op. cit.*
10. Charles D. Weller, "On 'FTC Sings the Blues' and Its Respondents," *Journal of Health Politics, Policy and Law,* 7(2), Summer 1982: 547–558.
11. H. E. Frech and Paul Ginsburg, "Competition Among Health Insurers," in Warren Greenburg, ed., *Competition in the Health Care Sector: Past, Present, and Future* (Germantown, Md.: Aspen Systems Corporation, 1978).
12. Mark V. Pauly, "Competition in Health Insurance Markets," *Law and Contemporary Problems,* 51(2), 1989: 237–271.
13. Stephen E. Foreman, John A. Wilson, and Richard M. Scheffler, "Monopoly, Monopsony and Contestability in Health Insurance: A Study of Blue Cross Plans," *Economic Inquiry,* 34(4), October 1996: 662–677.

14. The disappointment of many observers over the apparent ineffectiveness of cost containment techniques since the mid-1980s may have been the result of its effects being overshadowed by the underwriting cycle. Paul J. Feldstein and Thomas M. Wickizer, "Analysis of Private Health Insurance Premium Growth Rates: 1985–1992," *Medical Care,* 33(10), October 1995: 1035–1050.

15. James C. Robinson, "Use and Abuse of the Medical Loss Ratio to Measure Health Plan Performance," *Health Affairs,* 16(4) July–August 1997: 176–187.

16. Thomas C. Buchmueller and Paul J. Feldstein, "The Effect of Price on Switching Among Health Plans," *Journal of Health Economics,* 16(2), April 1997: 231–247.

17. Bryan Dowd and Roger Feldman, "Premium Elasticities of Health Plan Choice," *Inquiry,* 31(4), Winter 1994–1995, pp. 438–444.

18. For a more extensive discussion of community rating, see Pauly, "The Welfare Economics of Community Rating," *Journal of Risk and Insurance,* 37(3), September 1970: 407–418. See also David F. Bradford and Derrick A. Max, "Implicit Budget Deficits: The Case of a Mandated Shift to Community-Rated Health Insurance," Working Paper Series (National Bureau of Economic Research: Cambridge, Mass., March 1996).

19. *Health Care Insurance Regulation Program: An Assessment of Effectiveness,* Executive Office of the Governor, Lewis Cass Building, Lansing, Mich., March 1973, p. 11. Also see Dana P. Goldman, Arleen Leibowitz, Joan Buchanan, and Joan Keesey, "Redistributional Consequences of Community Rating," *Health Services Research,* 32(1), April 1997: 71–86.

20. "New York Finds Fewer People Have Health Insurance a Year After Reform," *The Wall Street Journal,* May 27, 1994, p. A2. See also Karen Pallarito, "Commissioner Berates Actuarial Report," *Modern Healthcare,* 24(43), October 24, 1994: 40.

21. Paul J. Feldstein, Thomas M. Wickizer, and John R. C. Wheeler, "Private Cost Containment: The Effects of Utilization Review Programs on Health Care Use and Expenditures," *New England Journal of Medicine,* 318(20), May 19, 1988: 1310–1314.

22. Mark V. Pauly, "Paying the Piper and Calling the Tune: The Relationship between Public Financing and Public Regulation of Health Care," in Mancur Olson, ed., *A New Approach to the Economics of Health Care* (Washington, D.C.: American Enterprise Institute for Public Policy Research, 1981), pp. 67–86.

23. Lawrence G. Goldberg and Warren Greenberg, "The Emergence of Physician-Sponsored Health Insurance: A Historical Perspective," in Warren Greenberg, ed., *Competition in the Health Care Sector* (Germantown, Md.: Aspen Systems Corporation, 1978).

24. For early examples of such activities, see "The American Medical Association: Power, Purpose, and Politics in Organized Medicine," *Yale Law Journal,* 63(7), May 1954: 938–1022.

25. "Embers Glow Through Ashes of Washington State's Reform," *Medicine and Health Perspectives,* (Washington, D.C.: Faulkner and Gray, April 1, 1996); and Bill Richards, "Perils of Pioneering: Health-Care Reform in the State of Washington Riles Nearly Everyone," *The Wall Street Journal,* April 5, 1996, p. A1.

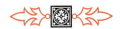

CHAPTER

Market Competition
in Medical Care

THE EMERGENCE OF COMPETITION IN MEDICAL CARE

The delivery of medical services in the United States changed dramatically in the 1980s. The trend in the late 1970s was toward increased regulation. An increasing number of states were moving toward rate regulation of hospitals, hospital investment was being regulated by both the state and federal governments (certificate of need legislation [CON]), and there were discussions in the literature of granting hospitals public utility status. Yet, rather than moving in the direction of increased regulation, market competition became the dominant force affecting hospitals and health professionals. This change was not anticipated.

The emergence of market competition was not the result of any legislative objective on the part of Congress or the administration. How it evolved is instructive for understanding the reasons for change in the medical sector.

When Medicare and Medicaid were enacted in the mid-1960s, they were designed in such a way that one of the outcomes would have to be inefficiency. Hospitals were reimbursed their costs plus 2 percent, physicians would be paid their usual and customary fees, and neither capitation payments to HMOs nor selective contracting with specific providers were permitted, since the American Medical Association (AMA) insisted that "free choice" of provider be available to all Medicare and Medicaid beneficiaries. The price constraints facing Medicaid patients were removed and were greatly reduced for Medicare patients. The government was committed to paying for the medical services for the aged and poor, regardless of the cost of those services. Further, it was not possible to change the method of payment, fee-for-service for physicians and cost-based for hospitals. As a result, providers had minimal incentives to be concerned with expenditures under these programs.

As a consequence, government expenditures for Medicare and Medicaid greatly exceeded their original projections. Medicare's actuaries stated that Medicare would cost only $2 billion a year. However, because Medicare was an entitlement program, its benefits and beneficiaries were defined by law; no limit was placed on its overall expenditures. Federal expenditures under both of these programs increased from $3 billion in 1965, to $31 billion by 1975, to $111 billion in 1985, and to $304 billion by 1995. State expenditures under Medicaid also increased sharply, from $4 billion in 1965 to $89 billion in 1995.

Rising inflation in the late 1960s served to stimulate the demand for employer-paid health insurance, which was not considered taxable income to the employee. As incomes increased due to inflation, employees moved into higher income tax brackets (as high as 70 percent) and unions bargained for increased health benefits. As insurance coverage in the private and public sectors increased, consumer concern with health costs diminished. Health providers were able to increase their prices with little fear of decreased demand. In a growing economy with rising inflation, business firms were able to pass on their higher labor costs by increasing the prices of their goods and services. Expenditures in the private sector went from $28 billion a year in 1965 to $487 billion in 1995.

These massive increases in medical expenditures by both the public and private sectors were equivalent to a huge redistribution of wealth, from the taxpayers to those working in the medical sector.

Early attempts at reducing the rise in medical expenditures came from the federal government. As Medicare expenditures were about to exhaust the Medicare Trust Fund, Social Security taxes were continually increased to fund the hospital portion of Medicare. (The physician portions of Medicare and Medicaid are funded from general tax revenues and increases in these programs assumed greater importance in subsequent years when the federal deficit became a political issue.) As it became politically difficult to continually request additional Social Security taxes, successive administrations developed a concentrated interest in halting Medicare's rapidly escalating expenditures.

Few options were available to any administration for limiting Medicare expenditures. Asking Congress to reduce Medicare benefits or to have the aged pay more would have cost any administration a great deal of political support from the aged and their supporters. If taxes were not to be continually increased nor benefits to the aged reduced, then the only alternatives for limiting the increase in Medicare expenditures, which were rising by approximately 15 percent a year, were either to limit payments to providers or to place controls on utilization of services.

The federal government started chipping away at the cost-based reimbursement of hospitals in 1969, when it removed the plus 2 percent from the cost plus formula. In 1971, because of rising inflation, President Nixon placed the entire U.S. economy under a wage and price freeze (the Economic Stabilization Program). The rest of the economy was removed from this freeze after one year. However, the health sector remained under price controls until April 1974. Following the removal of these controls, physician and hospital expenditures increased very rapidly.

Additional regulatory approaches were tried but each one failed or had unintended consequences. Physician fee increases under Medicare were limited by the Medicare Fee Index; the result was that increasing numbers of physicians declined to participate in the Medicare program, thereby reducing the aged's access to care. In 1974, Congress enacted the National Health Planning and Resources Development Act (CON), which placed limits on hospitals' capital expenditures. (Existing hospitals used the capital controls to limit entry by new hospitals into their market and prevented free-standing outpatient surgery centers from being established.) Utilization review programs (professional standard review organizations) were legislated by Congress in 1972. Again, empirical studies failed to find significant savings in hospital use or expenditures as a result of these programs. (Physicians had no incentive under fee-for-service arrangements to limit patients' use of the hospital.)

In 1979, President Carter made hospital cost containment his highest legislative priority—and it was rejected by Congress, whose members were mostly from the same political party. His proposed legislation would have placed limits on the annual percent increase in each hospital's expenditures.

From the mid-1960s through the 1970s, price competition among medical providers did not occur. There was little demand side pressure for providers to compete on price. Patients had little incentive to be concerned with medical prices since they had comprehensive health insurance, either from the government, Medicare and Medicaid, or from their employers. Free choice of provider was mandated under public programs, information on provider prices was unavailable (and in many places prohibited by medical societies), and physicians, through their medical societies, colluded on their prices when negotiating with insurance companies. Further, large employers (e.g., autos and steel) were not very concerned with the effect of rising insurance premiums since they could increase their product prices with little fear of import competition.

Given the size of the U.S. population, differences in income, willingness to pay for health care, and so on, it would be expected that a variety of payment and delivery systems, in addition to fee-for-service indemnity insurance, would have emerged. However, the number of HMOs and their growth was, for many years, very small. If the medical services market were competitive, a demand for such organizations would have existed, particularly if HMOs could provide medical care of a quality comparable to that of the fee-for-service system and be price-competitive. Since HMO growth did not occur for many years, this slow growth should be examined to determine whether it was due to insufficient demand and/or reasons for an inadequate supply response.

One way to determine the potential demand for HMOs is to examine what percent of the population enrolled in an HMO when it was offered in competition with traditional fee-for-service insurance. Several HMOs, such as Kaiser, required that potential enrollees have a choice between their plan and an alternative, such as Blue Cross and Blue Shield. Based on studies where consumers have had this dual choice option, 20 to 60 percent of the subscribers chose the HMO. It would therefore be expected that a larger percentage of the general population would have been enrolled in such plans. To determine why the growth in such plans in previous years did not keep up with their potential demand, it is necessary to examine the supply side of this market.

Unless HMOs were as efficient as the fee-for-service delivery system, they would not be expected to increase their market share. However, comparative data of HMO premiums relative to those in the traditional fee-for-service system indicated that HMOs could compete effectively on price.

The reasons for the very slow growth of HMOs must therefore be found in nonmarket barriers that have inhibited their development. The first such barrier was attempts by state medical associations to deny hospital privileges to participating physicians, thereby denying HMOs access to hospitals (1). If an HMO could not provide its potential subscribers with hospital care when needed, the plan could not effectively compete with fee-for-service physicians in the community. According to Kessel, HMOs represented a lower-priced substitute to fee-for-service physicians because the premium was the same for all persons regardless of their income. Since fee-for-service physicians attempted to price discriminate according to a patient's income, a plan that charges all patients the same premium is a form of price cutting for those with high incomes.

Previously, state and county medical associations successfully prevented the growth of many HMOs by revoking the membership of, or refusing to grant membership to, physicians who desired to join them; such memberships had been prerequisites for hospital privileges. Therefore, to survive, an HMO such as Kaiser had to have its own hospitals. Although various medical societies subsequently lost antitrust suits, their anticompetitive actions were sufficient to raise the cost to potential HMOs to prevent their large-scale development.

In addition to the above actions, state medical societies were successful in having legislation enacted at a state level that placed additional barriers on HMO development and on HMOs' ability to compete with fee-for-service practice. Restrictive legislation subjected HMOs to strict regulation by the state department of insurance, required physicians to be a majority of the controlling board of an HMO, required HMOs to permit the participation of any physician in the community, required HMOs to be organized on a nonprofit basis, and prohibited HMOs from advertising their benefits and premiums.

Prohibiting an HMO from advertising erects a major barrier to its growth. Consumer ignorance of HMOs was an important reason why potential subscribers did not join. Further, HMOs are subject to greater economies of scale than are solo practitioners. An HMO must have certain minimum facilities, an organization to enroll members, and possibly its own hospital. Unless an HMO is able to enroll a sufficient number of subscribers, it will be forced to operate at relatively higher premiums (i.e., the declining portion of its long-run average-cost curve). If an HMO were prevented from advertising, it would take longer to reach the number of enrollees required to make its premium competitive with the fee-for-service sector. The time and losses required were too great an obstacle for many HMOs. Restricting the HMO to nonprofit status further removed any incentives that might have existed for nonphysicians to risk their talents and capital to start an HMO.

Given the above constraints that existed on the demand and the supply side of the market, the development of market competition was not anticipated. There were a number of events that provided the preconditions for market competition, but only one that made it possible to occur (2).

Federal Initiatives

The Increased Supply of Physicians

For approximately fifteen years, through the 1950s and early 1960s, the supply of physicians in relation to the population remained constant, at 141 physicians per 100,000. During this period physicians' incomes were rising (relative to those of other occupations), as were the number of applicants to medical schools (see Tables 12.1 to 12.4). As the demand for physicians' services continued to grow, stimulated by the passage of Medicare and Medicaid and the growth of private health insurance, an increased number of foreign medical graduates came to the United States.

During this period there was constant talk of a shortage of physicians. Many qualified U.S. students who could not gain admission to the limited number of medical school spaces went overseas to receive a medical education. Many middle-class families were concerned that their sons and daughters could not become physicians, while, at the same time, there was increased immigration by foreign medical graduates. Congress responded to these constituent pressures and passed the Health Professions Educational Assistance Act (HPEA). Senator Yarborough stated the reasons for the passage of the HPEA in 1963. "It was when we were trying to give more American boys and girls a chance for a medical education, so that we would not have to drain the help of other foreign countries." And again, "To me it is just shocking that we do not give American boys and girls a chance to obtain a medical education so that they can serve their own people" (3).

It took a number of years before the full magnitude of this act took effect. New medical schools were built and existing medical schools increased their spaces. (The same occurred for other health professions.) By 1980, the supply of physicians had expanded to almost 200 per 100,000, almost a 50 percent increase from the early 1960s. The ratio continued to expand so that by 1995, the physician to population ratio reached 250 per 100,000 population.

In response to their constituent interests and over the objections of the American Medical Association, Congress enacted legislation that eventually created excess capacity among physicians. It was not Congress's intention to create competition among physicians. However, their actions in passing the HPEA set the stage for it.

The HMO Act

In the early 1970s, President Nixon wanted to enact an inexpensive (to the federal government) health initiative. His proposal was to stimulate the growth of prepaid health plans, renamed health maintenance organizations (HMOs).[1] Paying health plans a capitated amount per enrollee in return for delivery of comprehensive medical services was not new. It was proposed by the Commission on the Cost of Medical Care in the 1930s. Early examples of such organizations are the Kaiser Foundation Health Plan and the Group Health Association. Under capitation the HMO and its physicians have a financial incentive to minimize the cost of medical care provided to its enrollees.

When Congress passed the HMO act in 1973, it included two provisions helpful to the development of HMOs and one that was a hindrance. First, employers with twenty-five or more employees had to offer their employees an HMO option if there was a federally qualified HMO available in their area. Second, federally qualified HMOs were exempt from restrictive state practices described earlier. These provisions reduced the marketing expenses of HMOs and removed restrictions hindering their development. Unfortunately, to become federally qualified, the HMO was required to offer a benefit package that was more expensive than those offered by competing insurance plans.

The requirements necessary to become a federally qualified HMO discouraged many HMOs from taking advantage of federal qualification. It was not until several years later that this benefit requirement was changed following complaints from HMOs that these requirements increased their premiums so that they could not be competitive with regular health insurance plans. (Also, as part of the 1979 Health Planning Act, large HMOs [enrollment greater than fifty thousand persons] were exempted from the CON process. Rather than this being procompetitive legislation for all HMOs, however, the main beneficiaries were the larger, established HMOs.) Once these restrictions were relaxed, HMOs took advantage of the beneficial provisions of the HMO act. As enrollment in HMOs increased, the lower hospital use by HMO enrollees contributed to hospitals' excess capacity.

The 1979 Amendments to CON Legislation

The initial CON legislation established planning agencies whose purpose was to limit the increase in hospital capital expenditures. HMOs needed access to a hospital to provide a full range of medical services. HMOs with hospitals wanted to be able to expand them, while other HMOs wanted to construct hospitals. HMOs complained to Congress that the CON legislation was being used by existing hospitals to block their growth. HMOs represented a competitive threat to existing hospitals and physicians in a community. "HMOs were subjected to more extensive controls than fee-for-service providers. Although financing plans and provider organizations of other kinds could be established

---

[1]The originator of the term "health maintenance organization" is Paul M. Ellwood Jr. See his "Health Maintenance Strategy," *Medical Care,* May–June 1971.

without government approval, establishment of an HMO was subject to planning agency review" (4).

In 1979, Congress amended the CON legislation so that the act should not be used to inhibit competition. However, these amendments did not grant all HMOs a complete exemption from the CON act; it merely loosened the restrictions.

Except for the change in the CON legislation and the enactment of the HMO act and its amendments, Congress could not develop a consensus with the various health interest groups as to what legislative approach, if any, should be used to limit the rise in federal health expenditures.

Political Opposition to a Competitive Strategy

Some of the opponents of President Carter's cost containment legislation, such as Representatives Gephardt and Stockman, began to propose an alternative approach, the use of market competition. Various academicians, such as Enthoven, wrote on the virtues of market competition (5). However, if market competition had to depend on congressional action, it would not have occurred. Too many powerful interest groups were opposed to organizing the delivery of health services along competitive lines (6).

Organized medicine correctly foresaw that its members would be worse off under competition. Physicians would have to accept changes in their style of practice, restrictions would be placed on their behavior by utilization review, and price discounting would emerge. Hospitals also did not support a competitive approach. HMOs would decrease the demand for hospital care and competition would force hospitals to reduce costs and compete on price. Many hospitals preferred the security of a regulatory system. Commercial health insurers opposed the concept of market competition. They were unsure of their future role in a system of competing HMOs. Instead, insurance companies preferred some form of all-payer hospital rate regulation so that the Blue Cross discount would no longer place them at a competitive disadvantage. Blue Cross was also reluctant to favor a change to market competition. Blue Cross plans with high market shares and good provider relations would have had little to gain from such a change.

Business groups, who might be expected to favor competition, were, at most, lukewarm supporters of health care competition. Many companies believed that they had preferred risk groups and did not want to incur increased administrative costs by offering multiple health plans to their employees.

Unions were among the most vocal of the groups opposing a competitive delivery system. Although unions had been strong supporters of Kaiser, those same unions had a basic distrust of competitive markets. They preferred not-for-profit health plans and wanted the government, rather than markets, to be the regulator of provider and insurer performance. Unions also opposed legislative proposals to increase competition that would have taxed employer-purchased health insurance premiums. Large unions, such as the UAW, had comprehensive health insurance benefits and a tax limit on health benefits would have made their members worse off.

The beneficiaries of a competitive market are consumers. Their interest in procom-

petitive legislation, however, is diffuse; the potential benefits of competition were unknown and not viewed as being sufficiently large to warrant their involvement in the political process.

Elimination of "Free Choice" of Provider under Medicaid

It was not until 1981, under President Reagan, that additional cost containment legislation was enacted. In return for reducing federal Medicaid expenditures, Congress
amended Medicaid so as to provide states with greater flexibility in how they could pay
for their medically indigent (7). States were no longer required to offer their medically indigent "free choice" of medical provider. This meant that states could take bids and negotiate contracts with selected providers. Although the law was a potentially powerful
force for using market forces in the Medicaid program, many states moved slowly.

New Hospital Payment System under Medicare. Starting in September 1983, the Reagan administration introduced a revolutionary method for paying hospitals under
Medicare, fixed prices per admission, according to diagnostic-related groupings (DRGs).
The hospital and medical associations were powerless against a Republican administration intent on reducing federal expenditures for hospitals. As the incentives facing hospitals changed, lengths of stay for the aged declined and hospital occupancy rates began
falling. However, by the time hospitals began to experience the effect of Medicare DRGs
on their occupancy rates, the move toward market competition had already started in the
private sector. DRGs reinforced the downward pressure on hospital occupancy rates.

Private-Sector Initiatives

Approximately two-thirds of the population has private health insurance coverage, and
most private health insurance (85 percent) is purchased through the workplace. The
stimulus for competition started in the private sector.

In 1981, the nation was faced with a severe recession. In addition, the automobile and
steel industries faced increased import competition from foreign producers. These were
also the same industries that had the most comprehensive health insurance programs for
their employees. The recession led to unemployment, loss of income, and a decrease in
health insurance benefits, resulting in a decline in elective hospital admissions. The recession also lowered tax revenues for states. Consequently, many states cut back on their
Medicaid benefits, decreased the numbers of eligibles, and instituted cost containment
measures, such as prior authorization for admission. These factors, which led to a decline
in the hospital admission rate for those under sixty-five years of age, started in late 1981.

Once the recession ended, those industries engaged in competition with foreign producers found that the strength of the U.S. dollar relative to other currencies forced them
to further reduce their labor costs to remain competitive.

President Reagan's tax cuts in 1981, which reduced the high marginal income tax rates
for employees from 70 percent to the mid-30s, provided employees with an incentive to

reduce their medical expenditures. A greater portion of any savings from lower insurance premiums could be used to increase their take-home pay.

Industry began to examine ways in which they could contain the rise in their employees' health insurance costs. Business began to pressure health insurers to hold their premiums down and to institute new cost-saving programs. Also, an increasing number of firms started their own self-insurance plans. The firms believed that they, rather than insurance companies, would be better able to control their employees' health care use. Businesses also added deductibles and co-insurance to their employees' health plans, thereby increasing their employees' price sensitivity. A survey of 1,185 companies found that the percentage of firms requiring deductible payments for their employees' inpatient care rose from 30 percent in 1982 to 63 percent in 1984; similarly, the percent of firms requiring preauthorization for hospital admission increased from 2 percent to 26 percent over that same period (8).

One of the most important changes firms (or insurers acting on their behalf) introduced was a change in the benefit package. Insurance coverage for lower-cost substitutes to hospitals was introduced. Previously, even though it was less costly to perform surgery in an outpatient setting, if this service was not covered by insurance, it became less costly *to the employee* to have the surgery performed in a hospital. Thus by adding outpatient surgery to the benefit package the insurance premium paid by the business could be reduced.

Private-sector initiatives had two effects. First, as purchasers of health care benefits, they demonstrated that they were concerned with health care costs. This concern was transmitted to their health insurers, who in turn included low-cost substitutes to hospital care in their benefit packages and began to undertake hospital utilization review. Prior authorization for admission, concurrent review, and second opinions for surgery were instituted as a means of reducing the insurance premium. Insurers, particularly the Blues, began to change their relationship with providers and became more adversarial. They began to place greater pressure on hospitals to limit their cost increases.

The second consequence of business's concern with their employees' medical costs was that hospitals developed excess capacity. Efforts to reduce hospital utilization, such as utilization controls, the growth of HMOs, and coverage of care in nonhospital settings, were succeeding. Occupancy rates in short-term general hospitals declined from 78 percent in 1980 to 64.8 percent by 1985. As excess capacity increased, hospitals were willing to participate with and become part of alternative delivery systems.

The Enforcement of Anti-Trust Laws

While demand side pressures for lower health care costs and the excess capacity among hospitals and physicians were important preconditions for competition, had it not been for the application of the anti-trust laws, it is unlikely that market competition would have occurred.

Medical societies and state practice acts inhibited market competition by erecting barriers to the development of competing delivery systems; limiting advertising, fee splitting, corporate practice of medicine, and delegation of tasks; and engaging in boycotts. Blue Cross and Blue Shield maintained the principle of "free choice" of provider; that is, their enrollees were not given a financial incentive to choose between providers on the basis of price. Blue Cross enrollees had a service benefit policy. Regardless of whether the participating hospital had high or low costs, Blue Cross paid their enrollees' hospital bills in full; Blue Shield reimbursed participating physicians according to their usual fees (up to a percentile limit), thereby lessening their enrollees' incentive to shop around.

In the past, during the 1930s, the same preconditions for market competition had existed. Physicians and hospitals had excess capacity; patients and their insurance companies were concerned with the cost of health care. Yet market competition did not occur. For example, insurance companies in Oregon attempted to lower their insurance premiums by placing restraints on physician utilization; preauthorization of services and monitoring of claims were also used (9).

The response by the medical societies in Oregon to these cost control approaches was twofold. First, the medical societies threatened to expel from the society any physician who participated in these competitive insurance plans. Second, the medical societies started their own insurance plans that excluded these aggressive utilization control methods. With the growth of their own insurance plans, physicians were encouraged to boycott other insurance plans. To have physicians participate in their plans, these other insurance companies had to drop their aggressive cost containment efforts. The medical societies were thereby able to determine that the type of insurance programs that would be offered to the public were also those that were in the physicians' economic interests.

Thus, unless the anti-trust laws were applicable to the health sector, physician and hospital boycotts and other anticompetitive behavior could have prevented market competition from once again occurring.

Up until 1975, it was believed that the anti-trust laws did not apply to "learned professions," which included the health professions. In 1975, the U.S. Supreme Court ruled against the Virginia State bar association, which established a minimum fee schedule for lawyers, believing that lawyers were not engaged in "trade or commerce." The Supreme Court thereby denied any sweeping exclusion for the learned professions from the anti-trust laws. In another important precedent, the Supreme Court in 1978 denied the use of anticompetitive behavior by the National Society of Professional Engineers even if it was to prevent a threat to either the profession's ethics or to public safety. Encouraged by the Supreme Court decisions, the Federal Trade Commission (FTC) began to vigorously enforce the anti-trust laws in the health field. The FTC, in 1975, charged the American Medical Association and its constituent medical societies with anticompetitive behavior. In a 1978 decision, the FTC prevailed. The AMA appealed the verdict to the Supreme Court, but was again unsuccessful.

The Supreme Court's decision, rendered in 1982, was a clear signal to health providers that they would now be subject to the anti-trust laws. The FTC subsequently brought suit to prevent physician and dentist boycotts against insurers (Michigan State Medical Society and the Indiana Federation of Dentists), prevent physicians from denying hospital privileges to physicians participating in HMOs (Forbes Health System Medical Staff), enabled advertising to be used (FTC v. AMA), and enabled preferred provider organizations and HMOs to compete (10).

Anticompetitive behavior is illegal on either per se grounds or by virtue of the rule of reason. Price fixing, economic boycotts, tying arrangements, and division of horizontal markets are per se violations; these activities are believed to be obviously anticompetitive and their effects are clearly harmful to consumers. Price fixing occurs when two or more competitors agree on a price at which their service will be sold. An example is when a Medicaid agency requests bids and two providers agree to submit similar prices. It does not matter whether the fixed prices are minimums or maximums; they are both illegal. A boycott occurs when, for example, a medical society threatens to "departicipate" from Blue Shield or other third-party payer if their payment demands are not met. "Tying" occurs when a purchaser who wants to purchase one product is also required to buy a second product (e.g., operating room and anesthesiology services as well). When competitors agree to divide up geographic markets, consumers, or services, and not compete with each other, it is illegal.

Other forms of anticompetitive behavior are analyzed according to the rule of reason, which attempts to determine whether the anticompetitive harm caused by the restraint exceeds the procompetitive benefits of not permitting the particular activity. Examples of cases brought under the rule of reason are hospital mergers (whether competition among the remaining hospitals would be lessened), staff privilege issues (as when a cardiologist claims that she was denied privileges, thereby depriving her of the right to compete against current cardiologists on staff), and the formation of PPOs (whether the PPO includes so many physicians that it becomes a form of price fixing).

Activities by professional associations that provide increased information on the quality and characteristics of health care providers, such as specialty certification, are not anticompetitive since they do not limit either entry or choice of provider. Such actions may improve market performance by providing the consumer with more information. In the past, however, professional regulation resulted in limits on entry and on choice of provider, as well as other forms of anticompetitive behavior.

The application of anti-trust laws to the health field is based on the belief that competitive markets have desirable outcomes. As new delivery and payment systems emerge in the health field, anti-trust questions will be raised as to whether these new arrangements are procompetitive (e.g., take advantage of economies of scale) or whether they are a means of lessening competition among competitors. An appreciation of the economics of competitive markets is essential for understanding the probable anti-trust implications of these new arrangements.

After the removal of restrictions on HMOs, there was rapid growth in both the number of HMOs and in their enrollment during the mid-1980s. HMOs were believed by employers and others to represent the solution to rising medical expenditures and quality medical care. It was unfortunate that HMOs became synonymous with the concept of market competition, since many HMOs did not engage in price competition at that time.

Under the HMO act, employers were required to contribute an equal dollar amount (on behalf of employees) to federally qualified HMOs as they did to the traditional plan. Employers offered their employees a choice of health plans, however, because many employers paid the entire health insurance premium or because the HMOs set their premiums equal to that of the traditional indemnity plan, employees did not have to choose a health plan based on their relative premium contribution. HMOs and indemnity insurers competed on nonprice factors, such as the comprehensiveness of the benefits and ease of access to providers. Employers also became concerned that HMOs were receiving a lower-risk group of employees while receiving a premium based on the average risk of the entire employee group. As a result, employers found that they were not saving money by offering HMOs to their employees.

As HMOs began to increase their market shares at the expense of the indemnity plans, insurers began instituting managed care techniques, such as utilization review. As a result, inpatient admissions and length of stay declined. Hospital occupancy rates dropped and, with their growing excess capacity, hospitals began to engage in price competition to increase their volume.

Indemnity insurers also began to compete against HMOs by starting their own HMOs. In this manner the insurance company was able to offer different products to consumers with different elasticities of demand. Presumably, those subscribers with the least price elastic demand will continue to purchase fee-for-service insurance, which has the highest premium; those with the most price elastic demands would be expected to purchase the more restrictive health plans, such as HMOs.

Employers have also begun to limit the number of HMOs offered to their employees in an attempt to reduce selection bias. In some instances, a single insurer will offer employees a choice between an HMO, PPO, and a managed fee-for-service system, a "multiple-option" plan. In this manner the problem of selection bias is solved since the same insurer is also at risk should the higher risks remain in the indemnity plan.

In more recent years, as HMOs increased their market share, the HMO act was modified further. Employers no longer had to contribute the same amount to the HMO and non-HMO plan. Employer contributions to HMOs can now be less than their contribution to indemnity plans. For example, employers could use risk adjustment when determining their employees' HMO premium; this would reduce favorable risk selection by the HMO. These changes should lessen employer concerns that their total expenditures were increased because they paid the HMO the same premium as their traditional plan and HMOs received a preferred risk group. Employers can now require employees to make some contribution to an HMO. Some employers were concerned that when the HMO was at zero cost to employees, they would select the HMO even though they were covered under a health plan offered by their spouse's employer. Last, the dual choice provision was repealed.

The reasons for the emergence of market competition in medical care were the result of demand side changes and the applicability of the anti-trust laws. Business and the federal government each developed a concentrated interest in holding down the rise in their medical expenditures. As a result of the 1981 recession, severe import competition, and a lowering of marginal tax rates, business moved toward self-insurance; their increased concern with health care costs stimulated insurance companies to introduce cost saving innovations in their benefit packages. The federal government introduced DRGs as a means of controlling rapidly rising Medicare expenditures. Low-cost substitutes to traditional providers developed, namely, HMOs and outpatient surgery clinics.

The excess capacity among physicians and hospitals and the changed incentives in both business and government were important preconditions for market competition. However, it is unlikely that market competition would have occurred had it not been for the applicability and enforcement of the anti-trust laws.

The role of the health insurer changed as a result of business's demand for lower premiums. Previously, insurers had a passive role—marketing, enrollment, and paying claims. Under employer pressure, insurers became involved in decisions affecting the physician's practice. Through utilization management, the insurer determined whether the patient should be admitted to a hospital and for how long. By covering low-cost substitutes to the hospital, they determined in which setting the patient is to be treated. And by having hospitals and physicians compete on price to be included in their provider network, the insurer affects the patient's choice of provider.

By not recognizing the demand for cost containment, physicians and hospitals lost an opportunity to perform these functions themselves. Instead, new firms, such as HMOs, entered the market, decreased medical costs, and transferred revenues from the traditional providers to themselves.

CHARACTERISTICS OF MANAGED CARE PLANS

Managed care plans encompass a wide spectrum of health plans. At the least restrictive end of the spectrum are managed fee-for-service indemnity plans. Enrollees in such plans pay the insurer a premium and are then responsible for a deductible and co-insurance up to a maximum out of pocket expenditure each year. The insurer has added a utilization management component to the traditional fee-for-service plan. Patients are responsible for receiving precertification from the insurer for elective hospital admissions and the insurer, once the patient is admitted, reviews the patient's length of hospital stay. If the patient fails to receive preadmission certification, he can be financially liable for the hospital expense. The patient can use any provider and can self-refer to a specialist. These types of plans typically have the highest premiums. The cost control mechanisms used by the insurer are primarily patient financial incentives, utilization management, and deductibles and co-pays.

A somewhat more restrictive managed care plan is the above managed indemnity plan with an option to use a PPO. If patients use PPO providers, then their deductible is lower as well as their co-insurance rate (e.g., 10 percent versus 30 percent for a non-PPO provider). PPO providers are paid fee-for-service, are not exclusive to any one insurance plan, and are selected based on whether they are willing to provide the insurer with a discount on their fees and/or according to their utilization profile (i.e., lower or more appropriate prescribers of medical services). Again, the patient is provided with a financial incentive to use fewer services from less costly providers. Not all insurers create their own PPO network; they may "rent" one from another organization.

Indemnity plans often use "catastrophic case management" as an additional cost control mechanism. Once a patient's medical expense reaches $25,000, the insurer assigns a case manager to that patient to try and limit that patient's medical costs. The case manager has authority to provide additional benefits (e.g., installing medical equipment together with nursing care in the patient's home) if that will reduce the length of the hospital stay.

The most restrictive form of a managed care plan is an HMO. HMOs, however, also differ in their restrictiveness. Early HMOs were primarily based on the staff or group model, whereby the HMO either employed physicians (e.g., Group Cooperative of Puget Sound) or contracted with a group of physicians who had an exclusive arrangement with the HMO (e.g., Kaiser Permanente Medical Groups in California). Patients were not required to pay deductibles and only minimal co-payments (e.g., $5 a visit). The HMOs' benefits were typically more comprehensive than those offered by the indemnity plan. If patients used non-HMO providers, they were liable for 100 percent of the bill. Staff and group model HMOs typically relied on a "gatekeeper" primary care physician who provided primary care and who decided whether to refer the patient to a specialist or to a hospital.

The mechanism used by group and staff model HMOs to control use of services was placed on the primary care physician. Physicians were typically paid a salary plus bonus at the end of the year. Hospitals, which were owned by the HMO, were paid their costs.

Since the late 1980s, HMOs have found it easier to expand by contracting with community physicians and hospitals. This has reduced the need for many patients to give up their physician if they join an HMO. Group model HMOs, such as Kaiser, have in recent years changed; they no longer rely on their own hospitals or solely on their own physicians. In some markets they are similar to other HMOs in that they contract with community physicians and hospitals.

These other nonstaff HMOs may either contract (usually on a nonexclusive basis) with two or more independent groups (network model), directly with physicians in independent practices, and/or with one or more multispecialty groups (Independent Practice Association, IPA). (An IPA contracts with solo and small groups of physicians on a nonexclusive basis.) Providers in the above models may be paid in various ways, discounted fee-for-service, negotiated rates (perhaps with a small risk-sharing pool at the end of the year), fixed prices per admission, or capitation.

Capitation is a risk-sharing arrangement in which the provider group receives a predetermined fixed payment per member per month (PMPM) in return for providing all of the contracted services. A capitated provider group bears the risk that they can provide all the contracted services for their enrolled population at less than the capitation payment. The provider group has an incentive to accurately assess their enrollees' risk (actuarial accuracy becomes essential) and to provide care in a cost-effective manner.

The responsibility for cost control under nonstaff model HMOs depends on which entity bears the risk. Earlier HMOs paid their providers according to discounted fees and/or according to a fee schedule; the HMO bore the risk that the cost of medical services would be less than the capitation payment. The HMOs therefore undertook the utilization management function themselves. As more medical groups formed, increased in size, and gained experience in managing patients in a capitated environment, they began accepting capitation payments for medical services. The medical groups then became responsible for utilization review, quality assurance, appropriateness of care studies (including physician profiling, information feedback to their member physicians, and dropping overutilizers), and payment of their physician members, which may be according to fee-for-service or subcapitation.

As more medical groups, including IPAs, accept capitation, they are negotiating risk-sharing arrangements for reduced hospital utilization. Typically, a capitated medical group and a capitated hospital group will share a part of the hospital's capitation payment. In this manner, if the medical group is able to reduce hospital use, both groups share in those savings.

One variant of the above model is where a large medical group contracts with an HMO and receives 85 percent of the HMO's premium. The medical group then bears the risk for all of the enrollees' medical services and contracts with other providers for the services it does not provide. The HMO no longer bears any risk; it has all been shifted to the medical group. The medical group in turn has the incentive to innovate in improving the enrollee group's health status as well as in reducing their medical costs.

The last type of managed care organization is an HMO with a POS option. A POS plan is similar to an HMO except that the enrollee is allowed to see a non-HMO provider but must pay a significant out-of-pocket expense (e.g., 50 percent of the bill). The advantage of this option to enrollees is that they are not locked into the HMO. If enrollees make use of the POS option, it becomes more difficult to control medical expenses. Although POS plans have increased in popularity, out-of-plan use has been low because of the high cost sharing.

The premium in a typical HMO is allocated as shown in Figure 9.1. The HMO receives, for example, $100 PMPM. They retain $15 PMPM for administration (including enrollment and customer service), marketing, care received by enrollees outside the HMO's service area, stop loss insurance for certain catastrophic medical expenses, and profit. About $5 PMPM is used to pay for pharmacy benefits; typically the HMO has been at risk for this benefit. Approximately $45 PMPM goes for medical services, including primary care, specialty care, and ancillary services, such as laboratory tests. And $35 PMPM is for hospital and other facility services (e.g., outpatient surgery). Risk-sharing pools between the medical group and hospital are shown by the dotted lines.

Providers within these budgetary allocations may be paid in a variety of ways, as dis-

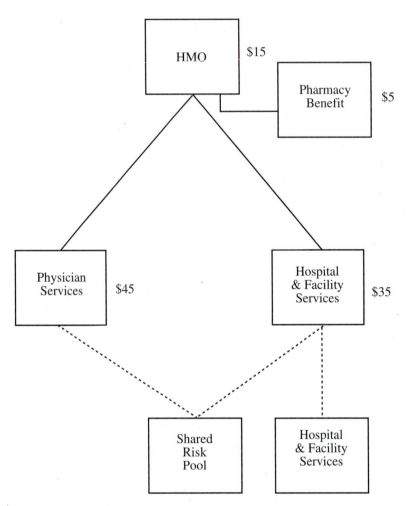

FIGURE 9.1 • Allocation of HMO premiums.

cussed above. Within a medical group, many arrangements have been tried and they are continually changing. Primary care physicians may be capitated or paid fee-for-service; similarly for specialists. When capitation is not used then there is usually a withholding of part of the fee, to ensure that there are sufficient funds at the end of the year.

Managed care organizations (MCOs), as discussed above, encompass both a variety of organizational models and a variety of managed care products. MCOs currently offer a diversified product line. In response to employers desiring more choice for their employees, HMOs have expanded their offerings to include, in addition to an HMO option, a POS plan, and a managed indemnity plan, including a PPO. (Having one insurer offer a spectrum of plans decreases the cost of adverse selection to an employer who would otherwise have to contract separately with an indemnity insurer.) For the same reason, previous indemnity insurers now also offer HMO and other options to large employers.

That part of the MCO industry that was primarily HMOs has been changing over time (11). For-profit HMOs have grown more rapidly than non-profit HMOs. (For-profit entrepreneurs have been quicker to see the profit from reducing hospital costs in high-use areas and have been more willing to enter new geographic areas, while nonprofits have been more concerned with serving a regional hospital system.). IPA model HMOs now have a majority of the enrollees and have increased their enrollments relative to staff and group model HMOs. (It has been easier for an HMO to expand and to enter a new area by contracting with local physicians than investing the time and money to develop a group.) The variety of products offered by HMOs, discussed above, has increased.

The industry has been consolidating, through mergers, to take advantage of economies of scale and to be able to receive greater discounts from provider groups. Recent studies indicate that economies of scale are essentially achieved once the HMO reaches about 115,000 enrollees (12). Since mergers are also occurring among large HMOs, it appears the main reason for such mergers is to benefit from being able to negotiate lower prices from the HMOs' suppliers, namely, hospitals and physicians.

The types of HMOs that have grown more rapidly are those that are larger and more well established. As shown in Table 9.1, the majority of enrollees are in HMOs that have been in existence for more than ten years. These older HMOs, which are also larger than the newer HMOs, have also had the most rapid growth in the past several years. The smaller and newer HMOs have experienced the most difficulty. HMO model type is also changing. The largest increases in enrollment are occurring in for-profit HMOs. IPA-type plans, which contract directly with physicians in private practice, have a greater percent of enrollees than other types of HMOs and are growing more rapidly than the others.

PERFORMANCE OF A COMPETITIVE MANAGED CARE MARKET

It has taken managed care plans a relatively short time to dominate the health insurance market and in doing so, they have received their share of criticisms. Limits have been placed on patient access and providers have seen their practices disrupted. An examination of the effect that managed care plans have had on market performance should therefore examine the following indicators of performance: First, has quality of care, health outcomes, and patient satisfaction been decreased? Second, has the growth in managed care lowered the rate of increase in health care expenditures? Before examining these two measures of performance, however, it is useful to review the differing incentives between a capitated and fee-for-service payment system.

The Incentives Underlying Capitation versus Fee-for-Service

The movement from fee-for-service to capitation changed the incentives facing providers. Under fee-for-service providers had an incentive to undertake only those services that were reimbursed. Further, given that the physician's time and effort were scarce, that effort was allocated according to those activities and services whose price (as determined

TABLE 9.1 Year-End Enrollment and Number of HMOs by Age of Plan, Size of Plan, Profit Status, and Model Type, 1986–96

	Total Enrollment		Percent of Total	Percent Change
	12/31/1986	1/1/1996	1/96	12/86–1/96
ALL PLANS	25,777,130	52,464,445	100.0	104
Age of Plan:				
<1 year	719,145	229,195	0.4	−68
1–2 years	3,313,588	1,276,697	2.4	−61
3–5 years	3,594,288	1,696,061	3.2	−53
6–9 years	4,976,512	10,672,506	20.3	114
10 or more	13,173,597	38,589,986	73.5	193
Size of Plan:				
<14,999	1,715,147	1,068,938	2.1	−38
15,000–49,999	4,859,863	5,957,919	11.3	23
50,000–99,999	5,463,426	6,943,111	13.2	27
100,000 or more	13,738,694	38,494,477	73.4	180
Profit Status:				
For-profit	10,735,498	31,021,082	59.1	189
Not-for-profit	15,041,632	21,443,363	40.9	43
Model Type [a]				
Staff	2,987,103	3,813,644	7.3	28
Group	6,822,759	14,330,235	27.3	110
Network	6,010,398	5,724,571	10.9	−5
IPA	9,956,870	26,696,532	50.9	168

Source: The Interstudy Edge (Interstudy: Excelsior, Minn., Spring 1987), p. 6, and The InterStudy Competitive Edge 6.2, *Part II: HMO Industry Report* (Excelsior, Minn.: Interstudy, September 1996), pp. 8 and 9, Table 3.

[a] The data for 1996 do not include 1,899,463 enrollees (3.6 percent of total). These enrollees were served by mixed model HMOs with unknown composition.

Staff = An HMO that delivers health services through a physician group that is controlled by the HMO unit.

Group = An HMO that contracts with one independent group practice to provide health services.

Network = An HMO that contracts with two or more independent group practices.

IPA = An HMO that contracts directly with physicians in independent practices.

by fee schedules) to cost ratio were highest. Services that the insurer did not cover, such as preventive care, changing a patient's lifestyle, or instituting a smoking cessation program, received little or no physician effort. Thus medical resources were primarily devoted to acute care services that were covered by insurance.

Fee-for-service payment also had several other incentive effects. Since providers, physicians and hospitals, were paid to deliver services, providers could increase their revenues by providing more services. Since (privately and governmentally) insured patients were less concerned with the price of their services, providers delivered services to the point where the marginal benefit to the patients of those additional services were very small. Thus the marginal benefit was less than the actual resource costs of those services. Overuse was a natural consequence of fee-for-service when patients were not financially responsible for the cost of those services.

The adoption of capitation had incentive effects opposite that of fee-for-service. The capitation payment, hence the insurance risk, may be at the HMO level or it may be shifted (all or in part) to one or more provider groups. The extent of the insurance risk depends on whether the HMO subcapitates different providers or not.

When the capitation payment remains with one organization, then they have an incentive to be concerned with the coordination of all the medical services provided. When the risk is subdivided among several different providers (e.g., medical groups and hospitals), then the financial incentives of the different groups are not aligned and could result in inefficiency and conflict. Since an incentive exists in a competitive market to eliminate inefficiencies, new organizational structures will evolve that result in a greater alignment of incentives.

Several of the positive incentives that result from capitation are as follows. When each provider (e.g., physicians) is paid separately under fee-for-service and they are not fiscally responsible for costs they impose on other providers (e.g., hospitals), there are no financial incentives to use the least costly setting for patient treatment. Under capitation, the capitated organization has an incentive to provide care in the least costly manner. When medically feasible, there will be greater use of outpatient services, fewer hospital admissions, and shorter hospital stays, with the remainder of the patient's convalescence provided for in another setting or in the patient's home. The emphasis is on minimizing the cost of treatment.

Capitated organizations also have an incentive to be concerned with the costs of their enrollees' hospital use. The HMO has an incentive to contract with those hospitals that offer lower prices, are located near their enrollees, and have a better reputation. To be competitive, hospitals must be efficient, take advantage of any economies of scale that exist, and eliminate unnecessary and duplicative facilities. Hospitals must first compete on price to be included in the organization's provider network before they can compete for physician referrals.

Capitation provides the medical group with an incentive to increase their physicians' productivity. One way would be to have nurse practitioners and physician assistants perform tasks currently undertaken by physicians. As long as the revenue produced by the additional auxiliaries exceeds their cost, it is in the interests of the medical group, if they are capitated, to substitute toward less costly personnel, as long as it does not diminish quality of care or patient satisfaction. Delegation of tasks might eventually also be based on the training and experience of individuals rather than, as under current practice, whether a profession has a monopoly on the performance of those tasks.

To the extent that preventive care delivered to an HMO's enrollees decreases future demand for more costly medical services, the capitated organization would be expected to provide a greater amount of those services than is provided under fee-for-service. Similarly, to the extent that enrollee health habits can be improved, such as through smoking cessation programs, future demands for medical care could be reduced. (The capitated organization is more likely to undertake preventive-type programs whose payoff is relatively soon rather than farther in the future, since, given the amount of switching between health plans, it is not clear how long that enrollee will be with the organization.)

It is in the economic interest of HMOs, assuming they are at risk for their enrollees' medical expenses, to prescribe less costly drugs. The HMO has an incentive to evaluate different prescription drugs to determine whether the marginal benefit of a more expensive drug exceeds its additional costs. Similarly, to the extent that prescription drugs decrease hospitalizations, the organization has an incentive to monitor its patients' drug usage. This is particularly true for the aged in Medicare HMOs.

Perhaps the most important incentive under capitation is to innovate in the delivery of medical services. Innovations are often threatening to current providers, since they may substitute for existing personnel and facilities, hence decreasing their demand. Previously, such innovations have been inhibited either by legal protections for the threatened providers or by anticompetitive actions by the professional associations. A capitated organization, however, has a strong financial incentive to be innovative in methods that reduce costs, improve outcomes, or increase patient satisfaction. Innovation is likely to occur in systems to aid patient diagnosis, improve treatment, improve patient compliance, encourage prevention, and adopt management techniques and information systems for decision making. Increased profit and/or increased market share provide capitated organizations with an incentive to seek out and quickly adopt (when economically feasible) new techniques with both medical and management applications.

There are, however, incentives in a capitated system that are a cause for concern. Since providers receive a lump sum per enrollee, there is an incentive to do as little as possible for the patient, since spending fewer resources means greater profits. Similarly, increasing the number of capitated enrollees without increasing the number of providers will result in decreased access to care. There is also an incentive to seek out lower-risk groups, if capitation payments are the same for all enrollees. Under fee-for-service, a high-risk patient would receive more services since the provider is paid according to the number and type of services provided.

Because of these incentives to reduce services and decrease access to care, it becomes essential that HMOs and capitated providers be monitored for access, quality of care, treatment outcomes, and patient satisfaction.

The Effect of Competition on Quality

There is a concern that market competition will reduce quality; this concern may be divided into two parts: the effect of the for-profit incentive on quality and the effect of incentives under capitation on number of services.

Many believe that for-profit organizations will sacrifice quality for profit. When nonprofit providers do not perform well, it is said that they at least meant well. However, nonprofit status by itself does not ensure high quality. It was found that tissue committees in nonprofit hospitals did not perform as they should have; county nursing homes are not necessarily noted for their high quality of care; state mental institutions and Veterans Administration hospitals are not centers of excellence. Outside the health field, nonprofit status does not necessarily lead to higher quality, nor is their sensitivity to the public interest greater than that of for-profit competitors. All public schools are not necessarily of higher quality than private schools; municipal governments are often greater polluters than for-profit firms; and when nonprofit unions manage their own pension funds, they do not often receive as high a rate of return as received by for-profit funds.

Similarly, it would be unfortunate if legislation restricted for-profit health plans. For-profit plans responded quickly to demands of the market for HMOs. They have been innovative and have forced the large nonprofit health plans to respond to preserve their market share. Nonprofit status per se does not guarantee ethical behavior, patient satisfaction, high-quality outcomes, or efficiency.

Rather than attempting to regulate for-profit plans or restrict innovations in medical practice, greater emphasis should be placed on health plan and provider outcome measures and accountability.

Nonprofit status alone should not relieve us of a concern for quality. Quality should be monitored directly. Consequently, it should not matter that for-profit providers compete. If only nonprofit providers are permitted, the effort to monitor quality will be less. The advantage of permitting for-profit providers to compete in the medical market is that, precisely because they are not trusted, a greater incentive exists to develop and apply strong quality review mechanisms. These quality review mechanisms should then apply equally to all providers. (For a debate on whether health providers should be expected to be different from "purveyors of other goods and services," the reader is referred an exchange of letters on this subject between Relman and Reinhardt [13].)

It might be argued that under capitation and competitively determined prices, for-profit HMOs in particular might be tempted to provide minimal medical services so as to retain as much of the capitation fee as possible. Although such a situation is unlikely for a number of reasons, several safeguards exist and others can be built into the system to ensure that it does not occur.

One such safeguard is consumer choice. Under the anti-trust laws, no organization, whether it be an HMO or a large medical group, can have a monopoly over the delivery of medical services in an area. Urban areas have multiple HMOs as well as a fee-for-service system. Consumers choose from among these alternative delivery systems and among HMOs and renew their choice annually. The various HMOs and alternative delivery systems have to compete for new subscribers as well as to retain their existing enrollees. Some consumers make their enrollment decisions based on limited information. Other subscribers, however, are more knowledgeable; for example, large purchasers, such as employers and unions, can afford to develop the necessary expertise to evaluate alternative health plans offered to their employees.

Business coalitions, such as the Pacific Business Group on Health (PBGH), and employers require health plans and their providers to collect data by which the health plans can be evaluated on the quality of their care and outcomes. The greater selectivity of better-informed groups benefits the less-informed subscribers. (All automobile purchasers are not equally knowledgeable, yet automobile companies compete on the basis of quality [e.g., increased warranty periods] as well as on price and styling, because part of their market is knowledgeable and willing to shift their purchases. The same occurs in the markets for other durable goods.) If several large employers were to no longer offer a particular HMO to their employees because of concerns over quality the HMO would have to change its benefits, accessibility, quality, or premiums if it is not to lose market share. The competition among health plans for the better-informed, large purchasers, those who are more likely to switch plans if quality deteriorates, helps those who are less well informed.

In addition to the above demand side responses when it is costly to gather information, providers respond by attempting to develop brand name recognition for their products. Consumers purchase two things when they buy a brand name product: the product itself and information on the company's reputation as to the quality of the product. Consumers with little information are willing to pay a higher price for a product that contains both of these components than a lower price for just the product itself. In the health field it is likely that health plans, physician groups, and multihospital systems will use brand name advertising for their products. (One interesting development in this regard is the purchase of university teaching hospitals by investor-owned chains; such investments are intended to provide a quality name recognition for the firm's health care activities.)

Large organizations or corporations expect to be in business for a long time. The expected long life of such organizations leads them to behave differently than small firms or those in business for a short time. Whereas an individual entrepreneur may go into business, mislead consumers, produce a poor product, and then quickly move on to another area, large corporations cannot afford such behavior. A large corporation cannot undertake those business practices that will maximize its present income at the expense of future business. It cannot afford purposely to produce a poor product. Because for-profit health plans and HMOs have their reputations at stake, pocketing the capitation fee and providing little or no service would adversely affect the reputation of the organization and decrease its future business. Poor business practices are more likely to be expected of smaller organizations, for which the costs of entering and leaving a market are lower. This is as true in the medical field as it is for corporations in general.

Just as the permanence of an organization leads to efforts to maintain or increase quality, so does the size of an organization. In a for-profit organization or in large medical groups, the quality of care practiced by any one physician in the group affects the reputation, hence the incomes, of the other physicians. This spillover effect helps ensure that poor medical care is not practiced by participating physicians. Under the previous traditional fee-for-service delivery system, physicians did not have any financial incentives to monitor one another or to impose sanctions against those physicians whose performance, when examined by utilization review and tissue committees, was revealed to be unacceptable. Quality of care is expected to be higher when physicians practice as part of a group than when they remain financially unaffected by the actions of an incompetent or unethical colleague.

Actions by large purchasers force insurers and their providers to respond to quality concerns. Several large employers and business coalitions have been placing a great deal of emphasis on measurement of patient satisfaction, quality of care, and health outcomes. Unfortunately, since there are few good indicators of health outcomes, most studies use process measures, that is, whether a woman receives a mammogram rather than the stage at which breast cancer is detected. Employers have taken the lead in requiring health plans to provide them with performance data. A great deal of research is being devoted to developing health plan "report cards," such as the Health Plan Employer Data Information Set (HEDIS). Initial report cards were based on unaudited data submitted by the health plan. Future report cards are to be based on standardized data, collected by independent organizations, and include data on various preventive services, consumer satisfaction measures, use rates by several diagnostic categories, and so on. These measures will be related to the health plan and to participating hospitals and medical groups.

The Pacific Business Group on Health (PBGH), a business coalition that spends $3 billion annually on its employees' health care has set aside 2 percent of the health plan's premium to provide the plan and its providers with an incentive to improve customer service and quality.

The publication of these report cards will eventually produce changes in the collection and reporting of data, quality, outcomes, and patient satisfaction, as well as in the delivery of health care. Although not all consumers will use that information in choosing their delivery system, some large, informed purchasers will use it. Other consumers will then benefit by the actions of these better-informed purchasers. The development of a broader range of quality measures should improve consumers' ability to choose among delivery systems on the basis of quality, outcomes, access, and price.

Greater use should be made of financial penalties when instances of poor quality are determined to exist. In the past, strong sanctions for poor quality, such as removal of a license to practice or of the accreditation of a hospital, have been considered so severe that they were rarely used. If less drastic measures such as financial penalties were available, it is likely that they would be applied more frequently to minor infractions of quality that would otherwise have gone unpunished.

Empirical Evidence on Quality of Care

Empirical evidence is beginning to accumulate on the effect that competitive markets are having on quality of care. Based on a review of the literature mostly covering the 1980s, Miller and Luft concluded that HMO enrollees received either better or equivalent quality of care results as fee-for-service enrollees (14). The studies reviewed included data on quality of care received by Medicare enrollees in HMOs and fee-for-service. The findings indicate that the quality of care received by Medicare enrollees in HMOs "was at least as equal to the quality of care received by beneficiaries in the fee-for-service sector in terms of the access beneficiaries had to treatment, the response of physicians to medical problems, the process of care provided to beneficiaries undergoing treatment, and the outcomes of treatment" (15).

Although patient satisfaction rates are typically high in HMOs, most managed care patients require little care. Current studies on access and satisfaction have therefore begun to examine how such organizations treat those who are chronically ill. A particular concern with HMOs is with regard to care of vulnerable populations, the poor and aged, who do not have large employers to act as their agents.

A recent study compared the physical and mental health outcomes of chronically ill adults, including poor and elderly subgroups, in HMO and fee-for-service systems (16). The types of chronic illness examined included hypertension, heart disease, and depression. Multiple HMOs of various structures (e.g., IPAs and multispecialty groups) were compared to fee-for-service practices. The findings from this study were as follows: For the average patient, physical and mental health outcomes did not differ between the HMOs and fee-for-service systems. However, physical health outcomes were, on average, more favorable for nonelderly patients in HMOs; elderly patients had more favorable outcomes in the fee-for-service system. Average changes in mental health for the elderly and nonelderly did not favor one system over the other. With regard to those who were on Medicaid, the only difference between the two systems were for those who were initially ill. Poor patients initially ill did better in the fee-for-service system.

This study points up the importance of examining those who are chronically ill and those in vulnerable population groups as better indicators of health plan performance. There are a great many health plans with different structures and with different provider incentive systems. The performance of each health plan, including those in fee-for-service, need to be continuously monitored.

Currently, there are no nationally accepted standards of care by which health plans and their provider groups can be evaluated. Competition has been based on price. Until reliable information becomes available on outcomes, patient satisfaction, and quality of care, and it is used together with premiums in choosing health plans, the public will be unable to make informed choices and providers who deliver higher quality of care and treat sicker patients will be at a competitive disadvantage.

The Effect of Managed Care Plans on the Growth in Medical Expenditures

Whether HMOs and managed care competition have reduced the rate of increase in medical expenditures may be subdivided into several parts: first, attempts of early studies to determine whether HMOs were a less costly system for providing medical services; second, whether HMOs provided a one-time savings or whether HMO expenditures also increase at a less rapid rate than indemnity insurance plans; and third, whether HMOs had a "spillover" effect (that is, did they reduce the rate of increase in indemnity insurance?) These issues are discussed below.

The early claims that HMOs were less costly than the fee-for-service system were based on data from a few of the larger HMOs, such as Kaiser and Group Health Association. Comparative data on fee-for-service were based on either utilization surveys of the general population or, in several instances, surveys of groups of employees whose insurance companies, such as Aetna or Blue Cross, provided them with a choice between an HMO and fee-for-service plans. A major problem with many of the early studies was subscriber selectivity; if subscribers with low utilization patterns selected an HMO, differences in utilization rates between HMOs and fee-for-service could not be considered the result of the HMO, nor would it be possible to extrapolate the potential savings if a much larger segment of the population were enrolled in HMOs.

The most well-known study to determine whether the performance of HMOs was due to biased selection or to the style of practice in the HMO was a controlled experiment by RAND Corporation (17). Also examined in the study was the amount of out-of-plan use by enrollees in the HMO, since favorable HMO performance could be a result of high out-of-plan use. Individuals were assigned to one of three groups: two fee-for-service groups (in one all services were free whereas in the other copayments were required) and one group assigned to the HMO (referred to as the HMO experimental group). The study also examined a group that already belonged to the HMO, referred to as the HMO control group. Expenditures were imputed for use of services in the HMO so that comparisons could be made to those in fee-for-service.

Imputed expenditures between those in the HMO experimental and control groups were very similar, although the experimental group had a slightly higher out-of-plan expenditure. Both HMO groups, however, had much lower expenditures (including out-of-plan) than those of the free fee-for-service group (23 to 28 percent less). The size of the expenditures in the HMO groups was comparable to those in one of the fee-for-service plans, which had a 95 percent co-payment up to a family maximum of $1,000 a year. Although expenditures for these groups were comparable, those assigned to the fee-for-service 95 percent co-payment group had fewer face-to-face visits than did the two HMO groups.

The large differences between the HMO enrollees and the free fee-for-service group occurred in their hospital use rates, which were approximately 40 percent lower for the HMO group. The authors attributed this lower use rate to the "style of practice" at the HMO, which is less hospital-intensive.

The findings from the RAND study were consistent with earlier studies on HMO performance (18). These other studies found that the total cost of medical care (premium plus out-of-pocket expenses) for HMO enrollees was 10 to 40 percent lower than for persons with comparable insurance coverage using the fee-for-service delivery system.

An important determinant of lower hospitalization rates in HMOs is the method by which physicians are compensated. Based on a review of studies that examined physicians' financial incentives and patient utilization, Hellinger states: "Some of the studies . . . compared the utilization on enrollees with the same disease across health plans, some studies compared the utilization of patients in HMOs and in the fee-for-service sector treated by the same physician, and one study investigated utilization in HMOs that reimbursed physicians on a fee-for-service basis to utilization in HMOs that reimbursed physicians on a per capita basis . . . in virtually every study, measures of utilization adjusted for available information on differences in type of enrollee, physician, and health plan were lower when when physicians faced incentives to control their use of resources" (19).

There is still concern, however, that HMOs have received a more favorable risk group. Based on a review of the empirical literature, Luft and Miller conclude that some HMOs have received a preferred risk group of enrollees. New enrollees in some HMOs were more likely to have lower health use and expenditures prior to joining the HMO (20). (Biased selection is also discussed in Chapter 6.)

There is also evidence that preferred risk selection has occurred among Medicare HMOs (21). Medicare HMO enrollees had better functional status and were less likely to report their health status as fair or poor compared to Medicare fee-for-service enrollees. Further, Medicare enrollees entering an HMO had costs 37 percent below average while those leaving the HMO had costs 60 percent above average. Persons who are ill or who have chronic conditions are generally reluctant to leave their physician and switch to an HMO. Under such circumstances the HMO will enroll those aged who are healthier and have lower expenditures. The government pays for the high-cost aged in the fee-for-service system, while HMOs enroll, at 95 percent of the average cost, those aged with lower average costs. It has been estimated that the government still overpays the HMO by 6 percent on average. Research continues to be conducted on developing a better risk adjustment measure.

Research has demonstrated, controlling for selection, that non-Medicare HMOs have 20 to 35 percent lower costs than comparable fee-for-service plans, which were primarily achieved by reducing hospitalization among HMO enrollees.

There had been controversy, however, over whether these lower expenditures per enrollee were a one-time savings or whether expenses for HMO enrollees also increased at a lower rate than for enrollees in fee-for-service plans. Early research did not indicate that HMOs experienced lower rates of growth in their premiums. HMOs were initially thought of as being synonymous with market competition; it was believed that HMOs would engage in price competition with insurance companies. The pressure to compete on price would force insurance companies and HMOs to select hospitals and physicians on the basis of their prices and quality of services. However, there was a lack of price competition among HMOs and other insurance plans until the late 1980s. (Employees did not have a price incentive to choose a lower-cost health plan since their employer either paid the full premium or the employee contribution was unrelated to the plan selected.) HMOs initially set their premiums just under those of the indemnity plan ("shadow pricing") and competed for an employer's enrollees by offering more benefits than the indemnity plan.

As employers required their employees to pay the difference in cost for more expensive health plans, employees became price sensitive to lower-cost health plans and plans began to compete on price. Evidence began to accumulate that HMO premiums were increasing at a lower rate than indemnity plans.

There was concern by 1990 that market competition was not having the cost-reducing effect on medical expenditures that its proponents predicted. Studies began to examine whether HMOs and managed care competition were reducing the rate of growth in indemnity health insurance premiums. In debates over health care reform in the early years of the Clinton administration, the Congressional Budget Office (CBO) was responsible for costing out the various reform proposals. CBO's cost estimates were crucial to the acceptability of various health reform proposals. As part of its analysis, CBO assumed that HMOs would not affect the future rate of growth in health care costs. This was the conventional wisdom at the time.

More recent evidence, however, determined that increased HMO competition, measured by HMO penetration in a market, does reduce the rise in health insurance premiums among non-HMO plans (the "spillover" effect) (22). Advocates of managed care competition believed that as employees are given a price incentive to choose lower-cost plans, higher-cost indemnity plans would lose market share. HMO and non-HMO insurance plans are substitutes for each other. The lower-cost growth of HMOs would increase the premium difference between HMOs and indemnity plans. To reduce the rise in their premiums and recover their market share, indemnity plans would begin to adopt managed care methods. The initiation of utilization management by indemnity plans was a response to the HMOs' lower hospital use rates. PPOs were also their response to HMOs closed provider panels.

Using data for the 1985–92 period, Wickizer and Feldstein found that indemnity insured groups located in markets with higher HMO penetration had lower rates of growth in their insurance premiums. Employee groups located in areas with low HMO market penetration had annual premium increases of 8 percent per year (inflation-adjusted) compared to 4 percent per year among employee groups with indemnity insurance located in areas with high HMO penetration. (Other factors affecting premium increases were controlled for, such as differences in health plan benefits, characteristics of the insured group, differences in the markets where the insured groups were located, and the insurance underwriting cycle.)

Given the high degree of price sensitivity across different types of health plans (see Chapter 8), large premium differences between plans have resulted in large shifts in market shares between types of plans. Unmanaged indemnity plans rely only on deductibles and cost sharing to control costs. As a consequence their premiums have increased much more rapidly than managed indemnity plans and HMOs. Unmanaged indemnity plans have lost a great deal of their once predominant market share and are likely to become a small niche-type of insurance plan.

HMO enrollment growth, relative to unmanaged indemnity plans, increased sharply starting in the mid-1980s. There was also a large increase in the number of new HMOs, as shown in Table 9.2.

Although the rise in medical expenditures has been greatly reduced, it is unclear how rapidly medical expenditures will increase in the future. Competition is continuing to reduce inefficiencies in the medical care delivery system. As these inefficiencies are eliminated, the rate of growth in expenditures will be determined by a number of factors. These include cost-saving innovations in the delivery of medical services, advances in medical technology, the aging of the population, government regulations affecting the cost of providing medical care, and rising population incomes.

Those providers and firms that are most innovative in reducing medical costs will experience growth in their market shares and profitability. New medical technology will be developed with the objective of reducing medical costs and permitting care to be delivered in lower cost settings. (Previously, under fee-for-service and comprehensive insurance, medical technology was demanded as long as it increased medical benefits without

TABLE 9.2 Growth in Number of HMOs and Their Enrollment, 1976–95

Year	Number of HMOs	Annual Percentage Increases	Enrollment (in millions)	Annual Percent Increase
1976	175	6.0		
1977	165	−5.7	6.3	5.0
1978	203	23.0	7.5	19.0
1979	215	5.9	8.2	9.3
1980	236	9.8	9.1	11.0
1981	243	3.0	10.2	12.1
1982	265	9.1	10.8	5.9
1983	280	5.7	12.5	15.7
1984	306	9.3	15.1	20.8
1985	393	28.4	18.9	25.2
1986	626	59.3	25.7	36.0
1987	650	3.8	29.3	14.0
1988	607	−6.6	32.7	11.6
1989	590	−2.8	34.7	6.1
1990	566	−4.1	36.5	5.2
1991	547	−3.4	38.6	5.8
1992	546	−0.2	41.4	7.3
1993	545	−0.2	45.2	9.2
1994	574	5.3	51.1	13.1
1995	591	3.0	56.0*	9.6

Source: Group Health Association of America, *1995 National Directory of HMOs* (Washington, D.C.: Group Health Association of America, Inc., 1995), pp. 21, 22.
*Estimated.

regard to cost.) The population is aging and an older population requires more care and more costly care. Government regulations that require health plans to include costly benefits and/or mandate how care to be be provided, either by types of health professionals or in which institutional settings, will increase health plan costs and premiums. And, medical care is income elastic; that is, an increase in income will result in at least a proportionate increase in expenditures on medical care. Quality is also income elastic. Thus as incomes increase, other things held constant, expenditures on medical care should also increase.

Thus, increased medical expenditures do not mean that market competition cannot reduce the rise in medical costs. Instead, given the above demographic and economic forces, market competition attempts to achieve the "appropriate" rate of increase in medical expenditures.

SUMMARY

Market competition changed the incentives facing the purchaser as well as the supplier of medical services by transferring financial risk. Purchasers, whether they are patients, employers, or health plans, have an economic incentive to search for those providers that can provide a given quality product at the lowest price. Purchasers also have an incentive to consider the trade-off between price and quality; increases in quality that are worth less than their increased cost are less likely to be purchased. Regardless of whether the supplier is for-profit or nonprofit, they have an incentive to minimize the cost of the product they are producing when they face a fixed price, either market- or government-determined.

Different institutional arrangements have emerged on the supply side of the market in response to the heightened concern over expenditures on the demand side. Initially, there was a large growth in HMOs. However, the latter half of the 1980s demonstrated that price competition, when it occurred, involved more than just HMOs. The growth in PPOs, the development of managed fee-for-service, and the change in HMOs (greater growth in IPAs and POS plans) is indicative of the market's attempt to match employer and employee preferences by offering them a choice between higher premiums and greater restrictiveness of the delivery system.

One advantage of competitive markets is that they provide for a diversity of preferences among purchasers in how much they are willing to pay for medical services and in types of health plans. This multiplicity of choices, however, has the potential for health plans competing on risk selection rather than on how well they can manage medical treatment.

Unless biased selection among health plans is controlled, cost differences among competing health plans may represent enrollment of lower-risk groups rather than differences in plan efficiency. When the employer or the government pays a premium, unrelated to the risk of the enrollee, health plans have an incentive to compete for lower than average risk groups rather than on efficiency in managing the patient's treatment. The result can be that employers and the government may end up spending more money when a choice of health plans are offered than if everyone enrolled in a single plan.

Paying a risk-adjusted premium to a health plan would limit biased selection. It would also provide an incentive for a health plan to seek out high-risk individuals since the plan could profit by innovating in the management of their care.

An important aspect of price-competitive plans is that participating physicians and hospitals become part of a "closed panel." As the market share of these closed panel plans grow, nonparticipating providers are "locked" out of a significant part of the market. A delivery system must be able to exclude certain providers if it is to have control over its costs, quality, and reputation. Closed panel plans also create price competition among physicians. Physicians are willing to discount their fees if they can increase volume.

(Some states have enacted "any willing provider" laws as a result of lobbying by those providers who are not part of closed panels. Such laws lessen price competition in that any physician could participate in an insurer's provider panel. This lessens the incentive for provider panels to reduce their fees in hope of gaining an increased volume of patients, since their patients would then be shared with other physicians who decide to participate.)

It is important to realize that price competition was not widespread during the 1980s. In fact, in the latter half of the 1980s only about one-third of total medical expenditures were subject to price competition. For example, hospitals do not compete on price for Medicare patients, although they do have an incentive under Medicare DRG payments to minimize their costs per admission. Medicare patients must pay the same hospital deductible regardless of the hospital they enter. Medicare HMOs similarly do not compete on price for Medicare patients. Through the 1980s few states used competitive bidding for allocating their Medicaid population among managed care plans and providers. Government expenditures for Medicaid and Medicare represent approximately 45 percent of total medical expenditures and there is limited, if any, price competition among providers for these patients.

In the private sector many employers paid all or most of their employees' health insurance premiums. Other employers did have the employee paid the additional cost of more expensive health plans. Thus the preconditions for price competition were not widespread.

Price competition among competing delivery systems should continue to increase in coming years. And it is likely that more Medicare and Medicaid enrollees will be enrolled in managed care plans.

There has always been a concern that quality of care would suffer under a price-competitive system. There is the fear that some physicians would engage in unethical behavior to increase their incomes or that HMOs and other providers would provide fewer services. As health plans enroll employees directly at the workplace, unions and companies provide an important oversight function. It is more difficult for the individual to detect poor quality, and as a consequence the costs to the provider of providing less-than-optimal service are decreased. This was of greater concern in the previous fee-for-service system. The current emphasis on outcomes research and appropriate care should provide purchasers with information on quality that will improve the functioning of a competitive market.

Although health plan performance measures are still primitive and report cards have yet to be widely available, the competitive system has made a great deal of progress. The rate of growth in health care expenditures has been reduced. Information systems are being developed to evaluate providers and to generate data on health plan performance, publicity is being focused on health plans and their performance, studies are being conducted on the appropriateness of various medical procedures, and consumers have more choice on health plans. Twenty years ago, expenditures were increasing rapidly and provider performance data were not available; hospital accrediting commissions would not release their findings on hospitals and no information was available on providers, such as medical groups and hospitals. The system has improved and is becoming more accountable.

Recently, as a result of anecdotes on undertreatment of care by managed care organizations, the federal and state governments have enacted legislation that effectively prescribes medical practice. Although there has been no objective evidence of a decline in quality of care between HMOs and fee-for-service, legislators have responded to media publicity and enacted legislation. One example is legislation requiring forty-eight-hour maternity stays if they are medically necessary. HMOs are currently required to provide all services that are medically necessary. If the intent of the law was to require a minimum forty-eight-hour stay for uncomplicated deliveries, then this will increase insurance premiums. The Congressional Budget Office has estimated that over four years this will cost the federal government $233 million and the private sector $745 million (23). Another recent example was legislators' response over outpatient mastectomies for treatment of breast cancer patients. Johns Hopkins University Hospital performed outpatient mastectomies because of its effectiveness and patient satisfaction, not because it was under pressure from managed care companies.

If legislatures enact laws each time there is some adverse publicity about a particular medical treatment, experimentation with cost-reducing innovations will become difficult.

It should be emphasized again that neither a market approach nor regulation alone will solve all of the concerns that people have with regard to medical care. Redistributing medical services requires government intervention; however, government involvement need not be direct. Government subsidies can be provided through a market mechanism, such as through the use of vouchers. For a given redistribution subsidy, a market approach to the delivery of services can more efficiently achieve the redistribution objective.

Key Terms and Concepts

- Capitation
- "free choice of provider"
- Independent Practice Association (IPA)

- Report cards
- "rule of reason"

- "Any willing provider" laws
- Applicability of anti-trust laws
- Capitation and fee-for-service incentives
- Certificate of need legislation (CON)
- Competition and quality
- Cost containment programs
- Diagnostic-related groups (DRGs)

Review Questions

1. What are the reasons that the health field changed from a nonprice-competitive market to a price-competitive industry in the 1980s?
2. Explain why advertising among physicians is expected to result in lower physician fees. Wouldn't the additional cost of advertising increase physicians' fees?
3. If advertising in the health field is expected to result in lower prices, why do firms producing breakfast cereals, soaps, and so on, undertake such extensive advertising campaigns?
4. If HMOs are such a good idea, why did their growth only start in the mid-1980s and not before?
5. "Free choice" of physician has been interpreted by organized medicine (and dentistry) to mean that a patient's choice of physician should not be restricted to those physicians participating in a particular delivery system. Under what circumstances has this interpretation of "free choice" resulted in anticompetitive behavior by organized medicine?
6. How can the existence of adverse selection and preferred risk selection by HMOs increase the cost to the government of Medicare risk contracts?
7. Explain the similarities and differences among managed care, HMOs, and PPOs in terms of who bears the financial risk, how providers are paid, and incentives for efficiency in the delivery of medical services.
8. What are the different incentives to providers of being paid on a capitated basis rather than fee-for-service?
9. Using an economic framework, analyze the rise that has occurred in medical care prices, and using the same framework, what would you forecast for the next several years? Be explicit regarding any assumptions underlying your analysis.
10. Choose two different methods of reducing the rising price of medical care and explain what their intended effect (both direct and indirect) will be. What change, if any, will occur as a result of each of your two proposals?

11. What are the potential concerns (or sources of market imperfection) with implementing a price-competitive policy?
12. How can selection bias among health plans affect an employer's total medical premiums?
13. Evaluate the following statement: "A competitive policy for medical care has been a failure because many of the poor are unable to receive needed care."
14. What should determine the appropriate rate of increase in medical expenditures? Be explicit regarding your assumptions.
15. What is the role of government in a competitive medical market?
16. Why was market competition able to develop in the 1980s, but not in the 1930s, even though physicians and hospitals had excess capacity in both periods?

REFERENCES

1. See Reuben Kessel, "Price Discrimination in Medicine," *Journal of Law and Economics,* October 1958. This article is discussed more completely in the chapter on the market for physician manpower.
2. For a more complete discussion of the reasons for deregulation in both the medical and nonmedical sectors, see Paul J. Feldstein, *The Politics of Health Legislation: An Economic Perspective* (Ann Arbor, Mich.: Health Administration Press, 1996), Chapters 5 and 6.
3. "Health Professions Educational Assistance Amendments of 1965," *Hearing before the Subcommittee on Health of the Committee on Labor and Public Welfare,* U.S. Senate, 89th Congress, 1st Session, September 8, 1965, 39–40.
4. For a complete discussion of CON and its legislative changes, see Clark C. Havighurst, *Deregulating the Health Care Industry: Planning for Competition* (Cambridge, Mass.: Ballinger, 1982), p. 222.
5. Alain C. Enthoven, *Health Plan* (Reading, Mass.: Addison-Wesley, 1980).
6. For a more complete discussion of these issues, see Donald W. Moran, "HMOs, Competition and the Politics of Minimum Benefits," *Milbank Memorial Fund Quarterly,* Spring 1981; Alain C. Enthoven, "How Interested Groups Have Responded to a Proposal for Economic Competition in Health Services," *American Economic Review,* May 1980; and John K. Iglehart, "Drawing the Lines for the Debate on Competition," *New England Journal of Medicine,* July 30, 1981.
7. *Medicaid Freedom of Choice Waiver Activities,* Hearing before the Subcommittee on Health of the Committee on Finance, U.S. Senate, 98th Congress, 2nd Session, March 30, 1984.
8. *Company Practices in Health Care Cost Management* (Lincolnshire, Ill.: Hewitt Associates, 1984).
9. Lawrence G. Goldberg and Warren Greenberg, "The Emergence of Physician-Sponsored Health Insurance: A Historical Perspective," in Warren Greenberg, ed., *Competition in the Health Care Sector* (Germantown, Md.: Aspen Systems Corporation, 1978).
10. For a review of anti-trust actions in the health field, see L. Barry Costillo, "Anti-trust Enforcement in Health Care: Ten Years After the AMA Suit," *New England Journal of Medicine,*

313(14), October 3, 1985. Also see *Statements of Anti-trust Policy in Health Care,* issued by the U.S. Department of Justice and the Federal Trade Commission, Washington, D.C., August 1996.

11. Jon Gabel, "Ten Ways HMOs Have Changed During the 1990s," *Health Affairs,* 16(3), May–June 1997: 134–145.

12. Douglas Wholey et al., "Scale and Scope Economies Among Health Maintenance Organizations," *Journal of Health Economics,* 15(6), December 1996: 657–684; and Ruth S. Given, "Economies of Scale and Scope as an Explanation of Merger and Output Diversification Activities in the Health Maintenance Industry," *Journal of Health Economics,* 15(6), December 1996: 685–713.

13. Arnold S. Relman and Uwe E. Reinhardt, "Debating For-Profit Health Care," *Health Affairs,* 5(2), Summer 1986. This exchange was initiated as a result of the authors' participation in the following report: Institute of Medicine, *For-Profit Enterprise in Health Care* (Washington, D.C.: National Academy Press, 1986).

14. Robert H. Miller and Harold S. Luft, "Managed Care Plan Performance Since 1980: A Literature Analysis," *Journal of the American Medical Association,* 271(19), May 18, 1994: 1512–1519.

15. Kathryn M. Langwell and James P. Hadley, "Evaluation of the Medicare Competition Demonstrations," *Health Care Financing Review,* 11(2), Winter 1989: 73.

16. John E. Ware Jr. et al., "Differences in 4-Year Health Outcomes for Elderly and Poor, Chronically Ill Patients Treated in HMO and Fee-for-Service Systems," *Journal of the American Medical Association,* 276(13), October 2, 1996: 1039–1047.

17. Willard G. Manning et al., "A Controlled Trial of the Effect of a Prepaid Group Practice on Use of Services," *New England Journal of Medicine,* 310(23), June 7, 1984.

18. Harold S. Luft, *Health Maintenance Organizations: Dimensions of Performance* (New York: Wiley, 1981). See also Harold S. Luft, "How Do Health Maintenance Organizations Achieve Their 'Savings'?" *New England Journal of Medicine,* 298(26), June 15, 1978: 1336–1343.

19. Fred J. Hellinger, "The Impact of Financial Incentives on Physician Behavior in Managed Care Plans: A Review of the Evidence," *Medical Care Research and Review,* 53(3), September 1996: 294–314.

20. For a discussion of these issues, see Miller and Luft, *op. cit.*

21. Gerald Riley et al., "Health Status of Medicare Enrollees in HMOs and Fee-for-Service in 1994," *Health Care Financing Review,* 17(4), Summer 1996; and "Risk Assessment and Risk Adjustment in Medicare," Chapter 15 in *Annual Report to Congress* (Washington, D.C.: Physician Payment Review Commission, 1996).

22. Thomas M. Wickizer and Paul J. Feldstein, "The Impact of HMO Competition on Private Health Insurance Premiums, 1985–1992," *Inquiry,* 32(3), Fall 1995: 241–251.

23. Congressional Budget Office, letter to Congress, cost estimate of S.969, Newborns' and Mothers' Health Protection Act of 1996, July 17, 1996.

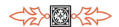

CHAPTER

10

The Physician Services Market

The emphasis of this chapter is on the efficiency with which physician services are provided rather than on the efficiency with which medical treatments, of which physician services are an important component, are produced and priced. Determination of the number of physicians and the market for medical education are discussed in separate chapters. Although these markets are closely related to the market for physician services, the rationale for discussing these subjects and the pricing and provision of physician services separately is that the determinants of the number of physicians are not identical to the factors that determine the quantity of physician services or how they are priced.

The interrelationship between these markets, the determinants of supply and demand in each market, and the different types of public policies that influence these separate markets are more easily visualized with reference to Figure 10.1.

The demand for physician services is determined by factors such as those discussed previously. There are noneconomic factors, such as need and cultural-demographic factors; the economic factors are the patient's income, the price the patient must pay for physician services (as well as the price of substitute and complementary services), the type and comprehensiveness of insurance coverage, and any time costs that are involved in the purchase and use of physician services.

The price of physician services, as shown in Figure 10.1, is determined by the interaction of supply and demand factors. Price, in turn, influences patient demand and the amount of services providers are willing to provide.

The supply of physician services is affected by the price received for physician services and by the cost of producing those services. The cost depends on input productivities and input prices. These are affected by the number of physicians, the number of hours they work, their use of auxiliaries, the capital and equipment available, and other inputs and

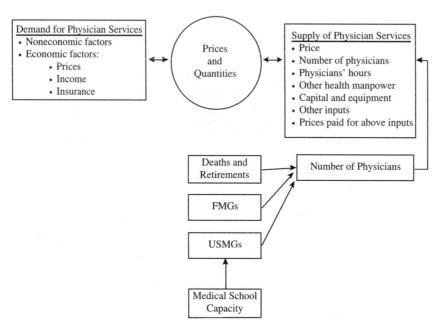

FIGURE 10.1 • The market for physician services.

expenses necessary to the provision of physician services, such as malpractice coverage. The number of physicians combined with other inputs determines the available supply of such services. Physician services may be provided using different combinations of physicians and other health manpower. Physicians may perform all of their tasks themselves or they may delegate varying amounts of those tasks to auxiliaries. With a greater degree of task delegation, physicians will be able to increase their productivity. The extent to which physicians delegate their tasks will affect not only the quantity and type of physician services available but also their cost.

In the short run, the output, physician services, can be increased by increasing all of the inputs except physicians. Physician hours, which can also be varied, are determined by the labor–leisure trade-off; what happens to the physician's hours of work as both the price received per hour of work and his income increases? Do physicians reduce their hours of work as their prices increase?

The long run is that period of time in which there can be an increase in the number of physicians. Changes in the number of physicians result from deaths and retirements, immigration of foreign-trained medical graduates and physicians, and increases in the number of U.S.-trained medical graduates. The number of U.S.-trained medical graduates is determined by the demand for and supply of medical education. The demand for a medical education is influenced by a number of factors, among which is the relative rate of return to such an education; as shown in Figure 10.1, the price and quantity determined in the physician services market (which is equivalent to gross physician income) is a component of that rate of return.

As shown in Figure 10.1, medical education is an important determinant of the number of physicians and, consequently, the supply of physicians' services. Separate chapters are devoted to an analysis of both the physician manpower and medical education markets, to include the development of their structural characteristics, their consequent effect on performance, and the relevant public policies within each market.[1]

Government policies have intervened at several points in physician markets. With respect to the demand for services, Medicare and Medicaid have served to stimulate the demand for services among specific population groups. In addition to the direct effects of these two programs, there were also indirect consequences: persons not subsidized by Medicare and Medicaid faced higher prices of physician services; controls on physician prices affected the quantity of those services, the hours physicians were willing to work, and the time patients had to wait to receive such services. Subsequent government policies attempted to limit the rise in Medicare physician expenditures; federal price controls between 1971 and 1974, the Medicare economic index, and the more recent Medicare resource based relative value scale (RBRVS), together with its annual updates, controlled the annual percent increase in physician fees.

Government policies on the supply side have, in the past, increased the number of physicians by providing subsidies for both the construction of new medical schools and for existing schools to increase their enrollments. Government loans and scholarships were provided (through the medical schools) to medical students, which, by lowering the cost of a medical education, increases its demand. Government policy has affected the inflow of foreign-trained medical graduates and physicians by its immigration policies. Also affecting the supply of physician services is state-level legislation that places limits on who can practice medicine and that defines the tasks that may be performed by various categories of health manpower.

In this chapter the performance of the physician services market is evaluated to determine, first, whether physician services are produced in the least costly manner and, second, whether the prices charged for such services are related to their costs of production. If the price of physician services were greatly in excess of their costs, fewer physician services would be purchased than if their prices were closer to the costs of production. Thus, a measure of how well the market for physician services performs is the relationship of prices to costs; because it is often difficult to measure costs directly, this price–cost relationship may be inferred through the method by which physician prices are determined. In relatively competitive markets, costs are minimized and prices approximate costs; in monopolistic markets, the seller's price may greatly exceed the cost of providing that service.

When evaluating the performance of the market for physician services, observed measures of performance will be compared with what might be expected to occur in a hypo-

---

[1]Quality-assurance mechanisms are placed, primarily, on medical inputs, such as the training requirements for physicians, and not on the services provided. The development of such "process" quality measures has had important effects on the structure of health manpower and health education markets. Alternative approaches to achieving quality assurance, and their effect on performance, are therefore discussed in chapters dealing with the manpower and education markets.

thetical competitive market. The reasons for any possible divergence between the observed and hypothetical outcomes will then be analyzed.

THE STRUCTURE
OF THE PHYSICIAN SERVICES MARKET

The structure of a market, such as physician services, is usually determined, first, by the extent of economies of scale to be gained by practicing in medical groups and, second, by barriers to entry into that market. As will be discussed in the chapter on medical education, there have been (and still are) barriers to entry into the medical profession. Physicians must graduate from an approved medical school, and they must be licensed. The number of spaces in medical schools has been restricted. However, even if entry into medicine is limited, given the large number of practicing physicians, it is still possible that the market for physician services could be competitive.

For more than one hundred years, the predominant form of medical practice was solo practice with fee-for-service reimbursement. The structure of the physician services market could have been characterized as competitive, except for various restrictions, such as limits on both physician advertising and on insurance companies' ability to negotiate discount prices among physicians. With the applicability of the anti-trust laws to the health field in the early 1980s, physician-imposed restrictions on advertising and price competition were eliminated. As competitive restrictions were removed and managed care organizations increased, physicians began to compete on price for HMO and insurer business. The structure of the industry began to change.

Economies of Scale in Medical Practice

A number of explanations have been offered for the shift from solo to group practice. The first and most obvious explanation is that physicians could increase their productivity and lower their costs if they were to take advantage of any economies of scale in group practice. The average cost of providing physician services is expected to decline from sharing inputs such as aides, equipment, and offices and from volume discounts on supplies.

Studies on economies of scale attempt to determine which size practices have the lowest cost per physician and to estimate the amount of inefficiency that exists by calculating the increase in productivity that would occur if existing sized groups were equal to the size that is estimated to be of lowest cost. However, unless these analyses are performed separately for physicians in urban areas and in rural areas, the extent of inefficiency for rural practices will be overstated. The optimal (least cost) size of practice in a rural area will be smaller since patient travel costs are higher, given the lower population density. The optimal size of a practice should consider not only practice costs but also patient travel costs. The larger the group size in a rural area the greater are patient travel costs. The optimal size practice therefore is one that combines both practice costs and patient travel costs, which would result in smaller practices in rural than urban areas (1).

A problem in estimating economies of scale in medical group practice is the definition and measurement of outputs and inputs. Large medical groups provide a greater variety of outputs than do small groups or solo practices. Larger groups are also more likely to own laboratories and x-ray facilities and participate in HMOs and insurance plans, which require additional administrative personnel. Unless outputs and inputs are measured accurately and adjustments made for differences in outputs, the results of studies may incorrectly conclude that large groups have higher costs and are therefore less efficient.

Detailed information on the quantity and mix of each of the services provided in a physician's office is generally unavailable. Empirical studies must therefore use proxy measures for physician services, such as annual gross patient revenues. Although this measure may reflect differences in quality and service mix among practices, it contains a serious problem in that higher patient billings may not reflect differences in output but may result from higher prices being charged for similar services.

Another often-used proxy for the output of a physician's practice is the weekly number of office visits, which implicitly assumes that quality does not vary by size of group. Physician productivity studies also generally assume that the mix of patient visits among different physician practices is similar. Over time, however, there have been important changes in the physician output mix. For example, the proportion of all physician services performed by specialists has increased.

The measurement of manpower inputs, with differing relative productivities, in production function studies can bias the results unless different manpower categories are separately measured. Physician extenders, such as physician assistants and pediatric nurse practitioners, are the closest substitutes for the physician and are more productive than are allied health workers (e.g., registered nurses), medical technicians (e.g., x-ray and lab technicians), and nonmedical assistants (e.g., clerical and administrative persons).

One other aspect that is important in interpreting the results of studies on economies of scale is whether there are selection biases in the types of physicians who join group practices. If certain types of physicians are more likely to join one form of medical practice than another and they are less productive, then differences in productivity (hence cost per unit of output) may be a result of the type of physician than the form or size of the practice.

Two types of studies have been undertaken to determine the extent of economies of scale in medical groups. The first examines whether patient revenues and/or visits per physician are higher in larger than in smaller practices. The second type of study is a "survivor" analysis, which assumes that the fastest-growing size of group is the most efficient.

According to empirical studies, the cost–size relationship appears to be U shaped; small groups appear to be more productive than solo practitioners but very large groups are less productive, per physician, than smaller groups. For example, using data from the late 1960s, Reinhardt concluded that physicians in groups generate about 5 percent more patient visits and billings than those in solo practice (2). The average number of weekly patient visits for general practitioners (GPs) in groups was 16 percent higher than for solo GPs. Two other studies, one using data on physician office visits from a 1978 national survey of group practice, the other using practice revenues, found that group size had a negative effect on the physician's hourly patient load and revenues; the larger the group, the lower the physician's productivity and/or office revenues (3).

In a recent study, Pope and Burge calculate optimum size of medical group by various categories, such as for single specialty groups (e.g., primary care, cardiology, surgery) and also for multispecialty groups. They find that the optimal size group varies by these categories, being largest for multispecialty groups, thirty-three physicians, with the other groups having about five physicians each. The amount of inefficiency that exists for each of these types of groups (which is the difference between their actual and optimal size and the increased productivity of being larger) varies, but generally being less than 10 percent (4).

Several of the above authors have attempted to determine the reasons for group practice economies of scale. These studies have attempted to determine whether physicians in different-size groups use the optimal number of aides. Early studies concluded that physicians hired less than the optimal number of aides.

Using 1965–67 data, Reinhardt determined that the average solo physician could profitably employ twice as many auxiliaries. Employing four rather than two auxiliaries, which was the average during 1965–67, would have resulted in a 25 percent increase in the number of patient visits per physician (5). Reinhardt calculated the optimal number of aides for a solo physician based on the price received per visit, the marginal productivity of an aide, and the weekly wage of the aide. (The marginal productivity of the aide, which is the additional number of visits produced by the aide, multiplied by the price received per visit is the marginal revenue product of the aide, or the additional value of that aide. The physician should be willing to pay a weekly wage, assuming no additional costs, equal to the additional value generated by that aide.) The employment of aides should increase as the price of the visit increases and decrease as the cost of aides increases.

Using 1976 data on office-based physicians, Brown reestimated the production analysis performed earlier by Reinhardt and found that physicians in group practice were 22 percent more productive than those in solo practice (6). Brown concluded that solo and group physicians used nurses efficiently but overutilized non-nurses, such as clerical and secretarial help. The increased productivity of group physicians was primarily due to greater use of physician assistants.[2] Brown found that the overall use of aides by physicians declined after 1978, attributing the decline to the rapid increase in the supply of

---

[2]For a group practice to determine whether they are over- or underutilizing aides it is necessary to have the following information: first, an estimate of the marginal productivity (MP) of each of the inputs used in producing a physician visit. (The marginal product of each input is derived from a production function for a physician office visit.) Next, the marginal product of each input is divided by its cost per hour. The resulting ratio is then compared for each of the inputs. For example, assume that the MP of a physician is 2.8 visits per hour and the MP of an aide is 0.8 visits per hour, their respective costs (wage) per hour are $75 and $18, and their ratios (MP/physician wage and MP/aide wage) are 0.037 and 0.044, respectively. Comparing the MP per dollar spent on physicians to the MP per dollar spent on aides indicates that aides (in this example) have a higher MP per dollar spent and are therefore being underutilized. Hiring an additional aide would increase the total number of physician visits produced but cause a decrease in the MP of that new aide (because of the

physicians after 1980 (with a consequent change in their wage relative to aides) and the changing specialty distribution of physicians (using a different number of aides).

As shown in Table 10.1 (which is an update of Brown's table), in the most recent ten-year period, 1985 to 1995, the per physician use of aides increased almost 50 percent, from 1.72 to 2.54. It is likely that this is the result of both the increase in number of physicians practicing in groups as well as increases in the size of groups in response to the more competitive managed care environment.

The second type of studies on economies of scale relied on survivor analysis. Survivor analysis is based on the premise that as a result of competitive market pressures, the most efficient size practice would expand while less efficient practices will contract. Survivor-type analyses implicitly incorporate patient travel costs, since patients would prefer to pay higher prices to go to smaller, higher-cost practices than traveling to larger, lower-cost practices located farther away.

Marder and Zuckerman examined changes in the size distribution of medical practices for three periods, 1965–69, 1969–75, and 1975–80 (7). The authors concluded that in the period up to 1975 solo practices (one to two physicians) were less efficient, all other size groups grew. In the later period, 1975–80, solo practice continued to decline, but by a very small amount, and there was very little change in the other single specialty size groups. For multispecialty groups, only large multispecialty groups (one hundred or more physicians) increased significantly and were therefore considered to be efficient. For single specialty groups, small-size groups appear to be most efficient.

These findings of economies of scale appear to be confirmed by more recent data indicating that more physicians are joining group practices. As shown in Table 10.2, in 1969, 21.7 percent of physicians were in group practice; by 1980, this had increased to 32.8 percent and by 1995 to 48.1 percent. The fastest-growing form of group practice during the 1980s was the single specialty form of practice, increasing from 10.9 to 20.1 percent of physicians between 1980 and 1995. It is interesting to note that while there are three times as many single specialty groups than multispecialty groups, multispecialty groups are much larger in average size, 25.4 versus 6.2.

Based on the above empirical studies, the observed increase in the number of physicians in group practice and the increase in size of each group suggest the following: group practice is a more efficient form of organization; the optimal size of group varies according to specialty practice; and the extent of inefficiency between actual and optimal size is

---

law of diminishing returns) from (for example) 0.8 visits to 0.67. Given their respective MPs and the same relative costs per hour, the use of aides is now optimal since the MP per dollar spent on physicians (0.037) is equal to the MP per dollar spent on aides (0.037). (For a given output level, the optimal use of inputs could have been achieved if the group practice reduced the use of the physician input, thereby moving up the physician's MP curve and raising the ratio of the MP/physician's wage.) Aides would have been overutilized in the earlier example if their initial MP was 0.5 visits per hour instead of 0.8, in which case their ratio would have been 0.027 compared to 0.037 for the physician input. Thus, to determine optimal use of inputs, it is necessary to know both the relative MPs and relative wage rates of each input used in the production of a physician visit.

TABLE 10.1 Physicians and Aides Employed in Offices of Physicians, 1970–95

	1970	1975	1980	1985	1990	1995
(1) Total employment in offices of physicians (thousands)	477	618	777	894	1,098	1,512
(2) Office-based practicing physicians (thousands)	188	213	271	329	360	427
(3) Aides = (1)–(2)	289	405	506	565	738	1,085
(4) Aides/physicians = (3)/(2)	1.54	1.90	1.87	1.72	2.05	2.54

Source: U.S. Department of Health and Human Services, *Health, United States,* various issues: *1983–1986,* and *1995:* Table 96, p. 217 and Table 99, p. 221; U.S. Bureau of Labor Statistics, *Employment and Earnings,* January 1996, vol. 43, no. 1; The number of nonfederal office-based physicians in 1995 comes from Lillian Randolph, American Medical Association, personal correspondence.

Note: Totals exclude persons in health-related occupations who are working in nonhealth industries, as classified by U.S. Bureau of the Census.

relatively small, less than 10 percent. Thus the trend toward group practice must be examined for reasons other than lower average costs resulting from economies of scale.

Additional Reasons for the Growth of Medical Groups

There are several reasons, unrelated to increased physician productivity, why both the size of medical groups and their number have increased.

Informational Economies of Scale

A distinguishing characteristic of the medical market is the lack of purchaser information on physicians, their accessibility, quality, bedside manner, and prices. Getzen uses this lack of patient information as an explanation for the formation of medical groups (8). Physicians are better able than patients to evaluate other physicians. There are therefore "informational economies of scale" to medical groups; it is less costly for the medical group to evaluate and monitor their member physicians than for consumers to do so. The higher patients' search costs, the larger is the optimal size of the group. Being a member of a medical group conveys information to patients regarding the quality of its members; it is equivalent to a "brand name" for physicians in that group.

A new physician entering a market is at a disadvantage compared to established physicians in that it takes time to develop a reputation among patients and to build a practice. (An established physician, relative to a new physician with an unknown reputation, would have a less elastic demand curve, hence able to charge a higher price relative to marginal cost.) By joining a medical group, the group's reputation is immediately trans-

TABLE 10.2 Number, Average Size, and Distribution of Office-Based Physicians by Group Affiliation, Selected Years, 1969–95

Type of Practice	Distribution of Physicians According to Type of Practice			Number of Group Practices			Average Size of Physician Group		
	1969	1980	1995	1969	1980	1995	1969	1980	1995
Total office-based physicians (Nonfederal)[a]	100.0	100.0	100.0	—	—	—	—	—	—
Individual practice[b]	78.3	67.2	51.9	—	—	—	—	—	—
Group practice	21.7	32.8	48.1[c]	6,371	10,762	19,636[d]	6.2	8.2	10.5
Single-specialty group practice	7.1	10.9	20.1	3,169	6,156	13,684	4.1	4.8	6.2
Multispecialty group practice	13.2	20.1	25.8	2,418	3,552	4,388	10.1	15.2	25.4
Family or general group practice	1.5	1.8	2.1	784	1,054	1,564	3.5	4.5	5.6

Sources: National Center for Health Statistics, *Health, United States, 1986,* DHHS Publication (PHS) 87-1232, Public Health Service (Washington, D.C.: U.S. Government Printing Office, December 1986), 163. J. N. Hung and G. A. Roeback, *Distribution of Physicians, Hospitals, and Hospital Beds in the United States, 1969,* vol. 2, Metropolitan Areas Center for Health Services Research and Development (Chicago: American Medical Association, 1970). P. L. Havlicek, *Medical Groups in the United States: A Survey of Practice Characteristics* (Chicago: American Medical Association, 1996), 44–46. The number of nonfederal office-based physicians in 1995 comes from Lillian Randolph, American Medical Association, personal correspondence.
[a]"Total office-based physicians" includes all patient care physicians except residents, interns, and full-time hospital staff. In 1995 there were 427,275 office-based physicians, which excluded 136,799 residents and interns as well as full-time hospital staff who provided patient care.
[b]The AMA defines a "group" as three or more physicians. Therefore, "individual practice" includes offices with a single physician and offices with two physicians.
[c]Excludes 5,298 physician positions in groups with unknown specialty composition.
[d]Excludes 151 groups whose specialty composition was unknown.

ferred to the new physician. The new group physician is able to receive patients from other, busier physicians in the group; they become better substitutes to established physicians but are not in competition with them. In return for transferring the reputation of a group to a new physician, the group usually extracts some of the new physician's income and places her on probationary status for two to four years before she becomes a partner in the group.[3]

The reputation of the group is more important to the patient for those physician ser-

---

[3]The group would be expected to add new physicians up to the point where the marginal revenue product of the last physician equals the average revenue product of the group. When MRP = ARP, then average income, which is equivalent to average revenue product, would be at a maximum.

vices that are less frequently used and that are more difficult for the patient to evaluate. It is for this reason that specialists are more likely to be part of a group than family practitioners. Patients are better able to evaluate the manner or style of a physician than the physician's technical ability. Finding a specialist involves greater search costs on the part of the patient (as well as by an insurer or employer contracting for physician services). Multispecialty groups offer greater informational economies of scale than do groups comprised of family practitioners.

Reduction of Risk and Uncertainty

The desire by physicians to reduce uncertainty and share risk is an another reason for their participation in medical groups (9). When physician compensation in a group is not directly related to the physician's productivity, the physician's risk is reduced. Physicians in solo practice are likely to experience greater variation in workload and income than are members of a group practice who share the workload. Risk-averse physicians are more willing to trade off the greater incentives of solo practice, whereby they receive the full return from their work effort and do not have to share their revenues, to become part of a group. The larger the size of the medical group, the smaller the uncertainty (variation) over one's annual income.

The trade-off with less risk is that productivity incentives decline as physicians receive less of their own marginal revenue. Gaynor and Gertler estimate that more risk-averse physicians are willing to sacrifice about 11 percent of their gross income compared to less risk-averse physicians. To the extent that large groups have greater sharing of revenues, such groups will be less productive than smaller groups, where compensation is more directly related to physician productivity. Disputes among group physicians over their compensation is an important reason why many physicians have not joined groups and why groups have dissolved.

Further, when physicians in a large group share the costs of inputs, each physician has an incentive to increase his use of inputs if the benefit they receive from the additional input use exceeds their share of the additional costs (10). And, as the size of the group increases, each physician's incentive to monitor the behavior of others in the group decreases since the benefits of monitoring must be shared among more physicians while the individual bears the costs of monitoring. To decrease inefficiencies arising from use of inputs, decision making in large groups is handled by physician committees and management rather than by individual physicians.

Increased Market Power

Large medical groups have greater market power than smaller groups, which enables them to increase their market share and/or receive higher prices. Large groups are better able to market their services directly to insurers, employers, HMOs, and hospitals. It is less costly (both administratively and in evaluating performance) for an insurer or employer to contract with a single large group than with many individual physicians. Further, a large medical group is more willing than smaller medical groups to accept capitation contracts from HMOs since they are better able to spread the risk of large medical expenses over a larger patient population. The HMO is thereby able to shift its risk to the large group.

Large medical groups also have greater leverage over hospitals. Such groups determine to which hospitals they will admit their patients. They are therefore better able than smaller groups to negotiate preferred arrangements with their selected hospitals, from having the hospital share some of its revenue with the group ("risk-sharing pools") to having the hospital invest capital to increase the group's productivity.

As shown in Tables 10.3 and 10.4, the number of physicians in group practice, 210,000, have steadily increased. The group size that has increased most rapidly has been the largest, those with more than fifty physicians. Such groups now include about 38 percent of all physicians in group practice. The percent of physicians in the other group sizes have either declined, the smallest groups, or have remained constant.

An indication of the ability of large groups to aggressively compete in the new managed care environment, as indicated by their contractual arrangements, is shown in Table

TABLE 10.3 Distribution of Groups and Group Physicians by Group Size

Group Size	Distribution of Groups			Distribution of Physicians		
	1969	1980	1995[a]	1969	1980	1995[b]
Total number	6,371	10,762	19,478	40,093	88,290	210,810
			Percent Distribution			
3–4	65.0%	55.3%	45.8%	34.6%	22.7%	14.7%
5–15	30.3	37.5	44.2	34.2	32.9	30.0
16–25	2.4	3.6	4.8	7.6	8.7	8.8
26–49	1.5	2.2	2.7	8.2	9.1	8.6
50+	0.8	1.4	2.4	15.4	26.6	37.9
Total	100.0	100.0	99.9[c]	100.0	100.0	100.0

Sources: Steve G. Vahovich, *Profile of Medical Practice* (Chicago: American Medical Association, 1973), Table 11; Sharon R. Henderson, *Medical Groups in the U.S., 1980* (Chicago: American Medical Association, 1982), Table 3-2; Penny L. Havlicek, *Medical Groups in the US: A Survey of Practice Characteristics* (Chicago: American Medical Association, 1996), Table 3-1.
Note: In 1980, 100+ group size totaled 18,899 (21.4%) physicians. In 1995, 100+ group size numbered 61,415 (33.3%) physician positions.
[a]Excludes 309 groups with unknown size.
[b]These figures represent physician positions. These figures were obtained by asking groups to report the number of physicians in their groups. Because physicians may practice in more than one group, some physicians may be counted more than once. Thus, these figures may overestimate the number of group physicians.
[c]Percentages do not sum to 100 due to rounding.

TABLE 10.4 Physicians' Contractual Arrangements by Size of Group, 1996

Practice Size	Percentage of Physicians with HMO Contracts	Percentage of Practice Revenues Capitated[a]	Percentage of Physicians Contracting Directly with Employers
1	63	25	8
2–4	72	22	12
5–9	80	21	12
10–24	86	16	20
25 or more	87	37	31

Source: David W. Emmons and Gregory D. Wozniak, "Physicians' Contractual Arrangements with Managed Care Organizations," in Martin L. Gonzalez, ed., *Socioeconomic Characteristics of Medical Practice* (Chicago: American Medical Association, 1996), Table 1, p. 8; Table 5, p. 15 and Table 7, p. 18.
[a]Among physicians with capitated contracts.

10.4. Physicians in large groups are more likely to have HMO contracts, a greater percent of their practice revenues are capitated, and they are more likely to engage in direct contracting with employers. Each of these types of contractual arrangements provide larger groups with greater opportunity to manage risk and to increase their revenues at the expense of smaller groups.

The advantages of group practice include economies of scale (to include the sharing of managerial expertise, technical personnel, claims processing, and marketing), informational (reputation) economies of scale to purchasers, reduced uncertainty and risk to physicians, and increased market power. The primary disadvantage of group practice lies in reduced efficiency incentives when compensation is not directly related to productivity.

The continued growth of medical groups and their size, some in the hundreds of physicians (in multiple locations), indicate that economies of scale and market power advantages of size appear to offset any diseconomies within a large group of designing fair compensation arrangements and monitoring other physicians' behavior with regard to quality and productivity.

The structure of the physician services industry has changed over time. It is consolidating. The image of the physician in solo practice has disappeared. More physicians are part of a larger economic entity, the average size of groups is increasing, and direct contractual arrangements with HMOs and insurers is crucial to their survival. Price competition among physicians (and their increasingly larger groups) for HMO and insurer contracts has intensified.

MARKET CONDUCT

The physician services market has been characterized by lack of patient information, extensive insurance coverage (private insurance, Medicare and Medicaid), and by a large number of competitors within a local market. To determine whether the physician firm has market power, given the lack of firm concentration in this market, it is important to examine the conduct of the physician firm. Monopoly power can be inferred through anticompetitive behavior. Examples of such behavior are monopoly pricing, price discrimination, and limits on advertising.

There are a number of imperfections on the demand side of the market that cause the physician services market to deviate from a purely competitive market. Consumers lack information on physicians (their quality, prices, accessibility, and medical treatment needed) and consumers have extensive insurance for physician services in both the public (Medicare and Medicaid) and private sectors. This lack of consumer information and their insurance coverage result in a less price elastic (downward sloping) demand curve facing competing physicians, which provides them with some monopoly power.

Monopolistic Competition

A perfectly competitive market is characterized by (in addition to free entry) many firms producing a homogeneous product. When variations in prices and increases in prices are observed, a competitive model relies on differences in costs to explain these price differences. When these variations in prices cannot be explained by just differences in costs, then an economist explores whether there are also differences in the price elasticity of demand for the services; this is called the monopoly explanation.

Certain peculiarities of the physician services market have, in the past, been more important than the extent of economies of scale in determining the number of physician firms, hence its market structure (11). Neither physicians nor their services are homogeneous; they differ not only in the variety of physician services offered but in the manner in which each physician provides that service. There are real as well as perceived differences in their quality, perhaps reflected in the medical school they attended and where they had their residency; they differ in their age and sex, in how they communicate with their patients, in how long patients must wait and the value the patient places on waiting time, the location of the physician's office, and so on.

Patients have had little information by which to choose and judge physicians. They have had to rely on their physician for diagnostic information and for advice on their treatment needs, which has resulted in an agency relationship between the patient and the physician. The physician is presumed to act on the patient's behalf.

In addition to lack of information, patients have had little financial incentive to be concerned with physician fees. As shown in Table 10.5, before the enactment of Medicare and Medicaid in 1965, consumers paid more than 60 percent of physicians' fees out of pocket, government paid for 7 percent, and private insurance paid for 32 percent of physician expenditures. After 1965, government and private insurance became the major payers of physician services. Currently, the government pays 33 percent and private insurance 48 percent of physician expenditures. A decreasing portion of physician expen-

TABLE 10.5 Distribution of Expenditures on Physician Services by Source of Funds, 1950–95

Year	Total	Consumer Direct	Third-Party Payers		
			Total	Private Insurance	Public Total
1950	100%	83.2%	16.8%	11.4%	5.2%
1955	100	69.8	30.2	23.2	6.7
1960	100	62.7	37.3	30.2	7.1
1965	100	60.6	39.4	32.5	6.8
1970	100	42.2	57.8	35.2	22.5
1975	100	36.7	63.3	35.3	27.7
1980	100	32.4	67.6	37.9	28.9
1985	100	29.1	70.9	39.9	29.3
1990	100	24.2	75.8	43.2	30.7
1995	100	18.3	81.7	48.1	31.7

Sources: R. M. Gibson and D. R. Waldo, "National Health Expenditures, 1980," *Health Care Financing Review,* 3(1), September 1981: 1–54, Table 3; U.S. Department of Health and Human Services, Health Care Financing Administration, Internet site http://www.hcfa.gov/stats/nhce96.htm, and unpublished data, 1996.

ditures is paid for out of pocket by the patient, less than 20 percent. As these third-party payments have increased, the patient's incentive to be concerned with the physician's fee in choosing a physician or in influencing the recommended treatment and the setting in which it is provided has been reduced.

(Physicians are currently feeling the effects of being included in managed care organizations' provider networks and by government payment methods.)

Lack of information on competing physicians results in other physicians being less substitutable to the person's own physician. There are always search costs involved in finding a particular physician. Since it is costly to gather information on different physicians, some patients who place a high value on their time will do less search and be willing to take a chance on paying higher prices. In fact, identical prices in a market such as physician services would be more indicative of collusion or price fixing than of competition. If prices for specified services diverge too greatly, however, some patients would be willing to shift to other providers. As the price differential increases, it will eventually exceed the value the patient places on particular providers and on perceived quality differences. Although prices for the same physician services are unlikely to be exactly the same, they would be expected to vary within a relatively narrow range.[4]

---

[4]The optimal search time is determined by both the costs and benefits of searching for lower prices. The benefits of search are greater the more expensive the service, the more frequently it is used, the greater the out-of-pocket price paid by the patient, and the less emergent the need for the service. The costs of search are greater for those with higher incomes (who are also more likely to have insurance). The above suggests that less price dispersion should be observed for visits to a family practitioner than for the services of a surgical specialist.

In contrast to a perfectly competitive market, a physician who raised prices would not lose every patient. Since the patient incurs search costs in finding another physician, whether the physician loses patients with an increase in prices depends on the magnitude of both the search costs and the price increase (12). When search costs are high, the individual physician's demand curve becomes less price elastic. More extensive insurance coverage also lessens the effect on the patient of an increase in the physician's price.

Since physicians differ and patients have limited information on other physicians, each physician faces a downward sloping demand curve for her services. As shown in Figure 10.2, there are two demand curves. *DD* is the overall market demand for physician services and *dd* is the demand curve facing the individual physician; *dd* has a more gradual slope (more price elastic) than *DD* since there are better substitutes for each physician than there are for all physicians' services. Thus empirical findings that the demand for physicians' services is price inelastic would refer to the overall market demand curve (*DD*) and not the demand facing the individual physician (*dd*). The *dd* demand curve indicates that if the individual physician lowered her price, and other physicians did not, the physician would receive an increase in market share. Similarly, if the physician raised prices and others did not, they would lose market share.

The physician services market is believed to be characteristic of "monopolistic compe-

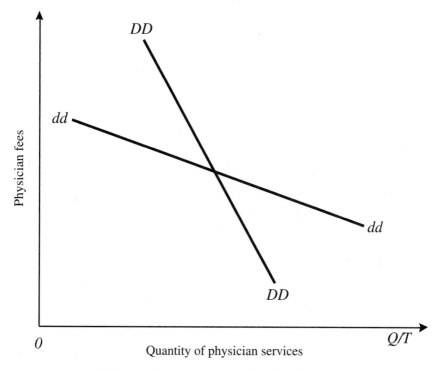

FIGURE 10.2 • Monopolistic competitive market for physician services.

tition" both because of the large number of competitors within a market and because each physician has a somewhat differentiated service, thereby providing each physician with a downward sloping demand curve.

A Monopoly Model of Physician Pricing

Given that physicians face a downward sloping demand curve for their services, a profit-maximizing physician would attempt to price as would a monopolist. A monopoly model of physician pricing behavior (physician prices in excess of marginal costs) can be used to explain increases in physician fees when there is a decrease in the price elasticity of demand for physician services. The effect on physician fees of a less elastic demand curve for physician services is shown in Figure 10.3. The initial demand and marginal revenue curves are D_1 and MR_1. The physician's marginal cost curve is MC, which, for simplicity, is assumed to be constant. The resulting price is P_1.

Increased insurance coverage for physician services would make the demand for physician services less elastic, shifting it from D_1 to D_2. The marginal revenue curve also shifts

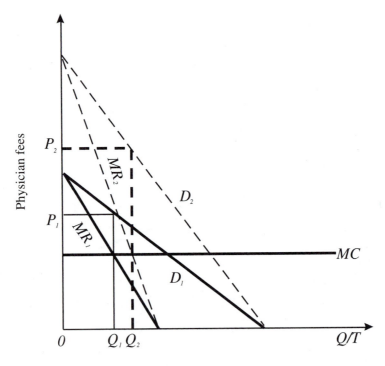

FIGURE 10.3 • The impact of insurance on physician services.

rightward. Thus, even though marginal costs have not changed, the intersection of the steeper MR_2 with MC results in a higher price, P_2, on the demand curve.

The method of reimbursement preferred by physicians has always been fee-for-service, according to their "usual, customary, and reasonable" (UCR) fees. Such a pricing strategy enables physicians to set what they believe is the profit-maximizing price. With the growth in private insurance for physician services and the passage of Medicare and Medicaid, the amount the patient had to pay out of pocket for such services was reduced. When physician fees are adjusted both for inflation and by the decline in the out-of-pocket price as a result of third-party coverage, the physician fee, *in constant dollars faced by the average patient,* has actually declined over the past thirty years. As the patients' responsibility for payment of physician fees declined and physicians charged third-party payers according to their UCR fee, physician fees increased rapidly. As more of a physician's fees were reimbursed by a third party, the constraints holding down physician fees were removed.[5]

Insurance coverage for payment of physician fees was not uniform among all physician specialties. The hospital-based specialties, such as radiology and anesthesiology, as well as surgeons (whose services were considered to be more costly), had the largest percent of their revenues covered by third-party payers. The decline in the patient's sensitivity to prices lowered the price elasticity of demand; rapidly increasing prices would be expected in such a situation. Those medical specialties that required less use of the hospital, such as pediatrics and psychiatry, had the smallest percent of their revenues covered by third-party payers. Not surprisingly, members of those specialties with the largest percent of their revenues paid by third-party payers also had the highest incomes. The usual market constraints, such as patients' seeking lower prices, disappeared as more of the physicians' fees were reimbursed by third-party payers.

Physician Pricing and Practice Behavior: Supplier-Induced Demand

An agency relationship exists between the patient and the physician. Given lack of knowledge regarding diagnosis and treatment needs, the patient must rely on the physician for advice on both. When the physician acts as a "perfect" agent for the patient, then the

---

[5]One explanation for rising physician fees has been the rapid increases in malpractice premiums. Malpractice premiums, however, are a fixed cost; they do not vary according to the number of deliveries or the number of surgical procedures performed. If a physician sets a profit-maximizing price (i.e., marginal revenue equal to marginal cost), changes in fixed cost should not have any effect on the physician's price. If physicians were able to pass on increases in their fixed costs, it is unlikely that they would spend their time in marches on their respective state capitols seeking legislative relief. Only in the long run in a competitive industry would increased fixed costs result in higher consumer prices. Since there is evidence that physicians were receiving above-normal rates of return during this period (see the chapter on health manpower shortages and surpluses), the long-run explanation is not applicable. Increased malpractice premiums may be used as a reason for increasing prices by physicians even though the more accurate explanation was a lessening price elasticity of the patient's demand curve; higher costs are a more palatable explanation than increased ability to pay.

physician's recommendation would be similar to what the patient would decide, if the patient had the physician's expertise. The physician would consider the patient's medical condition, income, insurance coverage, out-of-pocket prices for different treatment settings, preferences, and so on, when making a treatment recommendation.

The physician, however, is a supplier of both advice and a service. As such, there is a concern that because the physician has a financial interest in supplying services, the information provided to the patient could be biased. When the physician modifies the diagnosis and treatment recommendation to include a favorable effect on his own economic well-being, then the physician is an "imperfect" agent. In a fee-for-service payment system, this imperfect agency relationship has been referred to as "supplier-induced demand" (SID).

The lack of patient information together with extensive insurance coverage have reduced patients' sensitivity to physician prices and have given rise to the idea that physicians can both induce their own demand and set their own prices. In its simplest form, demand inducement is an extreme example of monopoly power.

The amount of SID undertaken by the physician who is an imperfect agent has been modeled in terms of a trade-off. The physician is assumed to be a utility maximizer; the physician receives utility from additional income and from practicing good medical care. The greater the quantity of induced demand, the greater the physician's income, hence utility. However, when the physician induces demand, it is assumed that the physician incurs a "psychic" cost or disutility. If the physician's income were to fall, either because of an increase in the supply of physicians or because of government limits on fees, the psychic cost of inducing demand is less than the marginal utility of the additional income it generates. At low levels of demand inducement, this psychic cost may be low in that additional follow-up visits might be justified and certainly not result in harm to the patient. At higher levels of induced demand the increased psychic cost to the physician of additional treatment (e.g., unnecessary surgery) exceeds the marginal utility of the additional income. The quantity of SID that the physician is presumed to induce is where the psychic cost of additional care equals the value of additional income.

Demand inducement is wasteful in that the expected costs to the patient from the additional care are greater than the expected benefits. Since the expected costs exceed the expected benefits, the physician, as the patient's (imperfect) agent, would be expected to induce demand only when facing declining fees and/or decreased demand for services.

One variant of how much demand a physician will induce is based on what "target-income" the physician desires (13). The target income is believed to be determined by the local income distribution, particularly with respect to the relative incomes of other physicians and professionals, such as dentists and lawyers, in the area. To forestall a decrease in income, according to this theory, physicians will either increase their fees or induce demand (shift the demand curve to the right) so as to enable physicians to maintain a target income.

Figure 10.4 shows the effect on physician fees and quantity of services of an increase in the supply of physicians using traditional economic theory as well as the target-income hypothesis. If market demand and supply were originally D_0 and quantity S_0, respec-

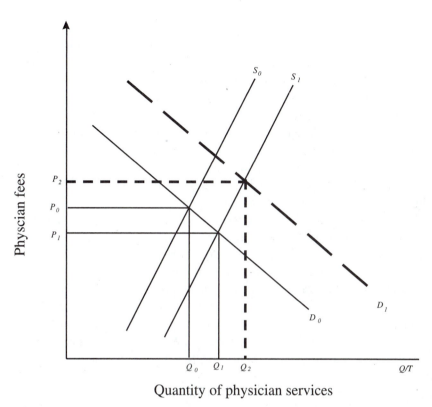

FIGURE 10.4 • An illustration of the target-income hypothesis.

tively, equilibrium will be at price P_0 and quantity Q_0. An increase in the number of physicians in an area would shift supply to the right, to S_1, which would, under traditional economic theory, result in a *lower* equilibrium price, P_1 and an increase in the quantity demanded (a movement down the demand schedule for physician services). The effect of an increased supply on physician incomes will be based on whether the market demand curve for physicians is price elastic or inelastic. If the market demand curve is price inelastic (consistent with empirical evidence), then total physician incomes would decline with an increase in the number of physicians. According to traditional economic theory, physicians would be unable to increase price or shift demand because as profit maximizers they have already set their fees to the maximum allowed by the market.

Under the target-income hypothesis, with an increase in the number of physicians in the community, to forestall a decrease in their demand and incomes, physicians induce an increase in their demand to D_1. The effect is an increase (or no change) rather than a decrease in physician fees. Proponents of SID do not necessarily believe that physicians can increase their fees and demand indefinitely. Because they are utility rather than profit maximizers, physicians are presumed to be to the left of (not on) their market demand curve, thereby able to increase demand as their incomes fall.

The SID hypothesis is based on empirical evidence indicating physician/population ratios are positively related to physician fees and/or use rates, after adjusting for other variables.[6] For example, in an early study on SID, Victor Fuchs found that a 10 percent increase in the surgeon/population ratio resulted in a 3 percent increase in per capita utilization. Also, opposite to what would be expected using traditional economic analysis, he found that prices were increased in this situation of induced demand. Thus, although the average surgeon's workload decreased by 7 percent, income per surgeon declined by a smaller amount. The extent of demand inducement, even among surgeons, is, however, limited, since "the average number of operations per surgeon . . . is far below the level that surgeons consider a full workload . . . and below the quantity that surgeons would be willing and able to perform at the going price" (14).

The literature on physician-induced demand is extensive (15). Rice found evidence of physician-induced demand in the Medicare market; he examined a change in the Medicare reimbursement mechanism in Colorado between 1976 and 1977, which resulted in a relative decrease in fees paid to urban physicians (their reimbursements rose by less than 5 percent) and a relative increase in fees paid to nonurban physicians (their reimbursements rose by approximately 20 percent) (16). He found that the lower the reimbursement rate for different services (medical, surgical, laboratory, and radiology), the greater was the intensity of the service provided. For example, a 10 percent decrease in the reimbursement rate for medical services led to a 6.1 percent increase in medical service intensity.

The change in the reimbursement rate for laboratory services also had a strong impact on the quantity of laboratory services provided; that is, the lower the payment rate for laboratory tests, the greater the number of tests ordered by the physician. (Limits on physicians' visit fees, however, are not necessarily demand inducement since such limits provide an incentive to the physician to substitute diagnostic tests for her own time.)

A more serious example of demand creation is unnecessary surgery. Patients are least able to judge whether a surgical procedure is necessary. The patient may be able to determine whether additional home and office visits are providing any benefits, but in the case of surgery, the consequences to the patient of being mistaken may be more serious. The types of surgery that were likely to result from demand creation are tonsillectomies, appendectomies, and hysterectomies. The physician might have rationalized that these surgical procedures were beneficial and did not affect the patient's ability to function. The patient would have no way of determining whether such surgery was useful, since his well-being would probably be unchanged after recovering.

A number of studies have shown that the rate of surgical procedures was higher when

---

[6]Robert Evans concludes that "the market for physicians' services is not self-equilibrating in the usual sense, that price does not serve primarily to balance supply and demand [but that] the primary role of price is instead as an input to supplier incomes, which are not themselves the product of explicit maximizing behavior, but rather of target-seeking through the manipulation of several control variables" (Evans [19], p. 173).

the physician was reimbursed on a fee-for-service basis (17). The rate of surgical procedures varied according to the method of physician reimbursement even though the two population groups being compared had similar characteristics and similar physician and hospital coverage. In one group, Health Insurance Plan of Greater New York (HIP), the physician was reimbursed on a capitation basis (the same rate of reimbursement regardless of the number of procedures performed); for the other group of patients, covered by Group Health Insurance (GHI) in Washington, D.C., the physician was reimbursed on a fee-for-service basis. The rate of hospitalized surgical procedures for HIP (capitated) enrollees was 4.38 per hundred persons per year; for GHI it was 7.18.

In another study of GHI and HIP populations no significant difference was found in surgical procedures among adult males, but they were found among adult females—6.56 in GHI and 4.97 in HIP. In a third comparative study of physician reimbursement under a capitation system (Kaiser) and a fee-for-service method (Blue Cross and Blue Shield and commercial insurance), when patients had identical benefit coverage under all three plans, it was found that the hospitalized surgical procedure ratios per hundred persons per year were 3.3, 6.9, and 6.3, respectively. A fourth comparison was of two groups of federal employees with the same benefits, where one group belonged to a capitation plan while the other group belonged to a fee-for-service system. It was found that the rate of hospitalized surgical procedures was 3.9 in the capitation plan and 7.0 in the fee-for-service system. One-third of this difference in the rate of surgical procedures was a result of differences in the rate of surgical procedures for appendectomies (1.4 versus 2.6), tonsillectomies (4.0 versus 10.6), and "female surgery" (5.4 versus 8.2).

There has been a great deal of debate over the validity of the empirical evidence on supplier-induced demand. Critics of SID find fault with both the logic and the empirical work on which it is based. For example, they contend that the empirical finding of a positive association between physician fees and physician/population ratios is the result of inadequately adjusting for differences in the physician visit, such as in patient time and quality of a physician visit, as well as in patient information. As the number of physicians in an area increase, there are decreased travel and waiting times to see physicians; this would result in an increase in the quantity demanded as the patient's time costs are lowered. Similarly, as the quality aspects of a physician visit are increased, as measured by the amount of physician time per visit and the length of the visit, the patient would be willing to pay a higher price for a physician visit.

Critics of SID believe that as it becomes possible to adjust physician prices for differences in the type of visit, particularly travel time, quality, and amenity differences among physicians, it should be possible to determine a negative relationship between physician fees and physician/population ratios. A number of studies have found limited, if any, demand inducement. For example, Rossiter and Wilensky used individual patient data from the National Medical Care Expenditure Survey (NMCES), which contains detailed health care utilization and expenditure information for 40,000 persons in 1977 (18). It was also possible to distinguish between patient-initiated ambulatory visits (57 percent of all visits) and physician-initiated ambulatory visits (43 percent of all visits), thereby permitting separate estimates of the impact of the physician/population ratio on each type of visit. The authors concluded that an increased physician/population ratio had no impact on patient-initiated visits, although it did have a positive impact on physician-initiated visits; the effect, however, was very small, that is, a doubling of the physician/population ratio, which would be a huge increase, would lead to only an 11 percent increase in physician-initiated visits.

For physician-initiated visits, the study found that the out-of-pocket money price and time price (time in the physician's office) had the expected negative effect on number of physician-initiated visits. That is, either patients or physicians or both are somewhat sensitive to the out-of-pocket price of services, while patients are sensitive to time prices. Visits for chronic conditions and other measures of disability were positively related to physician-initiated visits; this is consistent with a model of the physician as the patient's agent.

A study by McCarthy did not find evidence of induced demand for primary care physician services (19). McCarthy used data from a 1974 American Medical Association survey of 187 individual primary care physician firms in large metropolitan areas. McCarthy found that the physician/population ratio (squared) had a negative impact on the number of physician office visits. Patients were found to be sensitive to both time (in-office waiting) and money prices, both of which had negative relationships to office visits. Time and price both had price elasticities greater than −1. Moreover, the number of organized outpatient departments and emergency rooms per one hundred thousand population, which are measures of substitute sources of care, also had large negative impacts on physician office visits. (These results also support the premise of a monopolistically competitive market for physician services.)

While concluding that there is an absence of physician-induced demand *at the margin,* McCarthy acknowledges that there may have been demand inducement in the past. Reinhardt underscored this qualification, emphasizing that if an increase in the physician/population ratio leads to a decline in visits per physician, this simply indicates that physicians cannot *at the margin* induce demand to raise their incomes (20). This finding says nothing about what physician-induced demand occurred in the past and therefore how much money is currently being spent on physician-induced visits and tests.

It should be kept in mind that McCarthy studied primary care physicians, where the lack of patient information is not as great as when patients use specialists, who are used much less frequently; also, insurance coverage for primary care physicians is not as great as it is for specialists.

Using a traditional economic framework, Pauly and Satterthwaite attempt to explain the observed relationship between an increase in the number of physicians and fees in terms of a decline in consumer information, consequently, an increase in search costs (21). They analyze the situation among primary care physicians, where the patient's insurance coverage is less than for surgeons and therefore price incentives still exist. In choosing a physician, consumers depend on the recommendations of others rather than shopping, as they typically do in other markets. When there are few physicians in an area, each physician's reputation is known throughout the community. Consumers are likely to know people who have gone to each physician. However, when there are a large number of physicians in a metropolitan area, the consumer's knowledge of each physician's reputation is less. There is also less information on each physician's qualifications and prices.

An increase in the number of physicians in an area therefore increases the consumer's difficulty in finding out about each physician. As this occurs, the consumer becomes less price sensitive and the physician's demand curve becomes less elastic. Physicians (or firms in monopolistically competitive markets) will then raise their prices.

Thus, different theoretical models have been developed to explain the empirical evidence of a positive association between the physician/population ratio and higher fees and/or use rates. The SID model is based on the assumption that the physician is not an income maximizer but a utility maximizer. At some point the disutility to the physician of providing unnecessary care exceeds the marginal utility of the additional income earned; this limits the extent of demand inducement.

In contrast to the above, Pauly and Satterthwaite claim that it is the increased cost of search to consumers as the number of physicians increase that results in a less elastic demand curve and consequently higher fees.

The SID and traditional theories (physicians as profit maximizers with limited or no ability to induce demand) lead to quite opposite predictions. Under the traditional view, continued increases in the physician/population ratio are likely to result in a lower rate of increase in both physician fees and incomes (assuming the overall market demand for physicians is price inelastic).

Supplier-induced demand would predict that the consequences of an increase in the physician/population ratio would be a shift to the right in the demand for physician services and a faster increase in physician fees and use of services than in the past, as more physicians attempt to attain their target income. Increased expenditures on physician services (with doubtful effects on health status) would be expected to increase rapidly.

The policy prescription for proponents of the SID theory has been establishment of arbitrary limits on expenditures for physician services and on the increase in number of physicians.

Additional demand inducement in the private sector appears to be limited, as indicated by recent evidence. The movement away from fee-for-service payment by a disinterested indemnity insurer and patients with little information and price sensitivity toward managed care has changed the market for physician services. The continuing increase in the supply of physicians has not led to more rapid increases in fees and demand as would be expected if physicians were attempting to maintain a target income. Managed care techniques, such as the use of utilization review and case management, have placed constraints on physicians who attempt to induce demand. The increase in competing physician networks, whereby groups of physicians offer their services at a discounted price to insurance companies and employers, is indicative of a price-competitive market. The demand curve facing the individual physician has become more price elastic. As large purchasers of physician services are better able to monitor physicians in terms of their quality, price, and whether they induce demand, the negative consequences to physicians of demand inducement increase and are likely to severely limit the amount of demand inducement.

Physician-Patient Agency Relationships under Capitation

A physician who is an imperfect agent considers the effect on personal income when making a treatment recommendation. Under fee-for-service payment, an imperfect agent whose income is (or would be) low is likely to induce demand, since the gain in income exceeds the psychic cost of doing so. At higher levels of income, the marginal benefit of additional income is less than the psychic cost of inducing demand.

How is an imperfect agent expected to behave under a payment system that offers different financial incentives? Under capitation payment, the financial incentives are reversed. A physician who is capitated (paid an amount per enrollee regardless of the enrollee's usage) can increase his income if he has a greater number of capitated enrollees, while providing fewer services to each enrollee.

An imperfect agent who induces demand under fee-for-service would be expected to provide fewer services and/or decrease access to care (longer waiting times, fewer referrals, etc.) under capitation. This practice behavior is in contrast to a perfect agent who, under either type of payment system, would be expected to provide the same access and the same amount of care.

In addition to the agency relationship between the physician and the patient, there is also an agency relationship between the physician and the insurer. A physician's practice behavior can have financial effects on the insurer, either by increasing and/or decreasing enrollment.

It is because of imperfect physician agents that various types of monitoring mechanisms have been developed. Utilization management, preauthorization for admissions and for surgery, and physician profiling are methods insurers use to decrease the amount of induced demand under fee-for-service. When physicians are capitated, HMOs and insurers are concerned that if their enrollees are dissatisfied because of decreased access to care, the enrollees will switch to another HMO. It is for this reason that HMOs have developed enrollee satisfaction surveys and other monitoring mechanisms to mitigate the practice behavior of imperfect physician agents.

The Effect of Prohibiting Advertising on the Demand for Physician Services

Until the Supreme Court decision in 1982, advertising was prohibited by state codes that regulated ethics in the health professions. The penalties for violating such codes were severe, including suspension of the practitioner's license. An interesting question is why medical societies were opposed to advertising.

Prohibitions on advertising were in physicians' economic interest. Had medical societies permitted physicians to advertise, the effect would have been to lower the average price of physician services. This may not be intuitively obvious since advertising is an additional cost to the firm. The following discussion therefore attempts to explain why advertising of medical services results in lower prices for medical services and to provide supporting empirical evidence.

Until advertising was permitted in the 1980s, information on providers was almost nonexistent. Each medical provider therefore had a less elastic demand curve. A patient was usually unaware of different competitors' quality, accessibility, and price of medical services, thereby making these other providers poor substitutes for the patient's current provider. To determine the attributes of different physicians and the price of their services, the patient had to spend time and money.

Advertising of medical services performs three functions. First, it reduces the patient's search costs. When price information is unavailable, wide variations in prices will exist, since it will be up to the patient to search out the firms with the lowest prices. Because search is costly, patients will not keep searching until they find the firm that sells its services at the lowest price. Search will continue until the marginal benefit of increased search (lower prices) equals the marginal cost of additional search. When information is disseminated through advertising, travel and other costs are lowered. Differences in prices, as well as differences in quality and other attributes of the service, would continue to exist, but these differences would be smaller than previously.

(In a world of perfect information, prices charged for what is perceived to be the same product would be the same and differences in prices would reflect differences in their costs of production.)

"Price-dispersion is a manifestation of—and indeed it is a measure of—ignorance in the market" (22). Without provider information, the consumer may first have to purchase the service to determine its attributes as well as its price.[7] Although advertising is less effective when services are directly experienced, provider information on prices and qualifications still contributes to the information the consumer needs to make a choice. The consumer might then have to resort to additional sources, such as employee satisfaction surveys, provider report cards, and consumer groups for additional information on the provider.

Second, advertising that provides patients with information on the similarities and differences of services sold by different providers enables patients to evaluate the degree

---

[7]Nelson classified goods into two categories: search goods and experience goods. Search goods are those for which adequate information concerning their desirability exists prior to purchase (e.g., an airplane trip). Experience goods need to be purchased to be assessed (e.g., a dinner in a restaurant). Philip Nelson, "Advertising as Information," *Journal of Political Economy,* 82(4), July–August 1974: 729–754.

of substitutability of competing providers. The demand curves of the different providers are made more elastic.

The effect of advertising on prices is shown in Figure 10.5. With little information available to patients to judge other physicians, the physician's demand curve is less elastic, shown as D_1. Assuming that the physician firm wishes to maximize its profits, it will set its price at that point on the demand curve where the marginal revenue (MR_1) and marginal cost curves intersect. The resulting price will be P_1. With advertising, patients have more information with which to evaluate substitute physicians, such as physician qualifications, accessibility in terms of location and hours, and so on. Other physicians now become better substitutes for one another. As this occurs, the physician's demand curve becomes more elastic (the closer the substitute, the more elastic the demand curve). The new, more elastic, demand curve is D_2. For the sake of simplicity, the marginal revenue curves in Figure 10.5 were drawn so that they intersected the marginal cost curve at the same point. With the same marginal cost curve, a more elastic demand curve results in a lower price, P_2, instead of P_1.

The cost of advertising is not shown in Figure 10.5, since it does not increase the firm's marginal costs; instead, advertising increases the firm's average cost curve. Advertising costs may be considered a fixed cost, since they are unrelated to the cost of producing ad-

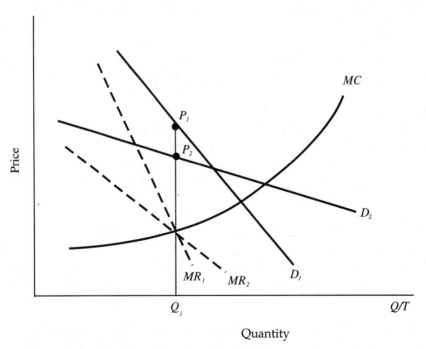

FIGURE 10.5 • The effect of advertising on the elasticity of demand and on the firm's pricing strategy.

ditional quantities of the particular service. Thus the cost of advertising itself does not affect the price charged by a firm attempting to maximize its profits. The price would be determined by the elasticity of demand and the marginal cost of producing that service. By causing the firm's demand curve to become more elastic, advertising is expected to lower prices.

In the nonhealth field, many products are already viewed by consumers as being relatively homogeneous. One firm's soap or aspirin is considered to be a good substitute for the same product produced by another firm. In these cases, advertising is used by a firm to differentiate its product from that of its competitors. As shown in Figure 10.1, if a firm is selling a relatively homogeneous product (demand curve D_2), it advertises to make consumers believe that other products are less substitutable for its own, thereby hoping to change its demand curve to D_1.

Third, a firm's inability to advertise has been used as a barrier to entry in a market. For example, large organizations, such as HMOs, are subject to economies of scale, that is, they must achieve a minimum enrollment size before their premium can be competitive with those of traditional insurance plans. Their previous inability to advertise required such plans to incur large losses; they had to price their premiums competitively, but since they had such small enrollments, their costs per enrollee exceeded their premiums. Advertising enables such plans to increase their enrollments quickly so that they can take advantage of economies of scale.

Health providers, particularly HMOs and hospitals, have now begun to advertise. Few studies, however, have been conducted to determine the effect of advertising on prices and price dispersion. Instead, evidence on the effects of advertising has been based on studies of optometrists.[8]

The FTC attempted to determine what happens to prices and quality of services among providers who advertise compared to those who do not. Data were collected from three types of optometrists: optometrists in cities where advertising of eye examinations and eyeglasses was prohibited, optometrists who did not advertise even though advertising was permitted in their areas, and optometrists who did advertise. The FTC used seven individuals with similar visual conditions who "were trained at two schools of optometry with regard to the components of an optometric examination. They obtained examinations, recorded price, time spent, and details on the various tests and procedures performed" (23).

The findings of this study were that "the presence of advertising causes substantial and significant declines in the prices of eye examinations offered by all types of optometrists."

---

[8]One study suggests that physicians might advertise to obtain less price-sensitive patients, thereby leading to higher prices, more time spent with the patient, and fewer total visits. The authors believe that, had they not controlled for selection effects, their findings would have been reversed. John A. Rizzo and Richard J. Zeckhauser, "Advertising and the Price, Quantity, and Quality of Primary Care Physician Services," *Journal of Human Resources*, 27(3), Summer 1992: 381–421.

Prices were reduced, but not by much, even for optometrists who did not advertise but who were located in markets where advertising occurred. Further, nonadvertising optometrists in advertising markets spent more time with their patients (a proxy for quality) than did advertising optometrists and even more time than did nonadvertising optometrists in nonadvertising markets.

The author concludes that advertising does not reduce quality by all practitioners in a market. In fact, enough nonadvertisers remain in advertising markets so that the overall market quality is higher. The removal of advertising restrictions was estimated to result in a 20 percent decrease in price without any decline in overall quality. Nonadvertisers in advertising markets compete on price and quality and apparently consumers are able to choose and differentiate among providers on the basis of prices and quality of service (24).

Another indication of quality, patient satisfaction, was based on a survey of retired persons undertaken after price advertising began in Florida. One of the test questions was: "All things considered, the next time you buy eyeglasses or contact lenses, would you return to the same place where you bought your last pair?" The responses were then matched to another question, which asked if the place of last purchase advertised prices. The issue, "Are consumers more dissatisfied with opticians who advertise?" was thus answered. "The results show that while 58 percent of the customers of nonadvertising opticians indicated a willingness to give the seller repeat business, 86 percent of the advertisers' customers indicated they would return . . . only 8 percent of the customers of advertising opticians said that they 'probably' or 'definitely' would not go back. A full 25 percent of the customers of nonadvertising opticians gave the same answer. . . . In brief, if there is a quality problem it is not with advertising opticians. Rather it would appear that it lies with those who refuse to advertise their prices" (25).

The strong desire health (and other) professions have had to maintain codes of ethics that prohibit advertising can be explained by the fact that professional control over information leads to higher prices.

PERFORMANCE OF THE PHYSICIAN SERVICES MARKET

Based on the earlier discussion of the structure of the physician services market, it was determined that it could be a competitive industry. However, the peculiarities of the physician services market, lack of information, and extensive insurance coverage for physician services resulted in a downward sloping demand curve for physicians. Physicians' market conduct exhibited monopoly power, as evidenced by monopoly pricing and induced demand.

When evaluating the performance of the physician services market, one must be aware that there has been a change in this monopolistically competitive industry. The growth in managed care and competition among physicians have limited physicians' ability to induce demand and have made their demand curves more price elastic. Under pressure from large employer coalitions, HMOs and their provider groups are being required to provide employees with data on their performance, such as frequency of preventive mea-

sures and medical outcomes. The availability of this information, together with information on access, referrals, and prices, will enable employees to make more informed choices, thereby making different physicians and medical groups closer substitutes for one another, and consequently, their demand curves more price elastic.

One of the measures used to evaluate the performance of a market is whether the output, physician services, is being produced efficiently (at least cost). As a result of the changing structure of the industry, more physicians are becoming part of groups and the size of groups is increasing. One reason for the increase in size of groups is to take advantage of economies of scale. Another finding is that physicians have apparently increased their productivity; physicians no longer appear to be underutilizing aides. While it is difficult to determine whether physicians are producing their services as efficiently as possible, it appears that the industry is no less productive and is likely more efficient than it was previously.

Related to the concern with efficiency is whether physicians' market power has decreased over time. Pricing closer to costs is an indication that physicians' demand curves have become more price elastic; hence their market power has diminished. The movement to managed care has not only provided physicians with financial incentives to become more efficient, but has also increased competition among physicians for managed care contracts, thereby increasing each firm's demand elasticity.

The increased competitiveness of the physician services market can best be demonstrated when data on expenditures, fees, and incomes are compared over time.

Trends in Physician Expenditures, Fees, and Visits

Physician expenditures have risen rapidly over the past thirty years. In 1960, $5.3 billion was spent on physician services; by 1990, as shown in Table 10.6, this increased to $146 billion, and by 1995 to $202 billion. On a per capita basis, expenditures have increased from 6 to 8 percent annually, much more rapidly than the rate of inflation. These increased expenditures are primarily the result of increases in services per capita, changes in the type of service provided, and increased fees.

After the passage of Medicare and Medicaid in 1965, physician expenditures per capita increased rapidly, twice the rate of inflation. The inflation rate rose in the late 1960s as President Johnson used an "inflation tax" to finance the Vietnam War. (Inflation moved more wage earners into higher marginal tax brackets, the highest being 70 percent.) President Nixon imposed price controls (referred to as the Economic Stabilization Program—ESP) on the economy in 1971 and removed it the following year; however, it was kept in place for the medical sector until 1974. Price controls slowed the rate of increase in physician fees, but not expenditures. Following the removal of those controls in 1974, physicians' fees and expenditures increased sharply.

Inflation remained high in the late 1970s and began to decline in the early 1980s. Although inflation diminished, annual rates of increase in physician fees and expenditures

TABLE 10.6 Annual Rate of Change in Total Physician Expenditures, the CPI, and the CPI for Physicians' Fees, 1960–96

| Year | Expenditures on Physicians' Services | | Annual Percent Increase in Prices | |
	Total (billions)	Annual Percent Increase	CPI	CPI Physicians' Fees
1960	$5.3	9.0[a]	2.1	3.3
1965	8.2	9.2[a]	1.3	2.8
1966	8.8	7.3	2.9	5.8
1967	9.9	12.5	2.9	7.1
1968	10.8	9.1	4.2	5.6
1969	12.1	12.0	5.4	6.9
1970	13.6	12.4	5.9	7.5
1971	15.0	10.3	4.3	6.9
1972	16.7	11.3	3.3	3.1
1973	18.4	10.2	6.2	3.3
1974	21.0	14.1	10.9	9.2
1975	24.0	14.3	9.1	12.3
1976	27.1	12.9	5.8	11.3
1977	31.4	15.9	6.5	9.3
1978	33.8	7.6	7.6	8.3
1979	38.8	14.8	11.5	9.2
1980	45.2	16.5	13.5	11.7
1981	52.2	15.5	10.2	11.0
1982	57.7	9.6	6.0	9.4
1983	64.6	12.0	3.0	7.7
1984	72.6	12.4	3.4	7.0
1985	83.6	15.2	3.6	5.8
1986	93.1	11.4	1.9	7.2
1987	104.1	11.8	3.6	7.3
1988	118.7	14.0	4.1	7.2
1989	131.3	10.6	4.8	7.4
1990	146.3	11.4	5.4	7.1
1991	158.6	8.4	4.2	6.0
1992	174.7	10.2	3.0	6.3
1993	181.1	3.7	3.0	5.6
1994	189.4	4.6	2.6	4.4
1995	201.6	6.4	2.8	4.5
1996	—	—	3.0	3.6

Sources: U.S. Department of Health and Human Services, Health Care Financing Administration, Internet site http://www.hcfa.gov/stats/nhce96.htm, and unpublished data, 1996; Bureau of Labor Statistics, *CPI Detailed Report,* various issues.
[a]Average of the annual percent changes, each year, 1955–60 and 1960–65.

remained high. The continual rapid increase in physician expenditures was driven by fee increases, increased use of services, and new procedures.

It was not until the early 1990s that annual increases in physician fees and expenditures became smaller, although still greater than the rate of inflation. Managed care began to affect more physicians during the 1990s and the new Medicare physician payment system also became more stringent. It is likely that these two forces will continue to lower the rate of increase in fees and expenditures in the years ahead.

When the annual percent increase in total expenditures is compared to the percent increase in physician fees, it appears that during different time periods, fee increases have accounted for between one-half and two-thirds of the increased expenditures. (Part of these fee increases represent different types of visits.)

To gain some better understanding for the rise in physician expenditures, over the above time periods, in addition to fee increases, the trend in visits per capita are examined. Per capita visits started to increase in the late 1960s with the enactment of Medicare and Medicaid and the start of the ESP program.[9] Since the early 1990s, as shown in Table 10.7, the visit rate has been constant. Also of interest is the decline in the number of visits per physician (per week) since the late 1980s.

One possible explanation for the decline in visits per physician is that the supply of physicians (see Table 11-2) was increasing more rapidly than demand. However, if this were the only event occurring, then physician fees should have increased by less than that shown in Table 10.7 for new and established patients. (Given the various contractual arrangements physicians have with different payers, these fees are likely to exceed the average amount the physician was reimbursed.) It is also likely that the composition of office visits and surgical procedures have changed over time. If this has occurred, then part of the increase in physician fees is due to more costly visits and procedures, including more specialty services as well as additional services per visit.

The decline in physician fees in the most recent period, particularly for new patients, is likely indicative of the increasing competitive pressures among physicians.

Unavailability of data makes it difficult to examine the changing composition of physician services over time. However, it is possible to examine what has been occurring to physicians' practice costs and whether increasing costs have been driving fee increases.

If physician services were a competitive market, then physician fees would, in the long run, be determined by the cost of providing those services. In the short run, prices would equilibrate supply and demand and exceed costs when demand is increasing as prices are raised to ration demand. In the long run, however, one would expect increased prices to reflect the costs of the output provided. Thus as the costs of producing a physician visit increase, as would occur when the wages of aides increase, physician fees will also increase.

---

[9]There are several possible reasons for an increased number of visits during the ESP period. Controls placed on physician fees during the ESP decreased the real price of physician fees, leading to a movement down the demand curve for physician visits. An increase in visits could also have occurred as the result of induced demand.

TABLE 10.7 Number of Physician Visits per Person per Year, Number of Visits per Physician per Week, and the Mean Fee for Office Visits for Established and New Patient, 1975–96

	Number of Visits		Mean Fee for Office Visits			
	Per Person per Years	Per Physician per Week	Established Patient	Annual Percent Increase	New Patient	Annual Percent Increase
1975–80	5.0	134.6	$15.10	11.3	$25.24	11.3
1980–85	5.1	124.2	23.12	10.2	40.51	12.6
1986	5.4	117.7	30.10	7.3	55.75	7.5
1987	5.4	119.3	31.82	5.7	59.69	7.1
1988	5.4	121.1	33.91	6.6	63.51	6.4
1989	5.4	121.6	37.09	9.4	68.52	7.9
1990	5.5	120.9	39.87	7.5	74.84	9.2
1991	5.8	118.4	42.08	5.5	83.04	10.9
1992	6.0	114.8	46.43	10.3	88.17	6.2
1993	6.1	112.4	52.89	13.9	91.77	4.1
1994	6.1	109.6	56.24	6.3	97.16	5.9
1995	6.1 (est)	107.6	59.39	5.6	102.75	5.8
1996	—	109.4	58.57	−1.4	97.32	−5.3

Sources: Column 1: National Center for Health Statistics, "Current Estimates of Health Interview Surveys," *Vital and Health Statistics,* Series 10 (Washington, D.C.: Department of Health and Human Services, various years); Columns 2, 3, and 5: Martin Gonzalez and David Emmons, eds., *Socioeconomic Characteristics of Medical Practice* (Chicago: AMA, 1986, 1996, and 1997), 1986: p. 56, Table 13; p. 86, Table 28; p. 90, Table 30; 1996: p. 61, Table 16; p. 77, Table 28; p. 79, Table 30; 1997: p. 71, Table 16; p. 81, Table 24; p. 83, Table 26.

Recent trends in physicians' expenses, fees, and incomes are shown in greater detail in Table 10.8. Physicians' expenses (col. 1) during the 1980s have been rising at a more rapid rate than the CPI (col. 6), which suggests that the CPI is not a good proxy for physicians' costs. The largest component of physician expense is for nonphysician payroll (34 percent of total expense), which had high rates of increase in the late 1980s and early 1990s. These expenses are now increasing at a low rate.

One expense that continues to receive a great deal of legislative interest is malpractice insurance, which represented 7 percent of total expenses in 1982 and 11 percent currently (as of 1996). After rising very rapidly in the mid-1980s, premiums then actually declined and do not appear to be the concern that they once were. (The remaining categories of expense are office, 27 percent; medical supplies, 8 percent; medical equipment, 3 percent; and other, 16 percent.) It is interesting to note that in the period when physician liability insurance and nonphysician payroll were increasing most rapidly (25 percent and 14 percent in 1985), physicians' fees rose by the smallest percentage amount during the 1980s. As a consequence, physicians' real incomes declined.

TABLE 10.8 Annual Percent Change in Professional Expenses, Fees, and Incomes of Physicians, 1982–96

Year	Mean Professional Expenses	Mean Nonphysician Payroll	Mean Liability Premiums	Physician Fee for Established Patients	Average Net Income	CPI
1982	7.8	—	—	—	8.7	6.0
1983	8.9	−3.7	19.0	6.9	6.6	3.2
1984	10.1	7.6	21.7	6.5	4.1	4.3
1985	9.3	14.1	25.0	4.9	3.5	3.6
1986	15.3	9.0	21.9	7.3	6.5	1.9
1987	4.5	9.5	17.2	5.7	10.7	3.6
1988	13.8	13.9	−2.5	6.6	9.4	4.1
1989	5.4	8.9	−2.5	9.4	7.7	4.8
1990	1.1	3.2	−6.5	7.5	5.5	5.4
1991	12.3	12.7	2.8	5.5	3.8	4.2
1992	8.9	10.6	−7.4	10.3	6.5	3.0
1993	−0.7	2.9	4.3	13.9	4.2	3.0
1994	0.5	2.0	4.9	6.3	−3.6	2.6
1995	10.1	2.0	−0.7	5.6	7.2	2.8
1996	—	—	—	−1.4	—	2.9
1985–90[a]	9.2	10.6	7.6	8.4	9.3	3.6
1990–95[a]	6.9	6.7	0.7	9.8	3.8	2.5

Sources: Martin Gonzalez and David Emmons, eds., *Socioeconomic Characteristics of Medical Practice* (Chicago: American Medical Association, 1989 and 1997), 1989: pp. 88, 102, 110; 1997: pp. 81, 89, 93, 99, 105; Bureau of Labor Statistics, CPI Detailed Report, various issues.
[a]Average annual percent change.

It appears that changes in fees follow changes in expenses by one to two years. If physician fees continue to follow this pattern, physician fee increases should remain relatively low in coming years.

Evaluating the reasons for the rise in physician fees and expenditures is difficult because the visit mix has been changing over time: there has been an increase in the number of specialists. In addition to changes in the visit mix, the population has been aging, thereby demanding more visits. The decline in patient direct payments has also increased the demand for services. And Medicare is still an unmanaged, fee-for-service payment system.

Trends in Physicians' Incomes

It appears from the above data that fees are somewhat related to changes in practice expenses. However, the relationship between expenses and fees is not sufficiently close to conclude that expenses are the main determinant of changes in fees. Further, the rise in physician incomes has continued to increase, providing physicians with increases in their real incomes.

In a competitive industry, profits may be higher than normal in the short run because of an increase in demand. Over time, however, entry and increased competition are likely to result in normal profits. To fully evaluate whether profits, or with respect to physicians—their incomes, are normal, it is necessary to compare medicine to comparable occupations; this is discussed more completely in the chapter on health manpower shortages and surpluses. Since there are still limits on entry into the medical profession, it is unlikely that physicians' incomes and incomes in comparable occupations without entry barriers would be similar. However, comparing physician incomes over time would indicate whether the new competitive environment has eroded physicians' monopoly power.

With the growth of private and government payment for physician services starting in the mid-1960s, the demand for physician services increased more rapidly than supply, visits per physician increased, and physician fees increased faster than the costs of providing those services. As a result, physician incomes increased rapidly. Between 1965 and 1975, physician incomes increased by more than 100 percent, which was a more rapid rate of increase than that of dentists, lawyers, and, most likely, any other profession. Except for psychiatry, the annual rate of increase in physician incomes exceeded that of the CPI, as shown in Table 10.9.

In the late 1970s, the supply of physicians expanded, inflation increased, and then, by the early 1980s, a severe recession occurred. As a consequence, physicians' real incomes (adjusted for inflation) declined. The largest decline in real incomes occurred for those physicians in primary care. Specialists' and surgeons' real incomes continued to increase. Incomes for primary care physicians were, in part, limited by tight Medicare fee controls while technological advances permitted specialists to perform more procedures at higher fees. As the economy expanded in the late 1980s, physicians' real (adjusted for inflation) incomes increased, with the largest increases occurring for OB/GYN physicians. Specialists experienced larger increases than primary care physicians.

In the most recent period, 1991 to 1996, two events began to impact physicians' incomes. First, managed care became more pervasive with its emphasis on discounting and greater use of primary care physicians (PCPs) relative to specialists. Second, the new Medicare physician payment system (discussed below) attempted to raise fees of PCPs at the expense of specialists. As a result of these changed economic conditions, the average annual percent increase in physician incomes slowed. Primary care physicians experienced more rapid increases in their incomes than did specialists (such as surgeons) and hospital-based physicians (such as anesthesiologists).

The movement toward managed care with its greater demand for PCPs has also begun to affect the demand for a medical education. As discussed in greater detail in the chapter on the market for medical education, the increased demand for PCPs has resulted in an increased demand by medical students for a career in primary care.

Due to the growth in competing physician networks, HMOs, ambulatory care clinics,

TABLE 10.9 Average Annual Percent Change in Net Income from Medical Practice by Specialty, 1965–95

Specialty	1965–75	1975–85	1985–90	1991–96
General practice	8.8	6.5	5.3	4.1
Internal medicine	9.6	7.2	8.3	4.0
Surgery	9.0	11.6	8.8	3.0
Pediatrics	7.3	6.5	6.6	3.0
OB/GYN	10.3	8.8	11.1	0.7
Radiology	6.7	8.4	8.7	3.3
Psychiatry	4.2	8.6	5.6	0.8
Anesthesiology	7.2	13.6	7.6	0.6
All physicians	9.2	9.0	7.7	2.8
CPI all items	6.4	9.1	3.6	2.5

Sources: Zachary Dyckman, *Study of Physicians' Income in the Pre-Medicare Period–1965,* U.S. Department of Health Education and Welfare, Social Security Administration (Washington, D.C.: U.S. Government Printing Office, 1976), 10; David Goldfarb, "Trends in Physicians' Incomes, Expenses and Fees: 1970–1980," in David Goldfarb, ed., *Profile of Medical Practice* (Monroe, Wis.: American Medical Association, 1981): 114, Table 1; Martin Gonzalez, *Socioeconomic Characteristics of Medical Practice,* 1986 and 1997 editions (Chicago: American Medical Association, 1986, and 1997), 1986: 106, Table 39; 1997: 105, Table 44; Bureau of the Census, *Statistical Abstract of the United States,* 1996, 116th ed. (Washington, D.C.: U.S. Department of Commerce): 483, Table 745.

and outpatient surgery centers, the private market for physician services has become more competitive over time. In 1981, there were fewer than ten PPOs. By 1994, there were more than seven hundred PPO plans. As the growth of PPO plans has increased, so have the percent of physicians participating in such plans. In 1983, 11 percent of physicians participated in PPOs; by 1996, this percentage had increased to 75 percent (26). In 1996, 72 percent of physicians contracted with HMOs and 36 percent of physicians had a capitated contract. As HMOs and PPOs increase their enrollments, more physicians are finding it necessary to contract with such organizations so as to not lose their patients. Thus although past expenditure and fee increases may have been more the result of physicians' market power, it appears that current competitive pressures are reducing that market power and that future increases in fees and income will be more related to cost increases, as occurs in a competitive market.

Small Area Variations in Use Rates

A third aspect of market performance is whether the appropriate output is being provided.

A disturbing aspect of physician practice behavior is the wide variation in treatment patterns for patients with the same diagnosis. Stimulated by John Wennberg's early research, numerous studies have documented wide variations in use rates for hospital admissions and in surgical procedures among different communities as well as for the same specialties. For example, the rate of coronary bypass operations in Utica, New York, was 45 percent greater than in Syracuse (0.83 per one thousand versus 0.57 per one thousand); were people in Utica being overtreated or were those in Syracuse being undertreated? Again, C-sections as a percent of all births were 38 percent in Oneida, New York, while they were only 18 percent in Rochester (27). Attempts to explain these variations have examined differences in demand factors. After adjusting for age, sex, and health status, as well as differences in insurance coverage and incomes, the large variations in use rates remain.

Comparisons have been made with other countries, such as Canada and England, and there are similarly wide variations in use rates. The demand-inducement hypothesis is also not helpful in explaining these wide variations. Community variations persist even when economic factors that might provide physicians with an incentive to induce demand are held constant. Further, there are no incentives for physicians to induce demand in Canada or England, yet similar variations exist in those countries. Supply factors that could influence demand were also examined; but even when they were held constant, variations in use by specialty still existed.

The inability of traditional supply-and-demand factors to explain the wide variations in use of medical services is a cause for concern in terms of patient health outcomes as well as for economic efficiency. If, after adjusting use rates by procedure, for the relevant demand factors, variations still exist, then some patients are receiving too much treatment while others may be receiving too little. Some patients' lives are endangered, and favorable medical outcomes could be achieved with fewer resources.

For example, the number of carotid endarterectomies has increased, from 15,000 per year in 1971, to 85,000 in 1982, to an estimated 108,000 in 1994. The purpose of the procedure is to reduce the risk of stroke or death in patients with extracranial vascular disease. In one study, the investigators determined that 32 percent of the Medicare patients examined (1,302 Medicare patients randomly selected in three regions in 1981 who had the procedure) had the procedure for inappropriate reasons. Another 32 percent had the procedure for equivocal reasons (28). These procedures carry with it a significant risk of complications and death.

A number of studies have been undertaken, showing wide rates of use for particular surgical procedures with no differences in patient outcomes. If low users are not low quality but have the same outcomes, then performance, in terms of expenditures and patient outcomes, can be improved.

Additional hypotheses offered to explain variations in use both between communities and even within a hospital for a given specialty, involve the school where the physician was educated, experience, length of time in the community, and community norms. For example, it was determined that Boston has a higher hospital admission rate than New Haven, both excellent centers for medical training. Further, physician practice styles within a specialty have been found to be more important than patient severity of illness in explaining variations in use rates.

The gains from providing information to physicians so as to decrease inappropriate use is shown in Figure 10.6. Differences in physicians' belief as to the efficacy of treatment are shown by the three demand curves, D_1, D_2, and D_3; D_2 represents the demand for a particular procedure in a community based on what the fully informed physician would recommend. Social, economic, and demographic factors, as well as morbidity, among the three communities represented by the different demand curves are assumed to be similar. The only difference among the communities (represented by the different demand curves) are differences in physicians' practice styles and beliefs. The cost of providing that procedure is assumed to be constant and is represented by MC. The "appropriate" use rate in the community is Q_2, at which point the marginal value of an additional procedure equals its marginal cost. Communities whose physicians place too great a belief in the treatment value of that procedure would have a use rate of Q_3. Similarly, "too low" a use rate is shown by Q_1.

Providing information to physicians whose practice patterns result in demand curves D_1 and D_3 would improve economic welfare in the following manner. Individuals living in communities whose physicians believe the efficacy of a particular procedure is less (D_1) than it actually is (D_2) would be better off if the use rate of that procedure were increased; the marginal benefits of that procedure exceed its marginal cost. This lost value is repre-

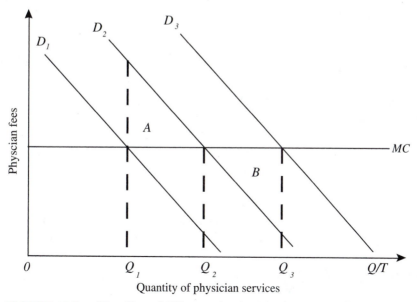

FIGURE 10.6 • The effect of differences in physicians' practice styles on procedure use rates.

sented by area *A*. Similarly, when the use rate is too high, the cost of that procedure exceeds its additional value; this excess of cost over its value is represented by area *B*.

Studies are being undertaken by managed care organizations and the federal government to determine the medical value or appropriateness of specific medical interventions. Such studies and the dissemination of their results can improve physician decision making and save enormous resources. One study attempted to estimate both the potential savings from reducing inappropriate medical use and for establishing priorities for undertaking studies on medical efficacy (29). The authors found that the annual welfare loss from variations in medical practice is approximately $8 billion (the average use rate is assumed to be the appropriate use rate). The present value of these savings would be 15 times the annual savings (at a real discount rate of 3 percent). The procedure that offers the greatest potential saving from reduced variations in use rates is coronary artery bypass graft. If the average use rate, which was the standard used, is too high, then the above savings would be even greater. These findings suggest that there are large potential savings for undertaking medical assessment studies and that priority should be given to studying those procedures that offer the greatest expected benefit in relation to the cost of the study.

Inappropriate use and wide variations among communities and physicians, within a given specialty, are indicative of important imperfections in the physician services market. Economic efficiency and patient outcomes could be improved if inappropriate use were reduced. Increased physician information on appropriate treatment should, together with appropriate incentives, improve the performance of the physician services market, with a consequent reduction in medical expenditures and improved patient outcomes.

PHYSICIAN PAYMENT UNDER MEDICARE

Physician pricing under Medicare is quite different than in the non-Medicare market. Medicare is such a large buyer of physician services, accounting for approximately 20 percent of total physician expenditures, that it is a monopsonist, that is, Medicare is a price setter because it can set the price it pays for physician services. The following is a discussion and analysis of how the government has used its buying power by examining past and current Medicare physician payment policies.

Physician Assignment under Medicare

When Medicare began, participating physicians had the option of accepting or rejecting assignment for payment of a beneficiary's claim. A physician accepting Medicare assignment was paid 80 percent of the approved fee by Medicare and the patient was responsible for the remaining 20 percent co-payment (in addition to a small annual deductible) which had to be paid directly to the physician. A physician not accepting assignment billed the patient for the entire fee, which was greater than the Medicare-approved fee. The patient then paid the entire fee directly to the physician and was reimbursed by Medicare for only 80 percent of the approved fee. Thus, the patient was responsible not only for the 20 percent co-payment of the approved fee, but also for the difference between the approved fee and the physician's charge. In addition, the patient had the increased burden of submitting the claim for payment before being reimbursed by Medicare for 80 percent of the physician's approved fee.

When the physician did not accept assignment, the difference between the Medicare-approved fee and the physician's fee was referred to as "balance billing." Balance billing increased the ageds' out-of-pocket price, thereby decreasing their access to physician services.

The number of physicians accepting Medicare fees as full payment was at 80 percent in 1996. Participating physicians now account for 90 percent of Medicare physician charges. This percentage has varied over time, its low being about 50 percent in 1976. The closer Medicare-approved fees were to fees in the private sector, the higher the assignment rate. In the 1980s, the increasing supply of physicians, the growing competition among physicians for patients, and an increase in Medicare fees to participating physicians made many physicians decide that it was in their economic best interest to accept assignment.

The assignment rate also varied according to region of the country, which reflected the market for physician services, and by physician specialty, which reflected the risk to the physician of not being paid by the patient. For example, surgeons, who had larger total charges, were more likely than primary care physicians to accept assignment. Also, patients were more likely to have to return to their primary care physician.

The following is an analysis of how Medicare reimbursement has affected physician assignment in the past. Assume that physicians have three types of patients: private-pay patients, which includes those with private insurance as well as Medicare-nonassigned patients; Medicare-assigned patients; and Medicaid patients. It is further assumed that the physician's fee is highest for the private-pay patients, lower for Medicare-assigned patients, and lowest for Medicaid patients. To maximize their income, physicians will serve patients paying the highest fees before serving other patients. How many patients in each category will be served by the physician will depend on the size of each market and the physician's marginal cost schedule.

The Medicare assignment problem can be described with reference to Figure 10.7 (30). The demand curve for physician services is D_1. The marginal revenue curve associated with that demand curve is MR_1. The downward-sloping demand curve assumes that physicians have some monopoly power. For private-pay patients the physician is a "price setter." The Medicare price is a horizontal line at PM. The physician is thus a "price taker" in the Medicare (and Medicaid) markets.

The physician will start by serving the private market. If the physician's marginal cost curve (MC) intersects the downward-sloping MR curve at a point above PM, such as A, this will determine the quantity of physician services to be produced and the price charged (the price charged will be that point on the demand curve directly above point A, which is where $MR = MC$). A physician in such a situation would not serve any Medicare-assigned patients. If, however, the physician's MC curve intersected MR at a point below the Medicare price (PM), the physician would serve that number of private patients given by the intersection of *MR* and *PM* (shown by Q_1). The physician would also serve Medicare-assigned patients up to the point where *MC* equals *PM*.

As shown in Figure 10.7, the physician would serve $0Q_1$ private patients and Q_1Q_2 Medicare-assigned patients. The marginal revenue of both private-pay and Medicare patients would be equal at that point. (If the physician served more than $0Q_1$ private patients, the foregone revenue from Medicare patients, *PM,* would exceed the *MR* of additional private patients.) The price for private patients would be P_1, while the Medicare price would be *PM*. The physician's *MR* curve is changed so that it becomes *MR* up to the point of intersection with *PM* and then it is horizontal (*PM*). (In this example the physician would not serve Medicaid patients, assuming that Medicaid pays a price less than *PM*.) A physician would enter the Medicaid market if the number of both private and Medicare patients is relatively small so that the physician's *MC* curve intersects the Medicaid price, which would be horizontal, as is the Medicare price, but presumably at a lower level.)

Several important factors affected the physicians' assignment rate. These may be classified as demand factors, supply factors, and Medicare policies. For example, an increase in private insurance that increased the private demand for physicians' services would shift the demand and *MR* curves to the right. If *MC* is unchanged, then *MC* would intersect *MR* at a point to the right of Q_1. The physician would serve more private patients and accept fewer assigned patients. The reverse would occur if there were a decrease in private demand. (Similarly, an increase in the supply of physicians would lead to a decrease in

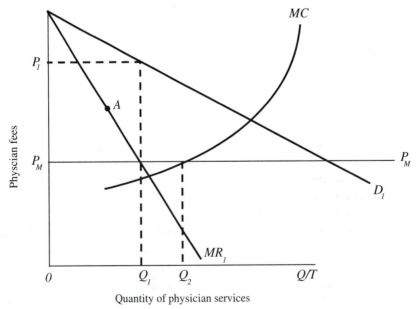

FIGURE 10.7 • Physician decision whether to accept Medicare assignment.

private demand per physician, thereby increasing assignment.) A change in the factors affecting the physician's *MC* curve, such as increased wages for personnel working in the physician's office, would also affect the assignment rate. With an increase in *MC*, the new *MC* curve would intersect *PM* to the left of Q_2. There would thus be a decrease in the number of assigned patients. Similarly, a decrease in *MC* would increase assignment.

Medicare policies also affect assignment. An increase in Medicare's price would raise *PM*. The higher *PM* would intersect the *MR* curve at a point to the left and higher than the previous point. Assuming that the higher *PM* intersected *MR* at point *A,* there would be a decrease in private-pay patients served (as well as an increase in their price) and an increase in the number of assigned patients. Other Medicare policies may have an effect on *PM* without explicitly changing it. For example, if Medicare makes it more (less) difficult for physicians to collect their fees for assigned patients, such as by delaying (speeding up) payment, this would be similar to a decrease (increase) in Medicare's net price. The consequence would be an increase (decrease) in the number of private patients served and a decrease (increase) in the number of assigned patients.

The above theoretical model for understanding assignment also contradicts the belief that physicians "cost shift" (charge private-pay patients more when government pays physicians less), is unlikely to occur and would not be a profit-maximizing strategy for physicians to follow. Recent empirical evidence supports the above theoretical discussion that physicians lower (raise) their prices to private patients when physicians' fees for Medicaid patients are reduced (increased) (31).

The factors affecting assignment rates noted above suggest alternative policies, with differing cost, that could have increased assignment. Medicare reimbursement rates could have been increased, physicians accepting assignment could have been reimbursed faster, and policies to lower the physician's *MC* curve could have been instituted.

Relative Value Scales, Balance Billing, and Expenditure Limits

In 1989, the Prospective Payment Reform Commission, in response to its congressional mandate to develop a new method of paying physicians under Medicare and to slow the growth in Medicare physician expenditures, proposed four significant recommendations. The first was to phase in, starting in 1992, a fixed fee schedule for Medicare physician payment based on a resource based relative value scale (RBRVS). The second was to limit "balance billing" among physicians, which is the amount beyond the Medicare payment that a nonparticipating physician can charge the Medicare patient. Third was to establish an overall expenditure target for Medicare physician expenditures, referred to as a volume-performance standard (VPS). Fourth was to fund research on medical effectiveness. These recommendations, which were historic changes in the payment of physicians under Medicare, were enacted by Congress in 1989 (32).

The impetus for changes in physician reimbursement came from two sources. The first, and most important, was the federal government, whose interest was (and still is) in reducing Medicare Part B expenditures, which is funded out of general revenues, and increases the federal deficit, an important political problem. The government, however, was constrained in achieving this objective by not having a large number of physicians drop their Medicare participation. The second impetus for change came from various physician specialties, third-party payers, and a number of academicians who believed that the previous Medicare payment system was inefficient and also resulted in inequities among physicians.

Background on Medicare Part B Financing

The financing of Medicare Part B and the distribution of expenditures under that program have been changing over time. Currently, 77 percent of Medicare Part B expenditures is financed out of the federal government's general tax revenues. The remaining 23 percent is paid for by premium contributions from the aged to that program. Federal contributions under Part B now represent one of our larger federal programs; Part B expenditures rose from $779 million in 1967 to over $40 billion in 1990 and to $75 billion by 1997. They are expected to reach $116 billion by the year 2002 (33).

Part B expenditures represented 22 percent of total Medicare expenditures before hospital DRGs were implemented in 1983; they have since increased to 36 percent. Physicians receive approximately 62 percent of all Part B payments (down from 75 percent five years ago); the remainder goes to other providers, such as hospital outpatient departments (24 percent—up from 19 percent five years ago) and to those providing home care (14 percent—up from 6 percent five years ago). The average annual rate of increase in Medicare expenditures to each of these three groups over the past five years was 6.6 percent, 12.8 percent, and 15.2 percent, respectively. Any reduction in these expenditure increases will make a significant contribution toward reducing the federal budget deficit.

Politics has restricted the choices available to the federal government for reducing the rise in Part B expenditures. Each choice imposes a cost on some constituency. Higher costs could be imposed on the aged, providers could be paid less, the nonaged could pay higher taxes (to subsidize the Part B premium), or future generations could bear the cost through a higher federal deficit.

The financial burden on the aged could be increased by raising the Part B deductible, originally $50 and currently $100. The co-payment, which is 20 percent, could also be increased. Higher deductibles and co-payments would reduce the demand for physician services, hence reduce federal expenditures. Also, the ageds' portion of the Part B premium, currently 25 percent, could be raised, thereby reducing federal expenditures. (Unless these increased costs to the elderly are income-related, an increased premium to all the aged would be equivalent to a regressive tax, which would be particularly severe on low-income elderly.)

Whichever political party proposes shifting a greater portion of the Part B costs to the elderly is likely to pay a "price." The elderly have high voting participation rates, associations representing their interests are quite active, and members of Congress run for re-election every two years. Thus, while some increase in the ageds' Part B premium contribution is likely to occur, the major reduction in the rate of increase in Medicare expenditures is likely to be resolved by shifting the burden to health care providers (lower payments) and to the nonaged (higher taxes) or future generations (greater deficits).

These latter methods were the approach previously used. During the Economic Stabilization Program in the early 1970s, provider payments were reduced; it was the basis of the Medicare economic index, which placed limits on physician fee increases; it was the method used to control Medicare hospital expenditures; and it continues to be the preferred federal approach to slowing the rise in Medicare expenditures.

The federal government is, however, limited in how little it can pay participating physicians, since it must ensure that a sufficient number of physicians are willing to participate in Medicare. While Medicare represents approximately 20 percent of total physician revenues, for some physicians and some specialties it is a sizable portion of their incomes. The loss of a significant number of physicians could cause access problems for the aged in some geographic areas. Once access begins to decline, Congress will be pressured by the aged to increase physician participation.

Fee-for-service results in two types of inefficiencies. First, the (imperfect agent) physician has an incentive to perform more services. Second, physician fees under Medicare were initially based on their fee profiles. As such, insured services were priced higher in relation to cost than other services. (Those services having a higher relative "profit" provide physicians with an incentive to perform a relatively greater number of these services.) Also, because of limits on Medicare fee increases over time and rigidities in Medicare fees, some services were priced much higher than others in relation to their cost. As procedures became routine and their costs fell with experience and volume, the fee for performing that procedure did not decline. The fee for coronary artery bypass surgery was initially established when the procedure required a great amount of a surgeon's time. As the surgeon's experience with this procedure increased and it became possible to delegate various aspects of the care for this procedure (e.g., pre- and postoperative care), the price for the procedure should have fallen, but Medicare did not decrease it.

Inequities also occurred among physicians because Medicare paid physicians according to their fee profiles but did not increase them frequently. Thus new physicians were able to establish a higher fee profile than older, established physicians in the same specialty. Further, large differences in fees for the same service between regions existed, unrelated to differences in cost of living. And fees charged by physicians for the same service varied depending on the physician's specialty.

Resource Based Relative Value Scales

These inefficiencies and resulting inequities in Medicare payment for physician services caused differences in physician incomes and affected physicians' choice of specialty and practice location. To correct these inefficiencies and resulting inequities, a number of academicians and physician organizations wanted a new fee structure.

The new payment system consisted of two parts. The first part, as described below, assigned values or weights to all services and procedures. Second, a conversion factor was applied to those relative values to translate them into dollars or fees. For example, if the conversion factor is $100 and a procedure has a relative value of 2.5, the fee for that procedure will be $250.

Since the main purpose of a relative value scale was to correct the inefficiencies and inequities of the Medicare fee schedules, the following principles should have been followed (34). First, there should be one price for each service regardless of the training and background of the person performing that service. Second, fees should be proportional to the costs of performing each service, so as not to bias the mix of services. Third, the costs of providing the service should be based on the most efficient method (i.e., lowest level of training required) rather than on averages of costs or charges.

Reimbursement for physician services according to the task performed rather than the level of training of the person performing it will eventually affect the specialty distribution of physicians. If a particular service can be performed equally well by a family practitioner, a specialist should not receive a higher fee for performing it. If specialists are not as busy as they would like to be, and they use their excess time performing services that nonspecialists can perform equally well, reimbursing specialists at a higher rate will provide them with a higher income than they would otherwise have.[10]

The relative value scale, developed by Hsaio et al., attempted to approximate the cost of performing each physician service (35). Its premise was that in a competitive market the price of a service will, in the long run, reflect the cost of producing that service. The cost-based approach to determining relative values is complex (relative values were established for over seven thousand services), required a great deal of analysis and data, must be continually updated, and involves a number of assumptions which, if different, could change the outcomes. For example, the calculation of the physician's time assumes that a certain amount of time is spent by the surgeon before and after the operation and it assumes an average length of time for the various tasks that the physician performs.

The total relative value for a service is divided into three components. First is the physician's work, to include the complexity of the service, so as to allow for differences in skill and effort required. Also included is opportunity cost, so that physicians with different training times can earn the same rate of return. Second are practice expenses, to include overhead expenses, such as office payroll and depreciation on equipment. Third is malpractice insurance, since its cost varies across specialties.

Two methods were used for estimating the complexity of a task: personal interviews

---

[10]The principle of establishing payment rates based on the lowest level of training required should apply to physicians and their aides as well as between physicians with different specialties, assuming the quality is the same. Under fee-for-service, a financial incentive to delegate is created if the same payment were made for a particular task regardless of whether it was performed by a physician or an aide. If the time of a lesser-skilled individual—a nurse or physician assistant, for example—can be substituted for a physician's time, the allocation of resources is improved. In the short run, the physician's time is freed for more complex tasks; in the longer run, if lesser-trained manpower takes over some of the tasks now performed by physicians, a smaller supply of physicians will be needed. Task delegation should occur automatically under a capitation system since physicians who did so would be able to treat a larger number of patients and earn greater net revenues.

and a modified Delphi technique in which each physician was able to compare her own estimate with the average of physicians within that specialty. Many assumptions were required, such as in calculating opportunity cost, that the years required for training in a specialty are the minimum necessary. Further assumptions were made regarding the lengths of working careers across specialties, residency salaries, hours worked per week, and an interest rate to discount future earnings.

Hsiao et al., performed a very useful service in calculating a relative value scale based on resource costs. In doing so data requirements and assumptions had to be explicitly defined. A number of criticisms, however, have been made of a cost-based relative value scale (36). For example, unless relative values include a quality factor high-quality physicians will decrease quality. Further, since there are constant changes in technology, equipment, office expenses, residents' salaries, and the time required to perform various services, unless the relative value units are updated, Medicare physician fees will diverge once again from market fees, creating imbalances between supply and demand for physician services and among specialties.

Relative value scales were also meant to redistribute income among the different physician specialties by realigning fees proportional to cost for all services. Fees for cognitive services were increased while fees for performing technical procedures were decreased. Primary care physicians gained at the expense of procedure-oriented specialists. For example, it was estimated that payments to family practitioners increased 37 percent, internists 16 percent, with declines of 21 percent for radiologists, 20 percent for thoracic surgeons, and 17 percent for ophthalmologists. The income redistribution among physician specialties explained their relative political positions on the new fee schedule.

Limits on Balance Billing and the Volume-Performance Standard

Two additional aspects of the new payment system were limits on the amount that could be balance billed and a target set for how fast Medicare physician expenditures were permitted to increase.

Physicians not accepting assignment could not charge more than 115 percent of the approved Medicare fee and are only paid 95 percent of that fee, therefore receiving, at a maximum, only 109 percent of the Medicare-approved fee. *Thus even physicians who decide not to participate in Medicare are restricted in how much they can charge for treating a Medicare patient.*

To control the increase in physician expenditures, the government annually updates the conversion factor which, when multiplied by the relative value scale, results in Medicare physician fees for the coming year. If the volume of physician services increased faster than expected, the conversion factor would increase less so that expenditures remained within the target.

The conversion factor update was designed to limit the growth in total Medicare physician expenditures rather than attempt to equilibrate the demand and supply of physician services in the Medicare market. As would occur with any government-imposed price, Medicare fees will be higher or lower than market-determined prices, which are established through supply and demand. Medicare physician fees are likely to differ from market prices regionally and by physician specialty.

A number of factors are likely to cause Medicare fees to differ from private market fees. For example, physician fees would be expected to increase over time as input costs, such as personnel wages, increase. Since Medicare determines its fees with an expenditure target as its objective, it may not match input cost increases, which would be reflected in private fees.

Similarly, increased demands for primary care physicians in the private and or the Medicare markets would result in their fees increasing relative to those of other physicians. If, over time, the government failed to raise physician fees for primary care physicians, as fees increased in the private, non-Medicare market, there will be a shift in supply to the nonregulated (private) market. Physicians would serve fewer Medicare patients (perhaps not accept new Medicare patients) and the aged would have to wait longer to see a physician. Access to care by Medicare enrollees will decline.

One method by which decreased access could be limited is to allow physicians to balance bill (charge the Medicare patient the difference between the regulated and market price). However, under the new system, the maximum amount that can be balance billed is 109 percent of the Medicare fee. Previously, an increase in the number of physicians who balance billed was an indication that Medicare fees were falling behind fees in the private market. Balance billing, however, was opposed by organizations representing the aged because it increases the aged's net price for physician services. As a result, balance billing under Medicare is virtually eliminated.

Assuming that private primary care physician fees increase more rapidly than Medicare physician fees, a shortage will occur in the Medicare market because price will be below the equilibrium level. Physicians will supply fewer services than patients will demand. (Regardless of whether the supply of physician hours is backward bending or not, the supply of physician services is positively sloped since the physician could substitute other inputs for his own time.)

To receive the same marginal revenue per hour of their time, physicians will shift more of their hours to the non-Medicare market, reducing the supply in the Medicare market and increasing supply in the private market. With an increase in supply, price in the non-Medicare market will increase less than it would have otherwise.[11]

---

[11]The probable effects on the Medicare and non-Medicare markets would be similar to the earlier discussion on Medicare assignment. With reference to Figure 10.7, limiting physician fee or payment increases will decrease the Medicare price over time. This lower price will intersect the physician's marginal cost curve to the left of Q_2, thereby reducing the quantity supplied to government-paid Medicare patients. Similarly, as the Medicare fee is reduced, it will intersect the MR curve for private patients to the right, at a lower point. Again, fewer Medicare patients will be served as the physician increases services to the non-Medicare market. Further, the physicians' price in the private market should decrease, as they increase their supply in that market. Whether price decreases or increases in the private market depends on whether one believes that physicians are limited in their ability to induce demand and increase their price at will (the neoclassical approach) or whether physicians will be able to "cost-shift" and raise fees in the private market (demand inducement or target-income theories).

Congress tried to achieve several contradictory objectives in enacting the RBRVS Medicare physician payment system. These were: first, to limit the growth in Medicare physician expenditures (because it contributed to the budget deficit) by limiting the conversion update factor; second, increase access to care for the aged by having a large number of physicians participate in Medicare (accept assignment); and third, reduce the aged's out-of-pocket expenditures by limiting balance billing. Limits on both balance billing and Medicare fee increases (conversion update) will eventually cause a significant shift of primary care physician supply to the non-Medicare market. If the gap between Medicare and private fees for primary care physicians becomes too large, the aged may find that their only access to care is if they join Medicare HMOs, where there are no restrictions on physician fees.

It is highly likely that there will be further changes in Medicare's physician payment policy in the years ahead as the conflict in objectives over limiting Medicare physician expenditures and access to care by the aged becomes greater. The federal government need not rely on a single payment method. A variety of approaches will allow both patients and physicians to move into those systems that are most preferable and these movements will provide information on how each of these systems performs.

Proposed Changes to the Medicare Physicians' Market

A number of proposals have been made to improve the equity and efficiency of physician services funded by Medicare. The following are two such proposals.

An Income-Related Premium for Medicare Part B

Currently, the aged pay only 25 percent of the Medicare Part B premium, the remainder being funded by general tax revenues. This subsidy is provided to all of the aged, regardless of their income or wealth. Making the premium income-related would have two effects: first, high-income aged would receive less of a subsidy, thereby decreasing the federal budget deficit or making the funds available to low-income nonaged. Second, reducing the subsidy to the aged would increase their cost of remaining in the current Medicare fee-for-service system compared to joining a Medicare HMO. This subsidy distorts the relative prices to the aged of their health plan choices. The increase in relative price of remaining in the fee-for-service system would cause more of the aged to switch to the HMO option.

Tax Medi-Gap Policies

More than 70 percent of the aged have purchased private health insurance ("Medi-gap" policies) to cover their out-of-pocket medical expenditures. The effect of such policies is to remove most of the cost-sharing provisions of Medicare, which include a 20 percent co-payment for physician services. Removing the co-payment increases the quantity demanded of physician visits with a consequent increase in Medicare expenditures. The premium for Medi-gap policies, however, is based only on the co-payment for those visits, not the Medicare portion of the expenditures. There is, in effect, an externality; those purchasing Medi-gap policies pay only a small part of their additional use of services, the taxpayers pay the remainder.

In addition to decreasing the price of physician services, Medi-gap policies reduce the patient's incentive to shop for lower prices and makes it more difficult for HMOs to compete for Medicare patients; Medi-gap enrollees have less incentive to join an HMO since they have access to an unrestricted choice of providers with almost full coverage at subsidized rates (37). Taxing Medi-gap policies to offset the increase in Medicare expenditures that result from such policies would decrease the demand for such policies, reinstitute cost sharing and provide incentives for shopping, and enable HMOs to better compete for Medicare patients.

SUMMARY

The structure of the physician services market is changing, from a predominance of solo practice to an increase in the number of physicians practicing in groups. Group size is also increasing. The movement to group practice and larger-size groups is due to economies of scale, reputational economies of scale, physicians' desire to reduce uncertainty and risk (although risk sharing reduces productivity incentives), and greater market power when negotiating with HMOs, insurers, and hospitals.

Along with the increasing size of groups is the change in physician composition within those groups. Previously, multispecialty groups were predominately comprised of specialists. With the movement toward large medical groups capable of contracting with and servicing managed care plans, on capitation risk contracts, there has been an increased demand for primary care physicians. Multispecialty groups have moved to an increased percentage of primary care physicians, such as 50 percent of each, and in some cases to 70 percent primary care.

Although the physician services market is not concentrated, it cannot be inferred that physicians do not have market (monopoly) power. There are certain peculiarities of this market that provide physicians with some monopoly power. Patients have limited information on physician practice styles, their fees, and their accessibility. Physicians differ in their technical ability as well as in how they relate to the patient.[12] In such a market situation, the costs of search are high and wide variations exist in fees, quality, and practice styles.

---

[12]Perfect purchaser information rarely exists in any market. Many consumers have little or no information on prices and quality of other consumer products, such as appliances, and yet these markets are relatively competitive. This lack of information is resolved in several ways. For example, brand name products often sell at higher prices than non-brand name items, since they consist of two goods: a firm's reputation and the product itself. In some markets, those consumers who are informed and are price-sensitive give the demand curve for that product its downward slope; even if ten people are not price sensitive with respect to the price of gasoline but several others are, the horizontal summation of all the individual demand curves for gasoline would be negatively sloped.

The lack of information has made it difficult for patients to determine how good a substitute other physicians are to their own physicians. Also making patients less price-sensitive was the growth in third-party insurance. With lower out-of-pocket costs, the patient has a decreased incentive to search for lower-priced physicians; their costs of search, primarily time and travel costs, are likely to exceed the marginal benefits of increased search, namely, lower net prices.

When physicians have downward sloping demand curves and the market structure is relatively unconcentrated, then the physician services market can be characterized as being monopolistically competitive.

Indicative of physicians' monopoly power is their market conduct. Before the antitrust laws became applicable to health care in 1982, physicians engaged in various forms of anticompetitive activities, such as insurer boycotts and bans on advertising. Physicians' pricing and practice behavior were also indicative of monopoly power. With a less price elastic demand curve as a result of lack of information and extensive insurance coverage, physicians were able to price as monopolists (always in the elastic portion of their demand curve) by setting their fees in excess of marginal cost. For example, McCarthy estimates that the price elasticity facing individual primary care physicians was −3, using 1975 data (19). This elasticity estimate is consistent with the physician firm having market power, although it is still quite price elastic. (An elasticity of −3 represents a price that is 50 percent above marginal cost.)[13]

One form of conduct was particularly indicative of monopoly power, namely, supplier-induced demand, which is the ability of physicians to shift their demand curves. It is not known how much demand inducement currently exists and there is still controversy regarding whether physicians are still able to induce demand by a significant amount.

The market for physician services has been undergoing major changes, which has been affecting its performance. The movement toward managed care, with both HMOs and indemnity insurance, has resulted in greater oversight of physicians' practice behavior. Utilization review mechanisms, emphasis on appropriateness of care, and physician profiling are reducing inappropriate use of services. Eliminating variations in medical services that are due to inappropriate treatment as a result of differences in physicians' practice styles would not only decrease expenditures but also improve patients' health. In coming years, as outcomes research expands, this information will be used by medical groups, hospitals, insurers, and self-insured firms to improve the efficiency of medical services. These actions should improve market performance.

There are, however, still concerns over physicians as imperfect agents. Under capitation, the physicians' financial incentives are opposite of those in fee-for-service. Patients (and purchasers on their behalf) are concerned that the financial incentives under capitation will result in imperfect agents providing too few services and decreased access to

---

[13]Assuming profit maximization (MR = MC), the physician would set price according to $P = MC(E/E + 1)$. Therefore, $P = MC(-3/-3 + 1) = 150$ percent of MC.

care and to specialists. Similarly, HMOs and insurers have an agency relationship with their physicians. HMOs and insurers are concerned that physicians' practice patterns under a capitated system may result in decreased patient satisfaction and, consequently, a decrease in the insurers' enrollments.

As the physicians' services market continues to adapt to the new competitive environment, physician groups can be expected to compete on the basis of both price and appropriateness of care for the business of large employers and insurance companies. The expansion of information systems to permit greater monitoring of physicians' practice patterns and the publicizing of these results offers promise that both inappropriate and insufficient care will be reduced. To be price-competitive, physician groups will seek to be efficient in their use of inputs as well as taking advantage of economies of scale. The demand curve for physicians competing for HMO, PPO, and employer contracts is likely to become more price elastic. Regardless of whether physicians have been previously able to induce demand for their services, their ability to do so in coming years will be lessened. Market forces are becoming increasingly stronger and are likely to improve market performance.

Key Terms and Concepts

- Balance billing
- Monopolistic competition
- Supplier-induced demand
- Survivor analysis

- Economies of scale in medical practice
- Income-related Medicare Part B premiums
- Market power of medical groups
- Medicare physician assignment
- Monopoly model of physician pricing
- Physician agency relationships under capitation
- Physician industry consolidation
- Resource-based relative value scale (RBRVS)
- Target income hypothesis

Review Questions

1. There are two contrasting theories of physician behavior. The first is the traditional model and the second is referred to as "physician-induced demand" or "target income."
   a. Explain each model and describe how these models differ in their assumptions regarding physician behavior and patient information.

b. What empirical evidence has been used to support the physician-induced demand theory? What alternative explanations support the observed data?

c. What would be the consequences of an increase in the supply of physicians on the price of physician services, the quantity of physician visits, and total physician expenditures of each of these theories?

2. What are some of the ways in which health insurers seek to compensate for the information advantage physicians have?

3. How do fee-for-service and capitation payment systems affect the physician's role as the patient's agent?

4. The price elasticity of demand for physician services has been estimated to be −0.2. Does this mean that each physician is a monopolist with a price inelastic demand curve?

5. What information would you need and how would you use it to determine whether physicians were over- or underutilizing aides in their practice?

6. Large variation in physician fees exists for the same type of service within the same market area. Provide two alternative explanations for this variation, one based on a competitive market model and the other using a monopoly framework. Do the same for the rise in physician fees over time.

7. What characteristics of the physician market provide physicians with market or monopoly power?

8. Why has the size of multispecialty medical groups been increasing in the past several years?

9. Explain the advantages and disadvantages to a physician for joining a group practice as compared to being in solo practice.

10. Explain how a resource-based relative value scale is used to determine physicians' fees.

11. Resource-based relative value (RBRVS) fees pay all physicians (within a specialty) the same fee for the same type of service. What are the similarities and differences between RBRVS fees and fees established through a price-competitive market? If relative value fees and market-determined fees differ, what are the consequences of using relative value fees?

12. Outline the structure of the physician services market. What features of this market differ from the purely competitive model? What changes, if any, would you suggest to change the performance of this industry?

13. The following statement appeared in the *Wall Street Journal:* "Most people who provide services say they're sorry that they have to raise prices, but they say they have no choice. Doctors say their fees have gone up because of whopping increases in malpractice insurance premiums." How would you use economic analysis to analyze this statement? Be explicit regarding any of your assumptions. (*Hint:* Are malpractice premiums a variable or a fixed cost?)

14. Explain how physicians decide how many Medicare patients to accept, the price they charge their private patients, and the effect on both of the above of a decrease in the price Medicare pays physicians for Medicare patients.

15. As demand for primary care physicians increases in the private sector, what would be the likely effect of the elimination of balance billing for all Medicare patients on: access to care by primary care physicians, the out-of-pocket price paid by Medicare patients, the supply of physician services to Medicare patients, and physician fees and supply of visits to the non-Medicare population?

REFERENCES

1. For an example of how economies of scale and patient travel costs are used to determine the optimal number and size of obstetrical units for Chicago, see Millard F. Long and Paul J. Feldstein, "The Economics of Hospital Systems: Peak Loads and Regional Coordination," *American Economic Review,* 57(2), May 1967: 119–129.

2. Uwe Reinhardt, "A Production Function for Physician Services," *Review of Economics and Statistics,* February 1972: 63.

3. Philip J. Held and Uwe Reinhardt, eds., *Final Report: Analysis of Economic Performance in Medical Group Practices* (Princeton, N.J.: Mathematica Policy Research, 1979), p. 440. See also Philip Held and Uwe Reinhardt, "Prepaid Medical Practice: A Summary of Recent Findings from a Survey of Group Practices in the United States," *Group Health Journal,* 1(2), Summer 1980: 4–15. Also see L. Kimball and J. Lorant, "Physician Productivity and Returns to Scale," *Health Services Research,* Winter 1977: 367–380.

4. Gregory C. Pope and Russell T. Burge, "Economies of Scale in Physician Practice," *Medical Care Research and Review,* 53(4), December 1996: 417–440.

5. Uwe Reinhardt, *op.cit.*

6. Douglas M. Brown, "Do Physicians Underutilize Aides?" *Journal of Human Resources,* 23(3), 1988: 342–355.

7. William D. Marder and Stephen Zuckerman, "Competition and Medical Groups: A Survivor Analysis," *Journal of Health Economics,* 4(2), June 1985: 167–176.

8. Thomas E. Getzen, "A 'Brand Name Firm' Theory of Medical Group Practice," *Journal of Industrial Economics,* 33(2), December 1984: 199–215.

9. Martin Gaynor and Paul Gertler, "Moral Hazard in Partnerships" (Unpublished manuscript, National Bureau of Economic Research, Cambridge, Mass.), April 1991.

10. Joseph Newhouse, "The Economics of Group Practice," *Journal of Human Resources,* 8(1), Winter 1973: 36–57.

11. For an excellent review of the physician services market, see Martin Gaynor, "Issues in the Industrial Organization of the Market for Physician Services," *Journal of Economics and Management Strategy,* 3(1), Spring 1994: 211–255.

12. David Dranove and Mark A. Satterthwaite, "The Implications of Resource-based Relative Value Scales for Physicians' Fees, Incomes, and Specialty Choices," in H. E. Frech, *Regulating Doctors' Fees* (Washington, D.C.: The AEI Press, 1991).

13. Examples of empirical studies lending support to the target-income hypothesis are Martin S. Feldstein, "The Rising Price of Physicians' Services," *Review of Economics and Statistics,* 52, May 1970: 121–133; and Robert G. Evans, "Supplier Induced Demand: Some Empirical Ev-

idence and Implications," in Mark Perlman, ed., *The Economics of Health and Medical Care* (New York: Halstead, 1974), pp. 162–173. For an excellent review of the target-income hypothesis and a reply to its critics, see Uwe E. Reinhardt, "Comment on 'Competition Among Physicians' by Frank Sloan and Roger Feldman," in Warren Greenberg, ed., *Competition in the Health Care Sector: Past, Present, and Future,* Proceedings of a Conference, sponsored by the Bureau of Economics, Federal Trade Commission, March 1978 (Germantown, Md.: Aspen Systems Corporation, 1978). Also see Uwe E. Reinhardt, "Commentary," *Medical Care Research and Review,* 53(3), September 1996: 274–287.

14. Victor R. Fuchs, "The Supply of Surgeons and the Demand for Operations," *Journal of Human Resources,* 13, Supplement, 1978: 35–56.

15. For further discussions on this issue, see Uwe Reinhardt, "The Theory of Physician-Induced Demand: Reflections After a Decade," *Journal of Health Economics,* 4, June 1987: 187–193; Roger Feldman and Frank Sloan, "Competition Among Physicians, Revisited," *Journal of Health Politics, Policy and Law,* 13(2), Summer 1988: 239–261; Roberta J. Labelle, G. Stoddart, and Thomas H. Rice, "A Re-examination of the Meaning and Importance of Supplier-Induced Demand," *Journal of Health Economics,* 13(3), October 1994: 347–368, and the response by Mark Pauly, pp. 369–372; John A. Rizzo and David Blumenthal, "Is The Target Income Hypothesis Economic Heresy?" *Medical Care Research and Review,* 53(3), September 1996: 243–266. Also see their references.

16. Thomas H. Rice, "The Impact of Changing Medicare Reimbursement Rates on Physician-Induced Demand," *Medical Care,* 21(8), August 1983.

17. For a more complete discussion of the foregoing studies and their sources, see George Monsma, "Marginal Revenue and Demand for Physicians' Services," in H. Klarman, ed., *Empirical Studies in Health Economics* (Baltimore: Johns Hopkins University Press, 1970).

18. Louis F. Rossiter and Gail Wilensky, "A Reexamination of the Use of Physician Services: The Role of Physician-Initiated Demand," *Inquiry,* 20, Summer 1983; and "Identification of Physician-Induced Demand," *Journal of Human Resources,* 19(2), Spring 1984.

19. Thomas R. McCarthy, "The Competitive Nature of the Primary Care Physician Services Market," *Journal of Health Economics,* 4, June 1985: 93–117.

20. Uwe Reinhardt, "The Theory of Physician-Induced Demand: Reflections After a Decade," *Journal of Health Economics,* 4, 1985.

21. Mark V. Pauly and Mark A. Satterthwaite, "The Pricing of Primary Care Physicians' Services: A Test of the Role of Consumer Information," *Bell Journal of Economics,* Fall 1981.

22. George Stigler, "The Economics of Information," *Journal of Political Economy ,* 69(3), June 1961: 213–235.

23. John E. Kwoka Jr., "Advertising and the Price and Quality of Optometric Services," *American Economic Review,* 74(1), March 1984: 211–216.

24. Using data from a previous FTC study in which the FTC trained nineteen professional interviewers to identify the equipment and procedures used in eye examinations, Haas-Wilson found that commercial practice restrictions used in various states in 1977 increased the price of an eye examination and a pair of eyeglasses by 5 to 13 percent, holding constant the thoroughness of the eye exam and the accuracy of the eyeglass prescription. Deborah Haas-Wilson, "The Effect of Commercial Practice Restrictions: The Case of Optometry," *Journal of Law and Economics,* 29(1), April 1986: 165–186.

25. Statement of the National Retired Teachers' Association and the American Association of Retired Persons on the Economics of the Eyeglasses Industry Before the Monopoly Subcommittee of the Senate Small Business Committee, U.S. Senate, May 24, 1977. Cited in Lee Benham, "Guilds and the Form of Competition in the Health Care Sector," in Warren Greenberg, ed., *Competition in the Health Care Sector* (Germantown, Md.: Aspen Systems Corporation, 1978).

26. David W. Emmons and Gregory Wozniak, "Physicians' Contractual Arrangements With Managed Care Organizations," in Martin Gonzales, *Socioeconomic Characteristics of Medical Practice, 1997* (Chicago: American Medical Association, 1997), pp. 7–20.

27. "Patient Data May Reshape Health Care," *The Wall Street Journal,* April 17, 1989, p. B1. For a review of small area variation studies, see Sherman Folland and Miron Stano, "Small Area Variations: A Critical Review of Propositions, Methods, and Evidence," *Medical Care Review,* 47(4), Winter 1990: 419–465.

28. Constance Winslow, David Solomon, Mark Chassin, Jacqueline Kosecoff, Nancy Merrick, and Robert Brook, "The Appropriateness of Carotid Endarterecomy," *The New England Journal of Medicine,* 318(12), March 24, 1988: 721–727.

29. Charles E. Phelps and Stephen T. Parente, "Priority Setting in Medical Technology and Medical Practice Assessment," *Medical Care,* 28(8), August 1990: 703–723. A recent study concluded that "Considerable variability exists among states in patient-level cost and length of stay for CABG surgery, after adjusting to the extent possible for clinical, demographic, hospital and regional characteristics. The lack of association at the state level between resource use and rates of mortality and hospital readmission suggests that costs could be reduced in many areas of the United States without compromising quality of care." Patricia Cowper et al., "Geographic Variation in Resource Use for Coronary Artery Bypass Surgery," *Medical Care,* 35(4), 1997: 320–333.

30. The discussion in this section is based on Lynn Paringer, "Medicare Assignment Rates of Physicians: Their Responses to Changes in Reimbursement Policy," *Health Care Financing Review,* Winter 1980. See also Donald E. Yett, William Der, Richard L. Ernst, and Joel Hay, "Blue Shield Plan Physician Participation," *Health Care Financing Review,* Spring 1981; Frank Sloan, Janet Mitchell, and Jerry Cromwell, "Physician Participation in State Medicaid Programs," *Journal of Human Resources,* 13, Supplement, 1978; and Frank Sloan and Bruce Steinwald, "Physician Participation in Health Insurance Plans: Evidence on Blue Shield," *Journal of Human Resources,* Spring 1978. The articles above also contain empirical estimates for the different factors affecting physician participation rates.

31. Mark H. Showalter, "Physicians' Cost Shifting Behavior: Medicaid versus Other Patients," *Contemporary Economic Policy,* 15(2), April 1997: 74–84.

32. John K. Iglehart, "The New Law on Medicare's Payments to Physicians," *The New England Journal of Medicine,* 322(17), April 26, 1990: 1247–1252.

33. Congressional Budget Office, unpublished data, 1997 and *Medicare and the American Health Care System, Report to the Congress* (Washington, D.C.: Prospective Payment Assessment Commission, June 1996).

34. Uwe E. Reinhardt, "Alternative Methods of Reimbursing Non-institutional Providers of Health Services," in *Controls on Health Care,* Proceedings of a Conference, January 7–9, 1974 (Washington, D.C.: National Academy of Sciences, 1975).

35. William C. Hsiao, Peter Braun, Douwe Yntema, and Edmund Becker, "Estimating Physicians' Work for a Resource-Based Relative Value Scale," *The New England Journal of Medicine,* 319(13), September 29, 1988: 835–841. Also see in same issue, W. C. Hsaio et al., "Results and Policy Implications of the Resource-Based Relative-Value Study," pp. 881–888.
36. The following book is devoted to an analysis of the Hsaio approach: H. E. Frech, ed., *Regulating Doctors' Fees* (Washington, D.C.: The AEI Press, 1991).
37. Thomas McGuire, "Paralyzing Medicare's Demand-Side Policies," in *Regulating Doctors' Fees, op.cit.,* pp. 174–192.

CHAPTER

11

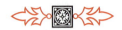

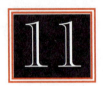

The Market for Hospital Services

BACKGROUND

The most important institutional setting to be analyzed is that of hospitals. In 1995, hospital expenditures totaled more than $350 billion, or 40 percent of personal health care expenditures. Hospital expenditures constitute the largest single health care expenditure category and have been rising at an annual rate that is more than twice as high as the consumer price index. The hospital is also the most expensive setting on a per unit of service basis, and it has been both the object and the beneficiary of much federal and state legislation. A great deal more emphasis is therefore devoted to hospitals than to the other institutional settings.

Hospitals are classified according to the major type of service delivered, length of stay, and control or ownership. A short-term hospital is one in which its patients, on average, have lengths of stay of less than 30 days. As shown in Table 11.1, of the 6,291 hospitals listed by the American Hospital Association, 5,519 are classified as short-term hospitals. The major types of services by which short-term hospitals are classified are general, psychiatric, and tuberculosis and other respiratory diseases. The general hospital is the predominant type of hospital; 5,220 hospitals have this service classification. Hospital control or ownership can be categorized as either governmental (i.e., federal, state, and local), nonprofit (i.e., voluntary or community), or for-profit.

Psychiatric, tuberculosis, and long-term hospitals have generally been public institutions, for welfare reasons and because of externalities, such as the contagiousness of tuber-

culosis, which led the state to provide care for such persons so as to protect the rest of the population. The demand for such public institutions, however, has decreased dramatically.

The decline in demand for tuberculosis hospitals has been the result of improved environmental conditions, widespread testing and earlier discovery, and improved treatment techniques. New treatment techniques for mental illness, including drug therapy, have shifted the demand for incarceration in a public psychiatric hospital to a demand for treatment in nongovernment psychiatric facilities with a shorter length of stay. Short-term general hospitals have also developed substitute facilities in the form of psychiatric units; these, together with outpatient treatment, provide psychiatric services that have left only the poor, the senile, and the incurable to the care of mental hospitals, which provide care of a different quality at much lower cost. The decline in demand for long-term hospitals is partly attributable to the development of substitute facilities (i.e., nursing homes), along with increased patient incomes and public insurance to pay for such care.

The demand for care in short-term general and other special hospitals, however, has increased over time, particularly since the 1960s. This increased demand resulted from changes in medical technology, which has made possible the provision of new services, such as heart transplants, as well as the growth in health insurance and an aging population. Since the mid-1980s, however, innovations in medical technology have made it possible to perform many surgical procedures on an outpatient basis. And insurance companies' interest in lowering the cost of hospital care has shifted the demand for many surgical procedures from the hospital to outpatient surgery centers. Continued advances in medical technology are leaving the hospital with "high-tech" type services while shifting the treatment of most other types of services to an outpatient setting.

The analysis of the market for hospital services emphasizes the performance of the short-term general hospital, and within that type of hospital, the voluntary, nonprofit institution. The predominant form of control and organization of the short-term general hospital is nongovernmental and nonprofit; these hospitals number 3,092. State and local governmental are next in predominance, numbering 1,350; then come the for-profit (investor-owned) hospitals, with 752. When one examines the data in Table 11.1 on admissions and the number of beds, the voluntary nonprofit short-term general hospital is even more predominant as the major institution involved in the delivery of hospital services. These institutions have 70 percent of the short-term general beds and admit 68 percent of the patients.

Table 11.1 reveals that the large majority of short-term general hospitals have fewer than two hundred beds, with 45 percent having fewer than one hundred beds. These same hospitals, however, account for only 11 percent of admissions. The vast majority of admissions, about 70 percent, occur in hospitals that have two hundred and more.

Hospitals not only differ in their size and ownership, but also in the services they offer. Hospitals are multiproduct firms. The services offered in a 500-bed teaching hospital are different from those found in a 150-bed community hospital. Further, while both institutions will offer some similar services, such as obstetrics, the larger teaching hospital

TABLE 11.1 Selected Data on Community Hospitals, 1995

Type of Hospital	Number of Hospitals	Percent 1975– 85	Change 1985– 95	Beds	Admissions	Percent Distribution of Admissions	Occupancy Rate[a]
Short-term						97.7	
General[b]	5,220	−3.3	−.8	874,286	30,966,019	93.0	62.8
State and local government	1,350	−10.4	−16.4	157,270	4,960,814	14.9	63.7
Voluntary	3,092	0.3	−8.1	609,729	22,556,693	67.8	64.5
Investor-owned	752	3.9	−6.6	105,737	3,427,850	10.3	51.8
Federal	299	−10.2	−12.8	77,079	1,559,089	4.7	72.6
Long-term[c]	772	−6.3	4.0	129,236	757,016	2.3	80.8
Community	5,194	−2.4	−9.4	872,736	30,945,357	100.0	62.8
Bedsize category							
6–99 beds	2,339	−11.8	−9.7	121,461	3,366,729	10.9	50.1
100–199 beds	1,324	3.2	−5.9	187,381	6,287,783	20.3	58.8
200–299 beds	718	9.0	−2.8	175,240	6,495,306	21.0	63.1
300–399 beds	354	16.1	−19.4	121,136	4,692,776	15.2	64.8
400–499 beds	195	3.9	−18.4	86,459	3,413,091	11.0	68.1
500+ beds	264	9.6	−17.2	181,059	6,689,672	21.6	71.4

Source: American Hospital Association, *Hospital Statistics* (Chicago: American Hospital Association, various editions): 1986 ed., text Table 2, 1995–96 ed., Table 3A, and 1996–97 ed., Table 3A.

[a]Ratio of average daily census to every one hundred beds.

[b]"Short-term general" includes community hospitals and hospital units of institutions. Community hospitals group consists of state and local government, voluntary and investor-owned hospitals.

[c]Includes general, psychiatric, tuberculosis and other respiratory diseases, and all others.

will, in addition, have facilities to provide care in greater depth, such as for high-risk pregnancies and neonatal intensive care units.

One indication of the multiproduct nature of hospitals is the high rate of technological innovation in new services. Examples of technological innovation in the 10 years, 1984–94, are shown in Table 11.2. The number of hospitals offering organ transplantation has risen threefold, from 244 hospitals in 1984 to 748 hospitals in 1994. (The cost of an organ transplant is approximately $200,000.) The percent of hospitals with new diagnostic equipment, such as magnetic resonance imaging (MRI) devices, has risen from 3 percent to 70 percent. Thus simple comparisons of hospital costs between hospitals or over time should be used with caution, since such comparisons do not allow for the vast differences in services offered or the introduction of new technology.

The picture that emerges of the hospital industry is of many small hospitals, likely located in rural areas, operating at low occupancy rates and serving a small percentage of the patient population. The growth in medical technology has been at the larger-sized

TABLE 11.2 Trends in Selected Medical Technologies Provided by Community Hospitals, 1984 and 1994

	1984		1994	
	Number of Hospitals	Percent of Total	Number of Hospitals	Percent of Total
Cardiac catheterization	942	17.7	2,033	44.2
CT scanner	2,555	47.9	4,252	92.5
MRI	166	3.1	3,200	69.6
Open-heart surgery	631	11.8	1,305	28.4
Organ transplantation	244	4.6	748[a]	16.3

Source: American Hospital Association, *Hospital Statistics* (Chicago: American Hospital Association, 1990), xii. Data for 1994 come from Lashelle Curry, American Hospital Association, personal correspondence.

Note: Data represent the number of hospitals providing the above services rather than the number of such technologies within the hospital.

[a] Data for transplant services.

hospitals, where most patients are treated and which are located in more urban communities (as will be discussed later.)

The above descriptive data illustrate the changes that have been occurring in the hospital sector. The short-term general hospital has increased in size and in the volume of services delivered; it has changed its product, and in turn there have been very large increases in the cost of its output. The large sums of money spent on hospitals make it important to determine the efficiency with which this market performs.

DETERMINANTS OF MARKET STRUCTURE

The market structure for hospitals can be characterized according to how many hospitals compete with one another. At one extreme is the competitive market, where there are many competitors. At the other end is monopoly, with only one hospital in the market. Two important factors determine how many hospitals compete in a market: economies of scale and barriers to entry. Entry barriers increase the market power, hence profitability, of those hospitals currently in the market. Such barriers have, at various times, proven to be significant in determining the number of hospital competitors. For example, Certificate of need (CON) legislation required that a hospital receive approval from a state agency before the hospital was able to build or purchase facilities or equipment that exceeded $100,000. New hospitals trying to enter a hospital's market were denied a CON. Existing hospitals also used CON legislation to prevent their competitors from adding services to compete with those offered by their own hospital.

Similar to entry controls have been quasi-controls, such as the (previous) refusal of an insurance company (e.g., Blue Cross) to pay for hospital care in certain types of institutions (e.g., for-profit hospitals). The price to the patient of going to a for-profit hospital was thereby increased relative to the patient's cost of going to a hospital where Blue Cross insurance paid for everything.

Although entry barriers have been important at various times in affecting hospitals' market structure, they have become less significant given the large amount of excess hospital capacity that exists. Certain entry barriers are, however, again being raised. Usually at the urging of nonprofit hospitals and their unions, a number of states have enacted legislation making it difficult for for-profit hospitals to enter a market by purchasing nonprofit hospitals. Nevertheless, the more important determinant of the number of competing institutions in a market are economies of scale.

The Extent of Economies of Scale in Relation to the Size of the Market

Economies of scale occur when average cost falls as the size of the firm is increased. For a given size of market, the larger the firm size required to achieve the minimum costs of production, the fewer the number of firms that will be able to compete. In a price-competitive market, when the most efficient size of firm is large, smaller firms with higher average costs will not be able to survive. Also determining the competitiveness of a market is the size of the geographic market (the larger the geographic market, the greater the number of competitors) and the closeness of substitutes.

Determination of market structure and the existence of hospital market power has become important in recent years because of an increase in hospital mergers. The FTC and the Department of Justice (DOJ) have been concerned that hospital mergers will lessen competition in the merging hospitals' market.[1] Crucial to the prosecution of the resulting anti-trust case are two important elements, both of which determine whether there are close substitutes to the merging hospitals: the definition of the relevant product market and the definition of the merging hospitals' geographic market (and the relative market shares of the merging hospitals within those markets).

Depending on the geographic (and product) definition of the market, a market structure can be either monopolistic or competitive. For any least cost size of hospital, the larger the geographic size of the market, the greater are the number of hospitals that are

---

[1] In addition to the argument that the merger does not lessen competition, the merging hospitals may also claim that the purpose of the merger was to achieve greater cost savings, by taking advantage of economies of scale, or to save a failing hospital, thereby preserving its assets for competition. Given the limited empirical evidence on economies of scale, it is difficult to prove large efficiencies as a result of a merger. In the latter case, the failing hospital should be acquired by the least competitive hospital so as to not be anti-competitive.

able to compete in that market. The geographic definition of the hospital's market determines which hospitals compete with one another.

When there are no close substitutes and the particular service is the only one in a particular geographic area, then the hospital with that service has market power, that is, it has monopoly power.

Market power is generally defined as a firm being able to act without suffering any economic harm. This means that the firm would not lose a significant amount of sales if it were to raise its price, for example, 5 percent, or provide less acceptable services. If a firm were to do either of these actions when close substitutes are available and other competitors are located nearby, their higher prices or less acceptable services could not be maintained; patients would either switch to competitors, to firms that offer close substitutes, or new competitors would enter the market. In a competitive market, price and other attributes of the service would reflect their respective marginal costs. Only with market power would a firm be able to raise its price above marginal cost without fear of competitors' actions.

In merger cases the relevant product and geographic markets as defined by the FTC are generally narrower than the definitions used by the analysts for the merging hospitals. A very narrow interpretation of the relevant product and geographic markets would find that there are no close substitutes to the hospital's service and that the geographic area is sufficiently small as to find few other competitors. Under this narrow definition, the merging hospitals would be found to have a high market share in both the product and geographic markets, thereby providing the merged hospitals with increased market power. Proponents of the merger typically develop broader interpretations of the geographic and product markets, thereby indicating a smaller market share for the merging hospitals.

Product or demand substitutability depends on a willingness of purchasers or patients to use alternative services. Alternative services should be reasonable substitutes, that is, have a high cross-price elasticity. Presumably, adult open heart surgery has low substitutability with other surgical procedures while inpatient cataract surgery has a high substitutability with outpatient cataract surgery. One indication of how close a substitute two products are is their price differential (assuming the prices are not regulated by government). If the price of one service is much higher than that of the other, then they are usually not close substitutes. Typically product market definitions have been less controversial in merger cases.

Determination of the relevant geographic market has been more difficult. Conceptually, the relevant geographic market would include: (a) suppliers who are currently in the market; (b) those firms in the market not currently providing the service but who could add that service in a reasonable time period; and (c) suppliers not in the market but who are capable of entering the market within a reasonable time. Entry by new suppliers into a geographic market is easier for services that are subject to small economies of scale, such as a competitor hospital offering a wellness screening program. More complex and costly programs, such as a transplant program, could only be introduced into a market after a number of years.

The patient's willingness to travel to other suppliers of the service will also define the geographic market. Patients might be willing to go to a smaller, more expensive hospital if the value of their travel cost and time more than offset the lower (explicit) costs of going to a larger hospital farther away. The total price of hospitalization is the relevant price to the patient, not just the hospital portion of that price.[2] Thus, when a high value is placed on patient travel relative to the cost of the service, such as for emergency care, then the relevant market is smaller than when the patient is willing to travel farther for more costly services, as is the case for elective surgery, such as transplants. One study found that distance has an important effect on hospital admissions for selected surgical procedures; a 10 percent decrease in distance increased admissions by 13 to 14 percent. Patients were less likely to go to more distant hospitals (1).

The relevant geographic market is also affected by the definition of the product market; the service area for wellness and transplant programs is not the same. The relevant geographic market thus depends on the level of care, with primary care services having a more localized market while tertiary care has a broader geographic market.

Controversy exists as to how the geographic market for hospitals should be empirically defined. Several empirical studies have used a specific geographic distance, such as a five- or fifteen-mile radius around a hospital (the hypothesis being that the patient's physician is unwilling to travel long distances to admit and treat the patient). Others have used government designations, such as counties or Standard Metropolitan Statistical Areas. (Geographic definitions, such as county, are usually larger than the hospital's actual market.) Other researchers have used patient origination data, defining the market as consisting of those zip codes from which a hospital drew a certain percentage of its patients (e.g., 75 to 90 percent of its patients). In such cases, a hospital was defined as a competitor if it admitted a certain percent (e.g., 5 percent) of its patients from that hospital's market (2).

Within a geographic area, researchers have classified the market as being more or less competitive based on the number of hospitals in that area; others have used the Herfindahl-Hirschman Index (HHI), which is the measure of concentration used by the De-

---

[2]In addition to providing information useful for determining hospital market structure, knowledge of hospital economies of scale is also useful for planning regional hospital systems. Planning such systems requires the same information that would produce the outcomes of a competitive market. In a competitive system, economic efficiency is achieved when both implicit as well as explicit costs are minimized. Thus, in addition to economies of scale (explicit costs), there are additional costs, such as patient travel cost and the cost of not having a bed (or service) when needed. For a discussion of the economics of health facilities planning and an illustration with respect to obstetric facilities, see Millard F. Long and Paul J. Feldstein, "The Economics of Hospital Systems: Peak Loads and Regional Coordination," *American Economic Review,* 57(2), May 1967: 119–129.

partment of Justice in its merger guidelines.[3] The advantage of this index is that it is sensitive to both the number of firms and their relative sizes (e.g., percent of total admissions). Thus for the same number of firms in the market, the index will indicate greater market concentration if a few firms have a high market share than if all the firms had the same share. The more concentrated the market, the easier it is for competitors to collude and to monitor their collusion.

When a merger occurs and the new HHI exceeds 1,400, the merger is likely to trigger an anti-trust investigation. The HHI, however, is not sufficient by itself to indicate whether the proposed merger will be anticompetitive; it is also necessary to determine the competitiveness of that market, how hospitals compete, and whether competition will be decreased as a result of the merger.

As the number of hospital mergers increase and more anti-trust cases are brought against such mergers, greater effort is being placed to define hospital geographic markets and whether mergers lessen competition in those markets.

Empirical Findings on the Extent of Economies of Scale in Hospital Services

The theoretical relationship between hospital cost and size is *U*-shaped. As the size of the facility (and its production) is increased, average cost per unit decreases, reaches a minimum, and then increases. The reasons for this expected relationship are several: with a larger facility there can be greater specialization of labor; further, licensure, as a means of assuring competent personnel in the health field, limits flexibility in delegation of tasks; thus larger institutions are able to more fully use licensed and specialized personnel than can smaller hospitals. Specialized equipment and facilities can also be used to their capacity in larger institutions. Finally, larger institutions are more likely than smaller institutions to be able to take advantage of quantity discounts in purchasing.

Offsetting these advantages of size is the greater proportion of time and effort required to coordinate and control work in large organizations. In general, for sufficiently small outputs, efficiency increases with size because the advantages that accrue from the use of specialized labor and equipment far outweigh the increased cost of management. As size increases, however, the reduction in per unit cost afforded by greater specialization begins

---

[3]The Herfindahl index is calculated by summing the squared market shares of each firm in the market. For example, if there are five hospitals in an area and each has the same market share, 20 percent, then the HHI is

$$20^2 + 20^2 + 20^2 + 20^2 + 20^2 = 2,000$$

If the five firms had unequal market shares, the HHI would be

$$40^2 + 30^2 + 10^2 + 10^2 + 10^2 = 2,800$$

to decline and is eventually outweighed by increased costs of coordination and control. Other things being equal, average hospital costs thus may be expected to decline initially and then rise as size is increased, as shown by the *U*-shaped curves in Figure 11.1. How rapidly these gains and losses from scale of operation occur is what determines the shape of the long-run average cost curve.

It has been difficult to empirically estimate the cost–size relationship of hospitals. Hospitals are not homogeneous in size or other characteristics. Hospitals are multiproduct firms. In addition to producing inpatient services, which differ in their quality, the type of patient treated, and the severity of the particular case, hospitals also produce outpatient services, education, training, research, and community services. Hospitals also differ in the prices they pay for their labor and nonlabor inputs as well as in their efficiency of operations. Studies have found it difficult to estimate the effect of size on average cost while holding constant all the other factors mentioned above.

For example, if larger hospitals are subject to economies of scale, but also treat more seriously ill patients, then it may appear that larger hospitals have *higher* per unit costs. This problem is illustrated in Figure 11.1. The hospital represented by the short-run average cost curve at point *C* is on a lower (different) long-run average cost curve than hospital B or A because it provides fewer services. If one were to examine unadjusted (for number of services) data on average cost and size, one would observe data points that represent the relationship between hospitals D and A. It would appear that hospital D,

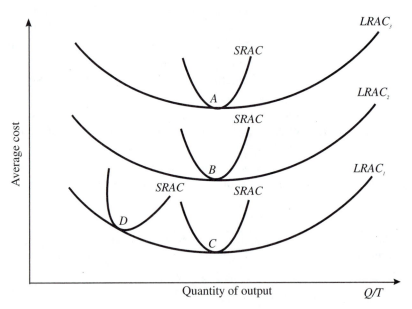

FIGURE 11.1 • Variations in average cost between hospitals.

which is smaller, has lower costs than hospital A, and that average costs increase as the size of the hospital is similarly increased.

If the different products offered by these two hospitals can be held constant, then it would be determined that hospital A is producing its output in the least costly facility (it is operating in a facility that is at the minimum point on its long-run average cost curve) on long-run average cost curve $LRAC_3$. Hospital D, however, is not only producing a different product (one that is less costly to produce than the one produced by hospital A), but it is also in a facility that is not least costly; it is at point D rather than point C.

Researchers have used two types of approaches to estimate hospital economies of scale. The first is a multivariate analysis where the different factors affecting hospitals' costs are included in the empirical analysis so as to be able to determine the net effect of size on average costs (3). Examples of measures that have been included in cost studies are the number and type of facilities and services, patient case-mix measures (the proportion of a hospital's patients classified into various diagnostic categories), quality (mortality rate, the probability that a patient will be turned away, or a patient's expected waiting time) (4), nonpatient care outputs of the hospital, such as teaching programs (and the impact that interns and residents have on hospital costs), outpatient services (which may share facilities and equipment with inpatient services in the hospital), and differences among hospitals in their physicians' contribution to the hospital's output (5). For example, teaching and community hospitals differ in their employment of staff physicians. Hospitals that employ physicians will include in their costs the physicians' salaries and consequently have higher costs than hospitals that do not employ physicians, although there may be no difference in either hospital's output.

To summarize the findings on economies of scale, there appear to be slight economies of scale: hospitals with approximately two hundred to three hundred beds appear to have the lowest average costs. The shape of this average-cost curve is shallow; that is, it does not fall sharply, nor is the minimum point much below that of hospitals on the ends of the curve.[4]

For highly specialized services, such as organ transplants, the extent of economies of scale can be used to indicate how many such services can be offered in a given area.

---

[4]To determine whether there are economies of scale, the output measure is allowed to be curvilinear; that is, either the variables are transformed into logarithms or a squared term is included for the output measure. For example, if the net effect of beds on average cost per admission is -0.04 BEDS $+ .0001$ BEDS^2, then the size of hospital with lowest average costs is determined by taking the partial derivative of AC with respect to BEDS, setting it equal to zero, and solving for BEDS.

$$\frac{\varphi AC}{\varphi(BEDS)} = -.04 + .0002 \text{ BEDS} = 0$$
$$+ .0002 \text{ BEDS} = +.04$$
$$\text{BEDS} = 200$$

Average costs per admission would be at a minimum in hospitals with 200 beds.

Hospital cost studies have found that the mix of patients in the hospital is an important determinant of hospital costs: in some cases, case mix explains more than 50 percent of the variation in average costs between hospitals. Since larger hospitals have a sicker mix of patients, unless case mix is held constant, it would appear that they are subject to diseconomies of scale. (Another implication of this finding is that accurate measurement of the hospitals' patient mix and the complexity of the cases is important in paying hospitals under any prospective payment system, such as Medicare and Medicaid).

The second type of study to estimate economies of scale are survivor analyses that examine changes in the size distribution of hospitals over time. Hospitals with the lowest average cost would be expected to gain market share while those that are either too large or too small would be expected to lose market share. Survivor analyses implicitly include all the factors that affect hospital costs, such as multiple outputs and services offered, as well as patient travel costs, whereas multivariate studies must attempt to include them and develop accurate proxy measures for each.

Survivor-type analyses have found that hospitals with less than one hundred beds have lost market share over time. Thus, similar to the multivariate studies, it appears that hospitals with more than one hundred beds, up to about three hundred beds, have lower average cost (6).

Lending support to the finding of economies of scale are data showing changes in the size distribution of hospitals over time, shown in Table 11.1. In the period before the onset of managed care (which created excess capacity among all size hospitals), the average hospital size had been increasing. The number of hospitals in the smaller bed size categories, less than one hundred beds, declined (they expanded in size) while the number of hospitals in the larger bed size categories increased. Since hospitals were reimbursed according to their costs during this period, this change in the size distribution of hospitals was not necessarily due to greater efficiency with increased size. (In the more recent past, part of the decrease in the number of small hospitals has been a result of their closure rather than increases in their size.)

In the more recent period (1985–95) hospitals were no longer paid according to their costs, price competition became more pervasive, there were greater incentives for efficiency, utilization declined as a result of utilization management, and technological advances permitted many types of surgical procedures to be performed in outpatient surgery centers. Many hospitals came under severe financial pressures. As some hospitals were forced to close and others to merge, the largest percent declines occurred among the larger-size hospitals (more than three hundred beds). The size distribution of hospitals appears to be compressing; hospitals at greatest risk of closure or merger appear to be both very large and small (rural) hospitals. The least-cost size of hospital now appears to be about two hundred beds.

Given the above findings regarding economies of scale, it becomes important to examine the geographic size of hospital markets to determine how many hospitals can compete within their markets, hence, the type of market structure.

The Extent of Hospital Markets

In 1995 there were 5,194 community hospitals. Of these, 2,958 were located in metropolitan areas and 2,236 were in nonmetropolitan areas. While 57 percent of the community hospitals are located in metropolitan areas, these hospitals contain 79 percent of the beds in community hospitals. Metropolitan statistical areas (MSAs) are government designations for geographic areas that represent an integrated social and economic area. A city with a population of at least 50,000 would be considered an MSA. MSAs would not necessarily be indicative of a particular market in which a hospital competes, since for some services the travel time might be too great while for other services (those subject to large economies of scale) the market may encompass multiple MSAs. However, the number of hospitals within an MSA provides a general indication of the number of competitors within a hospital's market.

As shown in Figure 11.2, in 1995, 152 MSAs (42 percent) have fewer than 4 hospitals and 74 MSAs (20 percent) have 4 to 5 hospitals. The remaining MSAs (38 percent) have more than 6 hospitals. However, these 38 percent of MSAs with 6 or more hospitals contain approximately 80 percent of the community hospitals that are located in metropolitan areas.

Based on the above calculations, it would appear that for the community hospitals that are located in MSAs (57 percent of all community hospitals and 79 percent of the beds), 42 percent of the MSAs have highly concentrated markets (less than 4 hospitals) and another 20 percent of MSAs are also quite concentrated (4 to 5 hospitals). (It is important to remember that the relevant geographic market for specialized services is likely to encompass more than one MSA.) However, these concentrated markets (62 percent of the MSAs) represent only 20 percent of the community hospitals located in metropolitan areas (MSAs). The large majority of community hospitals (and beds) are in less concentrated MSAs, with more than 6 hospitals per MSA.

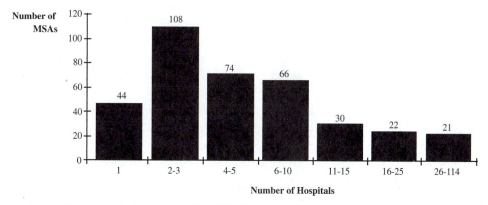

Source: Author calculation from *Hospital Statistics* 1996 to 1997 (Chicago: American Hospital Association) 1996, table 4.

FIGURE 11.2 • Hospital concentration in metropolitan statistical areas, 1995.

In concentrated hospital markets the market structure may be characterized as an "oligopoly," that is, the hospitals are mutually interdependent; each hospital is aware it is are affected by competitors' behavior. Oligopoly markets are typically less likely to engage in price competition since they would expect their competitors to match any price reductions. Nonprice competition is generally more likely to occur. However, in the current price-competitive environment with excess hospital capacity, and limited measures of hospital quality by which hospitals can differentiate themselves, it is likely that hospitals in oligopoly markets would also be expected to engage in price competition. Hospital mergers in oligopoly markets are likely to be closely examined by the anti-trust agencies.

The market structure of 38 percent of the MSAs, which contain 80 percent of the community hospitals in MSAs, could be characterized as "monopolistic competition." Hospitals in these markets are likely to engage in price competition and to try to differentiate themselves from other hospitals. It is likely that mergers and acquisitions will be used to consolidate hospitals in these markets so that they eventually represent oligopoly markets. While the number of hospitals will be larger than typically occurs in oligopoly markets, the number of hospital systems will be representative of oligopoly markets. Over time, oligopoly markets tend to be less price-competitive than monopolistic markets.

The increase in information on hospital outcomes and PPOs has expanded the size of most hospital markets. Travel costs for the patient and family are a small portion of total medical costs for complex treatments. The demand for highly specialized services is generally not of an emergency nature; the relevant market in which competition for such services occurs is much larger and for some specialized services, such as organ transplants, at a regional or national level. (Thus, even for highly specialized services, it is unlikely that a case can be made for treating them as a natural monopoly.)

The Growth of Multihospital Systems and Vertical Integration

The structure of the hospital market has changed over time. Until the late 1970s, hospitals were predominately nonprofit, independent institutions, generally competing in local markets, and providing inpatient services. The trend now is for hospitals to be part of a larger organization, a multihospital system, and to become vertically integrated, that is, provide an entire range of services, such as ambulatory care clinics, inpatient care, outpatient surgery, and home care.

Hospital affiliations and formation of what is referred to as "multihospital systems" has made the industry more concentrated. The types of multihospital systems vary widely. In some systems, the hospital affiliation agreements are relatively weak. The hospital and its medical staff are able to retain their decision-making authority over expenditures and investments. Weak forms of affiliation enable the hospital to take advantage of some economies of scale, such as in joint purchasing arrangements.

In stronger affiliations, hospitals are completely merged into the larger organization—the institution loses its autonomy. The reasons favoring this type of arrangement are also to take advantage of economies of scale, such as lower interest costs and greater access to the capital markets, lower administrative costs, as well as improved cash management and lower malpractice premiums. There are also economies in marketing a large network of providers to an insurer as compared to insurers contracting with separate facilities. Further, merging hospitals in the same market consolidates that market and increases the combined hospitals' market power; they are able to increase the prices they receive from insurers and HMOs. Each of these reasons requires the institution to be more tightly integrated with the other hospitals in the system. Hospitals facing declining occupancy rates, more stringent reimbursement policies, and declining profitability are more willing to give up their autonomy to survive.

Multihospital systems are comprised of investor-owned, secular nonprofit, religious, and public institutions and represent more than one-third of the total nonfederal short-term general beds. There has been a large increase in the number of nonprofit hospital systems during the 1990s. However most of these systems are relatively small, between five and ten hospitals each. The number of investor-owned systems declined from twenty-five to fourteen between 1990 and 1995, largely through mergers. As a result of mergers and additional acquisitions, investor-owned systems almost doubled the number of hospitals per system during this period, from thirty-four to sixty-two hospitals per system (7).

One important difference between investor-owned and the nonprofit systems is that the investor-owned are attempting to become national organizations for reasons of developing national contracting relationships with insurers as well as to take advantage of economies of scale (e.g., purchasing, lower interest rates, diversification of risk, etc.). The nonprofit systems have fewer hospitals per system because they are generally local as they attempt to increase their market share in a particular geographic area. To take advantage of purchasing economies, these systems have joined together in voluntary purchasing networks. These nonprofit systems are also exploring linkages among themselves to compete for statewide or larger contracts.

As independent hospitals experience financial difficulties, they are more willing, in the current competitive environment, to turn to large systems to manage their institutions. Part of the increase in number of hospitals per system by the investor-owned systems is the purchase of nonprofit hospitals. In 1995, Columbia/HCA alone purchased sixty-three nonprofits (8). Some members of the hospital industry believe that during the coming decade the unaffiliated community hospital will be the exception rather than the rule.

Vertical and Virtual Integration

The role of the hospital and its product line has been changing. Under the previous fee-for-service payment and delivery system, hospitals were the center of the medical delivery system. The most modern technology was housed in the hospital, hospitals competed for physicians based on their technology and services, and hospital administrators were concerned with filling their beds. As managed care grew, provider incentives changed and procedures began to be shifted outside the hospital. It became more profitable to keep capitated patients out of the hospital. Medical technology reinforced payment incentives by making possible greater use of nonhospital services, such as outpatient surgery, diagnostics, subacute care, and home care. Hospital utilization decreased. Hospitals now had to compete on price to be included in the insurer's provider network before they could compete for physicians. Hospitals became concerned that they were being moved from the center of the delivery system to its periphery.

As the entity with the largest investment in fixed assets and greatest access to capital, hospitals sought to preserve their centrality by changing their role. In addition to integrating horizontally to take advantage of economies of scale and to increase its market power in an area, hospitals have attempted to become vertically integrated organizations, also referred to as integrated delivery systems (IDSs). An IDS encompasses the entire production function for health care; it combines the successive stages of production and distribution of medical services into one organization. For example, in a capitated environment, the IDS will include services such as wellness care, acute care, recovery, and rehabilitation. All of the various institutional settings are included, from ambulatory care, inpatient care, outpatient care, to home health care.

A hospital can produce a particular service itself or purchase it from suppliers. Important to the hospital's decision of "make or buy" is whether there are economies of scale in the production of the service and differences in the transaction costs of these options. These transaction costs, in addition to the actual prices paid for supplies and labor, are part of the costs of producing a service. To be efficient, a firm must also minimize its transaction costs. When the transaction costs of dealing with suppliers exceeds the transaction cost of producing the service itself, other things being equal, then the firm is likely to vertically integrate the supply of that input.

A hospital's transaction costs, or the costs of controlling and coordinating the delivery of medical services, involves the collection of information about the different suppliers of each of the components of medical services, the negotiation of separate contracts with each set of suppliers, monitoring compliance with the contract, and the hospital's ability to enforce such contracts. The necessity for frequent negotiations with suppliers, uncertainty as to the suppliers' quality, and the difficulty of monitoring a supplier's behavior increase transaction costs to the firm.

When payment systems were cost based and each provider was separately reimbursed, there was little incentive for a provider to be concerned either with economies of scale or with transaction costs. They were not at risk for either their own or other providers' behavior.

As a result of the new competitive environment and fixed Medicare DRG prices, the dependence of hospitals on providers in other parts of the production process, particularly physicians, increased. Hospitals were placed at financial risk for their physicians' behavior. The hospital's referrals as well as its costs are affected by these other providers.

The shift to fixed DRG prices also increased the interdependency between hospitals and nursing homes. Under DRGs, hospitals have a financial incentive to discharge a patient early since they will not be reimbursed for the additional costs they incur on behalf of a patient. Many aged patients, however, can not be immediately discharged to their home but need to be in a nursing home. Nursing homes, however, are separately reimbursed by Medicare, and have an incentive to accept less severely ill patients since they are reimbursed according to maximum prices. Given the uncertainties of having adequate facilities to discharge their patients, some hospitals purchased nursing homes. It would be very costly for the hospital to negotiate customized contracts with the nursing home for each of its discharged patients, who vary in their care needs and discharge dates.

The dependence of hospitals on other providers and the difficulty of specifying contracts in great detail resulted in hospitals purchasing the separate components of the delivery and distribution system.

By coordinating care in different settings, the IDS expects to have a competitive cost advantage over less integrated delivery systems. Patients are able to move smoothly throughout the system and through different levels of care, with their medical information available to each provider, and without there being unnecessary duplication of services or tests. Essential to the success of an IDS are appropriate financial incentives among the various components of the system, primary care physicians, specialists, hospital administrators, and so on, capital to invest in developing an exclusive physician infrastructure, and an information system that enables coordination of patient care to occur without duplication of tests, and the like.

The governance of an IDS is typically shared between the hospital and medical groups associated with it. An IDS views ownership of each of the components of the production function for health as the preferred approach for organizing the delivery system.

Although a number of organizations have attempted vertical integration, there are few successful IDSs. Hospitals have purchased physician practices, only to find that physician productivity has declined as physicians no longer have the same financial incentives as previously. Other hospitals trying to develop an IDS have invested in medical groups, only to find that the medical groups do not share a common vision or that the group's financial incentives result in conflict with the hospital. Further, hospitals have been unable to develop the necessary information systems to coordinate care within the entire delivery system. Physicians have also been concerned with the governance of the IDS, believing that too much control rests with the hospital. The lack of a culture of cooperation between nonprofit hospitals and affiliated physicians have also been limiting factors in how closely the organization is integrated.

In addition to the above reasons for limiting the development and integration of an IDS, changes in physicians' market power relative to hospitals have resulted in a number of medical groups choosing to become independent of hospitals. These medical groups have decided that they can manage the production function for health care (produce medical services) less expensively by contracting with hospitals and other providers rather than integrating under a common ownership and governance.

"Virtually" integrated organizations have developed as an alternative to the vertically integrated system (9). Large medical groups may receive a capitation payment from an insurer or HMO for either all of the medical services, such as 85 percent of the premium, or for just the medical portion, for example, 40 percent of the premium, and share in the savings from reduced hospital use and cost. These large medical groups may sell their assets to physician management companies, which are publicly traded, and in turn receive capital for expansion, management expertise, information systems, and contracting assistance. These medical groups then rely on contractual relationships to provide all the medical services required by the patient.

Given hospitals' excess capacity, these large medical groups believe they can negotiate better hospital rates than if they had to purchase or use the hospitals within their own organization. Examples of the decline of vertical integration and movement toward virtual integration is Kaiser. Kaiser was composed of three entities: the health plan, the medical group, and hospitals. They recently decided to reduce their reliance on their own hospitals, not replace some, close others, and so on, and contract with existing non-Kaiser community hospitals. FHP International, an HMO (since merged with PacifiCare), also owned its own hospitals and had its own medical group as well as its own insurance products and HMO.

FHP divested itself of its medical group and hospitals, believing that purchasing hospital and medical services was less expensive than owning these inputs. Kaiser also concluded that hospital care could be purchased for less than it would cost in their own hospitals. Further, their own hospitals were not as geographically dispersed as were community hospitals. Separating from its medical group also permitted FHP to contract with other medical groups who might offer improved services and patient satisfaction, as well as lower prices.

Productivity and cost incentives were presumably improved when the HMO did not have to buy services from its own entities. The same reasons (as well as quality and patient satisfaction) appear to be the motivation for large medical groups engaging in contractual rather than ownership relationships with hospitals and other facility providers. In a virtually integrated organization, the HMOs and medical groups believe that the alignment of organizational incentives are improved in a contractual rather than in an ownership relationship.

As to which form of organization, vertical (IDS) or virtual integration, will become the dominant approach for organizing the production of health care depends, according to Robinson, on three factors: the method used to coordinate performance among the different entities in the delivery of care; the structure of organizational governance; and the approach for managing clinical innovation.

The different providers of medical services (e.g., hospitals and physicians) have divergent interests. What are the most effective incentives to be used so that providers will coordinate their activities? Two approaches that are used to improve performance are, first, cooperation between different providers (as occurs when all providers work for one organization) and, second, relying on financial incentives, as when different providers engage in contractual relationships. Each approach has advantages and disadvantages. Developing specific contracts to govern all aspects of a provider's performance is difficult, given differences among the patient population and their severity of illness. Alternatively, relying on provider cooperation entails weaker financial incentives for providers to be productive. Hospital managers, for example, may want additional facilities investment to increase their managerial responsibilities, hence incomes, at the expense of investments in other projects that offer higher returns for the organization. Alignment of financial incentives among mutually dependent provider groups is difficult to achieve.

With regard to governance structures, the for-profit model is clear in its objectives and results in quicker response to poor management. However, for-profit companies have a shorter time horizon in calculating their investment return; they may also have less of a commitment to their communities since a subsidiary may be closed or merged with another organization depending on its profitability. Conversely, nonprofit organizations are less accountable for their performance and slower to react to market changes.

Important to the future success of any organization is ability to innovate. Do vertically integrated systems have a greater commitment to maintaining their large investment in fixed assets and their current provider network than in developing innovations that threaten their existing stakeholders? Do virtually integrated systems have greater financial incentives to innovate than systems that rely on cooperative relationships? Which type of organization and which incentives offer the greatest encouragement to undertake risk? The rewards of risk and innovation in a large organization are diffused throughout that organization, while failure resulting from risk is more apt to be concentrated among several persons.

Organizational change is constantly occurring as the competitive market evolves. While it is difficult to anticipate new types of organizations, it appears that large, vertically integrated organizations, under common ownership, are less likely to be successful than virtual organizations, based on contractual relationships. Their governance structure, incentives for performance, and incentives for innovation appear to offer the promise of better performance.

HOSPITAL CONDUCT AND BEHAVIOR

To understand and to be able to evaluate the performance of the hospital industry, it is important to examine three aspects of this sector: the determinants of the industry's structure, payment systems and their effect on hospitals' incentives, and the objectives of hospital decision makers. Economies of scale and legal and regulatory restraints on entry are important determinants of the number of competing hospitals within a given market. The industry's market structure is typically an important factor determining the type of competition among firms as well as the performance of that industry.

Hospital objectives and the payment incentives facing hospitals, in addition to market structure, affect the type of competition among hospitals (and their consequent performance). Most hospitals are nonprofit organizations; thus, it is important to determine whether their market behavior is likely to differ from for-profit hospitals.

In a competitive system, the assumption that firms will attempt to maximize their profits makes it possible to predict what a firm's supply response will be to changes in demand and/or changes in its input prices. With entry into the industry permitted, firms would be expected to minimize their costs, and their prices will reflect the costs of production; there would be no internal cross-subsidization of patients or of users of different services. If prices are higher than production costs, new firms will enter the market and sell the service at a lower price. Because of the assumption of profit maximization and entry, prices would (in the long run) be expected to equal costs; the different mix of services provided would reflect what people are willing to pay for those services, which in turn would reflect their full costs. Competing firms would attempt to minimize their costs, and investment decisions would be based on profitability (i.e., demand and cost conditions).

Since hospitals are predominantly nonprofit, what does this difference in ownership imply for the behavior and performance of the hospital industry? Does it, as some persons have alleged, result in lower costs of production, since the hospital does not have to earn a profit and pay dividends? Or are the objectives of the nonprofit hospital decision makers such that nonprofit hospitals have poorer performance? Further, important for anti-trust issues is whether nonprofits act in the community's interest and therefore should not be subject to the same merger guidelines as for-profit hospitals. A model of the nonprofit hospital is needed to explain its past and current behavior.

Theories of Hospital Behavior

A Profit-Maximizing Model of Hospital Behavior

A number of theories have been developed to explain hospital behavior (10). The simplest model assumes that the nonprofit hospital acts as though it were a for-profit hospital but returns its "profits" to the community. (This profit-maximizing model with the profits returned to the community might also be referred to as a "public interest" view of the nonprofit hospital.) The nonprofit model will be examined with respect to how it would determine its price, output, and investment policy. Subsequent models vary the assumption of for-profit behavior as well as what the hospital does with its "profits."

Hospitals are assumed to have a downward sloping demand curve; each hospital has a somewhat differentiated product in that not all of its physicians have staff appointments at the other hospitals; its mix of services may differ, as does its location and reputation. To maximize profits, the hospital would select that price on the demand curve where its marginal cost curve intersects the marginal revenue curve; this is shown in Figure 11.3. The profit-maximizing price and output would be P_1 and Q_1, respectively, and the amount of profit would be the difference between P_1 and the average cost curve at that price, multiplied by Q_1.

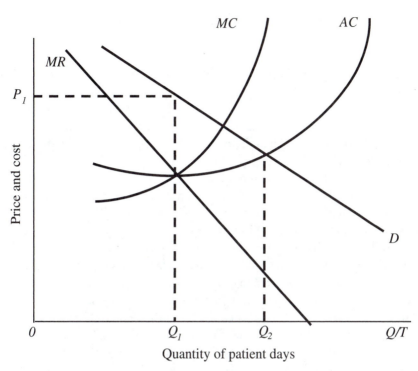

FIGURE 11.3 • Price and output policies of a profit-making hospital.

Further, since the hospital is a multiproduct firm with different payers, it can increase its profits by price discriminating according to the price elasticity of demand for each class of patient and type of service. (The ability of the hospital to practice price discrimination implies that the hospital has market power.) The hospital's room rate is more price elastic than is the demand for ancillary services because, once in the hospital, the patient cannot substitute other providers' ancillary services. The charges for ancillary services are also generally a small portion of the room charge. Thus the demand for ancillary services is believed to be less price elastic. To maximize its profits, the hospital will charge higher prices (relative to costs) for those services and that class of patients whose demands are less price elastic.

The profit-maximizing model of hospital behavior predicts that hospitals will increase their prices if demand either increases or becomes less price elastic, or if the prices of their inputs (i.e., the hospital's marginal cost curve) increase. Hospitals are also expected to minimize their costs of operation; otherwise they forego profits. Further, hospitals will invest on the basis of which investments offer the highest rate of return. Examples of the types of investments hospitals could undertake would be cost-saving technology or additional facilities and services. New facilities and services could be profitable in their own right or could serve to attract a greater number of physicians to the hospital's staff, thereby indirectly increasing the demand for the hospital's beds. According to this model, the hospital would determine its prices as would a profit maximizer, minimize its costs (since higher costs represent foregone profits), and invest only in projects that offer a profitable return.

With free market entry and price-sensitive purchasers, prices in excess of average costs and above normal profits could not persist in the long run. The performance of the industry would be similar to that of a monopolistically competitive industry; along with price competition and competition for physicians, hospitals would attempt to differentiate themselves from other hospitals. The prices of their services and classes of patients would, in the long run, reflect their respective average costs.

A nonprofit hospital, acting as a profit maximizer, would use its profits and contributions from the community to achieve the community's desires, such as engaging in altruistic activities like charity care to the poor.

A nonprofit hospital is not required to pay taxes or dividends to its stockholders, thereby providing the nonprofit form of ownership with a cost advantage over the for-profit hospital. If both types of hospitals behaved similarly and were equally efficient, then the nonprofit hospital would be able to drive for-profit competitors out of the market.

How well does a model of the nonprofit hospital as a profit-maximizing firm reflect past hospital behavior? There is evidence that nonprofit hospitals priced according to their price elasticity of demand. Prices have been much greater than marginal costs for those services believed to be less price elastic (ancillary services), but closer to marginal costs for those services believed to be more price elastic (room rates and delivery room) (11). Obstetric care has lower price–cost ratios since obstetric patients have the time to compare prices among hospitals.

After the introduction of Medicare in 1966, the aged represented approximately 40 percent of hospital patient days. The federal government reimbursed hospitals for their costs of providing services to the aged. The method used was the "ratio of charges to charges to cost." The hospital's charges to Medicare patients as a portion of its charges to all patients was the ratio of the hospital's total costs that would be reimbursed by the government. As the proportion of Medicare charges increased, so did the portion of the hospital's costs that would be paid for by the government. Anecdotal evidence indicated that many hospitals increased their charges for those services that were used predominately by the aged, such as bed railings. The effect of such policies was to increase the portion of the hospital's total costs that was reimbursed by Medicare. Medicare patients were only responsible for a deductible when they were admitted to the hospital; the patient had little incentive to choose a less costly hospital or to be concerned with the cost of her hospital stay.

Also during this period, hospital insurance coverage by the nonaged increased. As shown previously in Table 3-2, out-of-pocket payments by patients for hospital care decreased so that patients were, on average, responsible for less than 10 percent of their hospital expenditures. Patient sensitivity to hospital charges diminished. Other third-party payers of hospital care, such as Blue Cross, also paid hospitals according to their costs.

The effect of extensive government and private insurance payment lessened patient sensitivity to the costs of their care.

In late 1983 the federal government began to phase in over a five-year period a new method of hospital payment—DRGs. The hospital was reimbursed for each Medicare admission according to a fixed price. Also in the early to mid-1980s employers and unions became more concerned with their medical costs, particularly with the rising costs of hospital care, the largest component of medical costs. Insurers began to select hospitals into their provider networks based on which hospitals offered the lowest prices. As insurance companies and the federal government moved from cost-based payment to fixed-price systems, incentives facing hospitals changed.

Hospital incentives under a cost-based payment system are very different than when the hospital is paid a fixed price for its services or if it has to compete on price. Before the mid-1980s, under cost payment, nonprofit hospitals' behavior diverged from the profit-maximizing model with regard to the assumptions of cost minimization and the profitability of investments. Hospitals invested in facilities and services that were expected to result in substantial losses; cross-subsidies were provided to certain facilities and services to offset their losses rather than closing them. These money-losing facilities and services were not the sole source of such services in the community but were duplicative of others.

The assumption that hospital profits were returned to the community in the form of additional care to the poor was not supported by the data. Studies found that the amount of charity care, bad debt care, and percent of Medicaid patients served was similar to for-profit hospitals (12).

An additional problem with the profit-maximizing model of the hospital is that it excludes any important role for the physician. According to this model, the hospital competes for physicians, who then refer their patients to the hospital. In competing for physicians the hospital provides equipment and services to induce physicians to practice at that particular hospital. The only role for physicians is a passive one, to increase demand for the hospital. The model assumes that the hospital will attempt to keep adding physicians to its staff, whereas in the past the medical staff tightly controlled staff appointments and sought to limit rather than expand physician staff appointments.

Utility-Maximizing Models of Hospital Behavior

The next set of models incorporates some of the observed inconsistencies of the previous model. The first of these models suggests that the beneficiary of the nonprofit form of ownership is not the community but the decision makers, namely, the managers and trustees of nonprofit hospitals. These decision makers are assumed to have objectives other than just returning the "profits" to the community. One version of this model assumes that the managers themselves benefit (in terms of higher salaries) by being the administrator of the largest full-service hospital in the area.

According to this model, hospitals act as if they wanted to maximize their output or revenues. In the short run, hospitals attempt to maximize their profits and then invest those profits either in additional capacity, cost-saving technology, or facilities and services that result in the largest increases in their output. Hospitals still have an incentive to minimize their costs since to do otherwise is to forgo revenue, which could be used to increase output. With reference to Figure 11.3, an output maximizer would increase output to Q_2, which would represent the point on the demand curve where average cost equals price. This does not mean that for every service or class of patients price equals average cost, but it does in the aggregate. This model is similar to the previous model both in its predictions and in its lack of consistency with observed data.

A more sophisticated version of this model assumes that the decision makers have a utility function that includes some measure of the quality of the institution as well as its size. Greater prestige is associated with being an administrator or trustee of a large prestigious hospital. The quality of a hospital is not a well-defined variable; quality may include the type of facilities and services offered in the institution, the quality of its medical staff and its specialists, and the quantity and type of its labor inputs.

Under this "quality–quantity" behavioral model, the hospital will still seek to maximize its profits in the short run through its pricing strategy, but it will then attempt to invest that profit either in increased quantity (increased capacity, cost-saving technology, or facilities and services that result in an increase in quantity of patients) or in prestige/quality investments. Because quantity and quality are to some extent substitutable for one another in the utility function, the decision makers will have to make a trade-off according to the marginal increase in utility resulting from increased quality or from increased quantity.

The effect of adding quality to the decision maker's objective is to cause an increase in hospital costs, as shown in Figure 11.4. Assume that the hospital is operating on average-cost curve AC_1. Since it cannot keep any profits, its long-run price and output will be P_1 and Q_1, respectively. If the hospital invests in increased quality, the average cost curve rises to AC_2, but the increased quality also results in an increase in the hospital's demand, shifting its demand to D_2. The increase in demand may occur as a result of attracting additional physicians to the hospital.

After some point, increased expenditures for quality will result in small or negligible increases in demand (competing nonprofit hospitals will attempt to match these additional investments in quality); at this point the additional cost of increased quality may exceed the additional revenue resulting from the small increments in demand. Additions to quality beyond that point continue to raise the average cost curve to AC_3 but do not result in further shifts in demand. Since funds that are used to increase quality could be used to increase quantity by adding to capacity, the decision maker has to determine the relative weights to be placed on the quantity–quality trade-off.

The consequences for economic efficiency of a utility model of a hospital attempting to maximize both quantity and quality is that the price of hospital care will be higher than if quality were not continually increased. Continued increases in quality without increased demand will shift the average cost curve higher, possibly decreasing quantity and raising prices. Further, hospitals will be producing a higher-quality product than con-

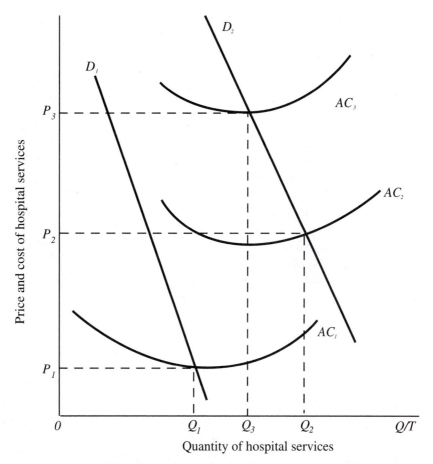

FIGURE 11.4 • The effect on hospital costs of increases in hospital quality.

sumers might be willing to pay for. Such a behavioral model could be accurate only if there were either some barriers to entry, such that lower-cost, lower-"quality" hospitals could not enter the market, or if consumers had an elastic demand with respect to hospital quality and the price of their care were subsidized.

In a market characterized by entry and price competition, consumers would select that combination of price and quality that corresponded to what they were willing to pay rather than to the quality–quantity preferences of the hospital administrator. In a price-competitive market, quality would increase in response to consumer demands for quality. If, on the other hand, barriers to entry existed or consumers did not have to pay the full price for hospital care, higher levels of quality could exist and would be determined by the preferences of hospital decision makers.

How consistent has the quantity–quality model been with observed behavior? This model still implies a profit-maximizing pricing strategy and cost-minimizing behavior since the forgone revenues could be used to increase quality or quantity. However, it does explain why hospitals might make unprofitable investments or maintain unprofitable services, as long as these services add prestige to the institution. This model also suggests that a hospital will invest in new technology as soon as it becomes available, not necessarily because of its effect on demand, but because of its effect on the perceived image of the hospital.

The quantity–quality model also suggests that hospitals with such objectives will be against the entry of for-profit hospitals into their communities. The nonprofit hospitals would be using internal cross-subsidization of their services to pay for the prestige services, which are money losers. For-profit hospitals, which do not have a prestige objective and do not have to resort to cross-subsidization of services, would not have to price their services as high as those of nonprofit hospitals. For-profits compete with nonprofits by lowering the price of the "profitable" services in comparison with the prices charged by the nonprofits. The nonprofits have claimed that for-profit hospitals "skimmed the cream" by not offering such money-losing services.

Critics of the extensive cross-subsidization of expensive services have claimed that the money-losing services were often duplicative and should not have been offered by multiple hospitals. Further, that quality and the number of expensive services offered were not synonymous. As evidence of this view, the number of hospitals with open heart surgery facilities are cited as an example of duplication of prestigious investments. In 1969, 23 percent of all hospitals with facilities for open heart surgery performed less than one surgery per month, and 71 percent performed less than one per week (13). Luft et al. found that for complicated types of surgery, the greater the volume of surgery performed, the lower the surgical mortality rates (after controlling for other factors that might affect mortality, such as the patient's age, sex, and health status) (14).

One of the drawbacks to the quantity–quality model is an expectation of cost-minimizing behavior. Including a "slack" variable in the manager's utility function assumes that hospital administrators are also interested in working in a pleasant environment, as defined by such amenities as additional administrative personnel and higher wages for employees so as to minimize conflict. This broader utility function of the hospital administrator predicts that hospitals would still price to maximize profits, and then spend those profits to achieve some combination of quantity, quality, and slack.

With the inclusion of slack in the manager's utility function, prices will be even higher than under the previous models. Under these circumstances, hospitals would compete with one another, but the competition would be to see which hospitals could become the most prestigious, while providing the administrative staff with a pleasant working environment. There would be a great deal of duplication within the industry, as well as excess capacity, high costs, and rapidly rising prices to finance the described behavior.

The survival of hospitals that act in such a manner depends on a situation where patients are responsible for paying even less of their hospital bill than under the previous models and where insurers and government, who are paying hospitals on behalf of the patients, are not concerned with hospital expenditures.

These models of hospital behavior explain some of the observed data in the period before the early 1980s. However, they attribute a passive role to physicians. Hospitals, under these models, attempt to attract more physicians to their staffs, yet physicians have attempted to limit additions to their staffs. The decision makers in the foregoing models are the hospital administrators and trustees but in reality physicians have had a great deal of control over the hospital, its pricing policies, and investment behavior.

A Physician-Control Model of Hospital Behavior

This profit-maximizing model of the physician assumes that the medical staff controls the hospital and that decisions undertaken by the hospital reflect the objectives of the physicians with staff appointments. Physicians, not the community or the administrative staff, were the major beneficiaries of the nonprofit form of hospital organization.

The physician is the manager of the patient's illness, with responsibility for deciding which components to be used in providing treatment. Under this model, the physician is expected to combine the treatment inputs in such a manner so as to increase his own income and/or productivity. The relevant price to the consumer (e.g., under indemnity insurance) is the total amount of out-of-pocket expenditure for a treatment, not the individual price of specific inputs, such as hospital care. The physician is able to retain more of the total price—thus, the less the patient has to pay for any one component, such as hospital care. Conversely, "the greater the supply price of the inputs, the smaller the return to the producer of a given quantity of the final product" (15).

Physician pricing and behavior, when the total price of medical care is the relevant price to the payer, can be illustrated with reference to Figure 11.3. The profit-maximizing price of the treatment is that point on the demand curve above the intersection of marginal revenue and marginal cost. The amount of profit is the difference between price and average cost. The higher (lower) the cost of other inputs, the less (more) profit available to the physician. For example, if two inputs are used in providing a medical treatment—hospital and physician services—then, the average cost curve represents the cost of hospital care. The difference between the price charged the patient (P_1) and the amount that goes to pay the hospital (AC at Q_1) is available to the physician.

The physician acts as a contractor, retaining the amount left over after all the other inputs have been paid. In this situation, the physician has an incentive to minimize the cost of providing the treatment, since higher input costs represent forgone revenue to the physician. (This situation is similar to when the medical group is capitated and has a risk-sharing bonus for reduced hospital use. The physician's incentive is to similarly minimize total treatment cost.)

Such profit-maximizing behavior on the part of the physician is not necessarily inconsistent with the physician's acting in the patient's economic interest as well. If hospital care is free to the patient (because of a Blue Cross hospital service benefit policy), while the patient must pay the full price for use of other components, it was in both the patient's and the physician's interest to hospitalize the patient.

This profit-maximizing model of the physician explains the American Medical Association's political positions on a number of issues. When the demand for medical care increased, it was in physicians' economic interest that it was met by an increase in physicians' productivity, which would increase physicians' incomes, rather than by an increase in the number of physicians. For example, with reference to Figure 11.5, physician and hospital services are two inputs in a production function. With an increase in the demand for medical care, the increased output, represented by the highest isoquant, can be produced with different quantities of either physician or hospital services. At the initial amount of medical care being produced, isoquant Q_{MC1}, the combination of physician and hospital care is Q_{MD0} and Q_{H1}, respectively. As the quantity of medical care to be provided increases to isoquant Q_{MC4}, the number of physicians and the quantity of hospital care can be increased in the same proportions as previously. It will, however, be in the economic interest of physicians if their number remains the same while the quantity of hospital care is increased. With the same number of physicians, Q_{H4} of hospital care will be required. Since the quantity of medical care produced is greater, even though the number of physicians has remained unchanged, their marginal productivity has increased; correspondingly, the marginal productivity of the hospital has fallen. The higher the physician's productivity, the greater the income.

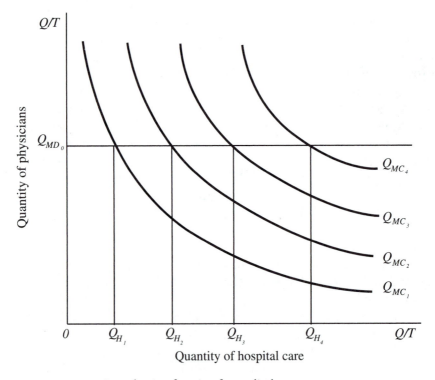

FIGURE 11.5 • A production function for medical care.

(Increasing output by expanding one input while keeping the quantity of the other input constant is the concept of the law of variable proportions. The marginal productivity of the variable input—in this case the hospital—will eventually decline, while that of the fixed input—physicians—will increase.)

With increased demands for medical services, physicians would be expected to favor increases in their hospital's capacity so as to increase their productivity, such as by increasing the number of interns and residents, who provide physician services for which the physician can charge the patient; additional facilities and services, such as an excess of operating rooms and obstetric facilities, so the physician does not have to wait or be inconvenienced; and facilities and services that are available in their hospital so that the physician does not have to refer a patient to another hospital and physician, thereby risking the loss of the patient and her fee. Physicians who do not have appointments at other hospitals would favor investment by their hospital, even though it may be duplicative for the community, because it increases their productivity and income.

Physicians would also prefer some hospital slack, if it enables them to economize on their own time.

Physician control over hospital investment policies results in economic inefficiency. It is a more costly approach for producing additional output (increased demands for medical care). The price to physicians for these other inputs is zero, particularly if they are paid in full by some third-party payer or the government.

Before the mid-1960s, when hospital insurance was not as extensive as it is today, the physician was more concerned with the hospital's costs, since the greater the patient's financial burden for hospital care, the lower would be the payment available to the physician. In large hospitals, however, the effect of inefficient behavior on the part of the hospital on any one physician's income would be small. Only in smaller hospitals, with correspondingly fewer physicians, would physicians be expected to be concerned with the efficiency of the hospital's operation.

As insurance coverage for hospital care became more widespread and as payment to hospitals was based on the hospital's costs, regardless of what they were, increases in hospital prices became less of a concern to the physician. As the out-of-pocket price of hospital care to the patient became smaller, physicians were able to increase their charges to the patient and were unconcerned with the rising costs resulting from the hospital's inefficiency and investment policy.

In the current managed care environment, physicians are once again concerned about hospital costs. HMOs prefer contracting with physicians who can provide medical treatments at a lower total cost, and capitated payment systems often provide medical groups with a share of the savings resulting from lower hospital use rates.

The physician-control model also explains hospitals' pricing behavior. Prior to the widespread availability of hospital insurance, physicians preferred that the hospital assign relatively low prices to services that were complementary to the physicians' services; for example, the surgeons wanted hospital charges for the operating room priced at or below cost. Similarly, obstetricians preferred the same type of pricing policy for the hospital's delivery room. As the out-of-pocket price for hospital care declined, physicians favored hospital profit-maximizing pricing policies (as long as they did not conflict with their own pricing strategies), since such prices would result in greater hospital profits, which could then be invested internally according to physician preferences.

Physicians also wanted hospitals to have an outpatient department and for hospitals to provide health screening services, both of which might appear to be competitive with physicians. However, the outpatient department is a convenient way of avoiding the financial risk of caring for low-income patients and physicians are also relieved of providing emergency services. Physicians are thereby able to allocate more of their time to higher-income patients and for leisure. Similarly, when the hospital provides free screening services the physician's time is freed for acute services, which offer a higher return per unit of time. Patients with health problems are referred to physicians on the hospital's staff, thereby increasing demand for those physicians.

Physicians also had an economic interest in the size of their medical staff. The Pauly–Redisch physician-control model posits that physicians' incomes would be higher under a closed rather than an open staff model of the hospital. Under a closed staff model, physicians would be willing to add additional members to the staff as long as each additional physician increased the incomes of other physicians on the staff. (As long as the marginal revenue product [MRP] of additional physicians is greater than average revenue product [ARP], which is equal to average income, additional physicians would be added.) An open staff model would have a greater number of staff physicians and the average income of staff members would be less than under a closed staff. Physicians would have an incentive to join the staff as long as staff members' incomes were higher in that hospital than elsewhere. Thus each physician specialty (e.g., surgeons) is interested in limiting hospital privileges; too many surgeons would decrease the average surgeon's income. (If other inputs, such as hospital beds or residents, increase, then this would cause an increase in the MRP and ARP curves of the medical staff.)

To sum up the physician-control model, before the mid-1960s, when hospital insurance was not widespread and major medical insurance was more prevalent, physicians would have been expected to minimize the cost of all the medical inputs used in providing a medical treatment. Patients were concerned about the total out-of-pocket price for medical services and physicians received the difference between the cost of the inputs and the total price of medical care charged to the patient. As hospital coverage became more extensive and hospitals were reimbursed for their costs, physicians no longer had to be concerned with the cost of hospital care. Physician payment was separated from payment for hospital services and physicians were neither financially responsible nor accountable for their decisions. There were no constraints on how the physician used the hospital or influenced its investment decisions. (Planning efforts to reduce duplication of hospital facilities failed because they were contrary to both the physicians' and the hospital's interests.)

Starting in the early 1980s, with the applicability of the anti-trust laws to the health field, the increased supply of physicians, the emergence of market competition among insurance companies, the growth of HMOs, and the concern of businesses with reducing the rise in health insurance premiums, the incentives of the pre-Medicare period reappeared. Insurance companies, employers, and HMOs became interested in minimizing the total price of medical services per enrollee; pressure is being placed on physicians to minimize the total cost of producing medical services.

One implication of the renewed emphasis on the total cost of medical services per subscriber is that the managed care provider, whether HMO, insurer, or physician, can retain more of those funds if the medical treatment is produced efficiently. Thus, as the supply of physicians increases at a more rapid rate than in the past, its input cost declines relative to the hospital input, and it becomes economically efficient to substitute physician inputs for hospital inputs, less care will be provided in the hospital and more of it will be provided in the physician's office. (Refer to Figure 11.5, which shows that physician and hospital inputs are somewhat substitutable for each other.)

Similarly, as the cost of hospital care continues to rise more rapidly than other inputs, the managed care decision maker will begin substituting less expensive inputs, physician services as well as more outpatient services and care in the patient's home, in the provision of medical treatment. Reinforcing the trend to greater use of physician (and other) inputs in producing a treatment are the financial pressures facing hospitals. Competitive pricing and fixed hospital prices for Medicare patients provide hospitals with an incentive to reduce their costs and use of inputs. Providing free inputs to physicians means lower hospital profits or threatened hospital survival. As hospitals provide fewer inputs to physicians than in the past, physician productivity will decline, with a consequent decrease in physician incomes.

The Nonprofit Form of Hospital Ownership

Several hypotheses have been offered to explain the predominance of the nonprofit form of ownership for hospitals. The first two explanations, which are not mutually exclusive, may be termed the "public interest" rationale; the community is the primary beneficiary of the nonprofit hospital. The third explanation is based on the economic self-interest of physicians.

Arrow suggested that nonprofit hospitals were a response to consumers' inability to judge the quality of medical services. In markets where there is a lack of information (informational asymmetries), such as medical care, consumers might believe that a greater degree of trust can be placed in the nonprofit form of organization (16).

Weisbrod claims that nonprofit organization is likely to arise in two types of situations. Like Arrow, he notes that consumers may place greater trust in nonprofit organizations when performance is difficult to measure and monitor, such as quality. Second, nonprofit organization is likely to occur for those services that may be considered "collective goods," such as charity care (17). It is difficult for the government to monitor how well subsidies to the poor are provided. Measures have not been readily available on the low-income population's access to care and the quality of care they receive. By subsidizing the nonprofit hospital, the hospital is trusted to provide those services desired by the government. Three types of subsidies are received by the nonprofit hospital to enable them to provide charity care. Donations are tax-deductible; the hospital is exempt from property taxes, and from corporate income taxes.

A more cynical view of the nonprofit form of organization is based on economic self-interest, namely, the physician-control model. The advantages to physicians of nonprofit hospitals are several. For-profit hospitals would have to pay property, sales, and corporate income taxes as well as dividends to their shareholders, thereby leaving less of the total income available to the physician (18). Further, physicians did not have to invest their own capital to own and control the hospital, the community donated it.

Physicians favor subsidies to their inputs of production when they are concerned with the total price of care paid by or on behalf of the patient. Inputs in a for-profit hospital have to be paid their market price. When hospitals are nonprofit, they can become the recipient of philanthropic contributions (which are tax-deductible), accept volunteers (who provide services at no charge), and receive substantial government subsidies, such as the Hill–Burton program. The effect of these various subsidies is to cause hospital costs to be lower than they would be otherwise.

Another advantage to the physician is that the nonprofit hospital can only use surplus funds internally. A criterion other than profitability, such as prestige (which would also be consistent with the goals of the trustees and managers), would be used for the investment of funds. The institution would be more willing to invest in duplicative services and facilities, which would be advantageous to the staff physicians, than if it were accountable to stockholders.

Physician control also enabled physicians to enforce a cartel arrangement. In the past, medical societies have been viewed as being similar to a physicians' cartel. The individual producer in a cartel always has an incentive to increase output, since the costs of doing so are less than the cartel's profit-maximizing price. Unless the cartel can prevent its members from expanding their output, the monopoly price will fall. Since there are so many physicians, it is relatively costly to monitor the output of individual physicians in their offices (although the cartel can limit the use of inputs contributing to increased production, i.e., which personnel can undertake different tasks). It was far easier to limit the number of hospital beds per physician, which also acted as a constraint on the physician's productivity. By controlling the number of hospital beds, the medical society was able to limit competition among physicians for patients. Limiting the number of hospital beds, however, makes them a scarce resource. If physicians were to bid for these scarce inputs, it would transfer income from the physician to the hospital. To retain these monopoly profits for themselves, the physicians in control of the hospital used a form of nonprice rationing, either seniority or some other standard, to distribute the scarce hospital privileges among themselves (19).

Physician control over the hospital prevents the hospital from hiring physicians and jointly producing hospital and medical services. If it were able to do so, then the hospital would receive the difference between the average costs of production and the total price charged. Medical societies ensured that hospitals would not be able to compete with physicians by having many states enact legislation prohibiting the corporate practice of medicine; only physicians could practice medicine, not organizations operated by non-physicians. If patients required hospitalization, they had to have a physician on the staff of that hospital.

Empirical Evidence on Differences Between Nonprofit and For-Profit Hospitals

A number of studies have been conducted on the differences between for-profit and non-profit hospitals (20). These studies have attempted to determine whether for-profits are more efficient than nonprofits, whether nonprofits provide higher quality of care, and whether nonprofits provide more charity care.

Comparative studies are difficult since there are numerous measurement problems with regard to the hospital's output, namely, its case mix of patients, their severity of illness, quality of care, and amenities. Also affecting the comparison are the different time periods examined. Prior to the mid-1980s, nonprofit hospitals were reimbursed according to their costs; since that time their financial incentives changed. Thus nonprofits would be expected to be more efficient in the latter period.

The evidence on whether nonprofit hospitals are less efficient is mixed. One study using a matched sample of hospitals found that there was no significant difference in their costs per admission, adjusted for case mix, but that for-profit hospitals generally charged higher prices for their ancillary services than did nonprofits. One explanation for the higher markup prices by for-profits is that they have entered markets where the population is growing rapidly (e.g., the South and Southwest). Expanding markets typically have less price competition. Thus the association of higher prices with for-profit hospitals may have more to do with the characteristics of the markets in which they compete than with their form of ownership.

Currently, hospitals face fixed prices for their services under Medicare and compete with one another on the basis of price, quality, location, and so on. Under these demand conditions and with few restrictions on market entry, hospital ownership is less important for efficiency incentives than when hospitals were reimbursed according to their costs. The incentives faced by both types of hospitals are similar.

With respect to differences in quality of care, studies have again been inconclusive. However, when differences in quality are examined for nonhospital institutions, such as nursing homes serving long-term-care patients, then nonprofits have been found to offer a higher level of quality.

Given the current interest by large employers in requiring measures of the quality of care received by their employees, and the movement to report cards, the necessity to rely on the trust factor in the nonprofit form of organization is diminishing.

The amount of charity care provided by nonprofit hospitals compared to for-profits varies by state and varies greatly among the nonprofits themselves. Several studies have found that the amount of charity care, bad debt care, and percent of Medicaid patients served was very similar for nonprofit and for-profit hospitals. It is the large teaching hospitals that are located in urban areas amidst low-income populations that provide most of the charity care. For-profits are typically not located in areas with low-income populations. The large amount of charity care provided by nonprofit teaching institutions may be related to their location and need for patients for teaching purposes than just for their charitable motivations (21).

Competitive pressures are making it increasingly difficult for nonprofit hospitals to cross-subsidize patients or to behave differently from for-profit hospitals. Studies have indicated that in highly price-competitive hospital markets (relative to less competitive markets), care to the uninsured by nonprofits has sharply decreased (22). As tax-exempt systems merge and compete more aggressively with investor-owned systems, their tax-exempt status is being questioned. Some communities believe that their nonprofits are providing little, if anything, to the community in return for their tax-exempt status. To retain their favored tax-exempt status, several states have established standards as to the amount of charity care nonprofit hospitals have to provide. Similar legislation is being considered at the federal level.

Also driving the reexamination of hospitals' nonprofit status are the billions of new tax dollars that states and communities could receive if the tax-exemption rules were changed.

Hospital Competition

Competitive markets are expected to result in greater efficiencies, lower prices, and greater responsiveness to purchaser demands. Competition among hospitals would lead to prices equaling the costs of services and the mix of services, differences in prices for differences in quality would reflect the costs of different levels of quality, and levels of quality would be determined by purchaser demand.

If, in the above situation, the number of competing hospitals declined (their concentration increased), the remaining hospitals would have fewer substitutes and hospitals would be able to increase their prices. Unless the anti-trust laws were enforced, mergers that increased hospital concentration would result in greater monopoly power and, consequently, higher prices.

Before the early 1980s, however, competition among hospitals had quite different consequences. Hospitals were paid according to their costs or charges, purchasers of hospital care had little information on prices and quality, patients were not price-sensitive because of extensive hospital insurance, employers were not faced with much import competition and thus had little incentive to be concerned with rising hospital costs, and many state laws precluded insurers from establishing provider networks based on negotiated discounts.

Given the lack of concern by patients with the price of services and the payment of hospitals by insurers according to their costs, hospitals were not concerned with being efficient, too much care was demanded (in the sense that the marginal costs exceeded the marginal benefit to the patient of those additional services), and hospital prices were not indicative of different levels of quality. (Quality was also perceived in terms of process or structural measures, such as the latest technology, rather than by outcomes of medical services.) And hospitals competed among themselves for physicians.

Hospital price competition did not occur under these conditions. Instead, hospitals competed for physicians, hence their patients, and competition was based on services and quality, not price (23). Nonprice competition manifested itself in several ways. Hospitals in more competitive markets maintained more excess capacity than hospitals in less competitive (more concentrated) markets. Physicians were thus assured that by affiliating with a particular hospital their patients were likely to have a bed when one was needed. Greater amenities were provided to patients as well as to physicians (offices next to the hospital at below market rents). To increase the productivity of physicians on their medical staff, hospitals provided them with more support staff, such as interns and residents, and a higher proportion of registered nurses in their nursing units. Hospitals also purchased the latest in medical technology and added facilities and services. Physicians did not have to refer their patients (and possibly lose them) to other institutions. High-tech services also provided a means for the hospital to indicate to prospective patients that it was a high-quality institution.

Nonprice competition led to rapidly rising hospital costs. Using data from the 1972–82 period, Robinson and Luft found that in more competitive markets (a greater number of hospitals), hospital costs were higher, hospitals offered more services, and average length of stay was longer (24). More competitive hospitals were also reluctant to engage in cost containment activities for fear of losing their physician referrals.

The finding of higher costs in more competitive (less concentrated) hospital markets was contrary to the expectations of traditional economic theory, namely, that more competitive industries are more efficient. To eliminate "wasteful" competition and to take advantage of economies of scale, according to the advocates of increased concentration, it was necessary to encourage monopolization of the hospital industry. Further, the advocates of increased concentration claimed that encouraging mergers would increase quality since hospitals that performed a large volume of complex surgical procedures had better outcomes than hospitals that performed few such procedures.

In the 1980s hospital competition began to change. Large employers and their unions, threatened by increased import competition, pressured their insurers to limit rising medical expenses. Insurers instituted utilization review, changed their benefits to include lower-cost substitutes to hospitals, and instituted increased patient cost sharing. In 1982 the U.S. Supreme Court upheld the applicability of the anti-trust laws to the health field. And in late 1983 Medicare began to reimburse hospitals according to fixed prices per admission (diagnostic-related groupings). Hospital occupancy rates began to drop because of the changed incentives under both DRGs and private-sector efforts to reduce the use of the hospital.

With changes in purchaser incentives and excess hospital capacity, hospitals began to compete on the basis of their prices. HMOs and PPOs were able to negotiate lower prices among hospitals; form provider networks based on price, the provider's reputation, its location; and to then influence the patient's choice of provider by channeling patients to the insurer's network providers (25).

The change to price competition among hospitals was not uniform throughout the country. In some areas, such as California, competition developed much more rapidly than in other areas. In 1982 California legalized selective contracting, which meant that third-party payers could negotiate discount prices with a group of hospitals while excluding other hospitals from participating in the contract. Enrollment in PPOs in California grew rapidly. HMO growth in California, which was historically high because of Kaiser, also rapidly increased.

The effect of price competition on California hospitals produced dramatic results. Melnick and Zwanziger classified California hospitals according to the competitiveness of their markets (using patient origin data to determine hospital markets and then calculating an HHI index for each market). They examined data from the 1980–85 period, which encompassed the period before and after price competition, and controlled for the introduction of the new Medicare DRG system. They found that during 1983–85 the rate of increase in cost per discharge of hospitals in highly competitive markets was 3.53 percent less than the rate of increase of hospitals in less competitive markets (26).

In a subsequent study of California hospitals, Melnick et al. were able to examine actual prices paid to hospitals by California Blue Cross. It was thus possible to determine the effect of differences in hospital market structure on actual prices paid by a large purchaser. These data show that Blue Cross was able to receive greater discounts from hospitals located in more competitive markets; further, these discounts were larger the greater was Blue Cross's leverage within the hospital (as measured by Blue Cross's percent of that hospital's total revenue). Conversely, the greater the hospital's leverage over Blue Cross (as measured by the hospital's market share in Blue Cross's network) the higher the price charged to Blue Cross by that hospital (27).

As managed care spread to the rest of the United States, a 1997 study by Melnick et al., using data for the 1986–93 period, attempted to determine the answers to two questions: Did the differential growth in managed care in the United States lead areas with high managed care penetration to have a lower rate of increase in hospital costs? Did more competitive hospital markets have a lower rate of cost increase than markets that were less competitively structured (28)?

Using each hospital's HHI index as the measure of competition, the authors found the results shown in Table 11.3. This table shows the percent increase in hospital costs according to whether the hospital is in a high- or low-competition market and also whether the managed care penetration is high or low. An increase in managed care penetration re-

TABLE 11.3 Hospital Cost Growth in the United States by Level of Managed Care Penetration and Hospital Market Competitiveness, 1986–93

Level of Managed Care Penetration	Level of Hospital Competition		% Difference
	Low	High	
Low	65	56	16[a]
High	52	39	33[a]
Percent Difference	25[a]	44[a]	67[b]

Source: G. Melnick, J. Zwanziger, A. Bamezai, and J. Mann, "Managed Care, Competition and Hospital Cost Growth in the US: 1986–1993," unpublished paper, 1997.

[a]% Difference = [(High − Low)/Low].

[b][Low/Low (65) − High/High (39)]/[High/High (39)].

duces the rise in hospital costs. The reduction, however, is much greater for hospitals in more competitive markets. Further, holding the degree of managed care penetration constant, hospitals in more competitive markets had lower rates of increase than hospitals in less competitive markets. The largest reduction occurs for competitive hospitals in high managed care markets.

Managed care has, thus, resulted in a lower rate of increase in hospital costs. Moreover, hospital competition by itself is important, regardless of the degree of managed care penetration.

The above findings are important for anti-trust policy that seeks to prevent hospital mergers that lessen competition. Those who advocate permitting hospital mergers that tend to monopolize the market emphasize the early studies that indicate that more competitive hospital markets lead to greater duplication and higher costs. The above studies, based on data from the mid-1980s to the present, demonstrating that hospital costs and prices are lower in more competitive markets, provide definitive evidence that hospital mergers that lessen competition would result in higher hospital prices.

The applicability of the anti-trust laws, purchaser incentives to reduce the cost of hospital care, excess hospital capacity, and increasing physician/population ratios led to a change in the nature of hospital competition. There has been a shift from nonprice to price competition. In the period before 1983, hospitals competed largely on the basis of nonprice factors, such as technology, bed availability, services, and amenities. Studies based on data from this earlier period concluded that hospital competition led to higher rather than lower costs. While hospitals still compete on nonprice factors, they now also compete on the basis of prices. Large health insurers have negotiated prices with high-quality regional health centers for specialized services such as transplants. It is less expensive for such insurers to send patients and have the family accompany them to these regional centers for treatment than to purchase similar services locally. These regional centers are also likely to have better treatment outcomes than local institutions that perform few such complex procedures.

Research findings indicate that the more competitive the hospital market, the more likely it is that the rate of increase in costs will be lower. The behavior that was first observed in California is now becoming more prevalent in other competitive hospital markets around the country. How rapidly price competition spreads to these other markets is related to the number of competing hospitals in a market, their degree of excess capacity, the increase in physician/population ratios, and the market power of third-party payers. Anti-trust policy that prevents a lessening of hospital competition is likely to result in lower prices to third-party payers and their enrollees.

Cost Shifting

The practice of raising prices to privately insured patients because Medicare, Medicaid, or the uninsured do not pay their full charges has been referred to as "cost shifting." Many employers believed that hospitals increased their charges to privately insured patients to make up shortfalls from the government; private insurers, hence employers and employees, were used to subsidize those who did not pay their "fair" share. As an indication of cost shifting, its proponents point to the price/cost ratios of Medicare (about 0.9), Medicaid (about 0.8), and private payers (about 1.3).

Cost shifting would be an indication of market power; the hospital is able to increase its prices to certain classes of patients without losing a sufficient number of those patients to make the price increase profitable. To determine whether cost shifting occurs, it is necessary to understand a hospital's pricing objectives. Different objectives result in different pricing strategies.

If a hospital prices so as to maximize its profits, then the hospital will set a profit-maximizing price to each payer class. Assuming there are two types of patients, privately insured and Medicare patients, then the hospital will have two sets of prices, the fixed DRG price per admission for Medicare patients and a price for the privately insured. The hospital is a price taker in the Medicare market and a price setter in the privately insured market.

In the private market, the hospital will set price at that point on its demand curve where marginal revenue (MR) equals marginal cost (MC). As shown in Figure 11.6, this profit maximizing price will be P_1. (This price would change only if the hospital's variable costs [MC] change or if the elasticity of the demand curve changes, thereby changing the MR curve. Changes in fixed costs would not change the profit-maximizing price.) If for some reason Medicare pays the hospital less, the MC and MR curves in the private market will not change. Consequently the profit-maximizing price in the private market should not change.

If the hospital decided to increase the price to private patients, to P_2 from P_1, then the hospital would be worse off; they would be forgoing profit they could have earned (the

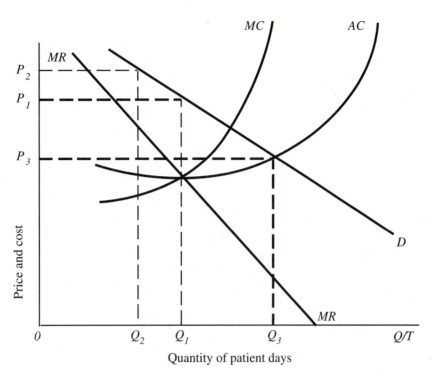

FIGURE 11.6 • Hospital cost shifting.

difference between *MR* and *MC*). Thus it is unlikely that the hospital would increase price if they are already at the profit-maximizing price.

Only if the hospital is not profit-maximizing could the hospital increase its price and make additional profits. If the hospital's price were at P_3, then increasing price to P_1 would increase profits. However, if the price were initially at P_3, then the hospital was not attempting to maximize its profits. For cost shifting to occur, the hospital's objective must have been to have a larger number of private patients rather than to maximize profits.

How likely is it that hospitals did not profit maximize so as to have more than the profit-maximizing number of private patients? As discussed previously, hospitals have certain objectives. If physicians are the dominant group in control of the hospital, they would prefer that any additional hospital revenues be used to increase their productivity and income. Increased numbers of hospital personnel, interns and residents, new equipment, or even lower charges for hospital services that are complementary to their own are examples of the opportunity costs of charging "too low" a price to private patients.

Even using a different behavioral model of the hospital, there is an opportunity cost of forgoing additional profit. Managers could be given higher salaries and more assistants, hospital staff could be paid higher wages, additional personnel could be hired, the physical facilities could be enhanced, or a greater amount of charity could be provided. Given the different ways in which the forgone profit could be used—namely, to charge private patients less or to forgo ways of achieving the hospital decision makers' objectives—it is more likely that the profit would be used by the hospital decision makers than for a group (e.g., private-pay patients or insurance companies) that is not as politically important to the hospital.

There is little empirical evidence to support the hypothesis that hospitals engaged in cost shifting (29). The few examples that were found came from the period before the mid-1980s when price competition occurred.

The observation that hospitals charge different prices (relative to cost) to different classes of patients is more likely to be indicative of price discrimination. A firm's ability to price discriminate depends on having purchasers with different elasticities of demand. (The condition that purchasers cannot resell their services is not applicable in this situation.) The class of patients with less elastic demands for hospital care will pay higher prices relative to costs than will those with more elastic demands (e.g., a large HMO that can shift its volume to a competitor hospital). For example, with reference to Figure 14.2, the two demand curves have different elasticities of demand. The group of patients represented by D_1 is less price elastic, hence has a higher price/cost ratio, than those represented by D_2.

Another example of price discrimination is with respect to privately insured patients and Medicare patients. The federal government, as a large purchaser of hospital care for Medicare patients, uses its market power and establishes a single hospital price for all Medicare patients. As shown in Figure 11.5, the hospital faces a horizontal demand curve for its Medicare patients. Assuming that private insurers do not have as much market power as the government, the hospital faces a downward-sloping demand curve by private (non-Medicare) patients. If the hospital sets its prices so as to maximize its profits, it will establish a price for private patients that will be higher than the fixed Medicare price; the private price will be at that point on the demand curve where the marginal revenues from both types of patients are equal. If the Medicare price were decreased, the profit-maximizing strategy for the hospital would be to decrease, not increase, the price to its private patients (assuming no change in the marginal costs of treating its private patients).

The above analysis is contrary to what many persons believe happens when the government reduces its payments to hospitals. The hospital may want to increase its price to private patients when it receives less from government. However, if the hospital is pricing to maximize its profits, then increasing its price beyond that point will reduce its profits. Only if the hospital's costs of serving private patients increase (e.g., inflation or a sicker mix of private patients) will the hospital raise its prices. As these costs increases and the prices to private patients increase, it may be thought to be the result of low Medicare payment; however, these increased prices would have occurred anyway. The hospital may say that it will raise prices to private patients if the government pays hospitals less; however, this may be more of an attempt by hospitals to scare private payers into lobbying with them against government reductions in Medicare prices.

The market for hospital services has become very price-competitive. Hospitals that did not profit maximize have found it difficult to increase prices to their privately insured patients. Hospital demand curves have become more price elastic as private insurers have formed PPOs and have chosen network hospitals according to their prices. Only those hospitals possessing market power are able to "cost shift," assuming that they are not currently pricing to maximize their profits. With increased price competition, hospital prices will reflect the cost of providing those services and it will not be possible for hospitals to raise prices when the government reduces its payments.

HOSPITAL PERFORMANCE

The major determinant of hospital conduct and performance after the enactment of Medicare in 1965 was not the structure of the industry but the methods used to pay hospitals. Medicare and Medicaid removed the incentive of the aged and the poor to be concerned with the price of hospital care. On the private side, insured patients had little concern over rising hospital prices. Reimbursement on a cost basis by government and private insurers removed any efficiency incentives hospitals may have had.

As the concern over prices was removed from patients and as budget constraints were removed from hospitals, the necessity of either party to make choices was eliminated. The responsibility for hospital performance was placed on the hospital's decision makers; their decisions were based on what objectives they hoped to achieve.

The physician played a decisive role during this period. As the patient's agent, the physician determined the hospital to which the patient was admitted. Therefore hospitals competed for physicians by offering them greater bed availability, the latest in technology, and increased staffing. The consequence was higher costs and duplication of expensive technology and facilities. Under a hospital cost-based payment system, physicians could serve the patient and hospital, as well as themselves, without any conflict.

The changes that occurred in the hospital market after 1965, when Medicare and Medicaid were enacted, are shown in Table 11.4. It was a period of rapid growth. Increased demands for hospital care resulted in a small increase in the number of hospitals, a much larger increase in the number of beds (thus an increase in average hospital size), as well as large increases in admissions, inpatient days, length of stay, occupancy rates, and outpatient visits. As demand increased, and there were few cost constraints on hospitals, total hospital expenses rose rapidly—20 percent per year until 1980. The rise in hospital expenses and charges greatly exceeded the economy-wide inflation rate, as measured by the CPI.

Although each of the cost measures in Table 11.4 is somewhat different from the others, all show similar patterns of increase over time. The trends in these measures of hospital costs suggest the following.

Prior to 1966, hospital costs rose about 6 percent annually. Hospital cost increases were 4 to 5 percent per year greater than the all-items CPI.

TABLE 11.4 Selected Characteristics of Community Hospitals, Measures of Hospital Costs, and Percentage Rates of Increase, 1960–95

Community Hospitals	1960[a]	1965[a]	1970[a]	1975	1980	1985	1990	1995	Percent Change 1985–95
Number of hospitals	5,407	5,736	5,859	5,875	5,830	5,732	5,384	5,194	-9.4
Total beds (thousands)	639	741	848	942	988	1,001	927	873	-12.8
Total admissions (thousands)	22,970	26,463	29,252	33,435	36,143	33,449	31,181	30,945	-7.5
Total admissions per thousand population	129	138	145	156	160	142	126	118	-16.9
Total inpatient days per thousand population	916	1,007	1,125	1,147	1,210	1,002	912	765	-23.7
Average length of stay (days)	7.6	7.8	8.2	7.7	7.6	7.1	7.2	6.5	-8.5
Percent occupancy	74.7	76.0	78.0	75.0	75.6	64.8	66.8	62.8	-3.1
Outpatient visits (thousands)	—	92,631	133,545	190,672	202,310	218,716	301,329	414,345	89.4
Total outpatient visits per thousand population	—	483	662	892	897	926	1,216	1,585	71.2
CPI all items (annual percent increase)	2.0	1.3	4.6	7.7	10.6	6.1	4.3	4.2	4.2
CPI semiprivate room charge (annual percent increase)	6.3	5.8	18.3	12.4	15.5	13.0	10.4	8.6	11.8
Expense per admission (annual percent increase)	6.4	7.1	18.7	14.9	16.4	16.7	13.5	8.3	13.7
Total expenses (annual percent increase)	10.3	10.3	22.8	20.0	19.4	14.0	11.2	8.0	11.9

Sources: American Hospital Association, *Hospital Statistics* (Chicago: American Hospital Association, various editions): 1996–97 ed., text Table 4, Table 1; 1991–92 ed., text Table 2; 1986 ed., Table 3, 4A. For data on CPI and civilian population: U.S. Bureau of the Census, *Statistical Abstract of the United States* 1996, 116th ed. (Washington, D.C.: U.S. Department of Commerce, 1996): Table 2, 745, 747; and CPI *Detailed Report,* various issues.

[a] Data for community hospitals are unavailable prior to 1972. These data represent total nonfederal, short-term, and other special hospitals. These data are roughly equivalent to those for community hospitals in the period studied.

A marked speedup in the rate of increase in hospital costs occurred after 1966 when Medicare, the federal program for financing hospital care for the aged, was implemented. The acceleration in hospital costs is strongly associated with the start of this program.

The growth of health insurance changed the financial constraints under which hospitals operated. The percentage of hospital revenues coming from private insurance, government, and direct consumer payments changed over time. In 1960, 50 percent of hospital revenues were paid for directly by consumers. Currently, about 90 cents of every dollar received by short-term general hospitals comes from either government or private insurance.

The annual rate of increase in hospital expenditures abated during the 1972–74 period as a result of wage and price controls imposed on the entire economy by the Economic Stabilization Program (ESP) in 1971. These controls were removed from the rest of the economy in 1972 and from the health industry in April 1974. After removal of the controls, expenditures increased rapidly and then returned to their more familiar post-1966 rates of increase.

The experience following the introduction of Medicare is consistent with the view that hospital utilization responds to changes in net price brought about by third-party coverage. At the time, insurance coverage for the elderly improved dramatically, while that of the rest of the population remained essentially unchanged. Survey data indicated that between the July 1965–June 1966 period and the year 1968, hospital admission rates decreased for every group except the elderly, for whom admission rates increased approximately 25 percent (30).

These findings are consistent with the following hypothesis, as depicted in Figure 11.7 (31). The total demand for hospital care can be divided into demand by the under-65 group and demand by the 65-and-over group. The older group received a substantial subsidy with the introduction of Medicare, thereby shifting its demand curve from D_2 to D'_2, while demand by the younger group remained essentially unchanged. The total demand curve thus shifted up, increasing equilibrium price (particularly if the supply of admissions was relatively inelastic). As price rose, there was some decrease in the quantity demanded, and the net effect was an increase in admissions for the 65-and-over group and a decrease for the younger group. One would expect the elimination of the least serious admissions in the under-65 group and a shortening of length of stay within case types. While case mix apparently did not change much for the elderly, stays for given case types were lengthened, and the latter phenomenon is consistent with the notion that demand for hospital care increases as net price falls.

Studies of hospital behavior under a cost-based payment system found that hospital costs were higher in more competitive hospital markets. Given the limited degree of price competition among hospitals in the late 1960s and 1970s, competition occurred on a nonprice basis.

Hospitals improved their financial positions after the introduction of Medicare, leading to a substantial increase in their net income/total income ratios (32). One study indicated that depreciation and interest expenses increased, on average, 29.5 percent per

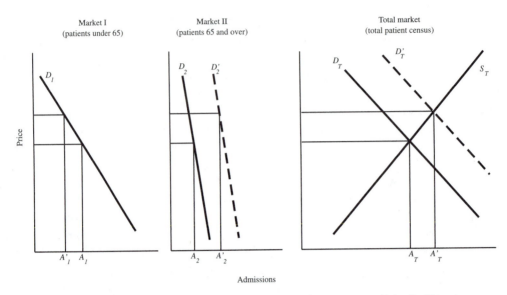

FIGURE 11.7 • The effects of Medicare on hospital use, by age group. (John Rafferty, "Enfranchisement and Rationing Effects of Medicare on Discretionary Hospital Use." Reprinted with permission from Health Services Research 10[1] [Spring 1975]. 52 Copyright 1976 by the Hospital Research and Educational Trust, 840 N. Lake Shore Drive, Chicago, IL 60611.)

year from 1966 through 1968. It appears that hospitals had changed their accounting methods to obtain greater reimbursements from Medicare and other cost payers. Evidence of this kind of behavior seems to suggest that in increasing their costs so rapidly after Medicare was introduced, hospitals and physicians were taking advantage of loosened financial constraints to accumulate funds to pursue their own objectives.

In the period after the enactment of Medicare, the incentives facing the decision makers were such that the output mix of the hospital industry was not optimal. There was a bias toward higher "quality," meaning more facilities and services, greater capital intensity, and a tendency to introduce new technology before its benefits were fully evaluated. The quantity–quality output mix of the hospital was different than what patients would have been willing to pay if they had to bear a greater share of the costs of hospitalization and had greater choice in this selection.

As a result of the hospitals' desire to enhance prestige and the physicians' desire to enhance their income by increasing their productivity, there was also unnecessary duplication of facilities and services; that is, to the extent that there are economies of scale in certain services, more institutions were operating at higher costs than necessary because of low use of facilities. There was system inefficiency, meaning that there were too many firms (facilities and services) operating in the industry. There was also firm inefficiency because of the desire for slack in the manager's utility function (and because the return to each physician declines, the larger the institution). When a large percentage of the population was covered by hospital insurance, with payment models based on each hospital's costs, it was less important for hospital managers to minimize their costs of operation. Finally, there were redistributive effects (both as a result of the methods used to set hospital prices, such as internal cross-subsidization, and the taxes that were raised to pay for the increase in hospital expenditures) in that income was redistributed from taxpayers to persons working in the hospital sector.

Corroboration of the redistribution that occurred between taxpayers (as well as the privately insured) and hospital employees under cost-based payment was investigated in a study by Doug Staiger (33). The marginal cost of higher wages to the hospital is reduced under cost-based payment, since the hospital could pass on the costs of higher wages to the government and private insurers. Once prospective payment (fixed prices) was enacted and hospitals became price-competitive, the marginal costs of higher wages increased since these costs are borne entirely by the hospital. To test whether hospitals paid their employees higher wages (in excess of the market wage) when the hospital did not bear the full cost of those wage increases, Staiger examined the effect on wages (in those occupations that were not specific to hospitals) when prospective payment was introduced. He concluded that under prospective payment hospitals had a greater incentive to reduce their costs and limit wage increases, with the consequent effect that wages were reduced by 5 to 10 percent.

Other studies have also shown that from 1969 to 1972 hospital workers made substantial gains relative to comparable workers in other industries as a result of cost-based payment (34). In fact, by 1969, registered nurses in hospitals earned on the average 13 percent *more* than other workers of the same sex, race, age, and schooling.

In the early 1980s hospital performance began to change. Early in the Reagan administration (1981), the economy went into a recession and the rate of inflation declined. The rise in total hospital expenses and expense per capita also began to moderate. As the economy began to recover, total hospital expenses and expense per capita increased at a decreasing rate. By the mid-1980s, the annual rise in these measures were similar to the pre-Medicare period. To limit its growing budgetary commitment under Medicare and Medicaid, the Reagan administration began to phase in price controls on hospitals, fixed prices per admission (DRGs), in October 1983, together with annual limits on DRG price increases.

Also in the mid-1980s the competitive environment facing hospitals began to change. Fixed prices under Medicare led to lower hospital occupancy rates, and pressure by employers on their insurers for lower premiums led to the use of utilization management by insurers, which also reduced occupancy rates. Faced with excess capacity and a desire by insurers for lower prices, so as to better compete on their premiums, price competition among hospitals changed their incentives. Regardless of the previous objectives of hospital decision makers, unless hospitals acted to minimize their costs, they could not compete on price.

Several measures are indicative of the changes that have occurred in the hospital industry since the new payment systems were introduced in the early 1980s. While the total population has been increasing, as well as the proportion of those 65 years of age and older, the total number of admissions to community hospitals started to decline after 1980, from 36.1 million in 1980 to 31 million in 1995. Along with the overall decline in admissions, the average length of stay has also declined, from 7.6 days in 1980 to 6.5 days in 1995. As both admissions and length of stay declined, hospital occupancy rates fell sharply, from 75.6 percent in 1980 to 62.8 percent in 1995. With the decline in admissions and length of stay, inpatient days per 1,000 dropped 37 percent, from 1,210 to 765. As a result, almost 40 percent of hospital beds are now empty.

Another indication of the changes occurring in the hospital industry was the movement toward outpatient care, which increased 89 percent between 1985 and 1995. The increase in hospital outpatient services occurred for four reasons. Third-party payers tried to decrease the use of the most costly component of care, the hospital, by expanding insurance coverage to the outpatient setting. In addition, insurers instituted utilization review mechanisms to ensure that surgical procedures that could be performed in less expensive outpatient surgery centers would not be performed in the hospital. (Hospital outpatient care was also more profitable than inpatient care in the 1980s because the emphasis by both government and third-party payers was to place limits on the price and use of inpatient care, but were unable to do so for outpatient care because of the greater number and different types of outpatient services.)

Third, provider financial incentives under capitation made it more profitable (less costly) to treat patients in an outpatient setting. And lastly, changes in technology occurred that permitted more procedures to be shifted from the hospital to an outpatient setting. As a result of these demand and supply factors, there has been a very large growth in outpatient procedures.

Decreased inpatient utilization and intense price competition have had an adverse affect on hospitals. As in any industry facing a declining demand and/or reimbursement, there has been an increase in the number of hospitals that have closed or merged with stronger institutions. Hospitals at greater risk of closure are those that are smaller, offer less specialized services, are located in inner cities or rural areas, and serve a greater portion of Medicaid patients.

Another motivation for increased consolidation of this industry is the attempt by hospitals to increase their market power. Some merger proponents claim that fewer hospitals will result in efficiencies that will be passed on by nonprofit hospitals in the form of lower prices. Opponents of this view claim that scale economies are relatively small and that nonprofit hospital boards do not have objectives that are necessarily in the community's interest; they may behave no differently in their pricing strategies than for-profit hospitals. Further, unless the anti-trust laws are vigorously applied to mergers that tend to lessen competition, hospital prices will increase more rapidly as hospitals gain increased market power.

The beneficial effects on hospital performance of increased competition, starting in the mid-1980s, has been documented in a number of studies discussed earlier. An indication of the slower rate of increase in hospital expenses is also shown in Table 11.4. All the measures of hospital prices have declined relative to the CPI from 1985 to 1995 as price competition increased. These slower rates of increase in expenses have occurred even though there have been continual increases in technology (see Table 11.2), an older patient population, a sicker patient mix, and treatment for illnesses for which little could have been previously provided.

SUMMARY

The structure of the hospital industry has been undergoing dramatic changes since the mid-1980s. Hospitals within a geographic area are becoming part of larger hospital systems and these systems are becoming vertically integrated. Large multihospital systems have also had a comparative advantage in contracting with large purchasers, as purchasers seek to contract with large networks of providers. Competition is likely to be between large provider systems. Individual hospitals will be at a competitive disadvantage. Changes in payment systems, declines in inpatient profitability, and advances in technology are moving hospitals into providing care in non-inpatient settings. As a means of increasing referrals to their institution, hospitals have attempted to develop stronger relationships with their medical staffs and physician groups. Many hospitals, in an attempt to forge physician relationships, have purchased physicians' practices. They have also lost large sums on these ventures as physicians no longer had the same productivity incentives as they did previously. Hospitals are still searching for ways to work together with physicians in a price-competitive environment.

To develop new sources of revenues, hospitals are moving into substitute product lines. Rather than lose the revenues from outpatient surgery centers, hospitals are providing these services themselves and forming joint ventures with their medical staffs. Changes in the reimbursement system are also moving hospitals into complementary product lines. Under a fixed-price reimbursement system, hospitals now have the incentive to discharge Medicare patients sooner. By discharging patients to other institutional settings, such as nursing homes and home care, however, the hospital can receive additional reimbursement for care in these settings. By vertically integrating into related products, the multihospital system is then able to approach employers and offer a complete product line with broad geographic coverage.

In addition to price competition, hospital systems will have to compete on quality, outcomes, and patient satisfaction. However, rather than using such imperfect proxies of quality such as whether the hospital has certain services, such as organ transplants, employers and insurers are developing sophisticated data systems that will enable them to determine the clinical outcomes for specific services within a hospital. In the years ahead, purchasers will have data on prices and clinical outcomes on which to base their decisions. A competitive market whereby competition is based on prices, outcomes, and satisfaction should lead to improved market performance.

A remaining concern as the hospital market becomes more price-competitive is who will serve the uninsured. Certain nonprofit teaching institutions located in low-income areas provided a great deal of charity care. This care was paid for through a system of cross-subsidies that are being eliminated through price competition and lower Medicare payments. Competitive markets cannot be expected to finance care for the uninsured; thus the issue of payment for the uninsured is becoming more visible and must be addressed by government.

Key Terms and Concepts

- Cost shifting
- HHI index
- Hospital's geographic market
- Industry consolidation
- Survivor analysis

- CON as an entry barrier
- Hospital economies of scale
- Hospital price discrimination
- Nonprice hospital competition
- Medicare diagnostic-related groupings (DRGs)
- Product or demand substitutability
- Profit-maximizing model of hospital behavior
- Physician control model of the hospital
- Utility-maximizing model of hospital behavior
- Vertical and virtual integration

Review Questions

1. What effect do economies of scale have on the market structure of an industry?
2. What are the difficulties with empirical studies that attempt to measure the extent of economies of scale in hospitals?
3. If you were an expert witness in an anti-trust case and were asked to show that a particular hospital had a low (high) market share in its product market, what would you emphasize to support your position?
4. Contrast the use of government determined areas, such as counties and metropolitan statistical areas (MSAs), with patient origin studies as a means of determining the geographic market of a hospital for use in hospital anti-trust cases.
5. Two models of hospital behavior are the profit-maximizing and utility- or prestige-maximizing models. Describe each model and then contrast their predictions and usefulness in two periods, the 1965–70s period and currently.

6. What are the advantages to physicians of hospitals being organized as nonprofit institutions?

7. In a "physician-control" model of hospital behavior, explain how the physician's incentive to minimize the cost of producing a treatment has changed over the three periods: before 1965, 1965–early 1980s, and currently.

8. Different combinations of physician and hospital services can be used to produce a medical treatment. If hospital services were essentially "free" to the physician and to the patient, such as occurs under Blue Cross's service benefit policy, what combination of hospital and physicians' services would be used by the physician to provide a medical treatment?

9. The move from cost-based payment for hospital services to payment based on DRGs was expected to change hospital behavior. Discuss what you would have expected to observe as the payment method changed.

10. What are the similarities and differences between DRG prices and hospital prices determined in a price-competitive market?

11. What are alternative explanations for the empirical observation that for-profit hospitals have higher prices than nonprofits?

12. What is "cost shifting"? Explain why an increase in a hospital's fixed costs or an increase in the number of uninsured cared for by the hospital will not change the hospital's profit-maximizing price. Similarly, why would a change in a hospital's variable costs change the hospital's profit-maximizing price?

13. Why are hospitals able to charge different purchasers different prices for the same medical services?

14. Under what circumstances can cost shifting occur?

15. How does cost shifting differ from price discrimination?

16. Hospitals have always competed with each other for patients. Contrast the effects of such competition (in terms of cost per admission, length of stay, services offered, and introduction of new technology) in the period of cost-based payment and the current price competitive market.

17. How are the following terms important for determining whether a hospital merger will be challenged on anti-trust grounds: Herfindahl index, failing hospital doctrine, economies of scale, entry barriers, and geographic and product market definition?

18. The economic forces affecting hospitals are changing. Within an economic framework, discuss the changing economic outlook for hospitals.

REFERENCES

1. Harold S. Luft et al., "Does Quality Influence Choice of Hospital?" *Journal of the American Medical Association,* 263(21), June 6, 1990: 2899–2906.

2. See the *Journal of Health Economics,* 8(4), February 1990 for several articles, editorials, and

comments and rejoinders on the subject of hospital geographic markets. The Spring 1988 issue of *Law and Contemporary Problems,* edited by James F. Blumstein and Frank A. Sloan, vol. 51, no. 2, is a special issue devoted to anti-trust issues in health care; included are several excellent articles on definitions of relevant hospital markets for anti-trust analyses. Also see Erwin A. Blackstone and Joseph Fuhr, "An Anti-trust Analysis of Non-Profit Hospital Mergers," *Review of Industrial Organization,* 8, August 1992: 473–490.

3. There have been a large number of hospital cost studies. See, for example, T. G. Cowing, A. G. Holtmann, and S. Powers, "Hospital Cost Analysis: A Survey and Evaluation of Recent Studies," in R. Scheffler and L. Rossiter, eds., *Advances in Health Economics and Health Services,* vol. 4 (Greenwich, Conn.: JAI Press, 1983); Thomas Grannemann, Randall Brown, and Mark Pauly, "Estimating Hospital Costs: A Multiple Output Analysis," *Journal of Health Economics,* 5(2), June 1986: 107–127; Freidrich Breyer, "The Specification of a Hospital Cost Function: A Comment on the Recent Literature," *Journal of Health Economics,* 6(2), June 1987: 147–157; and Martin Gaynor and Gerard Anderson, "Uncertain Demand, the Structure of Hospital Costs, and the Cost of Empty Hospital Beds," *Journal of Health Economics,* 14(3), August 1995: 291–317.

4. Paul L. Joskow, "The Effects of Competition and Regulation on Hospital Bed Supply and the Reservation Quality of the Hospital," *Bell Journal of Economics,* 11(2), Autumn 1980: 421–447.

5. Mark V. Pauly, "Medical Staff Characteristics and Hospital Costs," *Journal of Human Resources,* 13, Supplement, 1978: 77–111; and Gail A. Jensen and Michael A. Morrisey, "Medical Staff Specialty Mix and Hospital Production," *Journal of Health Economics,* 5(3), September 1986: 253–276.

6. Carson Bays, "The Determinants of Hospital Size: A Survivor Analysis," *Applied Economics,* 18(4), April 1986: 359–377; and H. E. Frech and Lee Rivers Mobley, "Resolving the Impasse on Hospital Scale Economies: A New Approach," *Applied Economics,* 27(3), March 1995: 286–296.

7. Jay Greene and Sandy Lutz, "Multi-Unit Providers Survey: A Tale of Two Ownership Sectors," *Modern Healthcare,* 26(21), May 20, 1996: 61–66.

8. Bruce Japsen, "Another Record Year for Dealmaking," *Modern Healthcare,* 26(52), December 23, 1996: 37–38.

9. For an excellent discussion of hospital integration, complete with full references, see James C. Robinson, "Physician-Hospital Integration and the Economic Theory of the Firm," *Medical Care Research and Review,* 54(1), March 1997: 3–24. Also see Douglas A. Conrad, Stephen S. Mick, Carolyn W. Madden, and Geoffrey Hoare, "Vertical Structures and Control in Health Care Markets: A Conceptual Framework and Review," *Medical Care Review,* 45(1), Spring 1988: 49–100.

10. The following is a representative list of articles dealing with hospital objectives. M. S. Feldstein, "Hospital Cost Inflation: A Study of Non-Profit Price Dynamics," *American Economic Review,,* 61(5), December 1971: 853–872; J. P. Newhouse, "Toward a Theory of Non-Profit Institutions: An Economic Model of a Hospital," *American Economic Review,,* 60(1), March 1970: 64–74; M. V. Pauly and M. Redisch, "The Not-for-Profit Hospital as a Physicians' Cooperative," *American Economic Review,* 63(1), March 1973: 87–99; Jeffrey E. Harris, "The Internal Organization of Hospitals: Some Economic Implications," *Bell Journal of Economics,*

8(2), Autumn 1977: 467–482; and M. V. Pauly, "Nonprofit Firms in Medical Markets," *American Economic Review,* Papers and Proceedings, 77(2), May 1987: 257–262.

11. Patricia M. Danzon, "Hospital 'Profits': The Effects of Reimbursement Policies," *Journal of Health Economics,* 1(1), May 1982: 29–52. See also Jeffrey E. Harris, "Pricing Rules for Hospitals," *The Bell Journal of Economics,* 10(1), Spring 1979: 224–243. Harris shows prices and long-run marginal costs for specific hospital services within one hospital for 1973. Major surgery (e.g., open heart) is generally priced below marginal cost while routine lab and x-ray are priced above their long-run marginal costs.

12. Frank A. Sloan, "Property Rights in the Hospital Industry," in H. E. Frech, ed., *Health Care in America* (San Francisco, Calif.: Pacific Research Institute for Public Policy, 1988), pp. 103–141.

13. Roger Platt, "Utilization of Facilities for Heart Surgery," *New England Journal of Medicine,* 284(24), June 17, 1971: 1386–1387.

14. Harold Luft, John Bunker, and Alain Enthoven, "Should Operations Be Regionalized," *New England Journal of Medicine,* 301(25), December 20, 1979: 1364–1369. See also Ann B. Flood, W. Richard Scott, and Wayne Ewy, "Does Practice Make Perfect? Part I: The Relation Between Hospital Volume and Outcomes for Selected Diagnostic Categories; Part II: The Relation Between Hospital Volume and Outcomes and Other Hospital Characteristics," *Medical Care,* 22(2), February 1984: 115–125; and Robert Hughes, Sandra Hunt, and Harold Luft, "Effects of Surgeon Volume and Hospital Volume on Quality of Care in Hospitals," *Medical Care,* 25(6), June 1987: 489–503.

15. Robert Rice, "Analysis of the Hospital as an Economic Organism," *Modern Hospital,,* 106(4), April 1966: 87–91.

16. Kenneth J. Arrow, "Uncertainty and the Welfare Economics of Medical Care," *American Economic Review,* 53(5), December 1963: 941–973. The nonprofit rationale for consumer protection would, however, also suggest that physician groups should similarly have a comparative advantage if they were organized on a nonprofit basis.

17. Burton Weisbrod, "Rewarding Performance That Is Hard to Measure: The Private Non-Profit Sector," *Science,* 244(4904), May 5, 1989: 541–546.

18. Tax exemption, by itself, is hypothesized to provide a significant reason for nonprofit organization. The value of tax exemption varies from state to state since states vary in their property, sales, and corporate income taxes. Henry B. Hansmann, "The Effect of Tax Exemption and Other Factors on the Market Share of Nonprofit versus For-Profit Firms," *National Tax Journal,* 40(1), March 1987: 71–82.

19. For a more complete discussion of this hospital control mechanism by physicians, see S. Shalit, "A Doctor-Hospital Cartel Theory," *Journal of Business,* 50(1), January 1977: 1–20.

20. Frank A. Sloan, "Property Rights in the Hospital Industry," *op. cit.,* 134–135; Mark V. Pauly, "Nonprofit Firms in Medical Markets," *op. cit.;* Edwin G. West, "Nonprofit Organizations: Revised Theory and New Evidence," *Public Choice,* 63(2), November 1989: 165–174; J. Michael Watt et al., "The Comparative Economic Performance of Investor-Owned Chains and Not-for-Profit Hospitals," *New England Journal of Medicine,* 314(2), January 9, 1986: 89–96; Bradford H. Gray, ed., *For-Profit Enterprise in Health Care* (Washington, D.C.: National Academy Press, 1986).

21. For a review of studies in this area, see Richard G. Frank and David S. Salkever, "Nonprofit

Organizations in the Health Sector," *Journal of Economic Perspectives,* 8(4), Fall 1994: 129–144.

22. Jonathan Gruber, "The Effect of Competitive Pressures on Charity: Hospital Responses to Price Shopping in California," *Journal of Health Economics,* 13(2), July 1994: 183–212.

23. James C. Robinson, "Hospital Quality Competition and the Economics of Imperfect Information," *The Milbank Quarterly,* 66(3), 1988: 465–481; and James C. Robinson and Harold Luft, "The Impact of Hospital Market Structure on Patient Volume, Average Length of Stay, and the Cost of Care," *Journal of Health Economics,* 4(4), December 1985: 333–356.

24. James C. Robinson and Harold S. Luft, "Competition and the Cost of Hospital Care 1972–1982," *Journal of the American Medical Association,* 257(23), June 19, 1987: 3241–3245.

25. David Dranove, Mark Shanley, and William White, "Price and Concentration in Hospital Markets: The Switch from Patient-Driven to Payer-Driven Competition," *Journal of Law and Economics,* 36(1), April 1993: 179–204.

26. Glenn A. Melnick and Jack Zwanziger, "Hospital Behavior under Competition and Cost Containment Policies," *Journal of the American Medical Association,* 260(18), November 11, 1988: 2669–2675.

27. Glenn Melnick, Jack Zwanziger, Anil Bamezai, and Robert Patterson, "The Effect of Market Structure and Bargaining Position on Hospital Prices," *Journal of Health Economics,* 11(3), October 1992: 217–233.

28. Glenn Melnick, Jack Zwanziger, Anil Bamezai, and Joyce Mann, "Managed Care, Competition, and Hospital Cost Growth in the US: 1986–1993," unpublished manuscript, 1997.

29. For a more extensive discussion of cost shifting, see David Dranove, "Pricing by Non-Profit Institutions: The Case of Hospital Cost-Shifting," *Journal of Health Economics,* 7(1), March 1988: 47–57. Also see Michael Morrisey, *Cost Shifting in Health Care: Separating Evidence from Rhetoric* (Washington, D.C.: American Enterprise Institute Press) 1994.

30. National Center for Health Statistics, *Hospital Discharges and Lengths of Stay—1972* (Washington, D.C.: U.S. Government Printing Office, 1972).

31. John Rafferty, "Enfranchisement and Rationing Effects of Medicare on Discretionary Hospital Use," *Health Services Research,* 10(1), Spring 1975: 51–62.

32. See Paul J. Feldstein and Saul Waldman, "Financial Position of Hospitals in the Early Medicare Period," *Social Security Bulletin,* 31(10), October 1968: 18–23; and Karen Davis, "Hospital Costs and the Medicare Program," *Social Security Bulletin,* 36(8), August 1973: 18–36.

33. Doug Staiger, "Regulation and Labor Earnings in Hospitals," Massachusetts Institute of Technology, July 1989 (unpublished).

34. M. Feldstein and Amy Taylor, "The Rapid Rise of Hospital Costs," in Martin Feldstein, ed., *Hospital Costs and Health Insurance* (Cambridge, Mass.: Harvard University Press, 1981), pp. 19–56; Martin Feldstein, "Hospital Cost Inflation: A Study of Non-Profit Price Dynamics," *American Economic Review,* 61(5), December 1971: 853; and Victor Fuchs, "The Earnings of Allied Health Personnel—Are Health Workers Underpaid," *Explorations in Economic Research,* 3(3), Summer 1976: 408–431.

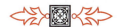

CHAPTER

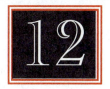

Health Manpower
Shortages
and Surpluses:
Definitions,
Measurement,
and Policies

Within the context of the overall market for medical care, the various categories of health manpower comprise separate submarkets. The health manpower professions are thus an *input* to the provision of medical services. Chapter 3 showed that the overall market for medical care consists of a set of institutional markets, a set of health manpower markets, and a set of markets in which the demand and supply of health manpower education occurs. With a change in the demand for medical care, perhaps resulting from an increase in the population with insurance coverage, there will be increases in demand for the institutional settings in which medical care is provided and, subsequently, an increase in demand by the different institutional settings for inputs used in the production of their services.

The demand for the different health manpower professions is, therefore, a *derived* demand, derived from the demand for medical and institutional services. These demands by the various institutions for different types of health manpower, together with the existing stock of trained health manpower, will determine the wages, the number of persons employed, and their participation rate (the percent of the available stock of each health manpower profession that is employed). The health education institutions determine the long-run supply or stock of health manpower in each profession. (The long-run supply is also influenced by immigration laws that affect entry by foreign-trained health professionals.)

How well the different health manpower and education markets perform has an effect not only on the wages and number of health professionals, but also on the price and quantity of medical and institutional services. Since the various submarkets are interrelated and feed into the market for medical services, the efficiency with which the health manpower market performs will affect prices and outputs in each of the other markets; the more efficient a market is, the greater will be its output. Thus an important reason for examining the separate health manpower markets for different categories of health professionals is to determine how well each market performs. If the markets are determined not to perform well, alternative approaches for improving their performance will be examined, giving due consideration to the reasons for inadequate performance.

The market for health professional *education* will also be examined to determine whether it is performing efficiently—that is, whether the quantity of health professional education has been "optimal" over different time periods and whether health education is being produced efficiently. The market for health professional education is important not only because it determines the long-run supply of health manpower, but also because it has been the recipient of a great deal of federal and state funding. Examples of federal and state health manpower legislation will be analyzed to determine both its purpose and how effective it has been in achieving its stated goals.

In addition to analyzing the efficiency, performance, and public policies of the separate health manpower and health professional education markets, alternative approaches for forecasting health manpower "requirements" will be examined. Historically, the physician and registered nurse markets have changed from one of "shortages" to "surplus." These definitions will be analyzed since, together with the approaches used for forecasting shortages and surpluses, they have served as the basis for much of the federal and state legislation dealing with health manpower.

DEFINITIONS OF A HEALTH MANPOWER SHORTAGE

For many years, public policy was concerned with reducing health manpower shortages. Various estimates were made as to the magnitude of these shortages and legislation was enacted to decrease these shortages. Currently, there is concern that there is a growing surplus of various health professionals and proposals are being made to reverse this trend. Essential to fully understanding the debate over shortages and surpluses, and consequently appropriate public policy, is their definition. The economic definition of a shortage or a surplus is often different than how it is defined by noneconomists. Further, a continuing disequilibrium in a market indicates that the market is not performing efficiently. Policies to improve market performance should therefore be based on the reasons for its inadequate performance. Thus unless there is agreement on what constitutes a shortage and a surplus, proposals for subsequent government intervention to improve market performance may be misguided.

This section therefore starts with a discussion of different definitions of shortage. Surpluses are discussed next. For each type of market disequilibrium various approaches used to measure shortages and surpluses are discussed together with appropriate policy prescriptions.

Normative Judgment of a Shortage

There are several *noneconomic* definitions of health manpower shortages. An example is the statement that the demand for physicians "ought" to be greater. It has also been said that the "need" for physicians is greater than the demand or that the price of physician services is "too high," thereby preventing people from consuming all the physician services they need. A normative judgment of a shortage is that there is a shortage of effective demand relative to what it should be. The noneconomic definitions of a shortage are based either on a value judgment of how much care people should receive, or on a professional determination of how much physician care is appropriate in the population.

Such normative judgments of shortage are based on a determination of "need" in the population, or on some professional estimate of health manpower requirements. For example, physician/population ratios in high-income states are contrasted with physician/population ratios in low-income states. The differences in the ratio are believed to indicate the "need" for physicians in low-income states, which is the number of physicians "required" to achieve a physician/population ratio equal to that of the high-income states. (The ratio technique is discussed in more detail below.)

The classic example of the use of professional determination to decide on the number of physicians "needed" was the 1930s study by Lee and Jones (1). Lee and Jones based their estimate of the number of physicians required on estimates of the incidence of morbidity and on the number of physician hours required to provide both preventive and therapeutic services to the population. The policy proposals resulting from normative definitions of a shortage of health manpower are generally the same: increase the number of trained professionals through increased federal funding.

In Figure 12.1 it is assumed that the initial situation is represented by the supply and demand diagrams S_1 and D_1, resulting in the quantity of physician services Q_1. The number of physician services for the population, based on either need or professional determination, is determined to be Q_2. The usual policy prescription to achieve an increase in

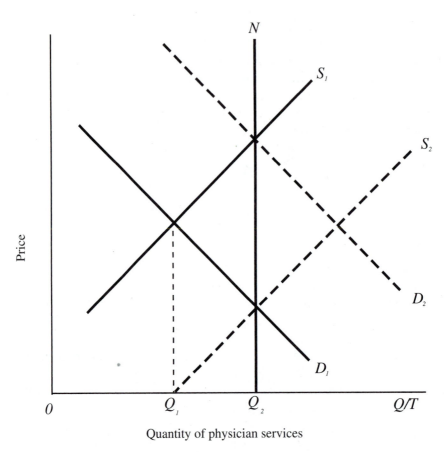

FIGURE 12.1 • Alternative policy prescriptions based on a normative shortage of health manpower.

physician services is to shift the supply of physicians to S_2, thereby increasing physician services to Q_2. The same increase in quantity, Q_2, of physician services can also be achieved by shifting the demand schedule to D_2. This would not require a shift in supply or in the number of physicians. (A shift in demand can be achieved through a demand subsidy, such as insurance coverage for physician services.)

Thus the normative judgment of a shortage of physician services, $Q_1 - Q_2$, can be alleviated either by increasing the number of physicians (shifting S_1 to S_2) or by subsidizing the demand for physician services (shifting D_1 to D_2) along a given supply curve. A movement along a given supply curve represents increased production by existing physicians; physicians either work longer hours or they use more auxiliary personnel.

Which policy alternative—the demand or the supply shift—is preferable depends on the cost of each proposal, the population groups receiving the benefits, and the length of time required to achieve the increase in services consumed. Normative judgments of a manpower shortage can be alleviated in various ways; however, these judgments of a shortage say nothing about how well the market for such health professionals is functioning. The market for physicians may be functioning efficiently, although some persons may believe there "should" be more physicians; conversely, the number of physicians may be less than would be produced in an efficiently functioning market. The basic policy prescription using a normative definition of a shortage, however, is always for federal funding to achieve an increase in the number of physicians.

If the market is not performing efficiently, there might be alternative ways of achieving an increase in the number of physicians or physician services *without* resorting to federal funding. Perhaps some legal barriers might be changed to permit an increase in the physician supply. To determine how well the market for health professionals is functioning, we must establish the economic definitions of a shortage and examine how such shortages may occur. Possible policy prescriptions for correcting these shortages will be an outgrowth of their analysis.

Economic Definitions of Shortages in Health Manpower

In a competitive market, market equilibrium occurs when the value placed on a good or service by its demanders (marginal benefit) equals the cost of the resources used in its production (marginal cost). When the value placed on that good or service exceeds its cost of production, too little of that good is produced, creating a shortage.[1] In freely operating markets, shortages can exist in the short run but not in the long run.

There are two ways of analyzing how an economic shortage can occur with respect to health manpower. First, the quantity demanded of a particular health profession (i.e., hospitals' demands for registered nurses) can exceed the quantity supplied at a given market price (wage). For this to occur, the wage would have to be below the equilibrium wage.

The second way in which a shortage can occur is when the income of a health profession (relative to other occupations) exceeds the additional costs of entering that profession. In this example, the income of a health profession reflects the value of the services that the profession produces. The costs of entering the profession include the out-of-pocket costs of training for that profession, as well as the value of the entrants' time, that is, their opportunity costs. (Since the time streams at which the income is earned and the costs incurred differ, an appropriate discount rate must be used in equating the two. It is also assumed that all other differences between occupations, such as variability in incomes, mortality risk, etc., are equal.)

The latter situation may be illustrated by use of Figure 12.2. D_1 is the demand by

---

[1] This situation also occurs when a monopolist establishes a price for its service greater than the marginal cost of producing that service.

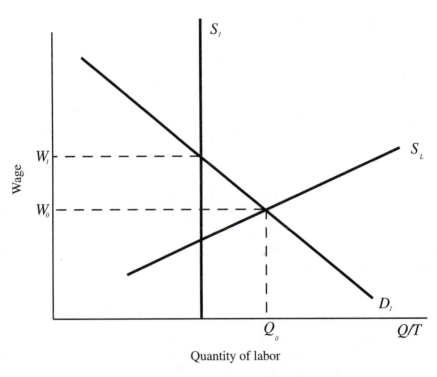

FIGURE 12.2 • A shortage created by restriction of supply.

firms for a particular health manpower occupation. S_L represents the long-run supply curve and is the number of persons willing to enter that occupation at different wage rates. S_1 is the current number of persons in that health profession. (S_1 could be more elastic since the supply of work effort from the current stock of trained professionals depends up the responsiveness of their hours worked and their participation rate to different wage rates.) With a supply equal to S_1 the wage will be W_1. If the market were operating freely, the wage would fall to W_0 as the supply of labor to that occupation increases. If the health manpower profession in question were able to establish entry barriers, S_1 would not shift to the right along S_L and the resulting wage would be W_1. Wage W_1 represents the value placed on that labor input by its demanders, and it exceeds the cost of inducing additions to the supply of that health profession.

Each of the two types of static shortage—the first example, where the wage is held below the equilibrium level, and the case just considered, where the wage exceeds the wage at which persons are willing to enter that occupation—is caused by market power on either the demand or supply side of the health manpower market. When the wage is prevented from rising to its equilibrium level, the demanders of labor are exercising monopoly power; in the latter case it is the suppliers of labor services that are the monopolists. In both types of shortage situation, the shortage would disappear with an increase in supply. Supply would increase in the first case if the price of the service were allowed to rise, and in the second case if more persons were allowed to enter the profession.

These discussions of economic shortage indicate what information should be examined to determine whether an economic shortage exists or has occurred. Since each of these approaches will be used with regard to different health professions (i.e., physicians and registered nurses), these approaches are discussed in more detail.

When quantity demanded exceeds quantity supplied at a given market price, as in Figure 12.3, the price will rise (to P_2) and there will be no excess demand. All who are willing to pay price P_2 will be able to purchase as much as they want of the commodity they are seeking. (There may be persons who cannot afford to buy as much of the commodity as others believe they should purchase at the new, higher price; however, such a normative judgment can still be handled using a market mechanism by providing subsidies directly to such persons.) An economic shortage would occur in the situation above if, with an increase in demand from D_1 to D_2, the price of the service were prevented from rising to its new equilibrium point P_2. With an increase in demand and a price of P_1 the demand would be for Q_3 units of service. However, at a price of P_1 the supply of that

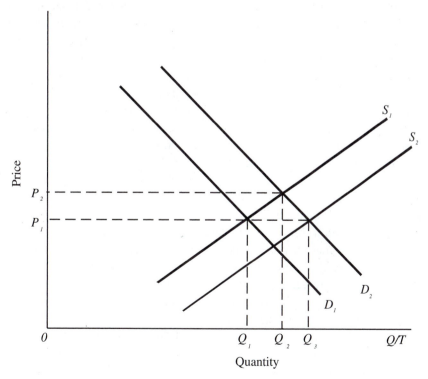

FIGURE 12.3 • An economic shortage.

service would be Q_1. The shortage would be the excess of demand over supply at the prevailing price of Q_3-Q_1.

There can be two types of economic shortage: a temporary (dynamic) shortage or a static (long-run) shortage. Both types of economic shortage are believed to have existed at one time or another in the health professions.

A Dynamic Shortage

A dynamic or temporary shortage occurs when, as in Figure 12.3, there is an increase in demand but the new price has not yet reached its new equilibrium point of P_2. Demand will exceed supply at the old price of P_1. Not everyone who is willing to pay P_1 will receive as much as she wants. In the long run, however, this form of temporary or dynamic shortage will work itself out; the price will rise to the equilibrium level and there will no longer be a shortage. If demand continues to increase, it will take longer to achieve the equilibrium situation. There will be continued claims of a shortage while the price is rising, although supply will also be increasing.

Increases in quantity supplied, as well as rising prices, distinguish a dynamic shortage from a static shortage.

How long will a dynamic shortage persist? In their article on dynamic shortages, Arrow and Capron claim that "the amount of shortage will tend to disappear faster the greater the reaction speed and also the greater the elasticity of supply (or demand)" (2). The reaction speed is the time it takes for a price to reach its equilibrium level given the excess of demand over supply. It will take time for firms to realize that there is a shortage at the old price and that they must raise wages to attract more personnel. Firms must also decide how many more persons they want in the event that they have to pay higher wage rates. It also takes time for employees to react to these higher salaries. If demand and supply are relatively elastic, it will take smaller price increases to bring about a new equilibrium situation. Thus, in a dynamic situation where demands are increasing, temporary shortages can exist. The magnitude of the dynamic shortage will depend on how fast demand is increasing, the reaction speed of increased prices to the excess demand, and the elasticities of supply and demand.

The policy prescriptions for a dynamic shortage differ from those for a shortage based on a "normative" judgment or for a static shortage. Increasing information to both demanders and suppliers in a market where dynamic shortages exist will make the equilibrium situation occur more quickly. Career information given to prospective applicants in professions where demand is increasing, and similar information given to prospective employers regarding the higher wages they will have to pay for such personnel, will bring about a quicker adjustment process. Massive supply subsidies to finance additional applicants entering those professions for which demands are increasing cannot be justified on grounds of economic efficiency. Such subsidies would have to be justified on the basis of other reasons, such as a normative shortage.

Static Economic Shortages

A static or long-run shortage occurs because supply does not increase; market equilibrium is therefore not achieved. In the typical case of a static shortage, prices are controlled and prevented from rising to their equilibrium level. If prices are not able to rise, the suppliers cannot pay higher prices to attract personnel away from other occupations. Similarly, a given health professional will not increase the amount of time that he is willing to work if the wage rate per hour does not increase; at some point the person will prefer leisure to more work. Thus suppliers will not increase the services they offer unless the prices paid for their services rise. The available supply in such situations is rationed by other methods: there may be long waiting lines to see a physician and only those willing to wait (those with low time costs) will see the physician; there may be a decrease in quality (i.e., physicians may spend less time with each patient); physicians may also refuse to see new patients.

It is possible that either a static shortage or a market equilibrium situation could exist in the physician *services* market, while in the market for physician *manpower* there could also be either an equilibrium or a static shortage situation. It is important to keep the analysis of these two markets—the services and manpower markets—separate. For example, in Figure 12.4, the left-hand diagram represents the market for physician services, while the right-hand diagram represents a typical firm (i.e., a physician in solo or group practice) within the overall market for physician services. Starting from an equilibrium situation in both markets, with price equal to P_0 and quantity of physician services equal to Q_0, the physician as a firm faces a price of P_0 and produces a quantity of services given by Q'_0, which is the intersection of the physician firm's marginal cost curve (MC) and the

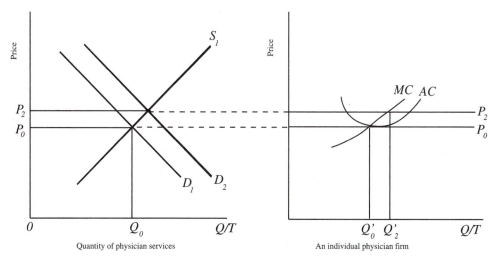

FIGURE 12.4 • The market for physician services and for an individual physician firm.

market price P_0. (For simplicity, we are assuming a competitive market in both the production and demand for physician services.) The physician firm is in equilibrium (physicians will neither leave the industry nor enter it) since they are earning a normal rate of return, with no excess profits, as shown by the position of the physician firm's average cost curve (AC) and the market price P_0.

Given the foregoing initial equilibrium position in both the services and manpower markets, let us assume that there is an increase in demand for physician services, possibly as a result of increased income in the population. The demand for physician services will increase from D_1 to D_2. Given the same number of physicians, physicians will either work longer hours or increase their productivity by hiring auxiliary personnel. This increased output is shown by a movement up the industry's supply curve (S_1), which is the sum of the physician firms' marginal cost curves. The market price will rise to P_2, and each physician will be making excess profits (the distance from P_2 to the firm's average cost curve at output level Q'_2). The increase in price and output in the market for physician services is the short-run reaction to the increase in demand for physician services.

In this situation there is no shortage in the physicians' services market. If there is an increase in the number of physicians (i.e., firms) in the long run in the manpower market because of excess profits, the industry supply curve will shift to the right (shown by S_2), and each physician firm will be producing at the point where the new price equals average cost and marginal cost. The increase in the number of physicians in the long run will also bring about an equilibrium situation in the manpower market, and no shortage will exist in either market.

If, however, with an increase in the demand for physician services the price is *prevented* from rising, a static shortage will occur in the services market. Equilibrium could still exist in the physician manpower market, since there will not be an excess of profits (or losses). Alternatively, if the price is allowed to reach its equilibrium level in the services market but new physicians are not permitted to enter the manpower market, a shortage situation will exist in the physician manpower market. Physicians will be earning excess profits and we would observe little, if any, addition to the number of physicians.

A static shortage in the number of physicians will be represented by high rates of returns [excess profits] to physicians and little or no entry into the physician market.

The policy implications for a static shortage situation are to allow the price to rise if the shortage is in the services market. If the shortage is in the physician manpower market, then easing the entry barriers will result in an increase in the number of physicians. With an increase in the number of physicians, excess profits per physician will fall until profits are "normal" and there will no longer be an economic shortage of physicians. If a static shortage exists because of barriers to entry, providing subsidies to the new entrants will not resolve the static shortage. The entry barriers are not eliminated by such subsidies. Subsidizing the limited number of new entrants will merely increase their return in a profession whose profits are currently considered to be excessive.

THE DEFINITIONS OF A SURPLUS
OF HEALTH MANPOWER

The above discussion defined a shortage in the physician manpower market as occurring when physicians earned an above-normal rate of return, or excess profits, on their investment in a medical education. A surplus of physicians would exist when the opposite occurs, that is, when physicians are earning a below-normal rate of return. (This would be characterized on the previous graph by the price being below the average-cost curve.)

A surplus situation can occur if one or both of the following situations occur. First, it could be the result of government regulation, so that the price of physician services is not permitted to rise as rapidly as the costs of providing physician services. Over time the relative rate of return to becoming a physician falls. The second way in which a surplus could occur is through a change in market conditions. The growth in managed care, together with HMOs limiting their enrollees' access to specialists, has decreased the demand for specialists. As a result, specialist fees and incomes have fallen. Exacerbating this situation is the supply of specialists, which is continuing to increase faster than the demand for their services.

Similar to the definition of shortages, surpluses are often defined in noneconomic terms. Typical approaches are to estimate the number of specialists, of various types, that are needed. For example, how many specialists would be needed if, for example, half of the population was enrolled in HMOs and the other half in fee-for-service, with their differing use of specialists. These needs or "requirements" for specialists are then compared to the number of specialists available. The difference is the surplus of specialists.

Surpluses are resolved more easily than static shortages (although there is a great deal of financial hardship to those in the surplus profession). As prospective applicants perceive a lowering in their rate of return to a medical education, fewer will apply to medical school; there will be a shift away from those specialties in greater surplus; some physicians may decide to retire earlier, while others move into management positions. Over time, the number of new entrants into the profession will be less than those exiting and the smaller increase in the physician supply will bring about a new equilibrium situation.

In a surplus situation as described above, the physician services market is in equilibrium (although fees are lower than physicians would prefer) and in the manpower market physicians are earning a lower rate of return than other professions. The professional societies seek legislative remedies (higher prices for their services, e.g., any willing provider laws, and decreased entry into the profession) to mitigate the financial hardship on their members.

Income redistribution occurs in surplus and shortage situations. When there is a surplus of physicians, incomes of practicing physicians decline while purchasers of physician services pay lower prices and have greater access to care. The fortunes of physicians and patients are reversed in a shortage situation.

THE MEASUREMENT OF HEALTH MANPOWER SHORTAGES AND SURPLUSES

In defining and distinguishing among normative, dynamic, and static shortages, it is clear that the latter two are different types of economic shortage, and that the normative shortage is based on either a professional determination or a value judgment of how many professionals of a particular type of manpower are needed. Similarly, there are economic and noneconomic definitions of a physician surplus. The alternative policy prescriptions for the different types of shortages and surpluses were also indicated. In this section the methods by which each of these types of shortages and surpluses have been measured is discussed. The measurement of a shortage or surplus is important since it enables us to distinguish between the different types of shortages or surpluses.

Professional Determination

Noneconomic shortages have traditionally been measured in one of two ways. The first is professional determination. The earliest approach, used by Lee and Jones, calculated the number of physicians required in the population based on an estimate of the number of physician hours needed, as determined by professional judgment, to provide medical care to the population. The authors developed a table of annual expectancy rates for diseases and injuries; they then asked leading physicians to determine the number of services required to diagnose and treat a given illness. The number of physician hours required to provide care for each illness category was then estimated. Finally, assuming a 40-hour workweek per physician, the authors translated these hours into a requirement for l65,000 physicians, or a proposed physician/population ratio of 135 per 100,000 population. The difference between the then current number of physicians and the number of physicians arrived at by the foregoing method was the "shortage" of physicians.

One of the problems with using such an approach for estimating shortages and for proposing government subsidies to increase the number of needed physicians is that the additional physicians do not necessarily go where they are most needed. Further, those persons most in need of physician services may not be able to pay for them even if they are made available.

The same approach has also been used to estimate a physician surplus. Concern by medical associations and educational institutions about a possible surplus of physicians led to the 1980 Graduate Medical Education National Advisory Committee (GMENAC) report to the secretary of health and human services on the future supply and requirements for physicians (3). The approach used by the GEMENAC committee was similar to the methodology used by Lee and Jones in the 1930s.

Estimates of future supplies of physicians were generated based on estimates of current numbers of medical school graduates, foreign medical graduates, residents, and deaths and retirements. No attempt was made to relate entry into medicine, entry into different specialties, or entry by foreign medical graduates to economic factors or to any other causal factors. Instead, it was implicitly assumed that such factors would not change over the period studied. Nor did this approach consider changes in physician productivity that might be occurring. It was a mechanical approach to generating future estimates of physicians and their specialty distribution.

The estimates of physician requirements were developed by combining data on current utilization and the "need" for physicians. Within each physician specialty, physicians were asked how many physicians were needed in that specialty. Again, such an approach does not explicitly consider patient preferences for care or economic factors such as changes in insurance coverage, factors that in the past have been important determinants of physician utilization.

The "desired balance" between physician supply and requirements in 1990 did not consider any equilibrating mechanisms such as changes in physician prices or hours worked. The GMENAC report stated that there would be a physician "surplus" of seventy thousand physicians by 1990.

At any given time there is an equilibrium price, resulting from the interaction of the demand for and supply of physicians. If the number of physicians exceeds the professionally determined estimate and if such a "surplus" of physicians were to be eliminated (a shift to the left in the supply of physicians), the consequence would be an increase in price and a decrease in quantity. If the price were a government-determined price and did not rise as the "surplus" is eliminated, then an *economic* shortage would occur (demand would exceed supply at the fixed price). The above methodology for estimating a surplus is silent on this issue, either because its adherents are unaware that this will occur or, more likely, they are aware of it and that is the reason for favoring an elimination of the surplus.

The Ratio Technique

The second and most popular approach to determining health manpower shortages and surpluses has been the ratio technique. When used to estimate a shortage, this method generally uses the existing physician/population ratio (or other health manpower/population ratio) and compares it with the physician/population ratio that is likely to occur in some future period. To calculate the future ratio, the proponents of this approach estimate the future population and then calculate the likely number of additional graduates to the stock of physicians, less the expected number of deaths and retirements. The difference between the existing physician/population ratio and the future physician/population ratio is the extent of the shortage that must be made up.

Until the late 1970s, studies using this approach consistently found the future ratio to be lower than the current ratio, meaning that an increased number of physicians were needed if the future ratio was to be at least equal to the current ratio. The policy proposal that was always prescribed based on the finding that increased numbers of physicians were needed was that federal subsidies should be provided to health professional educational institutions to produce more graduates.

There were variations in the use of the ratio technique for determining the number of needed physicians. For example, the highest regional or statewide physician/population ratio observed might be used as the ratio to be achieved for the entire country in some future period.

The ratio technique has served as the basis for much of the health manpower legislation in this country. It has been used for physicians, dentists, and registered nurses. Other health professional educational organizations also made use of this approach in their requests for federal subsidies. Since this approach has had such an important legislative role and has resulted in many billions of dollars of subsidies by both the federal and state governments, it deserves a critical evaluation.

One way of thinking of the physician/population ratio is that it is the outcome of an equilibrium situation. At any point in time there is a demand for physicians and a supply of physicians; the intersection of the demand and supply curves result in physician incomes and in a physician/population ratio. Attempts to change the physician/population ratio generally ignore the fact that this ratio is the result of demand and other supply factors. Any significant change simply in the number of physicians will cause changes in the demands for other inputs (substitutes for and complements to physicians) as well as in the demands for physicians themselves, which would mean a movement along the physician demand curve.

Three basic problems are associated with the use of the ratio technique for forecasting manpower requirements. The first problem is that the method does not consider any changes that may occur in the demand for physician (or other health manpower) services. If demand were to increase, then even maintaining an existing ratio is likely to result in an *increase* in the price of physician services (i.e., the shift in demand is greater than the change in the physician/population ratio). Demand changes could occur because of changes in financing care, such as Medicare, Medicaid, and tax-free employer-paid health insurance. Other demand factors include the aging of the population, changes in lifestyle factors that decrease the demand for medical services, and the increased use of other treatment inputs, such as pharmaceuticals.

Since the ratio technique basically ignores the demand side, differences between the future ratio of physicians to population and the ratio that would be demanded will be resolved through changes in the *price* of physician services. Some persons will be even less likely to buy physician services if the price of those services were to increase.

Thus, maintaining a given ratio says nothing about whether the future price of physician services will be the same; it may be higher or lower, but it is highly unlikely that it will be the same. Since the future price is likely to be different, what is the real purpose of maintaining a given ratio? If, under a projected "shortage" scenario, the objective were to provide more services to certain population groups or to the entire population, it would be important to lower the price of the service so as to increase consumption. The ratio technique and its basic policy prescription of changing the number of physicians does not even consider price or alternative ways to affect consumption of services.

The second problem with the use of the ratio technique is that it does not consider productivity changes that are likely to occur or that are possible to achieve. The ratio of farmers to the population has fallen drastically in the past one hundred years (from a ratio of 60 farmers to every 100 persons in 1860 to 3.5 per 100 persons today), yet few people would maintain that there is a shortage of farmers or that it would be desirable to retain the previous farmer/population ratio. Because of enormous increases in farm productivity, it takes fewer farmers today to produce food.

Although productivity gains in medical care appear to be more limited than what has occurred in agriculture, it is possible to achieve an increase in physician services without increasing the number of physicians. Lesser-trained personnel can be used to relieve physicians of many of the tasks they perform; delegation of tasks would permit an increase in the number of physician visits. If increased productivity is considered, a smaller physician/population ratio would be needed in the future. To alleviate a projected "shortage," increasing productivity is an alternative approach for achieving an increase in the quantity of physician services. Policies to increase productivity require smaller subsidies than do policies to increase the number of physicians.

(It is an indication of the real intent underlying the use of physician/population ratios that the subsidies should go to the medical schools, which would not be the recipients if the less costly approach of increasing physician productivity were used.)

The third problem with the use of the ratio technique is that no indication of the importance of the shortage of physicians is provided. For example, the Bane Report estimated that to maintain a specific physician/population ratio 15 years hence, an additional 11,000 physicians would be needed. These projections assumed that without federal support for medical education there would be 319,000 physicians, with a resulting shortage of 11,000 physicians (4). How much is it worth (in terms of governmental subsidies) to reduce this shortage to 7,000 physicians or to no shortage whatsoever? It is difficult, if not impossible, to use the ratio technique to compare the additional cost of decreasing the estimated shortage of physicians with their marginal contribution to medical care, increased health, or lower physician fees.

There are a number of other difficulties inherent in using the ratio technique that can cause variations in its estimates. It is necessary to exclude nonpatient care physicians from the physician/population ratio, to correct for the age distribution of physicians (since it may affect productivity), to adjust for the percent of female physicians who see fewer patients, to correct for the expected number of foreign medical graduates, to estimate the percent of the population in HMOs (which use fewer physicians per one thousand enrollees), to account for changes in the institutional settings where care is provided (hospitals use a greater mix of certain manpower than do ambulatory care settings or care in the home), and to develop an accurate forecast of the population in a future period.

However, the three conceptual problems inherent in this approach—no consideration given to demand or productivity changes and no understanding of the importance of the shortage estimate—are more difficult shortcomings to correct.

The Rate-of-Return Approach

In an equilibrium situation physicians earn normal profits. If there were an increase (decrease) in demand in the physician services market, physicians would, in the short run, experience higher (lower) prices, leading to above (below) normal profits, and in the long run, as a result of changes in the number of physicians, physician profits would return to normal.

This analogy of the physician as a firm is useful because it helps delineate what we expect to observe. Normal, above, or below normal profits mean that the rate of return to a medical education is either normal, high, or low relative to equivalent investments. Although not all, or even perhaps most, physicians seek a medical education because of its value as a remunerative investment, enough persons do so that if one profession becomes more lucrative than another, some persons will change their preference as to which occupation they wish to enter. This just means that as some professions and occupations become relatively more rewarding financially, some potential applicants who are relatively indifferent among one occupation or another will switch their preferences to the more rewarding profession. This switching between occupations and professions will, on average, equalize returns among different occupations. (Because there are always large variations in skills and abilities, returns *within* an occupation or profession will vary. In the long run, however, the average return should be similar among different occupations.)

When viewing medical education as an investment, the rate of return is calculated by estimating the costs of that investment and the expected higher financial returns achievable as a result of that investment. The profitability of a medical education can then be compared with alternative investments, educational and otherwise. The costs of purchasing a medical education are the direct outlays, such as tuition, laboratory fees, and book fees, and the forgone income had the student gone to work immediately upon graduating from college. These opportunity costs of the medical student's time are the more significant costs of securing a professional education. The financial return of an investment in a medical education is the higher income that a physician earns compared with the income of not having gone for a medical education. Since these higher incomes occur in the future, they are worth less than if they occurred immediately; the financial returns between being a physician as compared to not having gone on for a medical education must be discounted to the present. The comparison between these higher returns and the costs required to receive them is the rate of return to a medical education.

In similar fashion, the rate of return to a medical education can be compared to an investment in a legal education, a dental education, a Ph.D. degree, or an MBA. (More precisely, the internal rate of return is that discount rate which, when applied to the future earnings stream, will make its present value equal to the cost of entry into that profession, that is, the present value of the expected outlay or cost stream.)

A normal rate of return might be similar to the rate of return on a college education or on the return the individual could have received had she invested a sum of money comparable to what was spent on a medical education. It is necessary to compare the rate of return on a medical education with an alternative rate of return to be able to determine whether or not physicians are receiving a normal return.

Returning to our analogy of the physician as a firm, if physicians were receiving "excess" profits, this would be translated into a high relative rate of return to a medical education. If rates of return to medicine are higher than those received in other occupations, we expect to observe a greater number of applicants to medical schools. As the number of physicians increases over time, the rate of return to a medical career will become comparable to those of other occupations or investments.

With regard to shortages, to distinguish between a dynamic and a static shortage, it is necessary to examine the rate of return to a medical education, relative to some standard or to another profession, and also whether there is an increase in the number of physicians. A dynamic shortage would be characterized by a high relative rate of return in the short run, increases in the number of physicians, and eventually normal rates of return. A static shortage would also be characterized by a high relative rate of return, but it would persist since there would be little or no entry into the profession to drive these rates of return down. If rates of return remained relatively high and there was a large increase in the supply of physicians, this would be indicative of a persistent dynamic shortage.

The key difference between the dynamic and static shortage is whether additions to the stock of physicians occur over time. A dynamic shortage will eventually resolve itself; a static shortage requires intervention, since entry into the profession is prevented from occurring.

Similarly, a surplus of physicians would be indicated by a rate of return that is below that of a college graduate. As prospective medical students become more aware of the lower expected rate of return to becoming a physician, fewer students will decide to seek a medical education. With a smaller influx of new physicians, the rate of return will eventually rise so that it once again becomes "normal." How long it takes for a surplus to be reduced depends on growth in demand for physician services, the age distribution of physicians and how soon physicians decide to retire, the opportunity for physicians to move into managerial (or other) positions, how responsive prospective medical students are to the lower rate of return, and the size of the inflow of foreign-trained physicians. It is unlikely that a large surplus could be reduced quickly, since many physicians do not have the skills or opportunities to earn an income comparable to what they receive, even when it is at a below normal rate of return.

The main indicators of the performance of the physician market, as well as other health manpower markets, are data on relative rates of return and changes to the stock of physicians (or other health manpower). Changes in the use of various manpower categories, such as increases and decreases in the use of substitutes, are indicative of changes in the relative wages of such inputs rather than being indicative of a shortage or surplus of physicians. For example, if both incomes and costs of becoming a physician increased, the relative rate of return between occupations could still be similar but because there is a change in relative wages, substitution would occur. Thus the main method whereby different types of shortages are distinguished is in the use of relative rates of return and entry into the profession.[2]

EMPIRICAL ESTIMATES OF SHORTAGES AND SURPLUSES

Several studies have estimated the rate of return to a medical education. The earliest such study, undertaken in the early 1930s, was that of Friedman and Kuznets, who found that physicians earned, on average, 32 percent per year more than dentists (5). This higher income for physicians was, in part, offset by the 17 percent higher cost of becoming a physician. Friedman and Kuznets attributed part of the increased income of physicians to greater entry barriers into the profession. The greater return to physicians represented a relative shortage of physicians; that is, their marginal value as represented by their incomes exceeded the costs of producing additional physicians.

A subsequent study by Hansen found that by 1939 there was a slight *surplus* of physicians and dentists (their rates of return were below those of college graduates). However, by 1949, physicians and dentists had a 16 percent greater rate of return than did college graduates, indicating a shortage. By 1956 the shortage had decreased slightly: physician rates of return were only 10 percent greater than for college graduates; the comparable figure for dentists was 4 percent. These data are shown in Table 12.l, which is reproduced from Hansen's work.[3]

Several additional studies have estimated the internal rate of return to a medical edu-

---

[2]Another approach suggested for measuring whether or not a shortage exists is to examine changes in relative incomes. If one profession's income rises more rapidly than another profession's, a relative shortage is said to exist. (See, for example, Elton Rayack, "The Supply of Physicians' Services," *Industrial and Labor Relations Review,* January 1964.) The problem with this approach is that it does not consider differences in the relative costs of entering different professions. If training times have increased, or if there is a decrease in the number of working years, we would expect higher relative incomes for this profession in order for the relative rates of return to be similar. Another problem in using the relative income approach is that the base year for making comparisons among professions is quite important. Depending on which base year is used, the relative income approach can show a shortage or a surplus of the manpower in a particular profession. Finally, the relative income approach cannot distinguish between relative shortages in all professions and a shortage situation in only one profession.

[3]There is a difference in the method used by Hansen and the other studies. Hansen's income and cost streams begin at the first year of undergraduate college, and his forgone earnings are based on those of a high school graduate. The other studies are based on the forgone earnings of a college graduate and the income and cost streams begin at the first year of medical school.

TABLE 12.1 Internal Rates of Return to Male College Graduates, Physicians, Dentists, and Ratios of Internal Rates of Return of Physicians and Dentists to Male College Graduates, United States, 1939, 1949, and 1956

	1939		1949		1956	
	Rates	Ratios	Rates	Ratios	Rates	Ratios
Male college graduates	13.7	1.00	11.5	1.00	11.6	1.00
Physicians	13.5	0.98	13.4	1.16	12.8	1.10
Dentists	12.3	0.90	13.4	1.16	12.0	1.04

Source: W. Lee Hansen, "Shortages and Investment in Health Manpower," in *The Economics of Health and Medical Care* (Ann Arbor: University of Michigan, 1964), 86.

cation; these results are presented in Table 12.2 (6). (Unfortunately, there are no more recent studies that are comparable to those presented in Table 12.2.) The rates of return are shown for all physicians and separately for general practitioners. The "all physicians" estimate includes general practitioners as well as the various physician specialties. The rates of return to all physicians over the 1955–85 period were sufficiently high to make medicine a financially attractive profession. Between 1974 and 1985 there was a slight decline in the return to a medical education.

The rate of return to different specialties varies greatly, according to Marder et al., and Dresch, who find that in 1985 some specialties, such as anesthesiology and surgical subspecialties, earned 40 and 35 percent returns, while for pediatrics it was only 1.3 percent. Rates of return were typically higher for hospital-based specialties than for those in primary care. Dresch compared the rates of return to medicine with other professions and found that the rates of return varied greatly, depending on which occupation was compared to medicine. For example, the rate of return to a medical education was over 100 percent greater than that of a college professor.

What can we conclude based on the above rate of return data? In the pre–World War II period there appeared to be a slight surplus of physicians and dentists. The rate of return to a medical and dental education was lower than for comparable investments. After World War II, however, the rate of return to a medical and dental education increased. The rates of return during this period were sufficiently high to indicate a shortage situation. With increasing rates of return, increased demands for a medical education would be expected. If the stock of physicians were expanding rapidly, then it would appear that a dynamic shortage existed. If, however, the rates of return remained high, and in fact increased, and there were few or no additions to the stock of physicians, then one would have to conclude that a static shortage situation existed and that barriers prevented an adjustment process from occurring.

To determine whether a dynamic or static shortage of physicians existed throughout the post–World War II period, one must examine data on changes in the stock of physicians during these periods, as presented in Table 12.3.

TABLE 12.2 Internal Rates of Return, All Physicians and General Practitioners, 1955–85

Year	All Physicians		General Practitioners
1985	16.0[a]	—	4.1[b]
1980	—	14.0[c]	16.7[c]
1976	17.5[d]	13.3[c]	16.4[c]
1974	16.7[c]	—	—
1970	22.0[e]	14.7[c]	16.8[c]
1965	17.5[f]	—	21.4[g]
1962	16.6[f]	—	—
1959	14.7[f]	—	23.7[g]
1955	13.5[f]	—	29.1[g]

Sources:

[a]William Marder, Phillip Kletke, Anne Silberger, and Richard Wilke, *Physician Supply and Utilization by Specialty: Trends and Projections* (Chicago: American Medical Association, 1988), 79.

[b]William D. Marder and Richard J. Wilke, "The Value of Physician Time: Comparisons Across Specialists," in H. E. Frech, ed., *Regulating Doctors Fees* (Washington, D.C.: American Enterprise Institute, 1991).

[c]Phillip Burstein and Jerry Cromwell, "Relative Incomes and Rates of Return for U.S. Physicians," *Journal of Health Economics,* 4(1), March 1985: 63–78.

[d]Stephen Dresch, "Marginal Wage Rates, Hours of Work, and Returns to Physicians Training and Specialization," in Nancy Greenspan, ed., *Health Care Financing, Conference Proceedings: Issues in Physician Reimbursement* (Washington, D.C.: Department of Health and Human Services, 1981), 199–200.

[e]Roger Feldman and Richard M. Scheffler, "The Supply of Medical School Applicants and the Rate of Return of Training," *Quarterly Review of Economics and Business,* 18(1), Spring 1978: 91–98, Table 1.

[f]Frank Sloan, *Economic Models of Physician Supply,* unpublished doctoral dissertation, Harvard University, 1968, 164.

[g]Frank Sloan, "Lifetime Earnings and the Physicians Choice of Specialty," *Industrial and Labor Relations Review,* 24(1), October 1970: 47–56.

In 1950, there were 209,000 active physicians in the United States. By 1965 the number of active physicians reached 277,000, which is a rate of increase of less than 2 percent per year. When the increase in the number of physicians is adjusted for increases in the population, the physician/population ratio remained virtually unchanged between 1950 and 1963 (139 physicians per 100,000 population and 143 per 100,000, respectively). After 1963, the total number of active physicians began to increase at a slightly more rapid rate, averaging between 2.5 and 3.5 percent per year until 1975, when the annual

TABLE 12.3 Number of Physicians and Physician/Population Ratios, United States, 1950–96

Year	Active Physicians	Annual Percent Change	Physicians per 100,000 Population	Annual Percent Change	Foreign-Trained Physicians	Foreign-Trained Physicians as a Percentage of All Active Physicians	Physician/ Population Ratios Excluding Foreign-Trained Physicians (Physicians per 100,000 Population)
1950	108,997	—	139	—	—	—	—
1955	228,553	1.9	140	0.2	—	—	—
1960	247,257	1.6	139	−0.2	15,154	6.1	130
1965	277,575	2.5	145	0.9	—	—	—
1970	311,203	2.4	154	1.3	54,418	17.5	127
1975	366425	3.5	171	2.2	76,784	21.0	135
1980	435,512	3.8	193	2.5	91,826	21.1	152
1985	511,116	3.5	216	2.4	112,660	22.0	169
1990	559,988	1.9	226	0.9	122,823	21.9	176
1995	646,025	3.1	247	1.9	153,790	23.8	188
1996	663,943	2.8	251	1.8	158,282	23.8	192

Sources: U. S. Department of Health and Human Services, Office of Research, Statistics and Technology, *Health, United States, 1980,* DHHS Publication (PHS) 81-1232 (Hyattsville, Md.: U.S. Government Printing Office, 1980), 188; *Physician Distribution and Licensure in the United States Department of Statistical Analysis, Center for Health Policy Research* (Chicago: American Medical Association, 1977); *Physician Characteristics and Distribution in the United States,* 1981, 1986, and 1997–98 eds., Division of Survey and Data Resources (Chicago: American Medical Association, 1982, 1987, 1992); U.S. Department of Health and Human Services, Bureau of Health Professions, A Report to the President and Congress on the Status of Health Professions Personnel in the United States, draft, April 27, 1981, pp. 111–41, Table 7, pp. 11–143, Table 9; *Foreign Medical Graduates, 1986* (Chicago: American Medical Association, 1986); Bureau of the Census, *Statistical Abstract of the United States* (Washington, D.C.: U.S. Department of Commerce), various editions: 1970, 91st ed., p. 40, Table 48; 1985, 105th ed., p. 49, Table 72; 1995, 115th ed., pp. 8–9, Tables 2 and 3, p. 67, Table 82; 1997, 117th ed., pp. 8, 122, Tables 2 and 176.

increase was 3.5 percent. The physician/population ratio also began to show a gradual annual increase during this same period, reaching 171 physicians per 100,000 in 1975.

Part of the increase in physicians over this period was a result of increases in foreign medical graduates (FMGs). The Immigration Act of 1965 permitted large numbers of FMGs to enter the United States.[4] As a result, there was a rapid rise in FMGs between 1966 and 1976. During this period, approximately one-third of the permanent increase

---

[4]Before the 1965 act, immigration quotas were based on national origin (which limited Asian migration). The act eliminated quotas based on national origin and instead established a more flexible system of hemispheric quotas. (Migration from Asia represented the largest portion of the increased migration.) In addition, two new immigration categories—professional members with exceptional ability and workers in short supply (as determined by the secretary of labor)—favored foreign-trained physicians.

There are two main classifications of FMGs: those who have permanent immigrant status and those who

in physician supply was attributed to the inflow of FMGs. In 1960, 6.1 percent of the total number of active physicians were FMGs; by 1975, FMGs comprised 20 percent of active physicians. By the early 1970s, the number of FMGs entering the U.S. exceeded the number of U.S. medical graduates (USMGs). When the physician/population ratio is adjusted for the number of FMGs, the ratio of U.S. trained physicians was virtually unchanged between 1960 and 1975 (130 and 135, respectively).

Not all active physicians are involved in patient care. When the growth in the number of physicians is adjusted to determine those in patient care activities and the number of FMGs is excluded, the physician/population ratio for U.S. physicians engaged in patient care actually *declined* between 1960 and 1975, from 115 to 110 per 100,000 population.

The large increase in the supply of foreign-trained physicians benefited consumers while decreasing physicians' earnings (7). This effect is illustrated in Figure 12.5. The initial demand curve facing physicians is shown as D_1. The initial supply curve, S_1, is relatively inelastic over a short period because of the time it takes for medical schools to produce new medical graduates. (For simplicity, increases in physician productivity and hours of work are assumed to be constant.) In 1966 Medicare and Medicaid had increased the demand for physician services by both the aged and the poor. The demand for physician services in the private sector also increased as employers provided their employees with more comprehensive health insurance. This increased demand is shown by D_2. With the increased demand and the inelastic supply, price would have increased to P_2.

However, as a result of the 1965 law, which increased the number of FMGs, the new short-run supply of physicians (S_2) includes the rapid increase in FMGs and is very elastic. The new price, P_3, is the intersection of the increased demand and S_2.

---

have exchange visitor status. Exchange visitor FMGs are supposed to return to their own countries after they have received graduate medical training. In 1971, the requirement that persons with exchange visitor status had to spend two years overseas before being able to permanently immigrate to the United States was eliminated. This law further eased the migration of FMGs to the United States. The annual increase in exchange visitor FMGs exceeded the number of FMGs permanently immigrating up until the mid-1970s. Exchange visitor FMGs were an important component of total FMGs, and they were becoming a significant portion of all physicians.

In 1976 Congress changed the immigration laws affecting FMGs. Newly entering FMGs were now required to pass more rigorous medical exams, as well as exams in written and oral English. The legislation also restricted the number of FMGs who can remain indefinitely by requiring exchange visitor FMGs to return to their own countries after two years of U.S. graduate medical education. This legislation had its greatest impact on newly entering FMGs with exchange visitor status; their numbers decreased from 2,563 in 1976 to 544 in 1982. The number of newly entering permanent immigrants also declined. As a percentage of total new licensees, FMGs decreased from 36.0 percent in 1976 to 17.9 percent by 1985. In 1984 a more rigorous certification exam was introduced also, which reduced the number of FMGs being admitted to U.S. residency programs.

In 1991 the immigration laws were once again liberalized and the demand by teaching hospitals for residents resulted in a large increase in the number of foreign-born FMGs entering U.S. residency positions—from 2,201 in 1988 to 5,891 in 1994. See U.S. Department of Health and Human Services, Division of Health Professions Analysis, *Report to the President and Congress on the Status of Health Professions Personnel in the United States* (Washington, D.C.: U.S. Government Printing Office, 1981, 1986), pp. III-20, III-143; (1986): III-36, III-38. John K. Iglehart, *op. cit.*

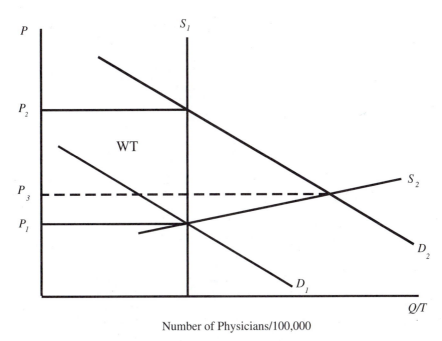

FIGURE 12.5 • An increase in foreign medical graduates on physician earnings and consumer benefit.

The benefit to consumers is the rectangular area or wealth transfer (*WT*) shown by P_1, P_3 and S_1, which is the area the physicians would have had but, as a result of the more elastic supply, the consumers were able to keep. Svorny estimated the size of *WT* for the 1966–72 period using different assumptions of demand elasticity. The size of *WT* was estimated to be 1 percent of total physician expenditures in 1966, increasing to 12 percent by 1972.

Svorny further estimates that physician earnings would have been 11 percent higher by 1971 had there not been any change in the 1965 immigration law.

It is not surprising, given these large wealth transfers from physicians to consumers as a result of the 1965 law, that the immigration laws affecting FMGs were changed in 1976.

Demand for physicians had been increasing during the 1950–65 period, as indicated by the relatively high rates of return to a medical education. We would therefore expect to observe large increases in the number of physicians. However, rather than increasing, U.S. physicians involved in patient care as a ratio to the population actually decreased during this fifteen-year period; the absolute increase in the number of U.S.-trained physicians was extremely small.

The small increase in the number of physicians was not a result of a lack of applicants to medical schools. As shown in Table 12.4, the applicant/acceptance ratio during this period was continually greater than 1.

In fact, the applicant/acceptance ratio appears to track changes in physician rates of re-

TABLE 12.4 Ratio of Applicants to Acceptances, 1947–48 to 1996–97

Year	Applicants/ Acceptance Ratio
1947–48	2.9
1950–51	3.1
1955–56	1.9
1960–61	1.7
1965–66	2.1
1970–71	2.2
1975–76	2.8
1980–81	2.1
1985–86	1.9
1990–91	1.7
1995–96	2.7
1996–97	2.7

Sources: American Medical Association, "Medical Education in the United States, 1971–1972," *Journal of the American Medical Association,* 222(8), November 20, 1972: 979, Table 12; "Undergraduate Medical Education," *Journal of the American Medical Association,* 256(12), September 26, 1986: 1561, Table 5, copyright 1971, 1986, American Medical Association; B. Barzansky, H. S. Jonas and S. I. Etzel, "Educational Programs in US Medical Schools, 1995–1996," *Journal of the American Medical Association,* 276(9), September 4, 1996: 716, Table 3.

turn fairly well. The high rates of return in the late 1940s (Table 12.1) show a correspondingly high applicant/acceptance ratio. As rates of return declined during the 1950s (Tables 13-1 and 13-2), the applicant/acceptance ratio similarly declined. With the rise in the rate of return during the 1960s and 1970s, the applicant/acceptance ratio also increased. The decline in the rate of return in 1985 was matched by falling applicant/acceptance ratios throughout the 1980s.

In 1965, Congress passed the Health Professions Educational Assistance Act in response to claims of a "shortage" of physicians and other health manpower. As a result of this legislation, which provided generous subsidies to health professional educational institutions, medical schools were required to increase their enrollments to qualify for federal funds. The effect of this legislation began to be felt by the late 1960s, when the number of U.S.-trained physicians began to increase at a more rapid rate.

By 1980, the total number of physicians per 100,000 population reached 193 and by 1995 it reached 247. Even when adjusted for the increase in FMGs, the physician/population ratio is greater than it has been for many years. The expansion in medical school spaces resulting from the previous manpower legislation continues to have an effect. The physician/population ratio should continue to increase since the annual percent increase in number of physicians exceeds the annual percent increase in the population.

Even with the increase in the physician/population ratio, the ratio of applicants to acceptances, which had been declining since 1975 (when it was 2.8) to 1.7 by 1990, started to increase once again, to 2.7 in 1996. Although there are no recent data on rates of return, the rising applicant/acceptance ratio during the 1990s is surprising since many believe there is a surplus of physicians during this period.

What can we conclude from the data on rates of return, physician/population ratios, and the ratio of applicants to acceptances to medical schools? During the entire post–World War II period, rates of return to medicine were high and rising. Based on these higher returns, greater entry by U.S.-trained physicians would have been expected. However, it appears that there was very little entry into the profession by U.S.-trained physicians. Although a large number of students demanded a medical education, as indicated by the applicant/acceptance ratio, very few additional physicians were produced. Even after the introduction of federal legislation that led to increases in the production of physicians, there was still an excess demand for a medical education. The only possible conclusion, based on the minimal increase in the number of U.S.-trained physicians until the mid-1970s, and the continued high rates of return, is that a static shortage situation existed.

(The mechanisms used by the medical profession to create and maintain a static shortage of physicians for so many years is discussed in the next chapter.)

Currently, there is a great deal of concern, particularly among medical professionals, that the rapid rise in the physician/population ratio together with the decreased demand for specialists by managed care organizations has caused a physician (primarily specialist) "surplus." If a surplus existed, one would expect to observe a decline in the relative rate of return to becoming a physician, fewer medical graduates taking specialty residencies, and a declining ratio of medical school applicants to acceptances, similar to the situation that existed in the 1930s, as shown in Table 12.1.

CONFLICTING ESTIMATES OF A PHYSICIAN SURPLUS

In one of the more detailed approaches using the ratio technique to derive an estimate of the physician surplus, Weiner, in a 1994 article, concludes that by the year 2000 there will be an overall surplus of 165,000 physicians, or 30 percent of the total number of patient care physicians (8).

Weiner's approach to estimating the "need" (or "requirements") for physicians and the available supply was to use data based on 10 large HMOs to determine the ratio of physicians to HMO members; he found a wide range of physician staffing within those HMOs, from 97 to 163 physicians per 100,000 members. He also examined the nonphysician staffing patterns, or the use of nurse practitioners and physician assistants per 100,000 HMO members. The range was also quite wide, from 0 to 37 per 100,000 members. Estimates were also calculated of the ratio of primary care physicians and specialists.

Weiner then made a series of adjustments to HMO staffing patterns, since the HMOs surveyed were less likely to serve the aged, those on Medicaid, and the uninsured. The purpose of these adjustments was to increase HMO staffing levels if HMOs were to enroll a more diverse population with higher care needs, as HMOs expanded to include a greater percentage of the population. Adjustments were also made for out-of-plan use by HMO enrollees. Several scenarios were used which varied the percent of the population that would be enrolled in different financing and delivery systems (e.g., HMOs, managed, and unmanaged fee-for-service). Different staffing patterns were also estimated for the fee-for-service sector.

Projections to the year 2000 were then derived for the likely number of physicians, by specialty. The difference between the need forecast and the number of physicians available was the likely surplus.

Although the above study was more detailed than previous ratio techniques and attempted to include many relevant factors in making a forecast of physician requirements, a sufficient number of problems remain that raise questions regarding the estimate of the size of the surplus. For example, the range in staffing patterns for physicians and non-physicians varied widely and the surplus estimate was sensitive to which estimate was used as the likely staffing pattern. In an increasingly price-competitive managed care market, continued innovation will occur in the use of physicians and methods to increase their productivity. Innovations in the use of technology to increase physician productivity will also occur in the fee-for-service sector as well as in HMOs. Such changes are likely to change the minimum cost staffing pattern and mix of primary care physicians (PCPs) and specialists.

According to Weiner's estimates, the need for PCPs was roughly in balance with future supply estimates but the number of specialists was likely to be about 60 percent greater than those needed. These surplus estimates, however, were also sensitive to the percent of medical students choosing a career as a primary care physician.

Also excluded from the analysis are the effect on HMOs and managed care organizations of recently enacted federal and state laws that prescribe medical practice (length of stay requirements), staffing ratios, and anticompetitive restrictions (any willing provider laws). These legislative restrictions not only increase the cost of delivering medical services, but also effectively increase the demand for physicians.

Perhaps of most concern regarding the study's projections is that no consideration was given to the effect of financial incentives on demands for care, physician productivity, or PCP/specialty mix. Choice of health plan and use of services are affected by enrollee co-premiums and co-payments. Changes in Medicare policy will greatly affect the elderly's behavior in this regard, similar to the way changes in financial incentives have affected employees' choice of plan and use of services. Physician fees will decline if the supply of physicians exceeds demand. Yet the effect of lower fees on an increased quantity demanded of physician services is ignored, as are the effects of lower fees on physician behavior, such as the decision to choose a medical career, specialty choice, and practice behavior.

As the surplus of specialists increases, more medical graduates are likely to choose primary care instead of a specialty. This shift from specialty to primary care will cause a decrease in incomes of primary care physicians as well, leading to fewer applicants to medical school.

The use of the above ratio technique simply assumes trends in supply and demand for physicians will continue and be unaffected by increases in physician productivity, the growth and use of nonphysician practitioners, such as nurse midwives, or changes in physicians' incomes.

Whether a physician (or specialty) surplus exists, or will occur, depends on the relative rate of return to a medical career. Unless the relative rate of return to a medical career falls below that of a college graduate (or comparable group of college graduates), there is no surplus.

Amidst all the concern about a growing physician surplus, other researchers claim that these fears are overstated. Schwartz et al. calculate the likely future supply of physicians, taking care to project only those engaged in patient care, changes in the supply of residents' services, and the fewer working hours of female physicians (9). With respect to the demand for physicians, the authors project the proportion of the population that will be enrolled in HMOs, the effect of the aging of the population on demand, as well as a per capita growth in demand based on prior periods. Based on these demand and supply projections, the authors conclude that it is unlikely that there will be any surplus. Based on which assumption the authors use of medical advances, there could even be a shortage of physicians.

The authors also contend that whereas a surplus would be indicated by a falling workload and declining physician incomes, during the late 1980s aggregate hours spent by physicians who provided patient care rose as did real physician incomes. These data indicate that demand has been increasing faster than physician supply and is contrary to the prediction by the Graduate Medical Education Advisory Committee that there would be a seventy thousand physician surplus by 1990.

Even if there is a slight surplus, the authors believe that it will largely remedy itself; physicians would become more involved in long-term care, move into administrative positions, or move to underserved areas.

The authors claim that one important way in which their study differs from those predicting a surplus is that they include estimates of increased per capita demands for medical care, based on past trends, that they believe will continue.

At this time there is no definitive evidence of a physician surplus, although there are indications that a surplus may be occurring among some specialties. In contrast to studies such as Weiner's, economic data do not yet indicate a surplus. While there is anecdotal evidence of drastically falling specialist incomes, data presented in the chapter on the market for physician services indicate that over the 1990–95 period physician incomes have increased faster than the CPI (Table 10.8). Physician incomes have, however, fallen in 1995, the most recent year in which data are available (Table 10.7). Is this possibly a trend? Data on the applicant/acceptance ratio have increased during this time, indicating that the demand for a medical education is strong and not indicative of a surplus.

Incomes of several specialties, however, have declined during the 1990s (Table 10.9). Anesthesiologists' incomes fell between 1990 and 1995, while surgeons' and radiologists' incomes did keep up with inflation. These data might be indicative of a growing surplus in these specialties.

Given the uncertainties as to whether there will be a physician surplus, particularly among specialists, what should be appropriate public policy, if any? Should reliance be placed on the market or on government intervention to adjust any imbalance between supply and demand?

PROPOSED POLICIES TO CORRECT IMBALANCES BETWEEN THE DEMAND AND SUPPLY OF PHYSICIANS

Both the medical profession and medical school educators believe that there is an increasing surplus of physicians, particularly among specialists. Medical societies, representing the economic interests of their members, are concerned with the effect of the increased supply on physicians' incomes. Medical schools have become concerned about their own survival, should there be a decreased demand for a medical education. The decline in the applicant/acceptance ratio in 1985 to below 2, for the first time since the early 1960s, lent credence to their fears. Further, several dental schools closed as their applicant pool diminished.

In 1980 GMENAC forecast a surplus of 70,000 physicians by 1990 (approximately 15 percent more than "needed") and 145,000 (or a 30 percent surplus) by the year 2000.

The forecasts by GMENAC of an impending surplus of physicians led to a number of proposals. One was for a reduction in the number of residency positions in each specialty; GMENAC proposed that an agency, such as itself, determine both the number and size of residency programs for each specialty. Another proposal was to phase out residency opportunities for FMGs. Reducing residency positions for USMGs, while more controversial, was also proposed. The Association of American Medical Schools proposed that medical school enrollments be reduced as a means of reducing future supply. Further, to offset the decline in medical school tuition as a result of having fewer students, the federal government should provide "decapitation" grants to medical schools.

The GMENAC study proved inaccurate in its forecast of a 70,000 physician surplus by 1990. Physician incomes in 1990, as described earlier, did not fall as would be indicated by such a large surplus nor did the applicant/acceptance ratio similarly fall. Factors that contributed to the inaccuracy of the GMENAC forecast were the following: the percent of physicians employed in HMOs is lower than forecasted; females as a percent of total physicians were underestimated, thereby overestimating (according to GMENAC) overall physician productivity (female physicians were estimated to have a 78 percent lifetime productivity of male physicians); GMENAC was also inaccurate with regard to its specialty requirements (e.g., the number of cesarean deliveries has been much greater than anticipated); GMENAC did not foresee the spread of AIDS and the consequent requirements for medical care, or the growth in transplants.

Not withstanding the inaccuracies of the GMENAC study, in 1986 Congress created the Commission on Graduate Medical Education (COGME) and charged it with the mission of analyzing trends in physician supply, specialty distribution, and financing graduate medical education (in addition to several other tasks). Based on their estimates of a growing surplus of physicians, particularly specialists, COGME issued a series of reports in the 1990s that included the following proposals. First, the number of residency positions should be reduced to 110 percent (or less) of the number of U.S. medical school graduates (rather than the current 140 percent). This policy would reduce the supply of new physicians by decreasing the number of residencies for foreign-trained physicians by seven thousand a year. Second, 50 percent of the residency positions should be for training generalists, thereby correcting the specialist imbalance. COGME proposed that teaching institutions that did not comply with these guidelines should be denied federal funding.

More recently, the PEW Commission recommended reducing medical school spaces by 20 to 25 percent by the year 2005 and reducing the number of residency positions to 110 percent of the number of U.S. graduates (10).

The intent of these proposals is twofold; first, to limit increases in the supply of physicians by reducing the number of medical school graduates and restricting residency opportunities for FMGs; second, to bring about a change in the specialty distribution of physicians. This discussion is concerned with the first of these objectives.

Medicare is the largest explicit source of funding for graduate medical education residencies and is included as part of Medicare's payments to teaching hospitals for care received by the aged. In 1993 the average Medicare payment per resident was $70,000 and in some East Coast hospitals as high as $200,000 (11). Medicare does not set any limits on the number of residencies it will support. These payments per resident to teaching hospitals increased their demand for residents. Since these hospitals could not receive enough U.S. medical graduates to fill all their residency positions, they recruited foreign-trained physicians. Thus Medicare policy provides an incentive to teaching hospitals to indirectly increase the supply of physicians. Further, Medicare policy provides an incentive for residents to be trained in hospitals (as specialists) and outpatient clinics rather than in primary care or managed care settings, since Medicare only supports training in the former settings.

The attempt to reduce the number of residencies has resulted in economic and, consequently, political conflict between the AMA and medical schools (and those interested in reducing Medicare expenditures) and teaching hospitals, who do not want to lose their financial support. About half of all FMG residencies are in four states—New York, New Jersey, Pennsylvania, and Illinois. Thus the political battle has been geographic rather than according to political party (12). Unless the teaching hospitals are somehow compensated for the loss of Medicare support, legislators from their states are unlikely to support reductions in residencies for FMGs.

Of interest here, however, is the question of how "appropriate" are COGME's and other commissions' policy proposals for reducing the physician surplus? In other words,

374 • CHAPTER 12

are the proposals likely to achieve the optimal number of physicians? Optimal is defined as when the marginal benefit of additional physicians equals their marginal cost. (This would occur when there is a normal rate of return to a medical education. Similarly, the optimal specialty mix occurs when the marginal benefit/marginal cost ratio of an additional specialist [of each type] equals the marginal benefit/marginal cost ratio of an additional primary care physician. This would occur when specialists and generalists earn equal rates of return—but unequal incomes [marginal benefit], since training times [marginal cost] differ.) The optimal number of physicians is discussed more completely in the chapter on the market for medical education.

The issue to be considered here is whether a regulatory policy, such as proposed by COGME, would be more effective in achieving the optimal number (and specialty mix) than a market-oriented approach (13).

Any policy that attempts to manipulate the number of physicians involves deciding what incomes physicians (as well as specialists) should earn. When COGME claims that there is a surplus of physicians, it is stating that physician incomes are or will be "too low." COGME has not explicitly discussed what physicians should earn. Would the criteria be the same as that of an economist, namely, a normal rate of return? Policies to determine physician and specialist incomes would be a very politically charged issue. Therefore it is unlikely that it would be resolved strictly according to economic criteria. Within any profession there is a wide range of incomes, based on skills, work effort, personality, and so on. Would COGME attempt to influence physician incomes, or would it also try to reduce the range of physician incomes? And if so, how? And what would happen if physicians were to increase their productivity and earn more than COGME believed appropriate?

Even if an appropriate level of income could be determined for each physician specialty, it is very difficult for a quasi-regulatory body, such as COGME, to correctly estimate changing demand conditions, productivity changes, and the effect of managed care competition to be able to maintain physician incomes at a given level. COGME would have to continuously monitor these market conditions so as to make appropriate adjustments to the number of medical students and their choice of specialty. Further, given the long training times to become a physician and a specialist, COGME would have to anticipate these market changes many years into the future so as to correctly change the number of new medical students and their specialties.

If the supply of physicians were to be determined by an agency such as COGME, then an error in forecasting would have much greater consequences in terms of the total number of physicians than if individuals forecast incorrectly. COGME's errors would result in much greater changes in the number of physicians than prospective students who differ on the outlook for physician incomes.

No other profession is subject to legislation establishing quotas or income levels to correct what that profession perceives as a surplus. The members of most professions probably favor less entry into their profession, hence less competition and higher incomes.

Given that researchers differ as to whether there will be a physician surplus, and if so how large, regulating future supply increases will have minimal, short-term effects on the supply of physicians. However, such policies can have significant long-run effects on access to care as well as physician incomes. Health manpower policy has overshot its mark in subsidizing the number of physicians that is now claimed to be in surplus. Future policy may be too restrictive with respect to new graduates. Previous manpower projections and policies have been far from accurate. Graduate medical education has emphasized training in a hospital setting while success in a managed care environment emphasizes practice in an ambulatory care setting. And government policy (Medicare payment for residents) has contributed to the "surplus" by providing hospitals with a financial incentive to recruit residents.

Given that medical educators act in their own institution's best interest, and that they have been unable to correctly anticipate future trends, it would appear to be unwise to continue to rely on a regulatory approach for determining the optimal number and specialty mix of physicians.

An alternative approach to economically defining and then correcting physician shortages and surpluses is to rely on market forces. The movement to managed care competition has already reduced the demand for specialists. This information has been quickly transmitted to medical students who have adapted by changing their career choices; fewer medical students are choosing specialty residencies. Allowing market forces, using prices of services and physician incomes as signals, to determine the number of physicians and the specialty mix will occasionally cause imbalances in the supply and demand for physicians. Physician incomes may temporarily increase and decrease as a result. However, these changes in signals will cause supply to adjust more rapidly than will a regulatory policy relying on widely differing projections as to future demand conditions.

It is unlikely that a market or a regulatory approach for determining the appropriate number of physicians will always be accurate. Permitting prospective applicants to decide whether they wish to enter medicine and, similarly, allowing the specialty decision to be made by residents places the burden as well as the benefits of that decision on the individuals rather than on a regulatory agency. Improved information would enable these individuals to make more informed choices. Individual decision making, based on professional and economic incentives, results in a rapid self-adjusting mechanism to changes in the marketplace. These adjustments are quicker and more accurate than if they were to be made by an agency whose constituency (medical schools and the medical profession) has its own economic objectives.

SUMMARY

A great deal of public policy has been directed toward the health manpower sector. Previously, public policy has been concerned with perceived shortages of various types of health manpower. Currently, there is concern over a possible surplus of physicians.

Whether a shortage or surplus exists depends on how they are defined. Noneconomic definitions often relied on the use of the ratio technique, that is, whether the physician/population ratio differs from specified ratio. Problems with the ratio technique include its failure to consider changes in demand and productivity, and an inability to indicate the importance of an estimated shortage or surplus, such as the changes in prices that would occur if the shortage or surplus were not eliminated.

Economic definitions of shortages and surpluses rely on the rate-of-return approach, namely, the rate of return to an investment in a medical education relative to that of a college graduate. Excess rates of return indicate an economic shortage while below normal returns are indicative of a surplus. Static, as compared to temporary, shortages are characterized by increased demand and rising prices, but limited entry into the profession. Entry barriers prevent the elimination of a static shortage.

Concern over a possible surplus of physicians has arisen as a result of the increase in the physician/population ratio and the movement to managed care. The various approaches used to define a surplus provide differing conclusions as to whether a surplus exists. While the physician/population ratio has greatly increased, the applicant acceptance ratio to medical schools is still greater than 1; unfortunately, recent data on rates of return to a medical education are unavailable. Although there is no definitive evidence of a overall physician surplus, a surplus may be occurring within certain specialties.

Proponents of reducing a possible physician surplus have proposed reducing the number of medical school graduates and the number of residencies. If implemented, these policies would increase physician prices and physician incomes, while decreasing access to care.

Having too many or too few physicians has costs and benefits to different groups. Using regulation to determine future supplies is likely to result in too few physicians because current physicians want to have high rates of return and medical schools want excess demand for their spaces. The representatives of these constituencies will dominate the regulatory body as they have with GMENAC, COGME, other commissions, and as they have in the past in determining the number of medical school spaces. Too few physicians imposes a cost on society; fewer physicians means that the prices of their services are higher, access to care by those with low incomes is reduced, fewer physicians locate in underserved areas, and fewer physicians are available to work in innovative organizational settings such as HMOs.

Unlike regulatory policy, relying on the market does not have to consider the political interests of those who may be adversely affected by changing market conditions. Often the economic interests of those affected will motivate the profession to seek legislative remedies that result in market inefficiencies.

Consumers bear the cost of too few physicians, whereas physicians bear the cost of too many. Thus whether greater emphasis should be placed on eliminating a surplus or a shortage depends on one's economic perspective.

The next two chapters describe how previous health manpower policies have been determined by the economic interests of the medical profession and medical educators. The mechanisms used by the medical profession to create and maintain a static shortage up until the late 1970s is discussed next.

Key Terms and Concepts

- Applicant/acceptance ratio
- Derived demand
- Physician/population ratio

- Definition of a health manpower surplus
- Economic definition of a shortage
- Normative judgment of a shortage
- Professional determination of shortages and surpluses
- Rate of return to a professional education
- Static and dynamic shortages

Review Questions

1. What is the difference between an economic and a noneconomic definition of a short-age? What are the consequences if public policy were based on a noneconomic defin-ition of a shortage?
2. Distinguish between the different economic definitions of shortage (e.g., dynamic versus static shortages), and describe the data you would need to differentiate between these different definitions. What might be appropriate public policies for each type of shortage?
3. What are the problems of using health manpower ratios to project health manpower "requirements"?
4. Through the 1960s, there was a shortage of physicians. A proposal to remedy this problem was to provide subsidies to prospective physicians (tuition, interest-free loans, etc.). Comment on the effect this proposal would have had on reducing the shortage of physicians. Be explicit regarding your assumptions.
5. "Trying to prove that there is a shortage of doctors by comparing their incomes to the incomes of lawyers only results in proving that there is a surplus of lawyers."
   a. How do you evaluate this statement?
   b. What does the relative income approach tell you about the supply of physicians?
6. Assume that a particular physician specialty association decides to limit the number of residencies in that specialty. Using diagrams, what would be the expected effect on that specialty and on other physician specialties? Should the physician specialty asso-ciation be concerned about Federal Trade Commission scrutiny?

7. How would be the various indications of a surplus of physicians? What would be the appropriate public policy to reduce such a surplus, if any?

8. Explain why physician incomes are not rising as rapidly as in the past. Distinguish among the different physician specialties.

REFERENCES

1. R. I. Lee and L. W. Jones, *The Fundamentals of Good Medical Care* (Chicago: University of Chicago Press, l933).

2. Kenneth J. Arrow and William M. Capron, "Dynamic Shortages and Price Rises: The Scientist-Engineer Case," *Quarterly Journal of Economics,* 73, 1959: 299.

3. *Summary Report of the Graduate Medical Education National Advisory Committee to the Secretary, Department of Health and Human Services,* vol. 1, DHHS Publication (HRA) 81-651, 1980: 48–56. Volume 2 contains a more complete description of the Modeling, Research, and Data Technical Panel.

4. *Physicians for a Growing America,* Report of the Surgeon General's Consultant Group on Medical Education, Public Health Service, U.S. Department of Health, Education, and Welfare (Washington, D.C.: U.S. Government Printing Office, 1959).

5. Milton Friedman and Simon Kuznets, *Income from Independent Practice* (New York: National Bureau of Economic Research, 1954).

6. The rates of return shown in Table 12.2 are unadjusted for the number of hours worked by physicians. There has been substantial debate about whether the internal rates of return, unadjusted for hours worked, adequately reflect the true internal rates of return to a medical education. Lindsay claims that because of her training a physician will receive a relatively high market wage. This high wage will induce the physician to substitute work for leisure; consequently, the physician will work more hours than someone with a lower market wage. Lindsay believes that there should be an adjustment for the number of hours worked before the income and cost streams are calculated. When Lindsay adjusts Sloan's data for hours worked (he assumes a sixty-hour week for physicians and a forty- to forty-five-hour week for the alternative occupation), the internal rate of return is reduced.

   Sloan's response is twofold: first, he claims that Lindsay overestimated the number of hours that physicians work; second, Sloan claims that being a physician provides intangible benefits, such as increased status in society, which compensate the physician for any additional hours worked. For this reason, Sloan argues, it is not necessary to take into consideration these extra hours when calculating the income and cost streams.

   For a more detailed discussion of the Sloan and Lindsay debate, see Cotton M. Lindsay, "Real Returns to Medical Education," *Journal of Human Resources,* 8, Summer 1973: 331–348; "More Real Returns to Medical Education," *Journal of Human Resources,* 11, Winter 1976: 127–130; and Frank A. Sloan, "Real Returns to Medical Education, A Comment," *Journal of Human Resources,* 11, Winter 1976: 118–126.

7. This discussion is based on an article by Shirley Svorny, "Consumer Gains from Physician Immigration to the US: 1966–1971," *Applied Economics,* 23(2), February 1991: 331–337.

8. Jonathan P. Weiner, "Forecasting the Effects of Health Reform on US Physician Workforce Requirement," *Journal of the American Medical Association,* 272(3), July 20, 1994: 222–230.

9. William B. Schwartz, Frank A. Sloan, and Daniel Mendelson, "Why There Will Be Little or No Physician Surplus Between Now and the Year 2000," *New England Journal of Medicine,* 318(14), April 7, 1988: 892–897. Also see William B. Schwartz and Daniel Mendelson, "No Evidence of an Emerging Physician Surplus," *Journal of the American Medical Association,* 263(4), January 20, 1990: 557–560.

10. The Third Report of the Pew Health Professions Commission, *Critical Challenges: Revitalizing the Health Professions for the Twenty-First Century* (San Francisco: Center for the Health Professions, University of California, 1995).

11. Robert B. Sullivan et al., "The Evolution of Divergences in Physician Supply Policy in Canada and the United States," *Journal of the American Medical Association,* 276(9), September 4, 1996: 704–709. Also see Marc L. Rivo and David A. Kindig, "A Report Card on the Physician Work Force in the United States," *New England Journal of Medicine,* 334(14), April 4, 1996: 892–896.

12. John K. Iglehart, "The Quandary over Graduates of Foreign Medical Schools in the United States," *New England Journal of Medicine,* 334(25), June 20, 1996: 1679–1683.

13. For an excellent discussion of this issue, see Uwe E. Reinhardt, "Planning the Nation's Health Workforce: Let the Market In," *Inquiry,* 31(3), Fall 1994: 250–263.

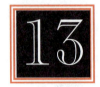

CHAPTER
13

The Market for Physician Manpower

ENTRY RESTRICTIONS IN MEDICINE

To better understand the development of the physician market, it is useful to examine how a shortage situation could have existed for so many years. The concern for consumer protection and quality of care was, presumably, the basis for the various restrictions that were developed to ensure that physicians were well trained. Also to be discussed is whether these measures improved consumer protection or whether they had the opposite effect.

In the previous chapter a dynamic shortage was differentiated from a static shortage according to whether or not there was entry into the market. Persistently high rates of return, it was suggested, could continue only if there were barriers to entry. Based on the small growth in the number of physicians until the mid-1970s, the continual excess of applicants to acceptances to medical schools, the rapid growth in foreign medical graduates, and the increasing number of U.S. students studying medicine overseas, it was concluded that entry barriers must have existed to prevent an equilibrium situation from occurring in the market for physician manpower.

Three entry barriers to the physician's market have been suggested: licensure, graduation from an approved medical school, and continual increases in training, such as the movement to a three-year residency program. There is, however, an alternative hypothesis to explain why barriers in medicine exist: rather than serving to increase the economic returns to physicians, the barriers increase the quality and competence of practicing physicians. It is rationalized that these entry barriers enhance the public interest in a variety of ways. Consumers have very little information on the quality and competence of physicians. Gathering this information is costly and the consumer may be irreparably injured if the physician is incompetent; licensure provides the consumer with protection by reducing the uncertainty as to the provider's training. Occupational licensure has also been rationalized on grounds of "neighborhood effects"; an incompetent physician may harm persons other than the patient being treated if, for example, the physician were to cause an epidemic. Licensure is thus a means of protecting others from bearing the costs of incompetent practitioners; that is, the social costs exceed the private costs (1).

Given these alternative hypotheses to explain the reasons for entry barriers to becoming a physician—namely, to increase physician incomes or to provide consumer protection from incompetent practitioners—which is the more accurate justification? If the barriers are reduced because they are believed to provide physicians with monopoly incomes, will the public lose its protection from incompetent providers? Similarly, if it is public policy to maintain such entry restrictions in the belief that they reduce consumer uncertainty and protect society from incompetent providers, but if in fact such barriers are meant to provide physicians with monopoly incomes, is the public really protected from incompetent practitioners? Could the public be better protected using other approaches, and at a lower cost?

To determine which hypothesis best describes the reasons for entry restrictions in medicine, one must determine how consistent each of these hypotheses is with regard to the assurance of quality or the achievement of monopoly power. If the restrictions are for consumer protection, the medical profession should also be expected to favor other measures that have the effect of improving quality or offering consumers protection from incompetent practitioners. If, on the other hand, the entry restrictions are meant to provide physicians with a monopoly, and to increase their incomes, the profession would only favor those quality measures that are in the economic interests of physicians; the profession would be expected to oppose quality measures that would adversely affect physicians' incomes.

BARRIERS TO ENTRY IN MEDICINE

The first step in controlling entry into a profession is to establish a licensure requirement. Each state has the authority to license occupations under the power granted to it to protect the public's health. A license to practice medicine, therefore, can be granted only by a state. Beginning in the mid-1800s, when the American Medical Association (AMA) was formed, and extending until 1900, the medical profession sought and received licensure in each state (2). The states, in turn, delegated this licensure authority to medical licensing boards, which have the authority to determine the requirements for licensure. These state licensing boards also have the authority to set the conditions for suspending or revoking a license once it has been granted. The conditions for licensure and for maintaining a license can be placed on the quality of care that the physician provides or they can be used to impose restrictions on who can practice, thereby limiting the number of persons entering the profession. The membership of the medical licensing boards in each state consisted of physicians who were either nominated by or were representatives of the state and county medical associations. It was in this manner that county and state medical associations influenced the conditions for licensure in each state.

The earliest requirement for licensure was an examination. Examination by itself, however, is a weak barrier to entry. A person might try to pass the examination many times, and the number of people taking the examination is not limited (3). A more effective barrier is one that raises the cost to those wishing to take the examination. Not everyone would be willing to bear this cost, particularly if there was uncertainty as to whether they would pass the licensure exam.

The second barrier to entry into the medical profession, therefore, was the imposition of an educational requirement and a limit on the number of institutions that could provide such an education. This stage began in 1904 with the AMA's founding of its Council on Medical Education. This group had the task of upgrading the quality of medical education offered by existing medical schools. Of the 160 medical schools in 1906, the Council on Medical Education found only eighty-two offering a fully acceptable medical education (4). To achieve greater recognition of its findings, the Council on Medical Education induced the Carnegie Commission to survey the existing medical schools and publish a report. The resulting report, popularly known as the Flexner Report, recommended the closing of many medical schools and an upgrading of the educational standards in the other schools. "Flexner forcefully argued that the country was suffering from an overproduction of doctors and that it was in the public interest to have fewer doctors who were better trained" (5).

The result of the Flexner Report was that state medical licensing boards instituted an additional requirement for state licensure: before taking an examination for licensure, an applicant had to be a graduate of an approved medical school. The approval of medical schools was conducted by the AMA's own Council on Medical Education. In the years that followed, as expected, the number of medical schools decreased, from 162 in 1906, to 85 in 1920, to 76 in 1930, to 69 in 1944. The number of physicians per 100,000 similarly declined.

The graduates of those medical schools that were closed continued to practice. No attempts were made to rectify any supposed inadequacies in their educational backgrounds. Whenever standards are raised, grandfather clauses protect the right of existing practitioners, regardless of their abilities.

The AMA now had control over entry into the profession in two ways. First, through its Council on Medical Education, the AMA was able to limit the number of approved medical schools and hence the number of applicants for licensure exams. Second, entrants into the profession then had to pass state licensure exams and any other prerequisites promulgated by the individual state medical licensing boards. Thus the AMA, through its Council on Medical Education, was able to determine the "appropriate" number of physicians in the United States.

The third method used by the medical profession to restrict entry, which is also meant to increase the competence of the new physician, is to lengthen the training time required for the student to become a practicing physician. Increased educational requirements increase the investment cost of becoming a physician, thereby decreasing the rate of return to entering physicians. Before entering medical school, a student has to have four years of undergraduate education. Medical school is four years, and the time spent in internship and residency programs continually increases; medical school graduates usually take a minimum three-year residency. For students desiring to enter certain specialties, more than three years is required. The effect of continually increasing the training required before entering a profession is to raise the costs to the entering student. Not only are tuition costs higher the longer the requirements for undergraduate and medical school education, but, more important, the income forgone because of the additional years of training is very large. These increased costs reduce the rate of return to prospective physicians.

The emphasis in terms of quality is always on the training of *entering* physicians and not on those currently practicing in the profession. It is in the economic interests of current practitioners that the costs of entering the profession continually increase; since the training of those currently practicing occurred in the past at a lower cost, they will receive higher prices and higher incomes in the form of economic rent (6).

Until the anti-trust laws were ruled to be applicable to health care in the early 1980s, more highly trained physicians were prohibited by the medical profession from advertising their additional training and more recent knowledge. Thus they could not receive a higher price for their services than physicians without this additional training. To prevent new physicians from receiving higher returns than existing physicians, who had less training, it was necessary for the medical profession to maintain the fiction that *all* physicians were of uniform quality. To enforce this impression among patients, the medical profession discouraged any intraprofessional criticism and, until recently, prohibited the advertisement of differences in training or any other quality differentials among physicians.

Whether a person was permitted to perform certain medical tasks depended on whether she was a physician. A physician was provided with an unlimited scope of practice; it did not matter whether the physician had specialized training. Anesthesiologists, for example, could be physicians who were board certified in anesthesiology, they could be physicians with additional training but not board certified, or they could be physicians without any additional training in anesthesia. Merely being licensed was sufficient to allow physicians to undertake tasks performed by other physicians who had additional training.

This third barrier to entry, which has taken the form of continual increases in the training costs for entering physicians, suggests that measures to increase the quality of physician services were independent of demands by consumers for increased quality and instead were related to the income considerations of the medical profession.

In addition to entry barriers, it was necessary for physicians to control productivity increases among themselves if they were to receive monopoly profits. Otherwise, it would be possible for some physicians to greatly increase their output, with a corresponding loss of business to other physicians, and consequently, a decrease in their rate of return. Productivity increases were (and, in some cases, still are) limited in two ways. First, only licensed physicians were allowed to perform certain tasks, thereby severely limiting the ability of physicians to increase their output by delegating tasks to other personnel.

Second, when new types of health personnel, such as physician's assistants, were trained to undertake certain tasks, previously the sole prerogative of the physician, state boards of medical examiners retained the authority to certify their use on an individual physician-by-physician basis. In this manner, a particular physician would not be able to hire a large number of such personnel and greatly increase his output. The medical licensing boards' control over physician's assistants can be used to approve their use in situations where demand for physician services has increased, or in areas where physicians are not available, such as in rural areas. Their employment can be limited in those places where physicians' practices, from the standpoint of the physicians, are underutilized.

The above barriers to entry and increased training costs, which have been used successfully by the medical profession to restrict both entry into the profession and productivity, have been adopted by other health professions as well. The American Dental Association (ADA), after successfully achieving state licensure of dentists, had a study conducted on dental education, which resulted in the Gies Report in the early 1920s. As a result of this report, applicants for state dental examinations had to be graduated from approved dental schools, with the accreditation being conducted by the ADA's own Council on Dental Education. The number of dental schools declined as standards, mandated by the ADA and carried out by its council, were increased. The length of the training time to become a dentist has also increased; and, as the number of dentists have increased, the ADA has called for an additional year of training in a hospital for new dentists.

The extent to which the price of physician services and physicians' incomes will rise in response to fewer physicians will depend on the elasticities of the demand and supply of physician services. Barriers to entry in the physician market are consistent with a monopoly model that would confer higher incomes on physicians.

Next is an examination of these barriers as a means of protecting the consumer from incompetent providers. For this hypothesis to be an accurate description of the justification for such restrictions, the medical profession, through its representatives in county, state, and national organizations, should favor *all* policies, not just entry barriers, to protect the consumer from incompetent practitioners. If the AMA only favors those quality measures that favorably affect its members' incomes, while opposing those that adversely affect its members' incomes, then it should be concluded that the real motivation for such measures is to enhance the monopoly power of its members.

If the AMA were in favor of protecting consumers from incompetent physicians, one measure the AMA would be expected to favor would be reexamination and relicensure of physicians. One justification given for increased training requirements for new physicians is that there has been an explosion of medical knowledge. Some physicians received their medical education thirty to forty years ago; reexamination and relicensure would ensure that existing physicians have kept up with this increase in knowledge. Reexamination for relicensure is required in other areas, such as for renewal of driver licenses and for commercial airline pilots.

There can be little justification for favoring increased training for new physicians but not for existing physicians, if quality and consumer protection are of concern to the medical profession. Yet the AMA is opposed to reexamination and relicensure. If reexamination and relicensure were required, then unless the passing level were set so low that everyone always passed, either a large number of physicians would fail the reexamination and be unable to practice, or different levels of licensure would be established to recognize what exists in practice. Namely, not all physicians are equally competent to perform certain tasks.

(For physicians to be board-certified, they must pass additional examinations. However, a physician does not need to be board-certified to perform various tasks. A primary care physician in California recently received a great of publicity when he started to perform liposuction and several of his patients died.)

Not all physicians should be permitted to undertake all tasks even though they are licensed. With the realization that licensure should exist by tasks or by levels would come the recognition that it is possible to prepare for different levels by using different educational requirements. It should be possible to have lower training requirements for some tasks; as the complexity of the task to be performed increased, so would the training requirements. One would expect, therefore, that the number of entrants would be greater the lower the training requirements.

If different levels of licensure were to exist, barriers to entry would be lowered and the incomes of practicing physicians would be decreased. Since such an approach to increasing quality among physicians would decrease the monopoly power of physicians, the AMA would be expected to oppose reexamination and licensure by task.

The emphasis on quality control in medicine is on the "process" of becoming a physician and not on the care that is provided ("outcome") once a person has become a physician. Controlling quality and competency of physicians through process measures, which require an undergraduate education, four years of education in an approved medical school, and a minimum of three years in residency, is consistent with constructing barriers to entry and raising training costs, thereby lowering the entering physician's rate of return. Once the physician has met all these requirements, there is no monitoring of the care that she provides.

Physicians may be well trained when they begin practicing, but this does not mean that they will be ethical. A number of studies have documented the amount of "unnecessary" surgery performed under the fee-for-service payment system; other studies showed that a significant portion of all surgery was undertaken by unethical or unqualified practitioners.

Virtually no quality control programs were instituted by the medical profession that were directed toward practicing physicians. It was for precisely this reason that in the

1970s Congress enacted the professional standards review organizations (PSROs) legislation in an attempt to develop peer review mechanisms to monitor the quality of care provided by physicians. The AMA opposed this legislation. If the medical profession were concerned primarily with quality rather than with monopoly power, the profession would place at least some emphasis on the quality of care provided by practicing physicians.

Requiring citizenship for physician licensure, as a number of states once did (it is now unconstitutional), is another example of the use of entry barriers to achieve monopoly power instead of promoting quality. If a prospective physician has met all the educational and licensure requirements, a citizenship requirement can *only* be viewed as a means of preventing entry into the profession by foreign-trained physicians. Although the quality of foreign-trained physicians varies, examinations and other procedures, such as monitoring of care, would be a more direct and accurate measure of quality than whether the person is a U.S. citizen.

Similar to citizenship is the requirement by some professional associations (e.g., state dental associations) of residency in a state before a person is permitted to practice. A year's residency is imposed on dentists who wish to locate in Hawaii. Such a requirement, which forces the practitioner to be without income for a year, decreases the attractiveness to dentists in other states of moving to that particular location. Such a barrier to entry is unrelated to quality, since it does not differentiate among the educational or performance backgrounds of the persons wishing to locate there. It is solely a device to enhance the monopoly power of the practicing professionals in that location.

It would appear, therefore, that the concern of the medical profession (as well as that of other health professions) with quality is selective. Quality measures that might adversely affect the incomes of their members, such as reexamination and relicensure, are opposed, as are any measures that attempt to monitor the quality of care delivered. The hypothesis that quality measures are instituted to raise the rate of return to practicing physicians appears to be consistent with the positions on quality taken by the medical profession.

It has been claimed that the selective approach to quality favored by the medical profession may actually have served to *lower* the quality of care available to the U.S. population (7). Once entry into a profession is restricted, the prices of those services are higher than they would be otherwise, and there is an increase in the growth and use of substitutes for that profession. Patients begin searching for lower-priced substitutes, such as faith healers. Patients also substitute self-diagnosis and treatment for the physician's services. Some of these alternatives may be of lower quality than if the restrictions on medicine were lower. Fewer, more highly trained physicians mean that a smaller percentage of the population will have access to medical care. When only physicians are permitted to perform certain tasks, even though other trained personnel might be equally capable of performing them, this will again mean that a smaller percentage of the population will have access to such services.

A relevant measure of the quality of care in society should not be confined to the care received only by those persons using physician services; it should also incorporate the population that does not receive any (or many fewer) physician services or that uses poorer substitutes.[1]

The current system of medical licensure, with its attendant requirements and emphasis on entry into the profession, imposes certain "costs" on society. The presumed successes of such a system of licensure in protecting consumers against unethical and incompetent practitioners are uncertain. What is desirable is the least costly system for alleviating consumer uncertainty and for meeting society's demand for protection.

Although there is still an excess demand for a medical education, the above entry barriers have become less important as a determinant of physicians' market power. In response to federal subsidies, medical schools expanded their number of spaces and the supply of physicians has been increasing.

Further, as discussed previously, there has been a change in the emphasis on quality of care, away from the process measures used in the past (requirements to become a physician) to measuring the outcome of care. Under pressure from large employers and business coalitions, HMOs, medical groups, and hospitals are being forced to collect and publish data on medical outcomes. Physicians are being profiled on the quality of care they provide and provider groups, such as medical groups, have their own quality assurance programs. Information on patient satisfaction, outcomes, and quality of care is being made available by business coalitions to assist their employees in choosing a health plan and their provider groups.

State medical licensing boards and medical societies have remained passive and reactive with respect to monitoring the quality of care practiced by physicians.

THE PHYSICIAN AS A PRICE-DISCRIMINATING MONOPOLIST

The establishment of barriers to entry and limits on physician productivity under FFS provided physicians with a greater rate of return than if such restraints had not existed. However, a monopolist can earn still greater returns if she were to become a price-discriminating monopolist. Profit-maximizing monopolists charge one price to all of their consumers; that price and the resulting output would be determined by the intersection of their marginal revenue and marginal cost curves. This situation is shown in Figure 13.1. The profit-maximizing price and output would be P_0 and Q_0, respectively.

---

[1]Milton Friedman has claimed that quality has been adversely affected because there was less experimentation in treatment, which tends to reduce the rate of growth in medical knowledge, since a person desiring to experiment in treatment must be a member of the medical profession. The profession also encouraged conformity in medical practice and discouraged malpractice suits against physicians by discouraging physicians from testifying against one another. This action also limited the consumer's protection against unethical and incompetent practitioners. The possibility of high malpractice awards would discourage incompetent practitioners from practicing, thereby providing protection to future patients.

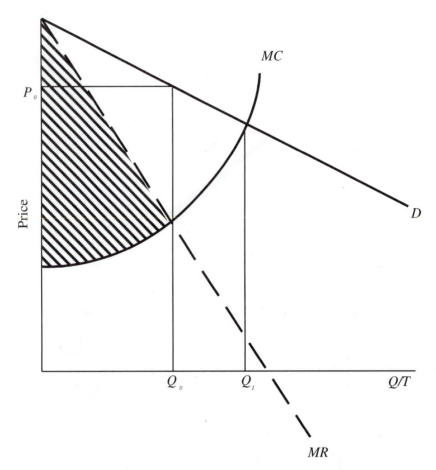

FIGURE 13.1 • Determination of price and output by a profit-making monopolist.

The amount of "profit" in this situation is the striped area between marginal revenue (MR) and marginal cost (MC). (The firm's profit is also the difference between price and average total cost per unit. But since in the diagram fixed cost and average total cost are not shown, the contribution to profit from each additional unit is the difference between the marginal cost and marginal revenue from each additional unit sold.)

When a monopolist is able to become a price-discriminating monopolist (e.g., first degree), thereby able to charge each patient a separate price, the monopolist's demand curve also becomes the marginal revenue curve. The profit per unit is the difference between the price along each point on the demand curve and the marginal cost curve at that price. To sell more services, the monopolist does not have to lower his price to all of his patients; just to those patients willing to pay a lower price. When the demand curve becomes the marginal revenue curve, then with the same marginal cost curve, the monopolist's profit will have increased: instead of being just the striped area, the profit now includes the entire area between the demand and marginal cost curve. The price-discriminating monopolist's output is also larger (Q_1), since he will produce to the point where the marginal cost curve intersects the demand curve, which is equivalent to the marginal revenue curve.

No single price is charged to everyone; the price-discriminating monopolist tries to charge each patient a different price. Because the profit can be greater if the monopolist can charge different prices to different purchasers for essentially the same service, we would expect monopolists to try to become price-discriminating monopolists.

Two conditions must be met if price discrimination is to be applied successfully in any market. The first is that the different purchasers of the service must have different elasticities of demand for the same service. Unless the elasticities of demand are different, the profit-maximizing price will be the same for each purchaser. The second condition is that it is necessary to separate the different markets in which the service is sold, so that the purchaser paying a lower price for the service cannot resell it in the higher-priced market. If such markets are not kept separate, prices will eventually become the same for all purchasers. Figure 13.2 is an illustration of price discrimination where the price elasticities differ between two purchasers or markets. Assuming a constant and similar marginal cost curve for serving each market, the profit-maximizing price would be higher in the market with a less price elastic demand curve, P_1, and lower when the demand curve is more price elastic, P_2.

Since price discrimination results in greater profits than would occur from setting the same price for each purchaser, it was hypothesized that physicians would attempt to maximize their "profits" by becoming price-discriminating monopolists. The necessary conditions for price discrimination are rather easily met in the physician sector. Patients

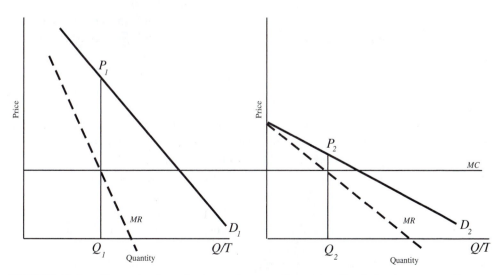

FIGURE 13.2 • Determination of prices and outputs by a price-discriminating monopolist.

paying lower prices for a physician's services cannot resell those services, thereby keeping the markets separate. The elasticities of demand for physician services differ, since persons with higher incomes are willing to pay more for the services than are persons with lower incomes.

Prior to widespread health insurance for physician services, physicians would price discriminate according to their patient's income. As insurance coverage among the population began to increase, the price-discriminating model would predict that physicians would still try to maintain their ability to price discriminate.

An alternative model used to explain physician pricing behavior postulates that differences in prices charged for the same services to different patients were because the physician was acting as a charitable agency. By charging higher prices to those who can afford them, the physician could provide services to persons with lower incomes who could not afford to pay as much. The physician thus acted as a charitable agency in determining who received care and for how much. The charity hypothesis was used by the medical profession to rationalize price discrimination. According to the charity hypothesis, however, as insurance coverage (both private and public) became more widespread among those with low incomes, there should no longer have been a need for the physician to price discriminate. There was less of a need for the physician to subsidize the care of the poor.

When public and private insurance coverage for physician services was examined, however, it was observed that physicians still practiced price discrimination. Until the 1980s, physicians had the option of accepting assignment under Medicare. Physicians could do so on a case-by-case basis. When the physician accepted assignment, she agreed to accept the Medicare fee schedule. For patients who had a greater ability to pay, the physician could decide not to be a participating physician. The patient would then pay the physician's fee and apply to Medicare for partial reimbursement. The physician received a higher fee from the patient while the patient paid a greater amount out of pocket than if the physician accepted assignment. (An illustration of this form of price discrimination was shown in Figure 9.4.)

The same method of price discrimination occurred among privately insured patients, such as those with Blue Shield coverage. The physician could choose to become a participating physician or to bill the patient directly.

To distinguish further between the two hypotheses and to test whether physicians acted as price-discriminating monopolists, the past behavior of county and state medical societies is examined. In this way it can be determined whether the societies' actions and political positions have consistently been directed toward maintaining a situation that enabled individual physicians to price discriminate.

Unless a cartel-like organization such as a medical society were able to enforce sanctions against price cutters, price discrimination could not have survived in what would otherwise be a price-competitive market. Even though entry barriers existed, there was still such a large number of physicians that the market could have been price-competitive. If one physician charged a higher price for a given surgical procedure, for example, other physicians could have been able to increase their market share by offering to sell the procedure at a lower price; price discrimination cannot exist in a price-competitive market. Patients with higher incomes, when charged higher prices, would seek out lower-priced, equally qualified physicians. Differences in prices for medical services would be related only to differences in the costs of providing those services, not to differences in the patients' price elasticity of demand.

To understand how price discrimination could have existed in what would otherwise have been a competitive industry, it is necessary to examine the *sanctions* that could have been applied to physicians if they priced their services competitively.

In his classic article entitled "Price Discrimination in Medicine," Kessel claimed that control over physician pricing behavior was related to the physician's need for hospital privileges and the prerequisite requirement of membership in the county medical society (8).

Internship and residency programs were once offered only in hospitals approved by the AMA. Physicians wanted the hospitals they were associated with to be approved for such programs, since interns and residents increase the physician's productivity, hence income. The availability of interns and residents in a hospital enables a physician to see more patients and to have more leisure time. Interns and residents are thus demanded by physicians. The hospital pays the salaries of interns and residents, while the physician receives the benefits of the services of a resident; the resident cares for the physicians' patients in the hospital. The Mundt resolution, which was declared unconstitutional in the mid-1960s, required that for the hospital to be approved for intern and residency training, the entire attending medical staff in the hospital be members of the county medical society.

Membership in the county medical society thus became important to physicians if they wanted hospital privileges, a necessity for almost all specialties of medicine. Membership in the county society was also a prerequisite if a physician wanted to take an examination to qualify for a specialty board. If a physician engaged in any form of competitive behavior that was branded "unethical," the county medical society, which determined its own rules for membership, could deny membership in the society, thereby denying that physician hospital privileges and access to specialty certification.

Those physicians who potentially offered the greatest threat to the existence of price discrimination were new physicians in the community. To establish a market, new firms must advertise their availability, competence, and specialty, and also offer lower prices to attract consumers away from established firms. To prevent such competitive behavior from occurring, county medical societies gave new physicians probationary membership. If the new physician engaged in any of the above "unethical" activities to establish a practice in the community, the county medical society would revoke membership and thereby deny hospital privileges to that physician. Probationary status was granted, not just to recent graduates, but also to physicians who had been in practice for a long time in another area (and were members of another county medical society) but had recently moved into the community.

After the invalidation of the Mundt resolution, medical societies developed other sanctions for use against physicians who wished to compete on price. Some states enacted legislation proposed by the medical society while other states delegated their authority to the medical licensing board, thereby enabling the board to determine the conditions for medical licensure. Included in state laws and licensing board rules were severe penalties for advertising and fee splitting. Although the mechanism for inhibiting price competition among physicians shifted from control over hospital privileges by county medical societies to state laws that prohibited such behavior, the effect was the same. Strong sanctions and penalties were available to organized medicine (which may be viewed as a cartel) to inhibit price competition, which would have eroded the physician's ability to price discriminate.

According to the above discussion, medical societies had the ability to control price discrimination. However, is there any evidence to suggest that medical societies used the above listed sanctions to maintain physicians' ability to price discriminate? Does the evidence indicate whether the sanctions were imposed for reasons of "quality," or whether they were consistently imposed on physicians who attempted to engage in price competition?

The AMA's position with regard to health insurance was the first evidence that Kessel examined in his test of the price discrimination hypothesis. Physicians would be expected to favor insurance coverage for physician services, since it would increase the demand for physician services. Health insurance, however, can vary with regard to the way in which physicians are reimbursed. Indemnity plans reimburse the patient a certain dollar amount (or percentage) and allow the physician to charge the patient whatever he believes the patient can pay. Such plans are the most conducive to price discrimination by physicians. Health insurance plans that guaranteed medical services, rather than dollars, would be opposed by the medical profession because high-income persons can purchase the same medical service at the same price as can a person with low income. Medical service benefit plans are also price-competitive with indemnity plans.

According to the charity hypothesis explanation of physician pricing, medical societies would not be expected to oppose medical service benefit plans. Thus the only conceivable reason for the medical profession's opposition to such medical service plans is that they undercut the ability of physicians to price discriminate. Examples of such medical service plans are HMOs, where the consumer pays a yearly capitation fee regardless of family income, and is then entitled to hospital and medical services when ill. It is interesting, therefore, to examine the sanctions that local medical societies have applied to prevent the development of HMOs, formerly referred to as prepaid health plans.

The opposition mounted by organized medicine against early HMOs was unaffected by the location of these plans or their sponsorship. The first type of sanction, aimed at putting such plans out of business, was to deny hospital privileges to physicians associated with such plans. If the physician was already a member of the county medical society, the medical society would disband and reestablish itself without including that particular physician. New physicians entering the area with the intention of joining an

HMO in the community would not be permitted to join the county medical society. Whether an HMO had its own hospital determined whether it was able to survive. It is for this reason that Kaiser Foundation, a well-known HMO on the West Coast, operated its own hospitals; otherwise, it could not have offered hospital care to its subscribers and would not have been able to compete. County medical societies leveled other tactics against the Kaiser Foundation. The State Board of Medical Examiners in California tried Dr. Garfield, the medical director of Kaiser, for unprofessional conduct and suspended his license to practice. In subsequent legal rulings the suspension was overruled; the board's action was considered arbitrary in that Dr. Garfield did not have a fair trial.

Another approach used by medical societies to inhibit the development of HMOs was to have a higher proportion of HMO physicians drafted during World War II. (The medical society played a strong role with regard to the drafting of physicians at that time.) A number of physicians serving during World War II were unable to qualify as officers in the Navy and had to serve as enlisted men because they could not obtain a letter from their county medical society stating that they were members in good standing. These physicians believed they were discriminated against because they were associated with HMOs. In other instances where local medical societies ousted physicians belonging to HMOs, successful lawsuits were brought against the medical societies under the Sherman Anti-Trust Act (9).

In addition to attempting to terminate HMOs through the use of sanctions against HMO physicians, medical societies attempted to legislate them out of business. State medical societies sponsored legislation in many states, and were successful in more than twenty states, in having restrictions placed on HMOs, thereby inhibiting their growth. These restrictive statutes permitted only the medical profession to operate or to control prepaid medical plans. (Federal HMO legislation enacted in 1973 specifically preempted federally qualified HMOs from such restrictive statutes.)

Another example of the medical profession's desire to maintain physicians' ability to price discriminate is the type of medical insurance plan favored by organized medicine. Blue Shield plans were developed and controlled by state medical societies and (during the 1940s and 1950s) offered physician coverage to consumers under the following terms. For subscribers whose income was less than a certain amount, generally $7,500 a year, the participating physician would accept the Blue Shield fee as full payment for physician services. However, if the patient's income was in excess of the stated amount, the physician was permitted to bill the patient an amount in excess of the Blue Shield fee for that service.

The medical profession favored Blue Shield because physicians would be assured of payment from low-income subscribers and would still be able to price discriminate among higher-income subscribers. If physicians were charitable agencies, there would no longer be any need for them to charge higher-income patients an additional amount once the lower-income patient was able to pay the full fee for their services (using Blue Shield). During the 1970s, to be competitive with other insurance plans, Blue Shield plans either raised the income limits or dropped them entirely. As a result, a number of medical societies dropped their sponsorship of Blue Shield plans since physicians could no longer price discriminate.

Additional evidence that the charity hypothesis is inapplicable for explaining physician pricing behavior is provided in the following statement by Kessel:

> Most of the "free" care that was traditionally provided by the medical profession fell into three categories: (a) work done by neophytes, particularly in the surgical specialties, who wanted to develop their skills and therefore require practice; (b) services of experienced physicians in free clinics who wish to develop new skills or maintain existing skills so they can better serve their private, paying patients; and (c) services to maintain staff and medical appointments which are of great value financially. The advent of Medicare has reduced the availability of "charity" patients used as teaching material, and has led to readjustments in training procedures, particularly for residents. (10)

The sanctions available to the medical profession for preventing price competition have changed over time. Advertising can no longer be prohibited by state practice acts. That the medical profession had been successful in inhibiting price competition is evidenced by the successful suit brought by the FTC against the AMA and several medical specialty societies (decided by the Supreme Court in 1982). The FTC claimed that the AMA's "Principles of Medical Ethics," which banned advertising, price competition, and other forms of competitive practices, resulted in a situation in which "prices of physician services have been stabilized, fixed, or otherwise interfered with; competition between medical doctors in the provision of such services has been hindered, restrained, foreclosed and frustrated; and consumers have been deprived of information pertinent to the selection of a physician and of the benefits of competition" (11).

The desire by organized medicine to maintain physicians' ability to price discriminate has influenced public policy on financing of medical care for many years. The AMA has always opposed any government program that required all physicians to participate according to a fixed fee schedule. The design of Medicare and Medicaid is indicative of the political power of the AMA. Both programs permitted physicians to participate on a case-by-case basis and to be able to bill the patient a higher fee when the physician did not participate ("balance billing"). The economic power of medical societies (the threat to boycott insurers) similarly influenced the design of private health insurance plans. Initially, private health plans also permitted physicians to balance bill the patient.

Both the political and economic power of organized medicine has declined in recent years as other groups, such as the purchasers of health care (employers, unions, and the government), sought to lessen their financial burden. And the applicability of the antitrust laws to health care eliminated medical societies' economic power.

The medical profession has been successful in acting in the economic interest of its members. The medical profession constructed entry barriers to the profession to limit the supply of physicians. Under the guise of controlling quality of care and eliminating unqualified practitioners, the medical profession emphasized "process" measures of quality control. Quality assurance was present only at the point of entry into the profession by means of requiring attendance at an approved medical school, licensure examinations, and longer minimum times spent in postgraduate training programs; virtually no quality control measures were directed at practicing physicians.

The continually high rates of return to an investment in a medical education and the excess of applicants to acceptances in medical schools are evidence of the successful strategies of organized medicine in creating a static shortage of physicians.

With the authority delegated to medical licensing boards by the state, the medical profession was able to go beyond the establishment of a simple monopoly. The medical profession, acting as a cartel to protect the economic interests of its members, was able to establish and enforce the necessary conditions to enable physicians to practice price discrimination. The sanctions used by the medical profession against members who participated in prepaid medical plans were sufficiently severe as to retard the development of such plans for many years. The consequences to society of these actions by organized medicine were that prices of medical services were higher than they would have been otherwise, the availability of such services was less, and, importantly, consumers were (and still are) not as well protected from unqualified and unethical practitioners as they have been led to believe.

PROPOSED CHANGES IN THE PHYSICIAN MANPOWER MARKET

The objective of proposing changes in the market for physicians is twofold: first, the demand for consumer protection should be achieved in the least costly manner possible; second, the market for physicians should perform efficiently. The key to improving market performance is to deal first with the issue of consumer protection.

Entry into the Medical Profession

If a prospective physician can pass the licensing examination, it is not clear why she also has to have attended an approved medical school. The only logical reason is that the licensing examination is not a sufficient assurance of the physician's knowledge. If this is the case, the examination process should be improved and less emphasis placed on the number of years of education required and on attendance at approved schools.

A second approach to lowering the cost of licensure, while also achieving a certain performance level of entering physicians, is to have "task" licensure. Currently, physicians are either licensed or they are not. Once licensed, they are permitted to undertake many tasks and practice the full scope of medicine, including a number of tasks for which they might not be well trained, such as in the case of the practitioner who is legally permitted to perform surgery and provide anesthesia services, as well as provide general medical care to the patient.

Physicians should be licensed to perform specific tasks. Such task or specific purpose licenses would recognize what exists in the real world: namely, even though physicians are licensed, the public would be better protected if they performed only those tasks which they are qualified to perform.

Task licensure would mean that all physicians would not need to take the same educational training; it might be possible to provide alternative levels of training (or train certain types of physicians) in a much shorter period. Different educational requirements would lower the costs of a medical education, since both educational and opportunity costs would be reduced. If physicians wanted additional specific purpose licenses, they could return to school and receive additional training before taking the qualifying examination for that license. (In this way a career ladder could be developed for medicine.) Under such a proposal, the training requirements to enter the medical profession would not be determined by the medical profession itself but would be related to the *demand* for different types of physicians and the least-cost means of producing them.

Continuing Assurance of the Quality of Physician Services

As discussed earlier, once a physician is licensed, the medical profession undertakes virtually no quality assurance mechanisms. Several proposals to deal with the issue of unethical and unqualified physicians should be considered. First, periodic reexamination and relicensure would require physicians to maintain their qualifications. Rather than mandating a certain number of hours of continuing education, reexamination would determine the appropriate amount and type of continuing education.[2] Reexamination would also be a more direct measure of whether the physician has achieved the objectives of continuing education. Periodic reexamination and relicensure would be consistent with the earlier proposal of task or specific purpose licensure. (Several physician specialty boards require reexamination as a condition for recertification, but the AMA has opposed requiring all physicians be reevaluated for relicensure.)

If physicians were reexamined and relicensed every few years for specific purpose licenses, the public would have greater assurance that physicians were practicing in the fields of medicine in which they were qualified.

Even with reexamination, however, there would still be a concern about qualified but unethical physicians who perform unnecessary services and charge for services not rendered. Continual monitoring of the care provided by physicians is essential. Physicians should be assessed financial penalties, which should vary according to the severity of their misbehavior. Penalties that remove or suspend the physician's license are usually considered to be so severe that they are rarely undertaken. Financial penalties would be more likely to be imposed for actions that are not sufficiently flagrant to call for removal of the physician's license but are in need of redress.

---

[2]After speaking to a hospital's medical staff on the "Economic Outlook for Physicians," I received a letter awarding me continuing medical education credits, which my audience had also received.

Unfortunately, the performance of state licensing boards in monitoring and disciplining physicians has been poor. Although there have been some improvements in certain states in recent years, the number of disciplinary actions against physicians varies greatly among states. As of 1994, the number of disciplinary actions per 1,000 practicing physicians was 11.4 in Florida, 5.7 in New York, 3.3 in Pennsylvania, and 3.8 in California (12). Many states had much lower disciplinary rates. These numbers, although inadequate in many states, still represent a great improvement over their previous state licensing board's performance. In 1982 the disciplinary rates were 7.4 in Florida, 0.5 in Pennsylvania, 1.1 for New York, and 2.8 in California. In 14 states the disciplinary rate was less than one per 1,000 physicians. In 1972 the disciplinary rate was only 0.74 per 1,000 physicians, which included a number of states that had not undertaken any disciplinary actions against physicians.

There is no reason to believe that unqualified or unethical physicians are concentrated (at a greater rate) in some states more than in others. Instead, it is likely that variations in disciplinary rates across states and over time is more a result of the diligence with which the licensing board decides to pursue complaints against negligent physicians.

It is difficult to develop appropriate incentive structures for these state regulatory agencies to act in the public interest. State medical societies are important contributors to state legislators, who would likely incur the displeasure of the medical association if they were to hold annual oversight hearings on the performance of the state licensing board. Thus other mechanisms must be relied on to monitor physician practice behavior.

Malpractice has been the traditional approach used against unqualified and unethical physicians. The purpose of malpractice laws should be twofold: to compensate the injured party as a result of the physician's negligence and to serve as a deterrent to future negligence. Damages to the injured party include economic losses (lost wages and medical bills) and "pain and suffering." Medical societies have, however, successfully lobbied many state legislatures in establishing financial limits ($250,000) on "pain and suffering."

Most instances of malpractice are not pursued. A 1990 study found that less than 2 percent of patients identified as victims of negligence filed a malpractice claim. And about 1 percent of patients injured through negligence received some compensation. Further, of those patients who did not file malpractice claims for negligence, about 20 percent of those negligent injuries were serious disabilities that lasted six months or more, including fatalities (13). Critics of the current system claim that the system does not deter physician negligence since only 2 percent of negligence victims filed claims.

Reliance on the malpractice system alone, therefore, is insufficient to provide the public with assurance that physicians performing the service are qualified and that they act in an ethical manner. Reforms are needed to the current malpractice system to enable it to achieve its twin objectives—deterrence of future negligence and compensation to the victims of negligence (14).

The performance of the medical profession, state regulatory agencies, and the malpractice system in protecting patients against negligent physicians has been inadequate.

One of the consequences of organized medicine's process approach toward quality and its sanctions for violating certain ethical standards was to prohibit the free flow of information on physician performance. Without the availability of data on physician performance, actions taken by state licensing boards, and comparative information on physicians, the public was less able to choose high-quality physicians.

It appears that reliance on a competitive health care market might well be the most useful approach to improving physician performance and providing consumers with the necessary information to make informed choices. Informed purchasers, such as large employers and business coalitions, are beginning to pressure managed care organizations to provide performance data on the health plan itself and on the health care providers with whom they contract. As employers make these data available to their employees in choosing a health plan, employees will become better informed. Competition among health plans will be based on premiums, as well as on other performance measures of the plan and on its provider network. Health plans and their provider networks are recognizing that they have a financial incentive to monitor the performance of their participating physicians.

The changes that have occurred in medical care since the mid-1980s have brought forth a new set of policy concerns. Incentives under capitation are different from fee-for-service. There is less interest in whether physicians can price discriminate as the anti-trust laws have eliminated the professions' anticompetitive practices to maintain such pricing behavior. And concern over a physician shortage has shifted to whether there is now a physician surplus. As the concern over a shortage has disappeared, so has the concern over barriers to entry.

It is important to understand the historical development of the physician manpower market. Many current policies are both the result of and reaction to previous behavior by medical associations. To understand the behavior of medical associations, in the past and present, as well as in the future, it is important to understand the causal relationship between the medical association's economic interests and their political positions.

SUMMARY

The entry barriers to becoming a physician are a licensing exam, an educational requirement met by attendance of an approved medical institution, and increased training times. These "process" measures of quality control have been justified in terms of consumer protection. An alternative explanation is that these entry barriers were designed to limit physician supply and provide physicians with higher incomes.

If the medical profession were primarily concerned with consumer protection, then the profession should be expected to favor all quality measures regardless of their effects on physician incomes. Favoring only those quality approaches that enhance (or do not decrease) physician incomes suggests that entry barriers are meant to increase physician incomes rather than protect the consumer from incompetent and unethical providers. In support of the latter hypothesis, it was noted that the medical profession's emphasis on quality control has been on the process of becoming a physician and not on the quality of care provided. The medical profession has not instituted any quality control measures that were directed toward practicing physicians. Quality measures that the profession should favor but does not are reexamination and relicensure.

Charging consumers according to their willingness to pay (differing price elasticities of demand) would increase physician incomes more than if all consumers were charged the same price. The historical sanctions used by the medical profession to maintain physicians' ability to price discriminate were examined, as were organized medicine's positions on physician payment under public programs.

To enhance consumer protection, several policies, such as specific purpose (task) licenses and periodic reexamination and relicensure were proposed. Further, reliance on a price competitive market in which large purchasers, such as business coalitions, require performance data from health plans and their providers appears to offer consumers more consumer protection than the previous system, which relied on inadequately performing medical licensing boards.

Key Terms and Concepts

- The Flexner Report
- Periodic reexamination
- Task licensure

- Charity hypothesis of physician pricing
- Physician market entry barriers
- Physicians as price-discriminating monopolists
- Process versus outcome quality measures

Review Questions

1. Why does price discrimination result in greater physician incomes than a single price to everyone?
2. What are the necessary conditions for price discrimination? How well have the conditions for price discrimination been satisfied in the case of surgeons? In the case of primary care physicians?

REFERENCES

1. A discussion of the reasons offered for licensure may be found in Thomas G. Moore, "The Purpose of Licensing," *Journal of Law and Economics,* 4, October 1961: 93–117; and Simon Rottenberg, "Economics of Occupational Licensing," *Aspects of Labor Economics,* National

Bureau of Economic Research (Princeton, N.J.: Princeton University Press, 1962), pp. 3–20. K. Leffler, "Physician Licensure: Competition and Monopoly in American Medicine," *Journal of Law and Economics,* 21(1), April 1978: 165–186, hypothesizes that the restrictions cited are in response to consumer demand. See also Lee Benham, "Licensure and Competition in Medical Markets," in H. E. Frech, ed., *Regulating Doctor's Fees* (Washington, D.C.: American Enterprise Institute Press, 1991), pp. 75–90.

2. Reuben Kessel, "Price Discrimination in Medicine," *Journal of Law and Economics,,* 1, October 1958: 20–53.

3. Milton Friedman, *Capitalism and Freedom* (Chicago: University of Chicago Press, 1962), p. 151.

4. Kessel, *op. cit.,* p. 27.

5. *Ibid.*

6. This aspect of licensing board behavior is discussed in Rottenberg, *op. cit.*

7. Friedman, *op. cit.,* pp. 155–158.

8. Kessel, *op. cit.,* p. 29.

9. This example of Group Health Association in Washington, D.C., and other examples cited are from Kessel, *op. cit.,* pp. 30–41.

10. Reuben Kessel, "The AMA and the Supply of Physicians," *Law and Contemporary Problems,* 35(2), Spring 1970: 267–283.

11. United States of America Before Federal Trade Commission in the Matter of the American Medical Association, a corporation, The Connecticut State Medical Society, a corporation, The New Haven County Medical Association, Inc., Docket 9064, p. 3, December 1975.

12. Communication with the Federation of State Medical Boards of the United States, Fort Worth, Texas.

13. A. R. Localio, et al., "Relation between Malpractice Claims and Adverse Events Due to Negligence," *New England Journal of Medicine,* 325, July 25, 1991: 245–251.

14. Patricia M. Danzon, "Liability for Medical Malpractice," *Journal of Economic Perspectives,* 5(3), Summer 1991: 51–69.

CHAPTER

The Market for Medical Education: Equity and Efficiency

PERFORMANCE OF THE MEDICAL EDUCATION SECTOR

In the previous chapter it was shown that barriers to entry into medicine have contributed to the high rate of return from becoming a physician. Perhaps the most important barrier to entry into the health professions is the requirement of having graduated from an approved educational institution. Since such educational institutions determine the number of new graduates, it is important to examine the performance of the medical education sector. Medical schools, dental schools, and other health professional education institutions are the main determinants of the number of health professionals in the United States. They have also been the recipients of large federal and state subsidies. Because of their combined role as the only approved health professional training institutions, as the determinants of the number of health professionals, and as the recipients of public funds, their performance should be examined in terms of (a) the economic efficiency with which this sector performs, and (b) whether there are any redistributive effects (the equity issue) in the manner in which this sector is financed.

THE ECONOMIC EFFICIENCY OF THE MEDICAL EDUCATION SECTOR

Every market performs certain functions. We are interested in two aspects of efficiency with respect to medical (and other health) education. First, is the industry producing an

401

"optimal" number of health professionals? The appropriate or optimal rate of output in medical (or other health professional) education is concerned with both the number of graduates and their type (i.e., the level of training). Second, is the output (a physician or other health professional) being produced at minimum cost? Efficiency in production is judged on the basis of the extent of economies of scale in medical education (the number of schools) and whether each school is minimizing its costs.

To establish an appropriate yardstick by which the performance of the medical education sector can be evaluated, a model of a purely competitive market is used. In examining the medical education sector as if it were similar to a competitive market, we look for any divergences between a competitive market and the current system of medical education to determine the reasons (and justification) for such differences. Using the yardstick of a competitive model and any possible economic rationales for differences between the two, we will evaluate the performance of the market for medical education and, if need be, offer proposals for improving its performance.

Medical Education in a Competitive Market

Both economic and noneconomic determinants affect the demand for a medical education. The major economic determinant of an investment in a medical education is the expected rate of return. One component of the rate of return is the price, or tuition, of a medical education. If other factors, such as physician incomes and the opportunity cost of attending medical school (incomes earned by college graduates), are held constant, a change in the tuition level would be a movement along the demand curve for a medical education. Shifts (to the right) in the demand for a medical education are caused by an increase in physician incomes or a decrease in the opportunity cost of attending medical school.

Tuition, in a competitive market, equilibrates the demand and supply of a medical education. In the short run, with a given stock of medical education capacity, changes in demand for a medical education would cause a shift along a given supply curve of medical education; the tuition level would rise, and at the higher levels of tuition all those demanding a medical education would receive it. The level of tuition would serve as a rationing device and there would be no excess demand (applicants over acceptances). The demand and the supply of medical education would jointly determine the number of enrollments and the tuition level.

The supply response in a competitive market would be as follows. In the short run, each medical school facing an increased demand for its spaces would raise its prices (tuition). The higher tuition levels would enable the schools to attract more resources, namely, to hire additional faculty by raising salaries. As a response to higher tuition levels, additional medical schools will be started (entry into the industry). The long-run effect of the increased tuition would be increased medical school capacity.

Each school would not necessarily increase its capacity as demand increases; some schools might prefer to remain small and offer a "higher"-quality product than other schools, such as more inputs per student or longer training times. Tuition levels in such schools would be higher than in schools that had much larger class sizes and lower training requirements. Whether such differences in types of schools could exist would depend on whether students demanded such differences in the quality of education.

Presumably, just as there are differences in tuition levels and in the perceived quality of undergraduate and graduate schools, there would be a demand for different types of medical education at different levels of tuition. In a competitive system, as in pre-Flexnerian days, the graduates of diverse educational institutions would have to pass a licensing examination. Some schools would have a much higher passing rate for their graduates than would other schools. Graduates from higher-quality medical schools would also find it easier to enter certain residency programs, achieve higher specialization, gain staff privileges at prestigious hospitals, have better liability experience, and be more sought after by certain medical groups. Presumably, the schools would advertise such differences as they would their tuition levels and other educational requirements.[1]

Not all schools under such a competitive situation would be for-profit. Some schools might be nonprofit and have objectives similar to those of medical schools today, such as prestige maximization. As long as entry was permitted into the medical education market, differences in a school's "product"—educational requirements, pass rate on licensing examinations, and perceived quality of that institution—would have to justify the higher input costs, which would, in turn, be passed on to prospective students in the form of higher tuition levels. Unless students (or their parents) were willing to pay for such differences in quality, these educational institutions would either exit from the industry or, more likely, change their product to conform to what was being demanded.

The supply side of the medical education sector, then, would consist of many firms; economies of scale in medical education, such as in library and clinical facilities, are not large enough to result in only one school's being sufficiently lower in cost to preclude competition from other firms. Further, it would be expected that the schools would take advantage of any economies of scale that might exist in medical education, since that would improve their competitive position.

Each school, in addition to moving to that size of operation that was of lowest per unit cost (for the type of product it was producing), would also attempt to minimize its own costs of operation. Again, the incentives for cost minimization would come either from the school's desire to increase its revenues or from competition from other schools offering prospective students lower tuition. Needless to say, schools would be forced to compete among themselves for prospective students.

Thus a competitive market in medical education, with the only entry barrier to the

---

[1]Not all professional schools are considered to be similar. Graduates from the Harvard and Stanford business schools are in greater demand than graduates from other business schools. The job opportunities for graduates of law school are also dissimilar. A similar quality spectrum would exist among medical schools.

profession being a licensing examination, would result in the following scenario. A variety of types of medical education (different training times, different input ratios of faculty to students, and so on) would be offered by different medical schools. Tuition levels would differ and reflect the minimum costs of producing different levels of "quality" of education. Medical schools would use different input ratios appropriate to the differing outputs they produce; they would seek to become economically efficient in producing their product; and they would become more innovative in their teaching methods, in curriculum design, and in the institutional settings where physicians are trained (e.g., ambulatory care settings rather than in a hospital setting as has been the practice). A price-competitive medical education system should result in greater efficiency in production, both for the individual school and for the system as a whole, a greater incentive for innovation, and greater responsiveness to demands for a medical education.

A competitive system in medical education, as just described, would produce an "optimal" number of medical school graduates, which, according to economic criteria, would occur when the benefits of a medical education to the student equaled the costs of that education. The demand for a medical education, at a given level of tuition, would represent the perceived private benefits of that education to the student; tuition would also reflect the costs of producing that education. As the equilibrating mechanism, tuition would reflect both the costs of producing the education and the benefits received from it. The resulting number of medical school graduates would therefore be optimal, inasmuch as the costs of education would equal the benefits from it.

It may be argued that the private benefits under such a system are less than the social benefits of having a greater number of physicians in society. Under such a circumstance the number of physicians would be too few. If there are external benefits to having a greater number of physicians (this will be discussed shortly), subsidies can be provided under a competitive system to increase the quantity of medical education demanded. The subsidies can be given directly to students, which, in lowering their tuition, would increase their demand, or they can be provided to the suppliers. When given directly to the students, students would have an incentive to seek out those medical schools that will provide them with the type of education they desire, at minimum cost.

The foregoing scenario describes how a competitive system for medical education would perform in achieving, at minimum cost, the optimal rate of output of medical school graduates and the different levels of quality in medical education. The crucial role of tuition in a competitive medical education market is to equilibrate demand and supply, thereby providing both the demanders and suppliers of medical education with price incentives as to the quantity demanded and the quantity supplied of medical education.

The Current Market for Medical Education

Tuition, under the current system of medical education, does not serve as an equilibrating mechanism. Medical schools receive, on average, less than 5 percent of their income from tuition payment, as shown in Table 14.1. (For public medical schools, tuition is only 2.8 percent of their income while for private schools it is 5.5 percent.) Since medical schools are not very reliant on tuition as a source of revenue, it is not necessary for them to respond to changes in demand for a medical education. Further, for many medical schools, the operating funds they receive from their university are unrelated to changes in their enrollment levels.

Medical schools are able to survive and to produce the type of medical education they want because they receive large, relatively unrestricted government subsidies. (Revenues from state and local governments represent 17.7 percent of public medical schools' unrestricted support, down from 33.9 percent in 1979–80.) The large educational subsidies received by the schools (and research grants and contracts that have also been used to subsidize educational activities) permit the schools to set tuition levels below actual costs of production.

According to several studies, tuition and fees covered less than 10 percent of the cost of education in 1972 and 15 percent in 1989 (1). (In 1989 this percentage was 27 percent for private schools and 8 percent for public schools.) When these figures are updated to 1995, tuition and fees were less than 20 percent of the cost of education (2).

Subsidized tuition causes demand for a medical education to be greater than it would be otherwise. This increased demand as a result of subsidized tuition, however, is not satisfied. The number of applicants admitted by medical schools is determined by the number of available spaces. The number of spaces, in turn, is unrelated to the demand for a medical education or to tuition levels; instead, the number is determined by the goals and objectives of the schools themselves. There is thus a continual excess demand for medical education by qualified students, given the high rates of return to a career in medicine and subsidized tuition.

This excess demand is shown schematically in Figure 14.1. With an initial demand for medical education shown by the demand curve D_1, and the supply of spaces shown by S, the amount of excess demand for medical school spaces would be $Q_1 - Q_0$, when the tuition level is T_1, which is below the equilibrium level. As physician incomes increase (or other demand shift variables change), there is an increase in the demand for a medical education to D_2. Again, since tuition does not serve its rationing function, the excess demand for a medical education increases to $Q_2 - Q_0$.

On what basis does the medical school ration its spaces, since it does not rely on tuition to perform this function? It is hypothesized that the medical school will select students who are most compatible with the goals of the school. Because all approved medical schools are nonprofit, they must have an objective other than trying to make the most money. It is hypothesized that their objective is one of prestige maximization, which is accomplished by retaining a faculty that is interested in research, a low student/faculty ratio that allows more time for research, and training medical students to be teachers and researchers rather than family practitioners.

The average medical school is likely to try and emulate Johns Hopkins and Harvard

TABLE 14.1 Patterns of Support for General Operations of Public and Private Medical Schools, 1968–69, 1979–80, and 1994–95 (Millions of Dollars)

	1968–69		1979–80		1994–95	
	Public Schools					
Number of medical schools reporting	47		73		74	
Total restricted support	$330	(52.0)	$1,102	(34.7)	$3,412	(22.5)
Total unrestricted support	305	(48.0)	2076	(63.5)	11762	(77.5)
State and local government appropriations and subsidies	171	(26.9)	1078	(33.9)	2691	(17.7)
Professional fee (medical service plan) income	38	(6.0)	359	(11.3)	5039	(33.2)
Recovery of indirect cost on contracts and grants	38	(6.0)	105	(3.3)	711	(4.7)
Tuition and fees	16	(2.5)	89	(2.8)	425	(2.8)
Income from college services	3	(0.5)	36	(1.1)	—	—
Endowment income	1	(0.2)	2	(0.1)	106	(0.7)
Gifts	2	(0.3)	31	(1.1)	222	(1.5)
Hospital and clinics	—	—	191	(6.0)	1774	(11.7)
Other income	36	(5.6)	185	(5.8)	795	(5.2)
Total public schools support	$635	(100.1)	$3,178	(100.0)	$15,174	(100.0)
	Private Schools					
Number of medical schools reporting	44		46		51	
Total restricted support	$450	(62.8)	$1,283	(50.9)	$3,781	(26.6)
Total unrestricted support	272	(37.2)	1240	(49.1)	10412	(73.4)
State and local government appropriations and subsidies	17	(2.3)	82	(3.3)	139	(1.0)
Professional fee (medical service plan) income	28	(3.8)	311	(12.3)	4737	(33.4)
Recovery of indirect cost on contracts and grants	56	(7.7)	215	(8.5)	1170	(8.2)
Tuition and fees	36	(4.9)	219	(8.6)	786	(5.5)
Income from college services	19	(2.6)	23	(0.9)	—	—
Endowment income	31	(4.2)	52	(2.1)	371*	(2.6)
Gifts	21	(2.9)	49	(1.9)	397	(2.8)
Hospital and clinics	—	—	189	(7.5)	2187	(15.4)
Other income	64	(8.8)	100	(4.0)	624	(4.5)
Total private schools support	731	(100.0)	2523	(100.0)	14193	(100.0)
Total medical schools support private and public	$1,366		$5,701		$29,367	

Sources: American Medical Association, *Journal of the American Medical Association,* 246(25), December 25, 1981: 2929, Table 34; J. Y. Krakower, J. L. Ganem, and P. Jolly, "Review of US Medical School Finances, 1994–1995," *Journal of the American Medical Association,* 276(9), September 4, 1996: 722, Table 3.

Note: Total restricted support includes federal appropriations plus direct part of federal and other grants and contracts. Other Income includes miscellaneous sources and parent university support.

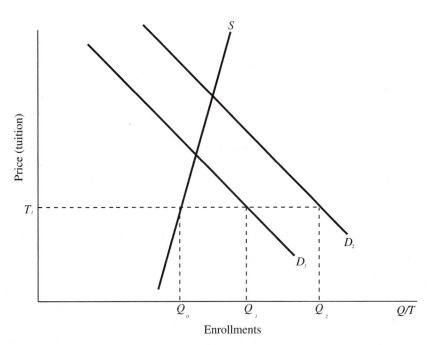

FIGURE 14.1 • The excess demand for a medical education.

medical schools, with their small class sizes, low student/faculty ratios, and emphasis on research. To achieve these goals, medical schools and their faculties want to select students based on high academic qualifications rather than on their future work preferences, such as desiring to work in rural areas. (There is little prestige among medical schools in having the highest percentage of its graduates become primary care practitioners in a rural area.) The excess of applicants resulting from setting tuition levels below the equilibrium level allows the faculty to select those students who most closely correspond to their goals.[2]

Attaining the goal of prestige maximization requires medical schools to be free from competitive pressures. If a school has to compete, then, as we have seen in the discussion of the competitive model, it will be forced to respond to the demands of students. Essential to freeing the school from competition are huge outside subsidies that relieve the school of reliance on tuition as a sole source of revenue.

---

[2]It has been claimed that the reduction in the number of medical schools as a result of the Flexner Report and the consequent excess demand for spaces enabled medical schools to discriminate against certain population groups in society (i.e., Jews, blacks, and women). Reuben Kessel, "The AMA and the Supply of Physicians," *Law and Contemporary Problems,* Duke University, Spring 1970: 270–272. In the 1970 Carnegie Commission Report on Medical Education, *Higher Education and the Nation's Health,* they suggest that medical schools "Refrain from discrimination on the basis of race, creed, or sex and also pursue positive policies to encourage the admission of members of minority groups" (p. 69).

Also important to achieving their goal are limits on entry into the medical school market by new medical schools that might have different objectives. The manner in which this restriction is achieved is through the accreditation process of new medical schools. It would be very difficult for a new medical school to start if its stated intention was to produce its graduates in a vastly shorter period, using a different curriculum and different input ratios to train its students. Because it might produce graduates at a much lower cost with the same probability of their passing the licensing examination, such a school would be a potential threat to other schools, and therefore it is in these schools' interests to prevent such a school from developing.

The Liaison Committee on Medical Education (LCME) accredits schools providing an MD degree and establishes the criteria the school must adhere to if it is to be accredited (3). For example, a minimum number of weeks of instruction and four calendar years for the instruction to occur are specified. An undergraduate education, usually four years, is required for admission to a medical school. Innovations in curriculum and changes in the length of time for becoming a physician (and to prepare for admission to a medical school) must be approved by the LCME. The LCME further states that the cost of a medical education should be supported from diverse sources: tuition, endowment, faculty earnings, government grants and appropriations, parent university, and gifts. By its concern that there not be too great a reliance on tuition, the LCME encourages the schools to pursue revenue sources and goals unrelated to educational concerns.

Medical schools must also be not-for-profit, if they are to be accredited. There is no incentive for private organizations (such as HMOs) to invest capital to start a new school by demonstrating that they could produce physicians at lower cost and of equal, if not higher, quality than many nonprofit medical schools.

It has been generally recognized for some time that medical schools are in need of reform. Since the 1960s there have been nine commissions to recommend changes to be undertaken by medical schools. A 1989 survey found that medical school deans, department chairs, and faculty overwhelmingly endorsed the need for "fundamental changes" or "thorough reform" in medical education (4). However, because faculty promotion and tenure are based on research productivity and clinical expertise, they do not have incentives to reform the educational process. Instead, the faculty emphasize the goals of their own academic specialty and department, rather than the educational goals of the school.

What are the consequences of the current system for producing physicians? On the supply side of the market, the educational requirements for producing physicians are determined by the suppliers themselves without regard to demands for such an education. The product is relatively standard and many years of education are required: four years of undergraduate education before admission to a four-year medical school. The product is relatively costly to produce and there are large variations among schools in their costs of production. There are strong indications, based on the wide variations in cost data, that the schools are not minimizing their cost of production, nor do they have any incentive to do so as long as they are the recipients of large government subsidies. It thus appears that efficiency in production is the exception rather than the rule.

It is also highly unlikely that the current system of medical education produces the appropriate number of graduates. Since tuition is only a small portion of the actual costs of education, the demand is much greater than it might be otherwise. (The price elasticity of demand for a medical education with respect to the tuition rate has been estimated to be approximately −0.4) (5). The demand for a medical education has continually exceeded the supply of medical school spaces, which have increased very slowly over time. As shown in Table 14.2, between 1946–47 and 1965–66, the number of medical school enrollments increased by less than 2 percent per year. Throughout this period there was a continual excess demand for medical school spaces.

The number of physicians produced was determined by the suppliers of education, either in conjunction with other organizations' requirements or solely in response to their own. The goals of medical schools appear to have been synonymous with the objectives of the American Medical Association. The AMA also prefers small additions to the stock of physicians. It is therefore in the AMA's interest that medical schools be nonprofit. The schools' incentive thereby changes from cost minimization and responding to increased demands for spaces to becoming prestigious.

The result of the constraint on the number of medical school spaces was twofold. First, there was a large demand by American students for a foreign medical education. Large numbers of qualified, but rejected, medical school applicants went overseas to study medicine and then reentered the United States to practice. These American students were willing to pay a much higher tuition level in places such as Guadalajara, Mexico, to spend additional years in residence (thereby increasing their opportunity costs), and receive an education considered inferior to that received in U.S. medical schools. Second, as a result of increased demands for medical care during this period, the rates of return for practicing medicine became even greater in the United States than in other countries, thereby providing FMGs with an even greater incentive to migrate to this country. These FMGs came predominately from less-developed countries to work on hospital staffs, and in many cases, they provided the medical care for the urban poor in the United States.

Congress responded to the demands by U.S. citizens to stem the inflow of foreign-trained physicians and enable their own children to have an opportunity for a medical education by passing the Health Professions Educational Assistance Act (HPEA) in the mid-1960s. The effect of this act was to increase the supply of medical school spaces. It was, therefore, the perception of Congress that the medical education market was not producing an appropriate number of physicians. To achieve an increase in the supply of physicians, funds were provided for new medical schools, and existing medical schools received capitation funds on the condition that they increase their enrollments.

Although the AMA and medical schools opposed mandatory enrollment increases, medical schools were in need of additional funds. These congressional financial incentives to medical schools proved to be effective. As a result of the HPEA legislation, enrollments and graduates began to increase. In 1965–66 there were 32,835 medical students in 88 medical schools. By 1980, the number of students had risen to 65,497 in

126 schools. (See Table 14.2.) (The consequence of this increase in medical school enrollment was a 50 percent increase in the number of physicians between 1965 and 1980.)

By the late 1970s, these large projected increases in the supply of physicians led to a concern, particularly among organized medicine and government, that "too many" physicians were being produced. As a result, the preferential immigration treatment for FMGs was removed, making it more difficult for FMGs to enter this country, and the HPEA financial assistance to medical schools began to be phased out in the early 1980s.

Between 1980 and 1996, as shown in Table 14.2, the number of students in medical schools has been approximately constant each year, regardless of the demand for such an education. This limit on the number of medical school admissions is expected to continue as decisions on the number of physicians are made by the suppliers rather than the demanders of a medical education.

Efficiency, Externalities, and the Optimal Number of Physicians

The optimal quantity of output in an industry occurs when the cost of producing the last unit equals the additional benefits from consuming it. The price that people are willing to pay for that output is an indication of the marginal benefits they hope to receive from consuming it. When price is equal to marginal cost, as would occur in a competitive mar-

TABLE 14-2 U. S. Medical School Enrollment, First-Year Students and Graduates, 1946–47 to 1995–96

Academic Year	Students Total	Students First-Year	Students Graduates	Number of Schools
1946–47	23,900	6,564	6,389	77
1950–51	26,189	7,177	6,135	79
1955–56	28,639	7,686	6,845	82
1960–61	30,288	8,298	6,994	86
1965–66	32,835	8,759	7,574	88
1970–71	40,487	11,348	8,974	103
1975–76	56,244	15,351	13,561	114
1980–81	65,497	17,204	15,667	126
1985–86	66,604	16,929	16,125	127
1990–91	64,986	16,803	15,499	126
1995–96	66,906	17,024	16,029	125

Sources: American Medical Association, *Journal of the American Medical Association,* 226, November 19, 1973: 910, copyright 1973; H. S. Jonas, S. I. Etzel, and B. Barzansky, "Educational Programs in US Medical Schools," *Journal of the American Medical Association,* 266(7), 1991: 916; B. Barzansky, H. S. Jonas, and S. I. Etzel, "Educational Programs in US Medical Schools, 1995–1996," *Journal of the American Medical Association,* 276(9), September 4, 1996: 716.

ket, the marginal private benefits equal the marginal private costs of production, and the optimal quantity of that good or service is produced (assuming no external effects). Those persons receiving the benefits of the good or service are paying the full costs of producing it.

When the concept of marginal benefits and marginal costs is applied to the number of physicians, the optimal number of physicians is produced when the cost of producing physicians is equal to the price (tuition) of a medical education. The price that a student is willing to pay for a medical education reflects the private benefits the student hopes to receive as a result of that education. If the price that prospective students are willing to pay for a medical education is greater than the price charged for a medical education, too few physicians are being produced. More resources should flow into that industry until the cost of producing additional physicians equals the price that students are willing to pay for that education.

Under the current system of medical education, however, the costs of producing physicians are greater than they would be in a system where there were fewer artificial educational requirements, such as minimum years required both before entering and during medical school, and where there were incentives for efficiency. Thus even if tuition were equal to the full costs of a medical education, too few physicians would be produced. Since the price is greater than minimum cost, demand would be greater. And additional physicians could be produced if the producers were more efficient and tuition reflected those lower costs of production.

It has been alleged, however, that in addition to the private benefits gained by the student receiving a medical education, there are benefits to the public at large from having a greater number of physicians (6). According to this argument, basing the demand for a medical education on just the private benefits to be received by students would result in too low an estimate of the demand for a medical education. The existence of additional (external) benefits, to be received by persons other than students, when added to the private demand by students would result in a greater demand for a medical education.

As shown in Figure 14.2, *MPB* represents the marginal private benefits received by students from a medical education. *MPC* represents the marginal private costs of producing additional physicians. The intersection of these marginal private benefit and cost curves would result in Q_0 number of physicians. Q_0 physicians is believed by some persons to be a nonoptimal number, that is, too few, because the external benefits to others from having physicians (*MEB*) are excluded from this calculation. If these external benefits are included, the sum of both the private and external benefits, shown by the line *MTB*, would intersect the *MPC* curve at a point to the right of Q_0 physicians; Q_1 would then be the optimal quantity of physicians.

The manner in which these external benefits would be included in the foregoing calculation would be to provide a government subsidy, the size of which would reflect the magnitude of the external benefits. To achieve the increased output, the government could provide a subsidy to the suppliers sufficient to shift the *MPC* curve down so that it

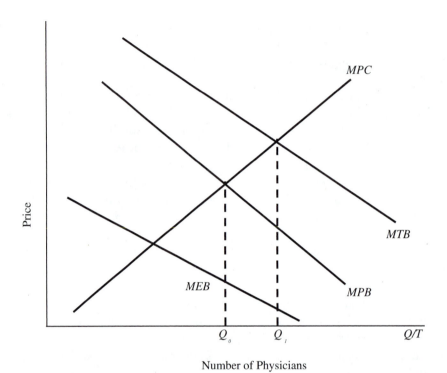

FIGURE 14.2 • An illustration of external benefits in medical education.

intersects the *MPB* curve along the dotted line to the point where *MPB* and the new *MPC* result in output Q_1. This government subsidy could be distributed either to prospective medical students, which would lower their tuition costs and increase the quantity demanded of a medical education, or, in a competitive market, the subsidy could be provided to the medical schools, thereby lowering their cost and, consequently, tuition.

It is important to determine whether there are external benefits (and, if so, their magnitude) from having additional physicians. If there are sufficient external benefits, this would justify government subsidization of medical education so as to achieve an optimal number of physicians. (It would still be necessary to calculate the size of the external benefits in order to calculate the number of additional physicians that would have to be produced and the consequent size of the government subsidy.)

Before attempting to answer the question of whether external benefits exist with regard to the number of physicians, an externality should be defined. When someone undertakes an action, such as purchasing or producing a good or service in the private market, and this action has side effects on other persons or firms that are not taken into account by the normal operations of the price system, an externality is said to have occurred. Since the allocation decisions of others are affected by the initial private decisions that created the externality, failure to consider these secondary allocation decisions would result in either too few or too many resources in the market. There are different types of external effects, both positive and negative, as well as externalities in consumption and in production.

For public policy purposes it is important to distinguish between technological and pecuniary externalities. The former are direct, nonmarket effects on others. For example, as a result of producing a product, a firm pollutes the water, thereby imposing a cost on those using the stream. Pecuniary externalities occur within the market; therefore they do not affect the market's ability to allocate resources. For example, as a result of an increase in demand by some participants in the market, the price is increased to all other participants in the market. Government intervention is required only when the externality occurs outside the market (technological externality) to correct what would otherwise be a misallocation of resources (7).

When externalities occur, the government, by calculating the extent of external costs and/or benefits and using a system of taxes and subsidies, should attempt to achieve the optimal allocation of resources. Such a process of nonmarket decision making would involve the use of methodologies such as cost/benefit analysis.

It is not easy to determine the extent of externalities, if any, in medicine. With regard to medical research, traditional public health programs, and water fluoridation, the case for externalities seems clear. Individuals undertaking medical research do not collect from all who benefit from such knowledge. And since all those who benefit do not contribute to the production of that research, too little research would be undertaken if it were based solely on support from those who contribute. The government should, therefore, calculate the size of external benefits, levy the appropriate amount of tax on those who receive the external benefit, and subsidize the production of medical research. Only in this manner would the optimal quantity of research be undertaken.

An example of external benefits in personal medical care occurs when an individual includes in her utility function the access to medical care by others. Government intervention in such a situation should seek to increase the consumption of or availability of medical care to low-income persons. This can be more directly achieved through some form of demand-increasing program to such persons rather than by indirectly subsidizing medical schools, which may have little or no effect on increasing the availability of care to such persons.

The issue is, are there external benefits as a result of having a greater quantity of medical education or a larger number of physicians? Is it possible to specify the benefits that accrue to others, or to society as a whole, in addition to those who purchase physician services? Without government subsidies to medical education, there would exist a certain stock of physicians, which would be determined by the private demand and private costs of producing them. Are there external benefits to having more physicians than would be provided under the private market? (The total contribution of physicians may be large, but their marginal contribution has been estimated to be small.)

The case for public subsidies as a result of externalities in education has generally been made with regard to grade-school education: everyone in a democratic society benefits from having a better-educated electorate. The case for public subsidies to higher education is weaker, and it is not at all clear that a case can be made for subsidies for a professional or technical education (8).

It is not enough to merely assert that there are external benefits to having a greater number of physicians and then to call for massive government support for medical schools. Even assuming that there are some external benefits of having a minimum number of physicians ("We all benefit by having physicians available in case we need them"), this would not justify government subsidies. The private market is likely to produce this minimum number. For example, with reference to Figure 14.2, if, when MEB and MPB are summed, their intersection occurs to the left of where MPB intersects MPC, then the private market will produce the optimal quantity of physicians. When the private market produces the optimal quantity, even though there are external benefits, it is referred to as "inframarginal" externalities.

Since there is neither clear evidence nor strong argument that external benefits exist in medical, dental, or veterinary education, the case for public subsidies to the health professions' educational institutions on grounds of externalities should be reexamined.

There might be other grounds for providing public subsidies to the health professions, such as attracting a certain mix of students, or having medical graduates locate in an underserved area. Such subsidies are based on societal value judgments rather than on externalities. The case for subsidies to medical education on other grounds will be discussed subsequently. These grounds include the improvement of equity in the distribution of medical care to the recipients, or the redress of possible market imperfections if medical education were to be financed through a full-cost tuition program. The equity of the current system of financing education (i.e., who receives the subsidies and who bears the cost) will also be discussed.

Some Proposals for Improving the Efficiency of the Current Market for Medical Education

An important defect in the current market for medical education is that there is no link between tuition and the role such a price variable should play on both the demand and the supply side of the market. When tuition acts as a price on the demand side, as would occur in a competitive market, then all who are willing to pay that price would have access to a medical education. There would be no need for thousands of Americans to pay higher costs to study medicine overseas. If medical schools were not provided with large educational subsidies, tuition would have to reflect all the costs of a medical education.

Allowing tuition to serve as a true price of medical education would encourage the suppliers to be efficient in production. If suppliers were inefficient and had to charge tuition of more than $100,000 a year, which is the educational cost per student per year in many medical schools they would have difficulty in filling their spaces. It is highly likely that educational costs would be greatly reduced in a competitive educational market. Tuition would become a more accurate signal for determining the optimal number of physicians when supply subsidies are either eliminated or sharply reduced and entry by new suppliers of medical education is permitted. Efficiency in consumption as well as in production would then occur.

If tuition reflected all the costs of education and prospective students had to pay all these costs, low-income students might be precluded from becoming physicians. Only students from high-income families would be able to afford what would be very high tuition costs (e.g., in excess of $400,000 for four years of medical school). However, in a price-competitive system (where quality is based on a number of examinations prior to entering the profession rather than on specific educational requirements prior to a licensure exam) full-cost tuition would be much lower than it is at present.

The cost per graduating student will be lower for two reasons. First, medical schools will have greater incentives to become more efficient and thereby reduce educational costs. Over time the medical school has evolved into an Academic Health Center (AHC), which includes a medical school and one or more primary teaching hospitals. AHCs have increased the number of medical school faculty and residency positions in response to their funding needs, grants for undertaking research, and payment for providing patient care, rather than for teaching medical students. Indicative of the AHCs' response to research and patient care funding sources is that while medical school enrollment has been relatively constant over the 1986–95 period, full-time clinical faculty have increased by more than 50 percent along with similar increases in faculty salaries over that same period.

It is likely that if medical education costs were accurately separated from patient care and research costs, together with the faculty engaged in each activity, education costs would be much lower than they are believed to be.

Pressures to increase efficiency at the medical school and the AHC are occurring because of the increase in managed care. Managed care is reducing medical schools' clinical patient care revenues (derived from faculty practice plans and teaching hospital revenues), which account for almost half of the schools' budget. Managed care plans emphasize primary care while medical school faculties have been predominately specialist-oriented. For the AHC to be price-competitive with other hospitals and to downsize as inpatient care declines, the AHC will be forced to reduce the number and type of clinical faculty.

Several medical schools are developing cooperative relationships with managed care plans to provide their students with an opportunity to work in a managed care setting and to learn about cost-effective alternatives without reducing quality. Medical schools will have to reduce their costs and reorient their educational objectives if they are going to survive in a managed care environment.

The second reason educational costs will be lower is because medical schools will also have an incentive to innovate in their curricula and teaching methods. As a result, the opportunity costs of entering the profession will be greatly reduced: Other countries, such as Great Britain, do not require a four-year undergraduate degree before entering a four-year medical school (9). Medical school deans acknowledge that the training times for entering the profession could be reduced by several years and the curriculum revamped. As one dean has said, "Despite the striking changes in patterns of physician education and practice, little change has occurred in the structure of the medical school curriculum since 1910." Further, there is "the rigidity of the established system that is sharply demarcated by four years of college, four years of medical school, and three to seven years of graduate medical education. The inflexibility of this structure has made it almost impossible to introduce new subjects into an already overcrowded medical school curriculum, which, in part, reflects redundancies between college science and medical school science, as well as between clinical experience in the last two years of medical school and clinical experience during three to seven years of graduate medical education" (10).

The opportunity costs associated with the long educational requirements to become a physician are more costly than increased tuition levels. In addition to receiving a physician's income three years earlier, the student would save undergraduate tuition and fees if he were to enter medical school after two years of undergraduate education and one less year of medical school.

Previously, the Carnegie Commission Report on Medical Education recommended reducing the number of years in medical school from four to three. Thus medical school tuition would be paid for only three years instead of four. If a starting physician were to earn approximately $100,000 a year, each year that the educational process could be reduced saves tuition and adds to the physician's income. Tuition could be greatly increased each year to offset the benefit to the student of entering practice one year earlier. If, as has been recommended, the student entered medical school after two years of undergraduate education and medical school were reduced by one year, the rate of return to a medical education would not be adversely affected by increased tuition.

An important concern to many persons, however, is that under a system of full-cost tuition the medical profession would be comprised of only children from high-income families. To determine whether such a concern is justifiable and, if so, how to alleviate it, it is necessary to examine the "equity" of the current system of financing medical education.

EQUITY IN THE CURRENT SYSTEM OF FINANCING MEDICAL EDUCATION

In the preceding section we were concerned with the economic efficiency of the medical education market. It was determined that under the current structure of medical education, it was highly unlikely that the optimal number of physicians would be produced, and that the production of medical education would be efficient. This section is concerned with the equity (i.e., who receives the benefits and who bears the costs) of the large governmental subsidies that support the current system of medical education.

Based on the estimate of the costs of medical education being at least $100,000 per year, as discussed above, and revenues from tuition and fees representing less than 20 percent of educational costs, the average annual subsidy for four years of medical education in 1995 was about $300,000. The size of this subsidy (which would differ according to whether the student went to a public or private medical school) has increased over time as educational costs have increased faster than tuition payments.

These subsidies are in addition to those received during the student's four years of undergraduate training, since higher education is also subsidized by government funds. The subsidies received by medical students are generally larger than those received by other students in higher education and in other professional schools. The reason is that the costs of medical education are greater than the costs in other departments within the university. With such large subsidies going to each medical student, it is legitimate to question how equitably these subsidies are being distributed. Do such subsidies have desirable redistributive effects, or are they neutral with respect to their effect on incomes in society?

Income redistribution is based on a societal value judgment that persons with lower incomes should be made better off by being subsidized at the expense of persons with higher incomes. The provision of such subsidies (and the taxes to finance them) may be direct, in the form of cash grants, or indirect, in the form of grants in kind, such as lower prices for specific goods and services. Education is an in-kind subsidy to all those using it. For an in-kind subsidy to have desirable redistributive effects, low-income persons should receive a proportionately greater share of the subsidy, while the taxes to pay for it should come from those with higher incomes.

Some redistributive schemes may have perverse effects, as when a greater proportion of the cost is borne by lower-income persons and a greater proportionate share of the benefits is received by higher-income persons. This occurs at times with Social Security, as when high-income aged receive benefits in excess of their contributions. A similar case occurs with high-income Medicare beneficiaries. In both cases, young, low-wage employees subsidize high-income beneficiaries.

In the typical market situation, when a person purchases a good or service, that person receives the benefits from the purchase and pays the cost of producing it. The benefits are fully received and the costs are fully borne by the purchaser, assuming no externalities. With regard to medical education, therefore, are the sizable subsidies that go to each medical student neutral in their redistributive effects, or, if not, which income groups end up subsidizing which other income groups?

Evidence suggests that subsidies to higher education, particularly to medical education, result in a large redistribution of income; however, the costs are borne by low-income persons and are used to subsidize the highest-income groups in society. Such redistribution is inequitable. Hansen and Weisbrod, in an examination of the financing of higher education in California and in Wisconsin, have shown that the size of the subsidy received by families that send their children to these state-supported schools is greater than the state taxes they pay for all state-supported services (11). These families have higher incomes, on average, than families that do not send their children to such schools.

As shown in Table 14.3, which is based on the Hansen and Weisbrod study, the average income of families with children enrolled in the University of California system was $12,000 in 1964–65. The average income of families with children enrolled in the California State College system was $10,000. The average for families without children in either system was $7,900. The average amount of state taxes paid by each of these families was $350, $260, and $182, respectively; the *net* subsidy to each of these family groups was +$1,350, +$1,140, and −$180. Because more children from higher-income families attended California's public higher education institutions, these families were subsidized by the remainder of the families, whose income, on average, was lower.

Hansen and Weisbrod make two additional comments that are relevant to our discussion on financing medical education. First, the additional state taxes paid by the subsidized students, once they begin working and earning higher incomes as a result of their subsidized education, are less than the value of the subsidy they received (on a present-value basis). Second, a number of subsidized students never repay any of their subsidy, since they leave the state. If these results have persisted over time (more recent data are unavailable) and if the evidence in other states is similar to what was demonstrated in California and Wisconsin, it is clear that prospective medical students (and others) receive substantial subsidies before they even enter medical school.

How are the subsidies in medical education distributed with regard to family income? Table 14.4 presents a comparison of family incomes for medical students with family in-

TABLE 14.3 Average Family Incomes, Average Higher Education Subsidies Received, and Average State Taxes Paid by Families, by Type of California Higher Education Institution, 1964–65

	Families without Children Enrolled in California Higher Education	Families with Children Enrolled in California Public Higher Education	
		University of California	California State College
Average family income	$7,900	$12,000	$10,000
Average higher education subsidy per year	0	1700	1400
Average state taxes paid	182	350	260
Net subsidy	−180	+1,350	+1,140

Source: Based on data in Table IV-12, p. 76, in W. Lee Hansen and Burton A. Weisbrod, *Benefits, Costs and Finance of Public Higher Education* (Chicago: Markham, 1969).

TABLE 14.4 Family Income of Medical Students, All U.S. Families, by Control of Medical School, 1974–75

Family Income[a]	Private Schools	Public Schools	All Medical Schools	All U.S. Families
Total	100%	100%	100%	100%
Less than $5,000	5	6	6	13
$5,000–9,000	10	11	11	23
$10,000–14,999	16	19	18	24
$15,000–19,999	14	16	15	18
$20,000–24,999	13	14	13	10
$25,000 or more	42	34	37	12
Estimated median	$21,972	$19,315	$20,249	$12,836

Sources: Reproduced from *Descriptive Study of Enrolled Medical Students, 1974–1975,* DHEW Publication No. (HRA) 76-97, prepared by the Association of American Medical Colleges, p. 26. Data for "All U.S. Families" came from U.S. Department of Commerce, Bureau of the Census, *Money, Income and Poverty Status of Families and Persons in the United States, 1974,* Series P-60, No. 99, July 1975.

[a]Based on students who supplied data.

comes in the rest of the population for the 1974–75 period. Based on data from this table, it is obvious that the family incomes of medical students were higher than those of all U.S. families. Three times as many families of medical students had incomes of $25,000 or more than there were in the population at large. Similarly, twice as many families in the population had incomes less than $15,000 than did the families of medical students. The estimated median income of families of medical students was almost twice as great as the median family income in the general population.

The large subsidies to medical students, therefore, were going to students whose family incomes were much higher than those in the rest of the population. It was also highly unlikely that state taxes paid by the families of medical students were, on the average, greater than the subsidies received. The redistributive effects of the subsidy method of financing medical education appears to be similar to the earlier examples of higher education in California and Wisconsin.

The redistributive effects of the medical school subsidies shown in Table 14.4 are actually an improvement over what they were in the past. In 1967, 20 percent of the medical students came from families with incomes greater than $25,000 a year, incomes that compared with only 2 percent of the families in the general population, a ratio of 10:1. Similarly, 42 percent of the families of medical students had incomes greater then $15,000, whereas only 12 percent of the families in the population had comparable incomes (12).

Data on family incomes of medical students published since 1974–75 are surprisingly misleading. According to a 1978 publication, the highest income level used was "$20,000 or more," which characterized 46 percent of all medical student families (13). Since inflation has been causing incomes to rise generally, a larger portion of the population also ends up in that highest-income category. Thus there is only a 50 percent difference in the proportion of families in that highest-income category. Had higher-income categories been used, the disparities in incomes would become much more obvious. A 1987 study tried to determine whether family incomes of prospective medical students relative to the population have been changing. After attempting to control for the problem of income categories, with the highest-income category being $50,000 and greater, the author concluded: "it appears that the incomes of families of students taking the MCAT (Medical College Admissions Test) have neither increased nor decreased to any substantial degree relative to the rest of the population over the period 1977–1983" (14).

Although it is undoubtedly true that some medical students came from families with low incomes, the major portion of the subsidy going to medical students goes to those with high family incomes. What is also interesting is that medical schools appear to show favoritism when it comes to admitting children of physicians (15).

Another factor bearing on the inequity of the current system of financing medical education is that once medical students graduate, they enter the top 10 percent of the income distribution in society. It would seem unnecessary to subsidize medical students through their undergraduate and medical education to enable them to enter the highest income distribution, but on top of that, the students who are being selected to receive the subsidy come from the highest-income families in the first place.

In light of the foregoing discussion, the proposals of the Carnegie Commission Report on Medical Education (1970), suggesting federal subsidies to medical students and medical schools to result in a uniform level of tuition for all schools of $1,000, would worsen rather than improve the performance of the current system of medical education. At such low tuition levels, the excess demand for medical education would become greater than before. Since schools would all charge the same tuition levels, there would be no competition among schools on costs to the students and this would favor the most costly, prestigious schools: if the price is the same, why not go to the "best" school? Such a system would also provide no incentives for schools to be concerned with their costs because they would receive sufficient subsidies to enable each school to charge only $1,000 tuition per year. A more desirable proposal could not have been developed by the deans of the most prestigious, high-cost, medical schools themselves.

Are there any justifiable reasons for continuing a method of financing medical education that has the effect of worsening rather than improving the income distribution? Three rationalizations are offered for continuing the present subsidy system. The first states that if it is a societal value judgment to have physicians locate in rural and underserved areas, it is necessary to subsidize medical education (16). Similarly, if a change in the mix of physicians is desired, subsidies to medical schools are necessary. Further, some persons believe that since medical students leave the state that provided them with a subsidy, to prevent the state that is acquiring them from benefiting, that state should also subsidize its medical students.

The common fallacy in each of the above arguments is the failure to recognize that subsidies can be provided on a selective basis. For example, only those physicians locating in a rural area would be subsidized by not having to repay all or part of their educational costs. Why should all physicians be subsidized, especially since most of them locate in high-income urban areas? Similarly, since only a portion of medical students are classified as minority students, why should the remaining medical students receive subsidies as well? If the purpose of state subsidies is to have its medical students remain in the state, then only those remaining in the state should be subsidized. By charging all students full-cost tuition, those medical students leaving the state would have paid their debt by having paid their full educational costs. Those remaining in the state could have, over time, all or part of their costs forgiven. This same argument could be applied to all persons, including lawyers, accountants, and teachers, who receive subsidized training and then leave the state to practice elsewhere.

A state should explicitly state the reasons it wants to provide a subsidy. The proposed subsidy would then generate discussion as to whether that is a value judgment with which others agree. Once a policy goal has been agreed on, that objective could be achieved much less expensively by providing the subsidies directly to persons fulfilling society's needs rather than by providing a generous subsidy to all medical students. Similarly, if the subsidies went only to those participating in a particular agreed-on program, more funds would be available to meet that objective.

A more sophisticated argument favoring subsidies to all students is that the sums of money required to pay for a medical education are so large that very few persons would be able to afford it. Banks would be unwilling to provide loans for tuition and living expenses with no collateral. Further, persons from low-income families have a higher rate of time preference (i.e., income today has a much higher value to the poor than income in the future). As a result, the poor will be less likely than those with higher incomes to invest in their own human capital (i.e., higher education). Also, undertaking an investment involves some risk that it will not pay off. Medical education is expensive, and future physician incomes may not be as attractive. If physicians have large debts to pay off, so some persons would say, they may select only the most lucrative forms of practice instead of serving certain population groups or perhaps undertaking research.

If all medical students were to be charged full-cost tuition, then such a policy would have to be accompanied by loan programs. A type of loan program that has been advocated by a number of persons is an "income contingent loan repayment plan" (ICLRP). The way in which an ICLRP would work is as follows. Students could take out a loan during the period they are in medical school to cover both tuition and living expenses. Once they have graduated and have started to earn an income, they would annually repay a fixed percent of their adjusted gross income. The fixed percent that would be assessed would depend on how much the student borrowed (17).

By relating the ICLRP to the income of the physician, the program would not distort the preferences of physicians as to the population they serve or the type of practice they enter. A loan repayment plan similar to the one described would also minimize the risk to the student as to the size of the loan that would have to be repaid.[3] Physicians' incomes have, in any case, been consistently high during the past fifty years. As investments go, an investment in a medical education would carry minimal risk and would be fairly predictable, as attested to by the continual excess demands for spaces and the willingness of large number of students to pay higher costs to receive such an education overseas.

What would happen to the demand for a medical education if medical students were charged the full cost of their education (and medical schools are no longer provided with education subsidies)? Would there be a large decrease in the number of medical school applicants? Assuming that full-cost tuition had been previously implemented, the results would have been as follows: The rate of return to a medical education was estimated to be between 15 and 22 percent in 1970 and between 14 and 17 percent in 1980; for many medical specialties, it was higher than that. It was estimated that the rate of return in 1976 would have declined to 13.5 percent with full-cost tuition (18). Even at this lower rate of return, an investment in a medical education would still have been very worthwhile in that there would still have been an excess rate of return to medicine. There have been no recent studies to indicate the effect on the rate of return of implementing full-cost tuition today.

In any case, if full-cost tuition were combined with a reduction in both the length of the undergraduate program and one year of the medical school, as discussed earlier, it should be possible to offset the increased tuition by the lower opportunity costs and the higher income as a result of entering practice three years earlier. There should be no diminution in the number of practicing physicians.

Medical schools would be forced to compete with one another for students if full-cost tuition were implemented. Once students have to pay a substantial cost of their education, they will become increasingly concerned with the school they select. Even if subsidies for medical education were provided to some students, the schools would have to compete for them. Medical schools would have to compete on the basis of their tuition, since it would affect the size of a student's ICLRP, and on their quality. It is likely that under such circumstances the schools will reexamine the number of years of undergraduate and medical education required.

Medical, dental, and other educational institutions much prefer that any subsidies go

---

[3]A problem with previous student loan programs was that former students nullified their debts by declaring bankruptcy. In 1977, however, "a new federal law went into effect that binds graduates to their student loan obligations even if they declare bankruptcy," *New York Times,* November 26, 1977, p. 25. A revolving medical student loan fund has been set up by Congress with the amount of funds available to medical students based on the repayment of previous loans. A General Accounting Office study found, however, that medical schools were ineffective in collecting loans from their graduates. "Doctors Lagging on School Loans: Senate Panel Staff Finds Many Higher-Income Physicians Fail to Make Payments," *New York Times,* December 7, 1981: p. 13. For a report on federal loan programs to medical students, see John K. Iglehart, "Federal Support of Health Manpower Education," *New England Journal of Medicine,* 314(5), January 30, 1986: 324–328.

directly to the school rather than to the student. By subsidizing the school, students have to go to that school if they are to receive subsidized education. It is for this same reason that schools prefer to distribute loans and scholarships rather than have the government or some other central agency distribute them. When the school distributes the funds, students can receive them only if they attend the institution distributing them. When students receive these funds directly and can then choose the school they wish to attend, the different schools are forced to compete for students.

SUMMARY

The economic efficiency of the medical education market was examined by contrasting its performance to that of a hypothetically competitive market. A competitive market in medical education would be more likely to produce an optimal number of physicians and at lower cost than does the current system of medical education.

One important difference between a competitive market and the current system is the role of tuition as both an equilibrating mechanism and as a source of revenue. The low levels of tuition as a result of large subsidies received by public medical schools and accreditation criteria regarding sources of revenue mean that medical schools do not have to compete on price. Further, since tuition is a small percentage of a medical school's source of revenue, medical schools have not been concerned with the costs of educating physicians.

Barriers to entry into the medical education market are a second reason for the current market's poor performance. The accreditation criteria inhibit the entry of innovative schools that would also reduce the time required to train a new physician.

The consequences of the poor market performance of the current system of medical education are that there is a continual excess demand for a medical education, there is limited curriculum innovation, educational costs are higher than if medical schools had to compete on price, and the time required to receive a medical degree is several years longer than necessary.

The equity of the present system of financing medical education was examined next. It was shown that medical students are subsidized through undergraduate education and medical school, and then enter the top 10 percent of the income distribution in society. These same medical students often come from the highest-income groups to start with. There is also no equity-based argument why medical students should receive greater subsidies than students in law or those studying for a Ph.D. degree. Proposals to improve the equity of the current system were suggested, such as having those students who benefit from an investment in a medical education bear the full cost of such an education. Specific value judgments of society, such as having physicians locate in certain areas, should be subsidized directly instead of rewarding all medical students regardless of whether they participate in the particular programs. A method to implement the concept of full-cost tuition, namely, income-contingent loan repayment plans, was suggested.

Eliminating medical school subsidies would also provide medical schools with the incentive to increase their efficiency and to innovate in teaching and curriculum if they are to survive. Once medical schools have to compete for students, bearing the full cost of their education, the length of the educational process would be reduced, students would be trained for the types of practice they enter (and what the managed care market demands), and the schools will have to develop quantifiable measures of the quality of their educational process.

Key Terms and Concepts

- Full-cost tuition
- Inframarginal externalities
- Prestige maximization goal
- Private and external benefits

- Income-contingent loan repayment plans
- Opportunity costs of a medical education
- Optimal number of graduates
- Tuition as an equilibrating mechanism

Review Questions

1. Describe the economic factors that affect the demand for a medical education. How are each of these factors likely to change in the coming years?
2. Evaluate the performance of the current market for medical education in terms of the number of qualified students admitted and the cost (medical education cost and foregone student income) of becoming a physician.
3. What would you hypothesize the consequences would be if medical education were to become a more competitive industry, like business and law schools?
4. What are the reasons for and against subsidizing all medical students seeking a medical education? How would you evaluate these reasons according to the criteria of economic efficiency and equity?
5. Currently, the public is protected from incompetent and unethical physicians by requiring graduation from an approved medical school, passing a one-time licensing exam, and continuing education. What are alternative, lower-cost approaches for achieving these objectives?
6. Evaluate in terms of both equity and economic efficiency: The Carnegie Commission Report on Medical Education (1970) recommends federal subsidies to medical schools and students in order to achieve a uniform level of tuition of $1,000 at all schools. (The subsidy would go to the schools.)

7. Medicare has been very generous in paying teaching hospitals for their residents. What would be the hypothesized effect on the demand for residents if Medicare reduces these payments?

REFERENCES

1. Institute of Medicine, National Academy of Sciences, *Costs of Education in the Health Professions,* Report of a Study, parts I and II (Washington, D.C.: National Academy of Sciences, 1974). Paul Jolly et al., "US Medical School Finances," *Journal of the American Medical Association,* 264, 1990: 813–820.
2. A rough estimate of the costs of medical education were calculated as follows: Based on Table 14.1, total unrestricted support for medical schools in 1994–95 was $22 billion and there were about 67,000 medical students during that year. Assuming that educational costs were at least one-third of the $22 billion unrestricted budget, then the average educational cost per student was in excess of $110,000. Further, dividing the amount of revenue generated by tuition and fees (about $18,000 per student on average) by the estimated cost of education ($110,000) results in tuition and fees representing, on average, 16 percent of educational costs. The difference between the educational costs and revenues generated by tuition and fees is the size of the student subsidy. The same approach was used to calculate the costs of education and the size of the student subsidy for earlier years.
3. *Liaison Committee on Medical Education, Functions and Structure of a Medical School* (Washington, D.C.: Association of American Medical Colleges and the American Medical Association, 1991).
4. C. Enarson and F. Burg, "An Overview of Reform Initiatives in Medical Education: 1906 Through 1992," *Journal of the American Medical Association,* 268, September 2, 1992: 1141–1143.
5. Thomas Hall and Cotton Lindsay, "Medical Schools: Producers of What Sellers to Whom," *Journal of Law and Economics,* April 1980.
6. Rashi Fein and Gerald Weber, *Financing Medical Education,* A General Report Prepared for the Carnegie Commission on Higher Education and the Commonwealth Fund (New York: McGraw-Hill, 1971), pp. 131–132.
7. For more discussion on this subject, see Edgar K. Browning and Mark A. Zupan, *Microeconomic Theory and Applications,* 5th ed. (New York: HarperCollins, 1996), pp. 576–585.
8. See Theodore W. Schultz, "Optimal Investment in College Instruction: Equity and Efficiency," *Journal of Political Economy* Special Issue: "Investment in Education: The Equity-Efficiency Quandry," 80(3), Part II, May–June 1972.
9. For some suggestions on how educational and opportunity costs might be reduced under a different system for providing medical education, see Reuben Kessel, "The AMA and the Supply of Physicians," *Law and Contemporary Problems,* Health Care Part I, School of Law, Duke University, Spring 1970: 276–278.
10. Robert H. Ebert and Eli Ginzberg, "The Reform of Medical Education," *Health Affairs,* 7(2), Supplement 1988: 5–38, quotes are on pages 15 and 19. Ebert was formerly dean, Harvard Medical School.

11. W. Lee Hansen and Burton A. Weisbrod, *Benefits, Costs and Finance of Public Higher Education* (Chicago: Markham, 1969), p. 76.

12. U.S. Department of Health, Education, and Welfare, *How Medical Students Finance Their Education* (Washington, D.C.: U.S. Government Printing Office, 1970), pp. 8–9.

13. W. F. Dube, *Descriptive Study of Enrolled Medical Students, 1976–1977,* final report from the Division of Student Studies, Association of American Medical Colleges for the Bureau of Health Manpower, Department of Health, Education, and Welfare (Washington, D.C.: U.S. Government Printing Office, February 1978), p. 55.

14. Paul Jolly, "Family Income of Students Taking the Medical College Admissions Test," unpublished paper, Association of American Medical Colleges, February 17, 1987.

15. Bernard Lentz and David Laband, "Why So Many Children of Doctors Become Doctors," *Journal of Human Resources*, 24(3), Summer 1989: 396–413.

16. An important reason why early loan forgiveness programs for physicians locating in rural and underserved areas were ineffective was that it was relatively inexpensive, given the heavily subsidized cost of education, for students to buy their way out of their contracted obligations.

17. The idea of an ICLRP is not new. It was proposed over thirty years ago as a means of financing higher education. Yale and Duke Universities have experimented with such plans. A good theoretical discussion of the ICLRP is presented in Marc Nerlove, "Some Problems in the Use of Income-Contingent Loans for the Finance of Higher Education," *Journal of Political Economy*, 83, February 1975: 157–183. The author also discusses the Yale Plan. A proposal to use such a plan for medical students has been proposed by Bernard Nelson, Richard Bird, and Gilbert Rogers, "An Analysis of the Educational Opportunity Bank for Medical Student Financing," *Journal of Medical Education,* August 1972. A computer simulation of such repayment plans to indicate their feasibility is performed in William C. Weiler, "Loans for Medical Students: The Issues of Manageability," *Journal of Medical Education,* June 1976. In 1986 Congress approved an ICLRP as a pilot project for ten universities.

18. Stephen P. Dresch, "Marginal Wage Rates, Hours of Work, and Returns to Physician Training and Specialization," in Nancy Greenspan, ed., *Health Care Financing Conference Proceedings: Issues in Physicians' Reimbursement* (Washington, D.C.: Department of Health and Human Services, 1981), p. 199.

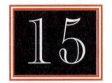

CHAPTER 15

The Market for Registered Nurses

ECONOMISTS' INTERESTS REGARDING THE NURSING MARKET

The market for registered nurses (RNs) has been subject to much analysis as well as government regulation and subsidies. Economists' major interests with regard to the nursing market have been twofold: first, an examination of the reasons for recurrent shortages of RNs, and, second, the effects of different market structures on nurses' wages and employment. Government policies to reduce nurse shortages and remedies to improve market performance have also been examined. At times, concern over nurse shortages and imperfections in the nurse market have been related; that is, imperfections have caused shortages. Because of the interrelationship between these two topics, a historical approach is used to review the market for nurses and the appropriateness of government intervention.

A FRAMEWORK FOR UNDERSTANDING THE PERFORMANCE OF THE MARKET FOR REGISTERED NURSES

To understand the various claims of a nurse shortage, as well as the different types of market imperfections, and the subsequent massive federal support for nursing education, it is useful to first examine how a competitive labor market for nurses would perform. If this market had been functioning well, then there would be no reason for government intervention to increase the supply of nurses. If such federal support occurred when the market for nurses was performing efficiently, then we must look for other reasons to explain the demand for subsidies to nursing education.

If, on the other hand, it is found that the market for registered nurses has not been functioning well, certain policy prescriptions might be called for. Depending on the particular reasons for its poor performance, federal subsidies might be one policy alternative; other forms of government intervention might also be appropriate. Only after examining the performance of the market for nurses can it be determined whether any justification for federal subsidies to nursing education exists. Also, by examining the effect of federal subsidies we might gain some insight into their intended as opposed to their stated purpose.

To understand the changing demand for RNs over time, it is necessary to understand the factors that both directly and indirectly affect the demand for RNs.

The demand for RNs is a derived demand; it is derived from the demand for the institutional settings where RNs are employed. As the demand for medical services increases, as a result of the growth in private and government insurance programs, the aging of the population, medical advances that can improve the patient's condition, and so on, there is a demand for those institutions, such as hospitals, outpatient clinics, skilled nursing homes, and home health care, where patients are treated. These institutions in turn have a demand for inputs used in providing care to those patients. In addition to capital for buildings and equipment, labor inputs, particularly nursing personnel, RNs, licensed practical nurses (LPNs), and aides, are also used.

The demand for these inputs is determined by the initial demand for each of these provider organizations, that is, the admission rate per one hundred thousand population and the price paid for an admission. Hospitals, which provide more intensive care for a patient than, for example, nursing homes, will use a different combination of inputs than will the nursing home. As the type of patient cared for (e.g., more severely ill) and the technology used in these settings change, so will the demand for the type of inputs used.

Also affecting the provider organization's demand for inputs is the relative productivity of each type of input and their relative wage. For example, as the wages of RNs increase relative to those of LPNs, then, other things held constant, the organization will begin to substitute LPNs for RNs. Similarly, as RNs are able to increase their productivity relative to LPNs, the organization will substitute away from LPNs to using more RNs.

The demand for an RN education is similarly derived from the provider organizations' demand for RNs. As the number of RNs demanded and their wage increase, the rate of return to becoming an RN increases relative to other occupations. The result will be an increase in the demand for an RN education. In addition to economic factors, there are also noneconomic factors that affect the demand for an RN education. Examples are increased opportunities for women in medicine and business. Demographics, that is, the size of the age cohort graduating from high school, is also important.

Over time both the direct and indirect factors affecting the demand for RNs have changed, each of which have affected nurses' wages and employment.

An efficiently performing market for nurses should perform as shown in Figure 15.1. Starting from an initial equilibrium point, with the demand for registered nurses (RNs) represented by D_1 and supply by S_1, the equilibrium wage would be W_1 and the number of RNs employed, Q_1. The assumption that the demand for RNs has been increasing over time would be represented by a shift in the demand curve to D_2. With a greater demand for RNs, wages would be expected to increase to W_2 and the quantity of RNs employed to increase to Q_2. The increase in RNs employed, along S_1, would come from an increase in the nurse "participation rate," which is the percent of the existing stock of RNs that are employed, as well as an increase in hours worked by currently employed RNs.[1]

Thus the short-run effects of an increase in demand on the market for nurses is an

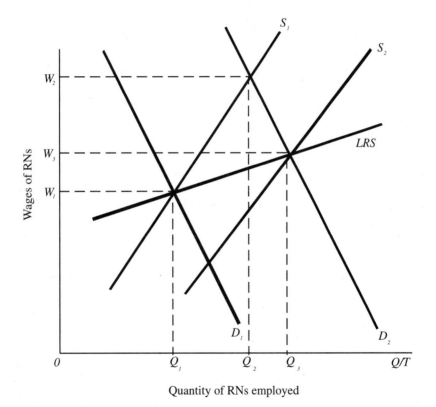

FIGURE 15.1 • The market for registered nurses.

---

[1]For the majority of trained nurses who are women, a number of factors influence whether they will seek employment. Wage is only one such factor. Whether a woman has young children and what her husband's income is are additional factors. However, if nurses' wages increase, while all other factors remain unchanged, some inactive nurses will decide to become active. The elasticity of the participation rate with respect to nurses' wages will indicate the percent increase in employment for a given percent increase in nurses' wages. This will be discussed in more detail later.

increase in their wages, from W_1 to W_2, and an increase in the nurse participation rate (and hours worked), from Q_1 to Q_2.

The long-run effect of the increase in demand, from D_1 to D_2, is an increase in the stock of nurses, which is shown in Figure 15.1 by a shift in the supply curve to the right, to S_2. The new supply curve represents a greater number of trained nurses; as the wage of RNs is increased, from W_1 to W_2, nursing becomes a relatively more attractive profession when compared with, for example, teaching. Assuming that all the factors that affect the demand for a nurse's and a teacher's education do not change, except for an increase in nurses' relative wages, some prospective teachers may instead decide to seek a nursing education. Changes in relative wages between professions do not have the same effect on all prospective students. Those who are "at the margin," that is, perhaps prefer each profession equally, are likely to be the ones who switch careers with a change in relative incomes.

Both S_1 and S_2 are short-run supply curves for nurses; each represents the supply of nurses for a given stock of nurses. The long-run supply curve for nurses is shown by *LRS,* which represents the number of persons who will become nurses over time in response to higher wages.

An efficiently performing nurse market would, in the short run, have the following outcomes following an increase in demand:

an increase in RN wages;
an increase in the rate of return to being an RN, both in absolute terms and relative to other occupations;
an increase in the nurse participation rate, leading to an increase in the number of RNs employed; and
an increase in the use of substitutes. As RN wages increase, RNs become more expensive relative to other types of nurses. Employers will substitute away from using RNs to greater use of other nursing personnel whose wages have not increased as rapidly.

Competitive markets, however, do not adjust immediately to an increase in demand. As observed in Figure 15.1, with an increase in demand from D_1 to D_2, wages would rise and the number of employed nurses would increase—in the short run through an increase in their participation rate, and in the long run through an increase in the number of persons becoming nurses (a shift to the right in the supply curve). Until the long-run supply adjusts, however, a dynamic shortage might occur. With an increase in the demand for nurses, the major employers of nurses may not know how much they have to increase nurses' wages to bring about an increase in their employment; similarly, it takes time for working nurses to learn which hospitals are paying higher wages and for inactive nurses both to learn of the increase in wages and to decide to become active again.

A dynamic shortage for RNs is illustrated in Figure 15.2. With the increase in demand from D_1 to D_2, the demand for RNs will initially be Q_2, which is at the old wage W_1 on the new demand curve D_2. Thus, in a dynamic shortage, until information becomes

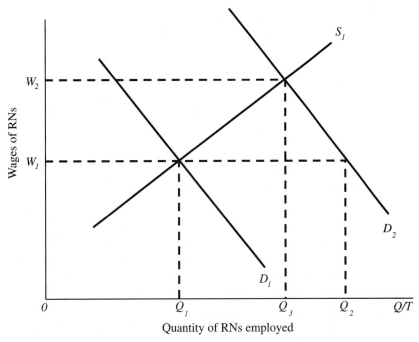

FIGURE 15.2 • A dynamic shortage in the market for registered nurses.

available to both nurse employers that they have to raise wages if they are to hire more nurses and to nurses that they could receive higher wages if they were to become active, there will be a shortage of magnitude $Q_1 - Q_2$. The indication of a shortage will be an increase in nurse vacancies, which are budgeted but unfilled positions. As RN wages increase and eventually reach W_2, the shortage will decrease, meaning that those employers who are willing to pay the higher price will be able to employ more nurses. The existence of a dynamic shortage is a temporary phenomenon and will disappear over time. Unless demand for RNs continues to increase faster than the supply of RNs, equilibrium will eventually occur.

Empirical evidence that a dynamic shortage existed (or continues to exist) would be nurse vacancies (generally greater than 5 percent), rising nurse wages, increased RN employment, an increase in RN participation rates, and greater use of substitutes. There is no economic justification for federal subsidies to increase the supply of nurses.

A more serious imperfection that might occur is a static shortage, in which nurses' wages are prevented from reaching an equilibrium level. Because the wages are below the market clearing wage, the shortage will not resolve itself as would a dynamic shortage. A static shortage can also be illustrated using Figure 15.2. With an increase in demand from D_1 to D_2, the quantity of nurses demanded at the old wage would be Q_2. If the wage is prevented from rising, the shortage, $Q_1 - Q_2$, will not disappear. In distinguishing between a static and a dynamic shortage, vacancy rates for nurses would be observed in both cases; however, in a static shortage increases in nurses' wages and in their participation rates will not occur. In both cases we would expect substitution away from the use of RNs to occur, since it is more difficult to employ as many RNs as the employers would like, in one case because nurses' wages have gone up and they have become relatively more expensive to employ, in the other because employers cannot hire all the nurses they would like to at the old wage.

Depending on the reason for a static shortage, some form of government intervention is required. At times the shortage may be a result of government action, such as the imposition of wage and price controls, as occurred during 1971–74. Had these controls not been imposed, wages would have risen and there would not have been a shortage. At other times, the anti-trust laws may have to be enforced to eliminate anticompetitive behavior causing the shortage. Again, it is difficult to justify providing federal subsidies as a means of reducing a static shortage. It would be more efficient, and less costly, to merely eliminate the market imperfection that prevents wages from rising.

As discussed in an earlier chapter, a nursing surplus will occur when demand is either shifting to the left, thereby causing a fall in wages, or supply is increasing faster (shifting to the right) than demand, also causing wages to fall. A surplus would therefore be indicated by wages and rates of return that are declining relative to other occupations. Vacancy rates would be very low as nurse employers are able to hire the number of nurses they want, there would be fewer students entering nurse education programs, and the nursing profession would seek political action to limit the supply of nurses or measures to stimulate the demand for nurses.

Having specified the measures of performance to be used in determining which of the foregoing market descriptions best characterizes how the market for nurses has operated in the past, we now turn to an examination of the data.

THE PERFORMANCE OF THE MARKET FOR REGISTERED NURSES

Nurses are predominantly employed in hospitals. As shown in Table 15.1, of the 2,115,815 registered nurses employed in 1996, 60 percent were working in hospitals. The remaining places of employment and their respective percentages were: nursing homes (8.1 percent), community or public health (17 percent), ambulatory care (8.5 percent), and other (6.3 percent). Thus what happens in the hospital sector has the largest effect on the employment of registered nurses.

The Market for Nurses Before Medicare and Medicaid

The demand for hospital care (hence the demand for RNs) has been changing over time, as described in the chapter on hospitals. Admissions and patient days in short-term general and other special hospitals (which have approximately 80 percent of all hospital ad-

TABLE 15.1 Number and Distribution of Active Registered Nurses by Place of Employment, 1996

Place of Employment	Number of Active RNs	Percentage of RNs
Hospitals	1,270,870	60.1
Nursing homes	170,856	8.1
Community or public health	362,648	17.1
Ambulatory care		
(physician or nurse solo or group practices and HMOs)	178,930	8.5
Other		
(nursing education, administrative offices or associations, and insurance companies)	132,511	6.3
Total	2,115,815	100.1[a]

Source: Health Resources and Services Administration, Bureau of Health Professions, *Advanced Notes I from the National Sample Survey of Registered Nurses, March 1996,* Internet site: http://www.hrsa.dhhs.gov/bhpr/dn/advnote1.htm, accessed on April 7, 1997.
[a]Percentages do not sum to 100 because of rounding.

missions) had been increasing (until the early 1980s) as a result of an aging population, rising incomes and health insurance coverage, and Medicare and Medicaid, started in 1966, which lowered the cost of hospital care to the aged and the poor. Advances in medical knowledge changed the nature of the hospital, from a place that provided chronic care to an institution that provides acute care. Also, medical technology increased demands for RNs per patient day—for example, in intensive care units. Thus there was an increase in the use of medical care, and more of this care was provided in hospitals. There was also a greater demand for nurses as a result of a shift to providing more of the nursing care by RNs. An increase in the responsibilities delegated to RNs for tasks that were formerly performed by physicians in hospitals added additional burdens.

As a result of the above forces, there was a 65 percent increase in the use of general duty nurses per patient (in nonfederal hospitals) between 1949 and 1966 (1).[2] With such a large increase in demand for RNs, a dynamic shortage would have been expected to occur. Increases in nurse vacancy rates, in nurses' salaries, in nurse participation rates, and substitution toward the use of non-RN nurses, would have been expected. According to

---

[2]A demand function for RNs in short-term hospitals was estimated by Donald E. Yett et al., and it was determined that the effect of a 1 percent increase in patient days would result in a 0.86 percent increase in RNs in hospitals of 200 or more beds. The effect of a 1 percent increase in RN wages would lead to a −1.75 percent decrease in number of RNs employed, and the cross-elasticity of demand for RNs with respect to the wages of aides was 1.43. D. Yett, L. Drabek, L. Kimball, and M. Intriligator, *A Forecasting and Policy Simulation Model of the Health Care Sector* (Lexington, Mass.: Lexington Books, 1979), p. 95.

the vacancy rate data shown in Table 15.2, nurse vacancy rates were high during the 1950s, reaching a peak of 23 percent in 1962. These data are consistent with a shortage.

Examining the other indicators of a shortage, however, provides inconsistent results. Over a longer time period, nurses' wages have risen by a similar amount as other comparable professions. When the increase in salaries both before and after the introduction of Medicare and Medicaid in 1966 are examined, nurses' salaries increased less rapidly than other professions between 1946 and 1966. However, after 1966, nurses' salaries increased more rapidly, with hospital RN wages increasing more rapidly than all RN wages over the longer period.

According to Table 15.3, between 1946 and 1966, the ratio of all RN salaries to those of teachers was approximately equal in 1946 at 1.03; for hospital RNs, it was 0.95. The comparable ratios of all RNs and hospital RNs to female professional, technical, and kindred workers was 1.05 and 0.97, respectively. Throughout the remainder of the 1940s, 1950s, and early 1960s, RN wages declined relative to these other occupational groups. These ratios declined to a low around 1963, where, for example, hospital RN salaries were only 0.73 of teachers' salaries. The same decline occurred for RNs relative to other occupations in which women were predominantly employed.

After Medicare and Medicaid were enacted, RN salaries began increasing faster than those of teachers or other female occupations. By 1972, RN wages, particularly hospital RNs, once again exceeded those of other female occupations, rising to 1.10 and 1.08, respectively, for all RNs and for hospital RNs. With respect to teachers, the hospital RN ratio was similar to what had existed in the 1940s.

Based on the above data on relative wages, it would appear that there was a relative surplus rather than a relative shortage of nurses before 1966! This is because the wages of other female workers increased more rapidly than those of nurses. This same observation is supported by data on relative rates of return to a nursing education when they are com-

TABLE 15.2 Vacancy Rates in Hospitals for General-Duty Nurses

Year	Vacancy Rate	Year	Vacancy Rate
1953	14.6	1967	18.1
1954	13.0	1968	15.0
1956	16.8	1969	11.2
1958	13.0	1971	9.3
1962	23.0		

Source: Reprinted by permission of the publisher, from Donald E. Yett, *An Economic Analysis of the Nurse Shortage* (Lexington, Mass.: Lexington Books, D.C. Heath, 1975); copyright 1975, D. C. Heath, p. 138, Table 3-13.

TABLE 15.3 Ratio of All Registered Nurses' and Hospital General-Duty Registered Nurses' Salaries to Those of Teachers and Female Professional, Technical, and Kindred Workers

Year	Female Professional, Technical, and Kindred Workers		Teachers	
	All RNs	Hospital RNs	All RNs	Hospital RNs
1946	1.05	0.97	1.03	0.95
1948	1.00	0.95	0.92	0.87
1951	0.97	0.92	0.86	0.82
1954	0.89	0.82	0.82	0.76
1957	0.91	0.85	0.79	0.74
1961	0.86	0.79	0.77	0.70
1963	0.90	0.87	0.75	0.73
1966	0.93	0.87	0.79	0.73
1969	1.02	0.95	0.87	0.81
1972	1.10	1.08	0.97	0.96
1975	1.08	1.08	0.96	0.96

Source: Donald E. Yett, *An Economic Analysis of the Nurse Shortage* (Lexington, Mass.: Lexington Books, 1975).

pared with "females with one to three years of college training." From 1946 the relative rate of return to nursing declined, reaching a low in 1961, thereby indicating a surplus of nurses; that is, women could receive a higher rate of return by entering an occupation other than nursing. By the late 1960s and early 1970s, however, the relative rate of return to nursing had increased.

What is of interest in the period before 1966 is that nurse wage increases were not uniform according to place of nurse employment. Wages (nominal) increased much more rapidly between 1946 and 1966 for nurse education (224 percent) and school nurses (215 percent) than for hospital-employed nurses (157 percent). After 1966 the opposite occurred, as hospital nurses experienced the largest percent increase in their wages.

When the increase in supply of nurses over this period is examined, the number of nurses employed in nonfederal hospitals increased by 109 percent between 1949 and 1966. However, as would be expected, the increase in the number of nurses employed in nurse education positions and in other areas that have had larger percent increases in their wages was much greater (254 percent) over the same period.

It thus appears that within nursing nonhospital-based nurses had more rapid wage increases. Similarly, the percent increase in nurse employment was greater in the nonhospital sector, which, at that time, employed only 23 percent of all nurses. The particular submarkets within nursing adjusted more rapidly than did the hospital sector; relatively large increases in nurses' wages in nonhospital markets led to correspondingly large increases in nurse supply. It was perplexing that nurses in the nonhospital sectors received higher wage increases. If there were no barriers to movement between the two sectors and if the training costs were similar, one would expect wage increases to be similar in both the hospital and nonhospital sectors.

Although the relative salary differential of RNs to other nurses (i.e., LPNs and aides) changed very little (until the mid-1980s), a great deal of substitution occurred (as shown in Table 15.4). From 1949 to 1966, the ratio of RNs to LPNs decreased, from 6.25 in 1949 to 2.22 in 1966. Substitution would be expected if salary differentials increased or if there was a change in relative productivity (if productivity changed, this should have been reflected in a change in relative salaries). There was, however, virtually no change in their relative salaries over this period. The downward trend in the use of RNs relative to LPNs began to reverse itself beginning in the early 1970s, with the use of RNs relative to LPNs increasing from 1.96 in 1970 to 2.70 in 1980 and to 6.5 by 1995. (The decline in the use of LPNs continued into the 1990s even though their wages relative to RNs also declined.)

Based on the above data, what can one conclude about how well the market for nurses was performing? Beginning in the late 1940s, the base period for comparison with changes over time and with other occupations, nursing appeared to be a relatively attractive profession from a financial standpoint. Its rate of return was slightly higher than comparable professions. From that base period to the mid-1960s, however, the relative fi-

TABLE 15.4 Ratio of RNs to LPNs in Nonfederal Short-Term General and Other Special Hospitals

Year	Employment	Year	Employment
1949	6.25		
1955	3.45	1975	2.17
1959	2.70	1980	2.70
1960		1985	3.70
1962	2.50	1990	4.76
1963		1995	6.25
1966	2.22		
1968	2.00		
1969			
1970	1.96		
1972	2.00		

Source: 1949–78: U.S. Department of Health and Human Public Health Services, Health Resources Administration, *The Recurrent Shortage of Registered Nurses: A New Look at the Issues,* DHHS Publication (HRS), pp. 3 and 6. Years 1980–95: derived from data in: American Hospital Association, Hospital Statistics (Chicago: AHA, 1980 through 1996–97, various pages).

nancial attractiveness of a nursing career declined. One possible interpretation was that although there was an increase in demand for nurses, it was smaller than the increase in demand for comparable occupations; therefore wages rose faster in other professions. With a smaller increase in wages and a decline in relative rates of return, few persons would be expected to enter nursing. Such a model would not explain a shortage situation but instead one characterized by a relative surplus of nurses.

This characterization of a surplus situation (i.e., demand increasing less rapidly than supply, resulting in a decline in the relative wage of nurses) does not coincide with what many people believed was occurring during this period. The common belief was that there was a shortage rather than a surplus of nurses. The indications of a shortage were the substitution of practical nurses for RNs and the increasing vacancy rates of RNs in hospitals. A dynamic shortage, whereby demand increased faster than supply, would re-sult in an increase in vacancies as hospitals found that they could not hire as many nurses as they would like at the prevailing wage, and substitution toward less expensive person-nel would begin. However, a dynamic shortage would also be characterized by rising RN wages and higher wages for RNs relative to practical nurses.

Thus the data on vacancy rates and substitution would be more characteristic of a dy-namic shortage except for the fact that hospital nurses' wages (and their rates of return) were not rising more rapidly.

There was no doubt by hospitals that there was a shortage. Throughout this period, hospital associations complained about the shortage of registered nurses. The evidence used to support such claims were data on vacancy statistics of unfilled nursing positions in hospitals and studies using the ratio of registered nurses to the population. For exam-ple, in 1956, it was estimated that there was a shortage of 70,000 nurses in the United States. By 1966 that estimate had increased to 125,000 and it was estimated (in 1963) that by 1970 the magnitude of the shortage would reach 200,000 nurses (2). Vacancy rates increased from between 13 and 16 percent in the mid-1950s to 23 percent by 1962.

As a result of these claims of a shortage of RNs, the U.S. Congress in 1964 passed the Nurse Training Act (NTA), which provided $300 million over a five-year period to alle-viate the alleged shortage. (The NTA was subsequently renewed and amended in 1966, 1968, 1971, and 1975. Concerns over a nurse shortage have periodically reoccurred, as will be discussed, in the late 1970s and again in the late 1980s, which again led to federal support for nursing. In all, almost $3 billion has been authorized by the U.S. government to alleviate the nurse shortage.)

Although it was generally accepted that there was a shortage, for policy purposes it is important to determine what type of shortage existed. Different types of shortages re-quire different types of policies.

The only type of market situation that logically incorporated the above contradictory data was a static shortage. The nurses' market was essentially in equilibrium during the 1946–49 period, as shown by the intersection of the demand and supply curves, D_1 and S_1, in Figure 15.2. As the demand for hospital care increased, bringing with it an increased demand for RNs, the demand curve shifted to D_2. If nurses' wages were kept below the new equilibrium wage, $Q_1 - Q_2$ would represent the size of the shortage (i.e., vacancies in hospitals). Hospitals would have had to substitute toward greater use of practical nurses because they could not employ all the RNs they wanted at the RNs' wage. Similarly, hospital RNs' wages, relative to those of RNs in other nursing employment, would increase less rapidly, if wages were held down in the hospital sector but not in other nurse employment sectors. As hospital RN wages were prevented from increasing, they would begin to fall behind those in comparable occupations and the RNs' relative rate of return would similarly decline.

A static shortage, where RNs' wages (increased in an absolute amount but) fell relative to nonhospital employed RNs and comparable professions, also explains why hospital nurse employment increased less than in the nonhospital sector.

Given that the data appear consistent with a static shortage in the hospital market for RNs in the period prior to Medicare, it is necessary to explain how such a static shortage could have persisted—namely, what mechanism would have prevented nurses' wages from reaching the equilibrium level, and second, why the static shortage disappeared in the period after 1966.

Imperfections in the Market for RN Services

The hypothesis offered to explain the static shortage of hospital RNs prior to 1966 was that hospitals acted as a cartel in setting nurses' wages. By acting collusively, hospitals set RN wages below the equilibrium level, thereby creating a static shortage.

As purchasers of nurses' services, therefore, hospitals had a great deal of market power; they employed 75 percent of all nurses (both hospital-based and private-duty nurses). Since there were few hospitals in any one area, it was relatively easy for them to collude in setting nurses' wages. Ten percent of all hospitals were the only hospital in an area, 31 percent of hospitals were located in areas where there were only one or two hospitals, and 47 percent of hospitals were in areas where there were fewer than four hospitals; more than 60 percent of hospitals were in areas where there were fewer than six hospitals (3).

In a competitive industry with many small firms, it is both difficult to organize a cartel and, if successful, to monitor firms to ensure that they do not violate the collective agreement. It is in each firm's interest to cheat, since by raising the wage slightly they can attract nurses from other firms. Hospitals, however, can quickly find out whether another hospital in the area has changed its wage policy. Also, since they employ almost all of the active nurses, it is difficult to attract nurses from other, nonhospital firms.

Hospitals believed that the short-run supply of nurses was relatively inelastic (i.e., increasing the wage would result in only a small increase in the number of nurses seeking work, either through a change in their status from inactive to active or from in migration from other areas) and therefore decided to hold down nurses' wages. RN wages also represented a significant portion of a hospital's budget; increasing the wage rate to attract new nurses would have required an increase in the wage to all existing RNs as well.

To test the hypothesis of hospital collusion in the setting of nurses' wages, Donald Yett conducted a survey of the thirty-one largest hospital associations to determine whether they had wage stabilization programs. Fourteen of the fifteen hospital associations that responded reported that they did have wage stabilization programs. (The one hospital association that did not have one asked how it could start one.) Additional evidence of the attempt by hospitals to fix nurses' wages in their area is the following statement that appeared in the *Los Angeles Times*: "The majority of hospitals fix wages for nurses on recommendations from the Hospital Council of Southern California. The Council's recommendations have always been accepted and are based on recommendations from the management consulting firm of Guffenhagen-Kroeger Inc." (4).

As hospitals found it difficult to hire more nurses during the pre-1966 period and vacancy rates continued to increase, they began recruiting foreign trained nurses and they lobbied for federal legislation to subsidize an increase in the number of registered nurses.

Before evaluating how effective the subsequent nurse training legislation was, it is interesting to examine what happened to the market for nurses in the post-1966 period.

The Market for Nurses in the Post–Medicare Period

In 1966, with the implementation of Medicare and Medicaid, the market for nurses changed. The demand for hospital care increased as the aged and the poor were provided with hospital coverage. At the same time, hospitals were reimbursed on a "cost-plus" basis. The effect was to increase the demand for RNs and, at the same time, to make the demand for RNs more inelastic with respect to their wage. When hospitals hired more nurses and increased their wages, these costs could then be passed on to the government (on a proportional basis, according to the "ratio of charges to charges to cost" of aged patients). Depending on what portion of their hospitalized population was covered under some form of cost reimbursement (e.g., government, Blue Cross, or other third-party reimbursement), hospitals were relieved from pressures to contain their costs.

Wage increases to hospital-employed nurses increased rapidly in the post–Medicare period, more rapidly than wage increases to nonhospital-employed nurses and to persons working in nonhealth occupations with comparable training. Nurses' wages, which were artificially held down for a number of years, were allowed to rise. Thus by 1969 rates of return to hospital-employed nurses were comparable to those of other occupations.

To sum up, then, hospitals were less inclined to act collusively in holding down nurses' wages after 1966 since Medicare and Medicaid reimbursed hospitals for the costs of caring for the aged and poor, regardless of how much that care cost. Nurses' wages consequently increased at a rapid rate. The effect of those wage increases was that nurse participation rates rose, hospitals were able to hire more nurses, and the vacancy rate decreased so that by 1971 the vacancy rate dropped to 9.3 percent from its high of 23 percent in 1962.

It appears, therefore, that there was a static shortage of registered nurses before 1966, created by the collusion of hospitals to keep nurses' wages from rising. Such a situation no longer exists. The appropriate public policy would have been to allow nurses' wages to rise, which would have increased hospital costs—a normal occurrence in an industry experiencing a rising demand for its services and facing a rising supply curve for its factor inputs. Claims of a "shortage" in this type of situation are merely a matter of employers not wishing to pay higher prices for their inputs. Allowing nurses' wages to rise would have brought forth an increase both in the stock of nurses and in their participation rate. Federal legislation to increase the supply of nurses would not have been necessary.

The Market for Nurses in More Recent Years

As a result of rising RN wages in the mid- to late 1960s, vacancy rates declined, nurse participation rates increased, and, within a few years, enrollments in schools of nursing increased. There is always a time lag as prospective students learn what is occurring in the nursing profession and adjust their career plans. Enrollments were sharply rising by the early 1970s, increasing the supply of RNs. There no longer appeared to be concern with a nurse shortage. In 1975 President Ford vetoed congressional renewal of federal funding for nurse education (but Congress overrode the veto).

The basis for another nurse shortage, however, began in 1971, when President Nixon imposed wage and price controls on the economy. Although these controls were removed from all other industries in 1972, they remained in effect for health care until 1974. These wage controls, together with the increased supply of RNs, began to have an effect by the late 1970s. Demand for RNs continued to increase throughout the 1970s, while the wage controls led to lower relative wages for RNs, and, by the mid-1970s, declining nursing school enrollments. By 1979 vacancy rates had reached 14 percent.

The 1979–80 shortage was short-lived. As shown in Figure 15.3, RN wages sharply increased at the same time the economy entered a severe recession in the early 1980s. The rising national unemployment rate caused more nurses to seek employment and to increase their hours of work. Since 70 percent of RNs are married, the loss of a job by a spouse, or even the fear of losing a job, is likely to cause RNs to increase their labor force participation rate to maintain their family income. Rising wages and the rising unemployment rate increased nurse participation rates, from 76 percent in 1980 to 79 percent by 1984. As a consequence of these forces, nurse vacancy rates declined to a low of 4.4 percent by 1983, essentially indicating that were was no longer a shortage. The (dynamic) nursing shortage was once again resolved through a combination of rising wages, an increase in the nurse participation rate, and a high unemployment rate nationally (5).

As nurse wages remained stable (and actually declined in real dollars) between 1983 and 1985, and the vacancy rate declined, nursing school enrollments dropped sharply.

Starting in the mid-1980s, the market for hospital services underwent dramatic changes, which affected the market for nurses. The trend by Medicare, private insurers, and HMOs to reduce the use of the hospital led to shorter hospital stays. Patients required more intensive treatment for the shorter time they were in the hospital. There was a greater degree of intensity of care being provided (e.g., a greater number of transplants and an increase in the number of low birthweight babies) to more severely ill hospitalized

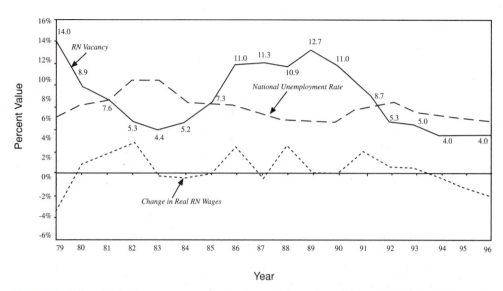

FIGURE 15.3 • RN vacancy rates, annual percent changes in real RN wages, and the national unemployment rate, 1979–96.
Source: Data compiled by Peter I. Buerhaus, Assistant Professor, Harvard School of Public Health, and director, Harvard Nursing Research Institute, and Douglas O. Staiger, Associate Professor, John F. Kennedy School of Government, and Research Associate, National Bureau of Economic Research, October 1997.

patients. (The Medicare patient case-mix index for all hospitals increased from 1.17 in 1985 to 1.39 by 1992.) The result was an increase in the number of RNs per patient. Nursing units were also being reorganized; their staffing patterns used a greater portion of RNs, as RNs could be used more flexibly, because of their training and state practice acts, than other types of nurses.

The greater demand by hospitals for RNs during this period is indicated by the following data: in 1975 there were 0.65 RNs per patient; it increased to 0.88 by 1980, and to 1.34 by 1990. The percent increase in RNs per patient exceeded the decline in patient days.

As demand for RNs increased more rapidly than supply in the latter part of the 1980s, another dynamic shortage occurred. Nurses; wages were slow to respond to these increased demands, the economy began improving, and nursing school enrollments had been falling until the mid-1980s. As a result, the vacancy rate increased from 5.1 percent in 1984 to 12.7 percent in 1989.

(As the nurse shortage has reoccurred over time, hospitals have lobbied for congressional subsidies for nurse training and for an easing of the immigration rules on foreign-trained nurses. The nursing shortage of the late 1980s resulted in Congress enacting the Nurse Shortage Reduction Act [1988] and the Immigration Nurse Relief Act [1989], which made it easier for foreign nurses to receive a working visa.)

As the economy began to weaken in 1990 and the unemployment rate increased in the early 1990s, nurse participation rates increased to 83 percent by 1992. Enrollment in nursing schools began to increase in 1988, two years after nurse wages and the vacancy rate began their increase. This increase in enrollments, which reflected the previous increase in demand, resulted in increased supplies of RNs. As a result of the increased supply of new RNs and the higher participation rate, nurses's (real) wages declined, as did vacancy rates, to 4 percent by the mid-1990s. There was no longer evidence of a shortage. Many in the nursing profession became concerned that there was a surplus. A further indication of a surplus was the decline in nursing enrollments by the mid-1990s.

Important to understanding future trends in the RN labor market is the effect that managed care is having on the demand for nurses. Buerhaus and Staiger recently examined the effect managed care has had on the nurse labor market by examining differences in demand for nurses in states with high and low managed care penetration (6). Although the proportion of all RNs working in hospitals has been declining, the effect has been much greater in high managed care states. As a result, there has been a shift in RN employment to nonhospital settings. This shift to nonhospital settings started earlier in the high managed care states. Also, RN employment grew more slowly in states with high HMO enrollment since 1990.

The effect of slower growth in demand for RNs and their shift to nonhospital settings has exerted downward pressure on RN wages; demand for hospital care decreased, therefore demand for RNs has increased more slowly than increases in RN supply. Further, as RNs moved to the lower-paying nonhospital sectors this has also slowed their wage growth. Although these effects are occurring in all states, they have been greatest in high managed care states.

If the effects of managed care continue in this direction, more hospitals will close and hospital demand for RNs will continue to decrease, with the consequence that RN wages will increase relatively slowly. Greater RN employment opportunities will be in the nonhospital sector. As wage growth for RNs diminishes, nurse enrollments will decrease, perhaps setting the stage for another dynamic shortage at some future time.[3]

Since the 1970s, nurse shortages were dynamic rather than static shortages and were resolved through increases in nurse wages. Higher wages brought an increased supply of nurses, by increasing nurse participation rates and through increased nursing school enrollments. It would thus appear that the market resolves these recurrent shortages and federal subsidies to support nurse education has been, and is, unnecessary. The most appropriate response to recurring dynamic nurse shortages is to facilitate the market's ad-

---

[3]The American Nurses' Association's efforts to change state licensure requirements for becoming a nurse could, if successful, drastically reduce the supply of nurses. According to the ANA, nursing graduates who wish to become a professional nurse should receive a BA degree. Those graduating from two-year programs would only receive a technical nursing license. To the extent the ANA is successful in changing state educational requirements for nurses in this manner, there should be a sharp reduction in the number of new graduates each year. Currently, graduates with a BA degree represent only 32 percent of new nurse graduates. If implemented today, this policy would result in a loss of two-thirds of nursing graduates. The effect of this policy would be an increase in salaries of professional nurses. These higher costs would, in part, be shifted to patients, government, and other third-party payers.

justment process. Better information to hospitals and to prospective nursing students about nurse labor market conditions would be helpful in eliminating the time lags in wage increases and enrollment that have resulted in these cyclical shortages.

MARKET STRUCTURE AND NURSE WAGES AND EMPLOYMENT

The earlier discussion on static and dynamic shortages of nurses assumed that the market structure for nurses was competitive. Hospitals were sufficiently small purchasers of RNs that they could hire all they wanted at the prevailing market wage, that is, hospitals faced a horizontal supply curve for nurses. Shortages occurred because of demand increasing faster than supply (dynamic shortage) or because of hospital collusion (static shortage).

A number of economists, however, have hypothesized that the market structure was not competitive. Instead, hospitals were monopsonists or oligopsonists with respect to the employment of registered nurses. Two conditions are necessary for this type of market structure to occur: first, there is only one or just a few hospitals hiring RNs; second, the hospital faced a rising (less elastic) supply curve for RNs. If one hospital raised nurses' wages, it was more likely to attract another hospital's nurses. Hospitals thus had an incentive to collude on setting nurses' wages. Preliminary evidence for this characterization of the nurse labor market is based on data showing that many markets consist of few hospitals within that market. Second, for monopsony to occur, nurses must also have limited mobility; otherwise they would move to those markets where wages are highest and labor supply curves would be more elastic. Particularly in previous times, diploma school graduates, married nurses who considered themselves secondary wage earners, and nurses with young children who preferred to work part-time were likely to be less mobile.

Thus monopsony and oligopsony market structure is an additional explanation for the existence of nurse vacancy rates and why hospitals claimed there was a shortage of nurses. Hospitals will demand more RNs than will be supplied at the going wage rate. Hospitals will therefore report RN vacancies and claim there is a shortage (7). Monopsony also results in lower wages and employment of RNs compared to a competitive market. Non-hospital settings (physician offices, outpatient clinics, etc.) employing RNs are small purchasers of RNs. These firms face a much more elastic supply curve for RNs and RNs represent a small portion of their total cost. These employers would therefore be able to hire all the RNs they want at or slightly above the prevailing wage.

The following discussion explains why a monopsonist reports vacancies and claims there is a shortage when an equilibrium situation exists.

A monopsonist, with a demand curve D_1, will face a rising supply curve for nurses described by S_1 in Figure 15.4. Since the monopsonist must pay a higher wage to all currently employed nurses each time it pays a higher wage for an additional nurse, it faces a marginal factor cost (*MFC*) curve that lies above the supply curve. The *MFC* curve represents the cost to the monopsonist of hiring an additional nurse. At each point on the

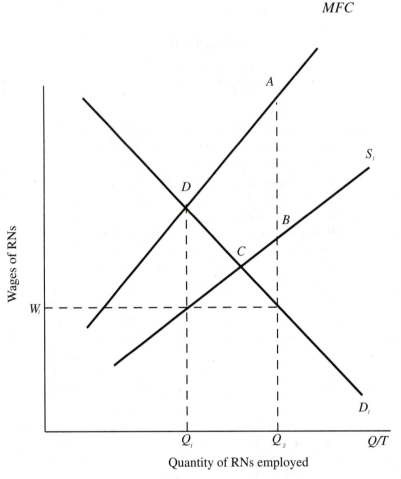

FIGURE 15.4 • An illustration of a monopsonistic market for registered nurses.

supply curve, the *MFC* curve indicates the additional cost in terms of higher wages that must be paid to all nurses hired previously. Thus the equilibrium quantity of nurses the firm will hire and the wage it will pay under such circumstances are given by the intersection of the demand curve and the *MFC* curve. Drawing a line down to the supply curve will indicate the wage the firm would pay and the quantity of RNs employed.

At the equilibrium wage, W_1, the monopsonist would be willing to hire Q_2 quantity of nurses, which is the point on the firm's demand curve. However, if the firm were actually to hire Q_2 number of RNs, it would have to pay a wage much higher than W_1 to attract them. The new wage would be at that point on the supply curve above Q_2 shown by *B*. The cost to the firm of that wage and Q_2 number of nurses would be point *A on the MFC curve.* Since point *A* on the *MFC* curve exceeds the firm's demand, the firm would not want to hire Q_2 nurses at a wage represented by point *B* on the supply curve. Thus

W_1 and Q_1 are equilibrium points for the monopsonist. However, at that wage, W_1, the firm will report $Q_1 - Q_2$ vacancies for nurses. These are the number of nurses it would be willing to hire at wage W_1.

Vacancies are thus expected and quite normal in a monopsony situation.

The effect of unionization in a market dominated by a monopsonist will be to eliminate the monopsonist's "shortage," since a prevailing wage will be established whereby the hospital could hire all the nurses demanded at that wage. The vacancy rate should decrease. Hospital monopsony power over nurses' wages is weakened by the growth (both actual and expected) of nurses' unions.

For example, if a union were formed and set a minimum (prevailing) wage for its employees, the supply curve for nurses would change. It would become horizontal up to the point of the minimum wage on the original supply curve. This would indicate that under the collective bargaining agreement, nurses cannot be paid below a certain minimum union wage. The hospital can hire all the nurses it wants at that wage. The *MFC* curve would also change. It would become equal to the new minimum wage, since there is no additional cost to the hospital as it hires an additional nurse; that is, it does not have to increase the wages of those nurses currently employed. Up to the point where the negotiated wage intersects the original supply curve, the hospital can hire all the nurses it wants at the negotiated wage. Beyond that point the hospital will again face a rising supply curve and a rising MFC curve; the hospital will have to increase its wages and also pay higher wages to its existing nurses.

In situations involving a monopsony purchaser and a union representing the employees, it is possible for the union to set a wage that is higher than the previous wage and also increase employment. See Figure 15.5. If the union sets a wage rate anywhere between A and B, it will raise the wage (since the current wage is W_1) and it will increase the number of nurses hired. Any wage between A and B will make the supply curve and the *MFC* curve horizontal up to that point. For example, a wage rate of W_2 is the point where employment of RNs is greatest. The new wage rate intersects the demand curve at the same point that the supply curve does. Therefore the wage rate (W_2) is the new *MFC* and supply curve up to the point where it intersects the original supply curve. To hire more nurses after that point, the firm will have to pay a higher wage and thus face a rising *MFC* and rising supply curve.

Point A on the demand curve is the highest union wage that can be set without decreasing employment of RNs.

With a union, nurse wages should increase and possibly employment as well. Whether increased employment will occur will depend on the union's objectives. If the union seeks to maximize wages for current union members, then there will be no increased employment of RNs.

Registered nurses employed in nonprofit hospitals were expressly exempt from the legal provisions of the National Labor Relations Act between 1947 and 1974 and therefore did not have legal protection of their rights to organize or support a union. Hospitals were under no obligation to engage in collective bargaining with their employees. (In

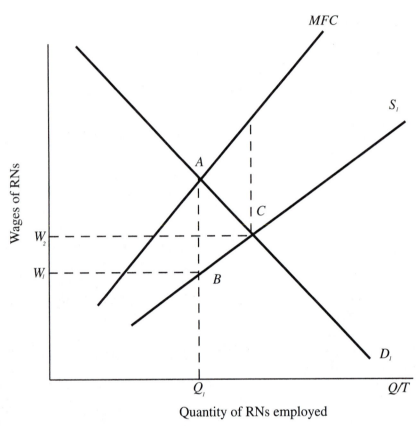

FIGURE 15.5 • Collective bargaining and a monopsony market for registered nurses.

1974, an amendment to the Taft–Hartley Act repealed hospitals' exempt status.) Collective bargaining on behalf of hospital nurses therefore started slowly. In addition to the impediments to collective bargaining contracts that legally permitted hospitals to refuse to bargain with unions representing hospital employees, the American Nurses' Association (ANA) had not been a strong proponent of unionization.

In 1970, approximately thirty-eight thousand RNs were included under collective bargaining agreements, representing about 5 percent of employed RNs. By 1977, two hundred thousand RNs, more than 20 percent of employed nurses, were included under collective bargaining agreements, a substantial increase over 1970. The growth in unionization has lagged behind the increased number of RNs, representing less than 20 percent of employed RNs (8).

The effects of collective bargaining agreements, however, are felt beyond the numbers of nurses covered. To forestall such agreements, hospitals are likely to offer higher wages to RNs.

A number of studies have attempted to estimate the degree of monopsony (or oligopsony) power in nurse labor markets (9). These studies have been of two types. One approach has been to estimate the potential for monopsony power by estimating the elasticity of the RN supply curve facing hospitals, an upward sloping supply curve being indicative of a monopsony market. The other approach used by researchers attempted to estimate the relationship between nursing wages and employment according to the labor market structure, monopsony being indicated by a positive relationship between wages and employment and more competitive markets. (Monopsonistic labor markets will have lower wages and employment.) Included in some of these studies have been attempts to measure whether unionization lessens monopsony power, as discussed above. These studies have also used data over different time periods.

Previous studies have generally found evidence supporting hospitals' monopsony power. It is likely that monopsony power was more prevalent in earlier periods. A greater percent of nurses graduated from diploma schools and were more closely tied to the hospitals where they were trained. Also, many nurses who were married and who had families considered themselves to be secondary wage earners and were therefore less mobile.

The increased number of hospital mergers and consolidation that are currently occurring increase hospitals' monopsony power and, consequently, can result in lower RN wages and employment. RNs should therefore favor the application of anti-trust laws to hospital mergers.

FEDERAL SUPPORT FOR NURSE TRAINING

To better understand the probable intent of the federal legislation to support nurse training and to determine how effective it was in achieving its stated goals of increasing the supply of nurses, it is worthwhile to examine the original Nurse Training Act in some depth.

The stimulus for the Nurse Training Act of 1964 was the 1963 report by the Surgeon General's Consultant Group on Nursing, appointed in 1961, that there was a serious shortage of nurses. The shortage forecast was made using the ratio technique and was thus unrelated to any economic definition of shortage. The forecast of a shortage was also unrelated to any analysis regarding the performance of the market for nurses.

Support for federal legislation to subsidize nurse training came from several groups: Congress recognized the potential political rewards of backing health legislation; the federal bureaucracy—specifically, the Division of Nursing in the U.S. Public Health Service—helped justify the need for the legislation with an eye toward an expanded role in administering it; hospitals favored it because they wanted an increased supply of nurses, thereby slowing down the rate of increase in nurses' wages.

The ANA also favored the legislation, but with different expectations as to its effects than hospitals. As a professional association, an important goal of the ANA is to increase its members' incomes. If the legislation were to have the effect desired by hospitals, namely, an increase in the supply of nurses, then the subsidy would limit the rise in nurses' wages, which would be the opposite of the ANA's objective. Instead, the ANA envisaged the educational subsidies as an opportunity to change the role of registered nurses. The ANA wanted the educational subsidies to be redirected toward producing fewer, but more highly trained nurses, who could increase their productivity by undertaking additional responsibilities. The effect of fewer nurses, with more training, would be an increase in nurses' wages.

Thus the reasons for federal subsidies for nurse education varied. Educational subsidies, either what the AHA or the ANA had in mind, would not have improved the functioning of the market for nurses. There was no economic justification for the federal legislation. The actual, as compared to the stated, intent of the legislation was to benefit either hospitals (by providing them with cheaper inputs) or nurses (by changing educational requirements and graduating fewer nurses capable of performing more tasks). By analyzing its implementation and its effects it becomes possible to determine who actually benefited from the legislation.

Two broad purposes were stated in the Nurse Training Act (NTA) of 1964: to increase the quantity of nurses and to improve their quality. These two goals matched the separate interests of the ANA and AHA. The goals and programs enacted in the NTA of 1964 were those recommended in the Surgeon General's report of 1963. To achieve both an increase in the quality and quantity of nurses, the NTA of 1964 provided four broad areas of federal support, which were continued in subsequent renewals and amendments to that act. The two most important areas, comprising 93 percent of the total funds expended on nurse training, were, first, a program of grants to schools of nursing for distribution in the form of scholarships and loans to students (40 percent of total funds were for this purpose). The second was for grants to the nursing schools for construction, planning or initiating programs of nursing education, or general financial support (53 percent of the funds went for this purpose).

The 1963 Surgeon General's report stated that with the federal support requested, 680,000 nurses would be a "feasible" goal by 1970. In updated estimates made in 1967, it was predicted that 1 million RNs would be needed in 1975. To achieve these increases in the number of nurses, it was proposed that schools of nursing increase the number of their graduates to 53,000 a year by 1969, which represented a 75 percent increase over 1961 (10).

Although it would appear that the nurse training legislation achieved its numerical goals (the number of nurses was as forecasted for 1970 and 1975), on closer examination it is unlikely that these achievements were a result of the federal support for nurse training. The number of graduates produced by schools of nursing in 1969 was only 42,196, not the 53,000 per year that was supposed to occur as a result of the federal program. In fact, the number of graduates was only 1,196 more than what the Surgeon General's report estimated would have been the case *without* any federal legislation. Since the funding of nursing schools and students did not achieve the increase in graduates believed necessary to achieve the numerical goals, how were the desired goals met?

An increase in the number of RNs employed can occur in one of three ways: (a) an increase in the number of nursing graduates, (b) an increase in the nurse participation rate, and (c) an increase in immigration of foreign-trained nurses. The federal program was directed exclusively at increasing the number of nursing graduates.

The federal program sought to increase the number of nurse graduates by: (a) funding new construction to increase the number of spaces in nursing schools, (b) the loan and scholarship programs to induce people to enter nursing who would otherwise not, and (c) financial assistance to the nursing schools, which could have resulted in either more attractive facilities or lower tuition rates to attract potential students.

Several economists estimated the increase in the number of nursing graduates as a result of the federal support for nursing education. It would appear that the federal subsidies led to an increase of fewer than 1,500 new graduates a year. Edgren estimated a total increase of 6,813 additional graduates (out of a total of 247,753 graduates) between 1966 and 1972 as a result of the federal subsidy program (11).

To understand why the increase in nurse graduates was so small, given the large federal subsidy program, it is necessary to examine the nursing education process. Nursing education is typically provided in one of three types of settings: three-year diploma schools associated with hospitals, community colleges offering a two-year associate degree, and four-year colleges offering a baccalaureate degree.[4] While attending classes, students in diploma schools worked in hospitals and received a stipend. Hospitals subsidized the cost of their diploma schools to assure themselves a supply of nurses upon graduation. However, as the mobility of nurses increased, hospital diploma schools became a diminishing source of nurses for the particular hospital subsidizing them. Hospitals were no longer assured that their subsidies to such schools would be repaid when the nurses left to work elsewhere. As tuition costs to the students in diploma schools rose, enrollments declined.

After World War II diploma schools of nursing declined rapidly. In 1950, there were 1,314 state-approved schools of nursing. Of these, 1,118 were diploma schools, 195 were BA programs, and 1 was an associate program. By 1966 there were 1,266 programs; of these, 788 were diploma schools, 280 were BA schools, and 198 were associate degree schools. By 1995, the total number of programs increased to 1,484; of these, only 135 were diploma schools, 501 were BA schools, and 848 were associate degree schools (12).

Hospitals wanted the federal subsidies to be used to increase the number of nurses graduating from diploma schools of nursing. There was sufficient capacity in those schools to accommodate increases in enrollment. However, the American Nurses' Association stated in 1965 that they wanted nursing education to occur in institutions of higher learning. The National League for Nursing (NLN) was designated as the accred-

---

[4]Of the approximately 2.1 million employed RNs in 1996, 24 percent graduated from diploma nursing schools, 35 percent from associate degree programs, 32 percent from a four-year baccalaureate degree program, and 9.1 percent from master's and doctorate programs.

iting agency for dispensing federal support to schools of nursing; its goals were, of course, similar to those of the ANA. Until 1968, payment to diploma and associate degree schools under the NTA fell short of what Congress authorized (50 percent), while payments to baccalaureate programs were approximately equal to what was authorized.

Although the number of diploma school programs declined, graduates from these programs still made the largest contribution to the number of new active nurses until 1972. Since then, more nurses have graduated from associate degree programs. These graduates represented 3 percent of graduates in 1960, 9.6 percent in 1965, 31.4 percent by 1970, and 60.5 percent currently. The large growth in associate degree programs began before the funds for the NTA became available. The percent of graduates from each of these programs is shown in Figure 15.6.

In administering the NTA no attempt was made to maximize the number of nurse graduates. If that had been the goal, the funds would have been allocated differently according to the types of nursing schools. Instead, there appears to have been a conscious decision to favor growth in the number of nursing graduates from baccalaureate degree programs, which coincided with the ANA's goals. Graduates with a BA degree were more likely to take on additional responsibilities and there would be a smaller increase in the number of nurses. Both effects would result in an eventual increase in nurse wages.

From the ANA's perspective, unless BA graduates were subsidized, fewer prospective nurses would choose a four-year school. A graduate from a baccalaureate school spends more time in school compared with graduates from associate degree or diploma schools, yet the wage differential does not compensate baccalaureate graduates for the additional training time or forgone income. Studies confirm that the rate of return to the nurse with a baccalaureate degree working in a hospital setting is less than for a nurse with only a two-year associate degree (13).

(To further make the BA degree a more attractive option to prospective nurses, the ANA has proposed a two-tier licensure system, one for graduates with a BA degree and the other for associate and diploma school graduates. The ANA has been successful in having such legislation enacted in several states. Presumably the differential licensure system will be more informative to employers [who would otherwise be unawares] as to the capabilities of nurses trained in different settings.)

The growth in demand for associate degree education was related to its relatively high rate of return compared with comparable occupations. It is thus likely that associate degree programs would have grown without federal NTA support.

If the federal subsidies for nurse education produced few additional nurses, then how were the quantitative goals for the number of nurses achieved? Based on an econometric model of the nursing sector, which was used to simulate changes that have occurred in nurse employment over time, one author concluded: "the achievement of the 1969 level of nursing is to be attributed to the increase in participation rates and the change in the age distribution of the stock of nurses, as well as increased graduations, and none of these events are even remotely influenced by the existence of the subsidy programs in question" (14).

It has been estimated that the sources of the net increase in employed RNs between

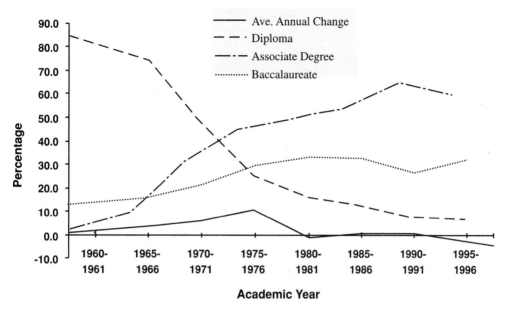

FIGURE 15.6 • Percent distribution of nursing graduates by type of nursing school program and average annual change in total graduates, 1960–95.
Source: Data from National League for Nursing, *Nursing Data Book* (New York: National League for Nursing), various years.

1966 and 1977 were: a change in the participation rate and in reinstatements (RNs who have renewed their lapsed licenses), 33.9 percent; foreign-trained RNs, 9.1 percent; and new graduates, 57.1 percent (15). The higher nurse participation rates during the period that the federal subsidy program was in effect were in large part due to the increase in nurses' wages, which resulted from the enactment of Medicare and Medicaid. Labor force participation rates for nurses increased from 55 percent in 1960 to 65 percent in 1966, to 70 percent in 1972, to 76 percent in 1980, and to 83 in 1996 (16). It appears, therefore, that the achievement of the employment goals underlying the NTA of 1964 was primarily the result of increased nurse participation rates rather than the federal subsidy program itself, which resulted in a very small increase in graduates compared to what would have otherwise occurred.

An alternative subsidy approach to increasing the supply of RNs would have been to subsidize RN wages directly. For example, it was estimated that the number of additional nurses employed as a result of the federal support to nursing schools was approximately 1,500 nurses per year or 24,000 for the 16-year period 1965–81. The estimated federal expenditures under nurse training legislation during that time period were $1.57 billion. This comes to $65,000 per employed nurse as a result of the federal subsidy program. If a direct wage subsidy were instead provided to all employed nurses, the federal subsidy dollars required would have been several times less.

Calculating the cost of increasing the supply of nurses as a result of a wage subsidy program requires an estimate of the elasticity of the participation rate with respect to nurse wages. Several studies have derived elasticity estimates ranging from a negative elasticity to an elasticity of 2.8 (17). In our example, a wage elasticity of 1.0 is used; that is, a 1 percent increase in nurses' wages leads to a 1 percent increase in the number of active nurses. It would thus require a 1 percent increase in nurses' wages, multiplied by all the employed nurses, to achieve a 1 percent increase in the number of employed RNs.

In 1963 there were approximately 550,000 active RNs receiving an annual wage of $4,714. A 1 percent subsidy to increase their wage would be $47 per nurse multiplied by 550,000 active nurses, for a total subsidy cost of $25 million. This would result in a 1 percent increase in the number of active RNs, or 5,500 additional nurses. The federal subsidy per additional nurse employed under this program comes to $4,545. As the number of active RNs increases, so does the annual number of subsidy dollars required to produce an additional active RN under this approach—from $4,545 per active RN in 1963 to $7,936 per active RN in 1969. To produce an equivalent 24,000 nurses through a wage subsidy program would have taken approximately four years at a total subsidy cost of $120 million, for an average cost of $5,000 per additional nurse.

When compared with the cost of $65,000 per active RN produced under the actual nurse training legislation, the cost per active RN under this alternative subsidy program is approximately 10 times less expensive (18). Even if one were to vastly change the assumptions used in these calculations (i.e., the elasticity of the nurse participation rates or the number of nursing school graduates produced under the NTA), this alternative subsidy program is still less expensive. For example, if a 0.25 elasticity estimate were assumed, a wage subsidy program would have been about half the cost of the program adopted by the government. (The attractiveness of this program would be increased further if the subsidies were discounted.)

Other advantages of the direct wage subsidy program are that the increase in active nurses would occur much more quickly and that the federal government would not have to make a continuing financial commitment to support nursing schools. A new constituency for continuing federal support has been created and it is difficult to reduce support even though there may no longer be a nursing shortage.

Paradoxically, the more successful the federal government is in increasing the number of nursing graduates, the lower will be the increase in nurses' wages. An increased supply of new nurses would hold down potential increases in nurses' wages; this dampening effect would have an adverse impact on the participation rate. Thus the subsidy to nursing schools could well have been self-defeating!

Although a wage subsidy program would have been less expensive and would offer quicker results than the education subsidy, there is no economic justification for this program either. It is inefficient to subsidize the cost of one input, since hospitals will then increase rather than decrease their relative use of RNs. Similarly, since any supply subsidy is unlikely to improve economic efficiency, it should be evaluated in terms of whether it is more efficient than a demand subsidy for increasing access to a those with low incomes (presumably the purpose of a value judgment to redistribute medical care).

AN ECONOMIC ANALYSIS OF COMPARABLE WORTH

Since nursing has been predominately a female profession (93 percent), nursing associations had been in the forefront of the movement to legislate "comparable worth" throughout the country. It was seen as a mechanism by which nurses' wages could be increased. Although these legislative efforts have been less active in recent years, it is instructive to examine this concept since it clarifies the determination of wages in a market system. The crux of the debate regarding comparable worth is over the appropriate mechanism for setting wages.

According to the 1964 Civil Rights Act, a person must receive equal pay for performing equal work; discrimination in employment is illegal. Comparable worth goes beyond that concept; its proponents want equal pay for work of comparable value. If two people are performing different jobs, but if a government agency determines that their work is of equal value, they should be rewarded equally. The proponents of greater pay equity base their argument on the empirical observation that certain jobs that are filled predominately by women are paid less than jobs that are filled predominately by men. The value of each job should be determined, not by the marketplace, but by fact-finding commissions.

Comparable worth is analyzed by first reviewing how wages are determined in a competitive market and, second, the effects on wages and employment of noncompetitive restrictions. Two alternative theories are then used to explain observed wage disparities between males and females. Next, the consequences of using comparable worth to achieve pay equity are discussed, and finally, alternative strategies to increase nursing salaries are presented.

The Determination of Wages

In a competitive market, wages and employees' incomes are determined by the firm's demand for employees and by the number or supply of those employees. The wage is the equilibrating mechanism; it is the price of labor. At higher or lower wages, the firm would be willing to hire fewer or more persons, respectively. Also, the higher the wage or income, the greater are the number of people willing to enter that occupation or profession. (A change in the wage represents a movement along the firm's demand curve and a movement along the supply of labor curve.)

The value of an employee's output also determines how many employees a firm will hire. The value of an employee's output consists of two parts: the productivity of the employee (i.e., how much output each additional worker can produce) and the price at which that output can be sold in the marketplace. (Changes in either employee productivity or the price of the output cause shifts in the demand for labor.) An employee's productivity is affected by her education, skill, and experience. Thus even within a given profession, differences in income exist because of differences in productivity. The higher the price at which the output can be sold, the greater the market value of the employee producing that output. For example, if a nurse practitioner is reimbursed for performing a physical exam at a lower fee than a family practitioner, the value of the output produced by the nurse practitioner is lower.

In a competitive market, therefore, a person's income depends on three things: his productivity, the price at which that service is sold in the market, and the number (supply) of people in the profession.

Market restrictions may either increase or decrease employees' incomes. Restrictions limiting entry into the profession will increase the incomes of those in the profession while decreasing the incomes of those who must work in other occupations that do not have such restrictions. These restrictions are often sanctioned by the government, such as with licensing, or by nongovernment groups, such as unions, when they determine, for example, who can work as a plumber. The effect of these entry restrictions is to have a smaller supply of professionals in the restricted market and a larger supply in the unrestricted market, causing a wage differential between the two markets.

Restrictions on the tasks that health professionals may perform have similar effects. There often are tasks that a person is capable of performing (either by experience or training), but the profession is prohibited from doing so by state practice acts. A professional prohibited from performing highly remunerative tasks thereby produces an output that has a lower economic value (the demand for her services is shifted to the left).

Another type of restriction is when employers collude on the setting of wages, as apparently occurred during the 1950s and early 1960s, when hospitals colluded in the setting of nurses' wages. The effect of such monopoly power by the purchasers of services was to hold down the rate of increase in nurses' salaries.

Finally, if a firm does not face competition in the sale of its product, then the firm does not have to be as concerned with its costs of production (i.e., the wage rates it pays or whether it employs the best people for the job). This would happen, for example, in regulated companies (such as utilities) or in state and local governments. Similarly, prior to enactment of prospective payment legislation (DRGs), hospitals were not constrained to produce in cost-minimizing ways. Medical schools that are heavily subsidized and that have excess demand for their places can also be less efficient.

A firm that is a monopolist in the sale of its product can pass on higher wages and the additional costs of hiring less competent personnel. It is precisely in such situations that firms can also practice discrimination in hiring. In a competitive industry, if a firm paid higher wages or hired less competent workers than its competitors, its costs would be higher. The firm could not compete on price and would either be forced to go out of business or to change its employment practices. Discriminatory practices are therefore more likely to occur in industries or among firms that are less concerned with their costs (19).

Theories to Explain Wage Disparities

Women, on average, earn less than men. Some occupations are also filled predominately by women. Why does this occur?

According to the "crowding" theory, women are channeled by either their own expectations or by those of others into certain professions that are predominately female. The exclusion of women from higher-paying male-dominated jobs causes a surplus of women within particular jobs, thereby leading to lower wages in the female-dominated jobs. Little evidence seems to exist to support the premise that women's occupations, such as nursing or clerical work, are more crowded than men's occupations. Moreover, for the crowding theory to be a valid explanation of differences in male/female wages, the market would have to be noncompetitive in some manner. Otherwise, some women would enter male-dominated professions to receive a higher rate of return. The mobility between occupations would equalize wages.

The most accepted explanation by economists for wage disparities is based on the theory of human capital (20). There are nonmonetary reasons why people select certain jobs; preferences as to the type of work and location may have an influence on a person's employment preferences. Wages reflect these differences in preferences. Second, individuals have different abilities, resulting in different incomes. However, an individual's productivity is not fixed; it can be increased with additional training and education. Therefore, wages also differ according to the individual's investment in education, training, and experience. Thus if females anticipate leaving the workforce, they may invest less in education; married women who have undertaken traditional home responsibilities have found this to be an obstacle in making a full commitment to their careers.

How well does the above explain male/female wage differentials? According to empirical studies, most of the differences in male/female wage ratios can be explained by differences in the total number of years of work experience, the years of tenure on the current job, and the pattern or continuity of previous work experience (21). These studies do not deny that discrimination may exist; however, it is not an important determinant of observed wage differences.

As differences in human capital between males and females lessen, so should differences in their wage rates. Career patterns and expectations have changed significantly since the 1960s. For example, in 1970, females represented 9.4 percent of medical school applicants and 8.4 percent of the graduates. In 1995, 42 percent of the applicants were female as were 38 percent of the graduates. This percentage should continue to increase. As educational levels, work roles, and work expectations of males and females become similar, so should their relative wages.

Determination of Wages Through Comparable Worth

What is likely to occur if wages were based on comparable worth instead of being left to the marketplace? Consultants and committees would be used to conduct job evaluations on each position within an organization or firm. These evaluations would involve assessment of the relative worth of each position according to skill required, effort involved, working conditions, and level of responsibility. Points would be assessed for each of these factors and salaries would be determined by the total number of points in each position.

The implementation of a comparable worth-based wage-determination system would result in a number of problems. First, the complexity of categorizing people would be tremendous, particularly if one were trying to establish a nationally applicable system affecting tens of thousands of jobs in hundreds of thousands of places. Further, these job evaluations would have to be updated as tasks and job conditions change. The implementation cost of such a system would be enormous, not only in terms of the time involved but also the cost of hiring the consultants and establishing job evaluation committees. An additional very large cost would be that arising from the resolution of identified pay inequities. This may well be in the billions of dollars.

Second, wage equity under comparable worth would not be achieved by lowering wages in job classifications in which job evaluations indicated that certain groups were being overpaid. Individuals in those groups would protest. Instead, occupations in which employees were currently being underpaid would have their wages increased. When the employer is a state government, the state can increase taxes to pay the increased costs; however, if taxpayers or their legislators are unwilling to vote for higher taxes, the effect would be similar to imposing higher wages on private industry. Less money would be spent on other programs or the employer would be forced to reduce employment in those occupations where wages were raised. Moreover, it is in female-dominated occupations that wages would be increased and, consequently, where fewer people would be hired. Although those remaining on the job would receive higher wages, some would be let go.

Third, wages determined by a commission would not reflect supply and demand conditions. Visualize a market with shifting demand and supply curves. The result would be shortages and surpluses of workers in different occupations. How would this be resolved? Will it be possible to increase wages in those occupations experiencing shortages? Jobs in surplus professions will have to be rationed since the wage would be above the equilibrium level. What criteria will be used? Rationing provides an opportunity for discrimination, as has previously been the case with medical school admissions.

In summary, while comparable worth may be conceptually appealing to those who distrust the market, its implementation would be costly and not likely to achieve the goals its proponents desire. Problems that would emerge are politicization of wage determination, a large bureaucracy for evaluating all positions in the economy, lower levels of employment for women in those occupations in which wages have been increased artificially, increased costs of services and a smaller output in those industries with a greater portion of women, a decreased incentive for women to move into other professions, and continual shortages and surpluses.

Alternative Strategies for Increasing Wages

Alternative strategies should be pursued to achieve greater pay equity. The first is the enforcement of current laws against discrimination; females desiring to enter male-dominated professions should be able to do so. A shift in the number of females from female-dominated professions to male-dominated professions should increase the wage in the former and depress wages in male-dominated professions. Differences in wages would more closely reflect either preferences for some types of occupations or differences in investment in human capital.

Next should be the elimination of the many restrictions that prevent labor markets from operating competitively. Legal restrictions that prohibit certain persons from undertaking tasks even though they are qualified to perform those tasks result in higher prices to society and in lower wages to those who are prohibited from performing them. For example, a nurse could receive increased income as a nurse midwife. However, when an insurance company refuses to provide malpractice coverage to obstetricians working with the nurse midwives or if an insurer refuses to pay the nurse midwife unless the bill is submitted by a physician, access by patients to nurse midwifery services is limited and nurses are prevented from increasing their incomes. In many instances, restrictive nurse practice acts unnecessarily limit the nurse's ability to perform certain functions.

The increasing trend toward competition in the delivery of health services should prove beneficial to the career goals of nurses. Managed care organizations must be price-competitive if they are to survive and grow. The managers of such organizations are more willing to look for less expensive methods of providing services, more willing to innovate, more responsive to patient concerns, and less bound to traditional tasks and roles than were not-for-profit hospitals reimbursed on a cost basis and state medical societies concerned with protecting their members' incomes. In a price-competitive system, nurses are moving into such new areas such as utilization review, case management for catastrophic care, and home health services, and performing additional tasks previously denied them.

The marketplace does not place the same value on people or services as many would prefer. However, years of experience with trying to control the market through wage and price controls have demonstrated that it is costly and eventually ineffective to try to do so. Therefore, an alternative approach to increase nurse wages is to understand the criteria used by the market to establish incomes and to use those criteria to help achieve the desired goals. Enforcing current laws on discrimination, removing economic restrictions, and providing access to educational and training opportunities would increase job opportunities and incomes for women while benefiting society through increased availability of services.

SUMMARY

The measures used to evaluate the performance of the nursing market were the rise in the number of hospital-employed nurses, their rate of return compared with other nurses and other occupations with comparable training, the increase in the number of nurses entering nursing, and the participation rate of nurses. In an efficiently operating market, as the demand for nurses increases so would their wages, their relative rate of return, the number of students entering nursing, and the percentage of trained nurses who are active.

Initially, in the late 1940s, the nursing market appeared to have been in equilibrium. However, up until the mid-1960s there was a shortage; the demand for nurses by hospitals exceeded the supply of nurses at the market wage. Based on an analysis of relative wages of hospital-employed nurses relative to other nurses, it appeared that a static short-age was created by hospitals colluding to prevent nurses' wages from rising. In an attempt to limit the increase in their nursing costs and a belief that increased wages would not in-crease the number of employed nurses, hospitals instead intensified their recruiting of foreign-trained nurses and substituted nurses aides for RNs. Hospitals also lobbied for federal subsidies to increase the supply of nurses.

The static shortage began to disappear when Medicare and Medicaid were enacted. As the demand for hospital care (and the consequent demand for nurses) increased, hospi-tals were able to pass on to the government both the increased costs of higher wages and of an increase in the number of nurses employed. Nurses' wages in the post–Medicare pe-riod increased rapidly, as did nurse participation rates. Nurses' employment and career decisions were more responsive to higher wages, in both the short and long run, than hospitals believed. The high rate of return to nursing led to increased enrollments in as-sociate degree programs. The rate of return to nursing again became comparable to other occupations. (The rate of return varied, however, depending on the type of degree re-ceived by the nurse.)

Federal legislation to support nurse training started in 1964 and continued for many years. The original manpower goals underlying the 1964 Nurse Training Act were achieved, although it appears that they would have been achieved without the federal sub-sidy program. In fact, had the federal subsidy program been very successful in increasing the number of nurse graduates, the increased supply of nurses would have led to a lower rate of increase in nurse wages, hence a smaller increase in the nurse participation rate.

There is no economic justification for the government to subsidize nurse education. If RNs desire to undertake additional roles, it is not the government's responsibility to sub-sidize their education to enable them to achieve their objectives any more than for any other professional group. Revision of state practice acts to permit nurses to undertake ad-ditional tasks for which they are trained and qualified to perform will result in an in-creased return from doing these tasks, which would justify increased investment by nurses for this training. Eliminating anticompetitive restrictions is a more appropriate policy. The goals used by the nursing profession to justify subsidies to nursing education should be made explicit so that it can be determined whether it is a goal agreed to by the rest of society and whether the proposed approach is the least expensive way to achieve it.

There have been recurrent claims of a shortage of nurses. These shortages, however, have been temporary or dynamic and have been resolved without government intervention.

The market for RNs has been changing with the advent of managed care competition. As substitution away from the hospital toward ambulatory care settings has increased, hospitalized patients are more severely ill. This has increased hospitals' demand for RNs. However, as the demand for hospitals has declined, so has hospitals' demand for RNs. The net effect of these opposing factors has been a slight increase in the number of hos-pital-employed RNs. In the past eight years, however, the percent of RNs employed by hospitals has declined from 68 to 60 percent. A larger percent of nurses are being em-ployed in ambulatory care settings, such as group practices, as well as undertaking new roles as nurse practitioners, and working with managed care organizations. It is likely that these trends will continue.

Nurse associations have sought various types of legislation to increase the roles, responsibilities, and incomes of nurses. These legislative remedies have included federal subsidies to nursing schools, comparable worth for setting nurse wages, minimum nurse staffing ratios in hospitals and other care settings, and efforts to prevent the merger and closure of hospitals.

Nurse aspirations of greater responsibilities and independence, along with higher incomes, are, however, more likely to be achieved in a competitive market than through government regulation. Managed care organizations and group practices, in their search for lower costs and increased quality, are less bound by traditional dividing lines between nurses and physicians. Several HMOs have begun contracting with nurse practitioners (who operate independently of physicians), paying them 80 percent of physicians' fees. The demand for different types of nurse education will be market driven, determined by the types of roles nurses will be engaged in, such as caring for more severely ill patients, greater responsibilities in primary care settings, as well as increased managerial responsibilities in managed care organizations.

Key Terms and Concepts

- Hospital collusion
- Nurse participation rates
- Nurse substitution
- Vacancy rates

- Comparable worth-based wages
- Derived demand for RNs
- Determinants of a firm's demand for employees
- Dynamic and static shortages
- Federal nurse education subsidies
- Monopsony and oligopsony in hospital markets
- Wage disparity theories

Review Questions

1. Various measures have been used to indicate that there has been a shortage of nurses. Evaluate the use of such measures to indicate the existence of a shortage. Second, what information would you use to indicate whether a shortage exists? Third, distinguish between a dynamic and a static shortage.
2. Contrast the market for registered nurses during the periods before and after Medicare. How well did the market for hospital-employed nurses perform in each of these two periods?

3. How have the past several shortages of nurses been resolved? How does an increase in nurse wages affect both hospitals' demand for nurses and the supply of nurses?

4. Why was the shortage of nurses that occurred before Medicare different from subsequent shortages?

5. Contrast the following two approaches for eliminating the shortage of nurses:
   a. Federal subsidies to nursing schools
   b. Providing information on nurse demand and supply to prospective nursing students and to demanders of nursing services, such as hospitals.

6. Nurses are restricted in the tasks they are permitted to perform. Also, certain nurse specialties (e.g., nurse midwives) would like to bill for their services on a fee-for-service basis rather than work for obstetricians. Using the theory of the demand for labor, explain how changes in each of the above would affect the demand for registered nurses.

7. You are an economic consultant to the American Nurses' Association. What would you expect the effects of changes in the health care markets, such as prospective payment for hospitals, growth in HMOs, the increased supply of physicians, and so on, to be on the employment and earnings of RNs? In your answer trace through the effects you expect on both the product and factor markets.

8. "Comparable worth" proponents seek equal pay for work of comparable value. What are the consequences of setting nurses' wages according to the concept of comparable worth? Describe the factors that determine wages in a competitive market (including those factors that cause shifts in the demand for labor). What are noncompetitive situations that have resulted in lower nurses' wages?

9. Nursing associations have proposed increasing the educational requirements to a four-year BA degree for all persons desiring to become professional nurses. What are the economic consequences of instituting such a change? Who would be expected to favor it, and who would be expected to oppose it?

10. How would unionization in a monopsony market for nurses' services increase both nurses' wages and hospital employment?

11. Would a more price-competitive hospital market result in higher or lower nurse wages?

REFERENCES

1. The discussion in this section is based on Donald E. Yett, *An Economic Analysis of the Nurse Shortage* (Lexington, Mass.: D. C. Heath, 1975), p. 110.

2. *Ibid.*, p. 19.

3. *Ibid.*, p. 221.

4. *Ibid.*, p. 221.

5. Peter Buerhaus, "Capitalizing on the Recession's Effect on Hospital RN Shortages," *Hospital and Health Services Administration,* 39(1), Spring 1994: 47–62.

6. Peter I. Buerhaus and Douglas O. Staiger, "Managed Care and the Nurse Workforce," *Journal of the American Medical Association,* 276(18), November 13, 1996: 1487–1493.

7. There have been a number of studies that have tested whether hospitals possess monopsony power with respect to RNs. Some studies have also estimated the effect of collective bargaining on wages in monopsonistic markets. One study, using data from 1979 to 1985, concluded that hospitals have a substantial degree of monopsony power; the labor supply curve is upward sloping with an elasticity of 1.25 in the short run (one year) and about 4 in the long run. Daniel Sullivan, "Monopsony Power in the Market for Nurses," *Journal of Law and Economics,* 32(2), Pt. 2, October 1989: 135–178. A recent study, using data from 1985 to 1993, does not find empirical support for the monopsony model; nurses' wages are found not to be related to hospital density and decrease rather than increase with respect to labor market size. Barry T. Hirsch and Edward J. Schumacher, "Monopsony Power and Relative Wages in the Labor Market for Nurses," *Journal of Health Economics,* 14(4), October 1995: 443–476.

8. Communication from the American Nurses' Association.

9. For one such study and a review of the literature, see Barry T. Hirsch and Edward J. Schumacher, "Monopsony Power and Relative Wages in the Labor Market for Nurses," *Journal of Health Economics,* 14(4), October 1995: 443–476.

10. For a discussion of the NTA, see Yett, *op. cit.,* p. 246.

11. John Edgren, "The Federal Nurse Training Acts," *Health Manpower Policy Studies Group Discussion Paper Series* (Ann Arbor, Mich.: School of Public Health, University of Michigan, 1977).

12. Data for 1950 are from *Source Book of Nursing Personnel* (Bethesda, Md.: U.S. Department of Health, Education, and Welfare, Division of Nursing, DHEW Publication [HRA] 75-43, December 1974); data for subsequent years are from *Nursing Data Review,* National League for Nursing, New York.

13. Evelyn Lehrer, William White, and Wendy Young, "The Three Avenues to a Registered Nurse License," *Journal of Human Resources,* 26(2), Spring 1991: 362–79. This study also contains reviews of previous research in this area.

14. Robert T. Dean, "Simulating an Econometric Model of the Market for Nurses," unpublished doctoral dissertation, Department of Economics, University of California at Los Angeles, 1971, p. 218. A further discussion of the ineffectiveness of the NTA may be found in Robert Deane and Donald Yett, "Nurse Market Policy Simulations Using an Econometric Model," in Scheffler, ed., *op. cit.*

15. Edgren, *op cit.,* p. 39.

16. *The Registered Nurse Population: An Overview,* from The National Sample of Registered Nurses, November 1980, March 1984, March 1988, and *Advance Notes I from the National Sample Survey of Registered Nurses March 1996,* Division of Nursing, Bureau of Health Profession, Health Resources and Services Administration, Rockville, Md.

17. The reasons for the differences in the estimates relate to the types of data used (aggregate versus micro), characteristics of the nurses, and the econometric methods employed. For a further discussion of these estimates, see Peter I. Buerhaus, "Economic Determinants of the Annual Number of Hours Worked by Registered Nurses," *Medical Care,* 29(12), 1991:

1181–1195. Buerhaus's study, based on data from the 1984 National Sample Survey of Registered Nurses, estimates wage elasticities of 0.49 for all RNs and 0.88 for unmarried RNs. Also included is a review of previous studies.

18. For the 1974–83 period the cost of an additional nurse educated as a result of the Nurse Training Act was estimated to have fallen to between $35,800 and $43,550. Steven R. Eastaugh, "The Impact of the Nurse Training Act on the Supply of Nurses, 1974–1983," *Inquiry,* 22(4), Winter 1985: 404–417.

19. Gary Becker, *The Economics of Discrimination,* 2nd ed. (Chicago: University of Chicago Press, 1971).

20. Gary Becker, *Human Capital* (New York: Columbia University Press, 1964).

21. F. Levy and R. Murnane, "U.S. Earnings Levels and Earnings Inequality: A Review of Recent Trends and Proposed Explanations," *Journal of Economic Literature,* 30(3), September 1942: 1333–1381; and F. Blau and L. Kahn, "Rising Inequality and the U.S. Gender Gap," *American Economic Review,* 84(2), May 1994: 23–33.

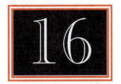

CHAPTER 16

The Role of Government in Health and Medical Care

GOVERNMENT INTERVENTION IN MEDICAL CARE

Government, particularly at the federal level, has a significant role in the financing, provision, and regulation of health and medical services. Federal expenditures for personal medical services have risen sharply since the passage of Medicare and Medicaid in the mid-1960s. Various levels of government are also suppliers of medical services, such as the Veterans Administration's (VA) system of hospitals and medical services supplied to military dependents in military facilities under the auspices of the Department of Defense. Different levels of government also provide indirect subsidies for medical services in the form of subsidies for medical research, for hospital construction (under the Hill–Burton Act), and for health manpower under federally supported programs, and subsidies by states for health professional education.

At least as important as financial involvement of government in medical service is the less obvious role of government in setting the rules under which medical services are paid for, organized, and produced, and the protection provided to patients through mechanisms such as licensing. Although government has long been involved in establishing the rules of the game for medical care, its role in financing medical care, particularly with regard to national health insurance, has been more controversial.

Some people view this increasing involvement of government in the medical sector as inevitable and beneficial; to others it is improper and the cause of inefficiencies. To clarify the debate over the increasing involvement of government in medical care, it is useful to review the traditional criteria for the role of government in a market system and to apply these criteria to medical care. Differences in opinion over the role of government in medical care can then be separated into differences regarding: (a) whether the traditional criteria for government involvement are appropriate; and (b) given the appropriateness of the criteria, whether such criteria warrant government involvement in medical care.

The appropriate criteria for justifying government intervention involve value judgments on the role of government. The sooner these differences are recognized as such, the sooner the participants will be able to focus the debate on whether there are more appropriate alternatives to the traditional criteria for government involvement. Then, given an agreed-on set of criteria for government intervention, the government role is more easily resolved because the existence of certain situations in medical care can be determined empirically. The evaluation of government's role in medical care, therefore, depends both on appropriate criteria for government involvement and on the applicability of such criteria to medical care.

There are two traditional areas where government is acknowledged to have a role in a market-oriented system (1). Each of these areas is briefly discussed.

MARKET IMPERFECTIONS

In a competitive market, economic efficiency on the demand and supply sides cannot be achieved when the assumptions underlying competitive markets are violated. The most important assumptions that are not fulfilled in medical care are the following: consumers and providers (physicians) have perfect information; there is complete mobility of resources;[1] and patients and providers have an incentive to minimize their costs of purchasing and providing medical treatment.

Consumers have insufficient knowledge regarding their medical diagnosis, treatment needs, the quality of different providers, and the prices charged by different providers. Patients' ignorance as to their medical needs, diagnosis, and treatment requirements have enabled physicians to induce demand for their services. The empirical evidence indicating demand inducement consists, for example, of differences in rates of specific surgical procedures according to methods of physician payment. The agency relationship between patients and their physicians has not always worked well. Different mechanisms

---

[1]Another imperfection would be with respect to the capital markets. If full-cost tuition were charged to medical students, students would not be able to borrow from banks based just on their prospective earnings and without collateral. This type of market imperfection exists for all forms of higher education and is not peculiar to medical or dental education. At present, however, other market imperfections in the health education market, such as barriers to entry, are of greater overriding concern, since they prevent full-cost tuition from being instituted.

have arisen to compensate for supplier-induced demand, such as utilization review. However, problems regarding the agency relationship still exist under both fee-for-service and capitation.

Lack of provider information is indicated by wide variations in use rates unrelated to differences in physician payment (discussed in Chapter 10). (Studies on appropriateness of care for different diagnoses, undertaken by HMOs and also funded by the government, are an attempt to increase physician knowledge.)

There are several types of barriers or restrictions on the mobility of resources. There are limits on entry into health manpower professions as a result of nonprofit medical schools and the accreditation criteria for those schools enforced by the Liaison Commission on Medical Education. The continual excess demands by applicants for a medical (and dental) education, continually high rates of return to the medical profession, and the willingness of U.S. citizens to bear higher costs and study for a longer period in foreign medical schools to become a U.S. physician are indications of barriers to entry. Second, many states still have certificate of need laws that bar institutions and even home health agencies from entering and competing in various markets within their state. And third, restrictions exist, unrelated to quality, on the tasks various personnel are permitted to perform.

Tax-free health insurance purchased by employers on behalf of their employees reduced patient concerns with costs of medical care. This health insurance continues to distort employees' choice of health plan and patients' use of medical services. Provider incentives to be concerned with their costs were lessened by the previous use of cost-based payment by third-party payers, including government.

Lack of consumer and provider information, barriers to entry and restrictions on tasks, and employer-paid health insurance have resulted in prices that exceed average costs and large variations in medical use rates. Excess insurance for patients and the previous cost-based reimbursement to providers resulted in inappropriate utilization, excessive duplication of facilities, rapidly rising medical costs, and a consequent concern for the efficiency with which medical care was produced.

The effect of barriers to entry and the lack of price competition was that patients paid a price for medical care that did not reflect their marginal valuation of using those services. Utilization of medical services by patients whose insurance is subsidized (either by the government or through tax deductions) exceeds what they would be willing to pay for that care if they had to pay the full price. Similarly, the price paid for medical care by third-party payers, the government, and patients (both through their out-of-pocket expenditures and through their taxes) exceeded the minimum costs of providing that care.

Thus it is apparent that there were (and still are) imperfections in the market for medical services. Many have been created by the government itself. To discuss the appropriate role of government in the face of these imperfections on both the demand and supply sides of the medical services market, it is first necessary to understand why many of these imperfections were originally instituted.

The tax exemption for employer-paid health insurance is a federal tax subsidy to increase the demand for health insurance. Instituted during World War II to prevent a strike for higher wages when there was a wage and price freeze on the economy, tax-free employer-paid health insurance was based on expediency; it was not an explicit redistributional policy to help those with lower incomes. Instead, its effect was the opposite. The main beneficiaries of this tax subsidy, as discussed in Chapter 6, are those with higher incomes who are in a higher tax bracket.

The *ostensible* reason for placing restrictions on entry, information, and price competition was to provide consumer protection. Given the technical nature of medical services and the potential harm that may be inflicted upon an uninformed patient by an incompetent provider, the government, working through the health professions and health institutions, placed its emphasis for consumer protection on nonprofit providers and on the process of becoming a health professional. Training requirements in nonprofit institutions were specified; licensure, carried out by the health professions, placed strong restrictions on who was permitted to practice and who was responsible for performing medical services; information on prices, quality, and accessibility was prohibited to prevent unethical providers from misleading the sick. Thus the very imperfections that prevented the medical sector from performing more efficiently were instituted under government auspices.

How can the demand for consumer protection[2] be satisfied while eliminating imperfections that cause inefficiencies in the medical sector? The U.S. Supreme Court ruling that the anti-trust laws apply to the health field have eliminated restrictions on advertising and price competition. The price-competitive market, under pressure from large employers and employer coalitions, is currently attempting to develop outcome, rather than process, measures of quality. Relying on outcome approaches for the training and, once practicing, the continued competence of health professionals would also be appropriate. Once licensed, physicians are not required to be reexamined. Only if they want to be board-certified are they reexamined. Relying more on examinations than standardized educational requirements, monitoring the quality of care provided, and reexamination are examples of outcome approaches. The competitive market, with its emphasis on monitoring mechanisms of physician behavior and practice patterns and outcomes information to improve consumer choice, is moving in the direction of greater consumer protection.

Consumer protection can be achieved more directly and more efficiently by an approach that actually monitors the quality of care provided. It would no longer be necessary to rely solely on proxy methods to accomplish this objective.

---

[2]A demand for consumer protection might be considered an externality; namely, if the government or some agency were to ensure that all providers are competent, all consumers would benefit from the lower risks and lower search costs when seeking a provider. The reason for including a discussion of consumer protection in this section rather than in the following one, which discusses externalities, is that whether externalities are in fact the real reason for the market imperfections mentioned, the proposed policy prescriptions are similar to what would be the situation if such imperfections were simply a result of monopoly behavior on the part of the providers.

Eliminating restrictions that cause market imperfections would enable market mechanisms to allocate medical resources more efficiently. Government subsidies to alleviate the consequences of imperfections of the type discussed, rather than eliminating the imperfections themselves, cannot be justified as a means of improving market efficiency. Entry and practice barriers decrease the availability of medical care by increasing its price. Government construction or manpower subsidies, which have as their stated goal an increase in availability of medical resources, merely mask the effects of the market imperfections. These subsidies would have to be justified on grounds other than as a means of improving market efficiency.

The appropriate role of government, when faced with imperfections in the marketplace, should be to eliminate restrictive practices and directly address the need that the restrictions were ostensibly imposed to meet (i.e., consumer protection).

Many people (particularly providers) oppose eliminating restrictions on information and on medical practice. Such persons also oppose a market approach for determining the quantity and quality of medical care to be provided. Their opposition to market competition is not based on grounds of greater economic efficiency, but is, instead, a result of a value judgment that such criteria are inappropriate in medical care. Patients, in their opinion, do not have sufficient information, nor are they rational enough to make competent choices as to the appropriate providers and correct amounts of medical care when they are ill. Such a decision should not involve the consumer at all but should be determined professionally; the professional determination, or allocation, of medical care should be based on medical need and not on consumer choice.

One of the criteria for economic efficiency in the demand for a service is that consumers will use a service until the price they pay for the last unit purchased (their marginal cost) equals the additional value they receive from it. When the marginal utility of the last unit consumed equals the price paid, consumers are maximizing their utility. Since the price they must pay represents forgone utility that could be received from other goods and services, consumers adjust their utilization when prices change so that the marginal value of their last unit equals the new price. Consumers use different quantities of services, even though they face the same prices, because the marginal utilities to them of additional units differ. Each consumer, however, is assumed to match the marginal utility of that last unit to the forgone utility of other goods and services. Further, when the consumer is the sole beneficiary of her purchases, it is said that her marginal private benefit is equivalent to marginal social benefit.

If consumers are not assumed to be rational, or if persons do not believe that consumer choice should prevail, the traditional demand curve does not represent marginal social utility. Under such circumstances, traditional economic policy, which favors removing imperfections so as to satisfy consumer wants, will not achieve the goals of those persons who do not believe in consumer choice and sovereignty in determining the amount of medical care to be provided.

Typically, those who oppose consumer sovereignty in medical care favor medical determination or prioritization of need for determining access to medical services. These approaches are difficult to operationalize. The criteria that government agencies would use for placing a marginal value on services so as to allocate resources would be very controversial. Not everyone would agree with the value judgment that a person should be prohibited from consuming something that he is willing to pay for (as long as it does not impose any negative effects on other persons). Based on their valuation of their time, some people may prefer to pay a higher price rather than wait for the receipt of a service. Substituting collective judgment for an individual's judgment to determine how much medical care is to be available represents a difference in values and is unrelated to whether a market system will be more efficient than an alternative system for achieving the same set of values.

This difference in values regarding how much medical care should be available, and to whom, is also related to another set of values. Those opposed to the use of consumer sovereignty in the demand for medical care are also opposed to the use of competition on the supply side. The proponents of market competition assume that when providers compete for consumers, they will minimize their costs, so as to better compete on price, and provide the services that consumers most desire. Persons who do not believe that providers should be responsive to consumer demands express similar disbelief in the ability of suppliers to compete with one another without harming patients; their preference is to substitute regulation and monopolization for competition.

Regardless of differences in values regarding who should determine the quantity and quality of medical services, it should be possible to allow different delivery systems to compete on the supply side. Allowing competition to exist and to be an alternative to a more controlled delivery system (e.g., a system of VA hospitals) would provide a fairer test of which approach is more efficient at achieving a level of output, whether it is established by government agencies or by consumers.

The reason for this discussion of differences in values in medical care is because the appropriate role of government is continually debated with regard to the values and criteria that underlie a market system. Much of the criticism of a market approach is not based on the market's ability to achieve the specified economic criteria. Instead, the disagreement is a result of differences in values and unspecified criteria, thus the discussion on the role of government and public policy alternatives would be sharpened if these distinctions were defined more explicitly.

MARKET FAILURE

There are certain situations where price competitive markets will not produce the optimal amount of output, which is defined as price equaling marginal cost. A "natural" monopoly in the provision of a particular service is one such situation. When economies of scale are very large, for a given size of market, it is less costly to have one firm produce that service. If multiple firms competed, one of the firms would be able to lower its costs by increasing its scale of production, thereby driving other firms out of business. Price competition cannot exist under natural monopoly, and the output is likely to be less than optimal because the monopolist will price according to where marginal revenue equals marginal cost; consequently, price will exceed marginal cost.

Natural monopolies, however, are relatively rare in the health field. Good substitutes exist for most medical services at a local level. While services, such as transplant units, may be subject to relatively large economies, these services serve a much larger market than is served by the hospital in which they are located. Thus the regional market served by such specialized facilities and services is sufficiently large for several units to compete with one another. Because few services in medical care appear to have the characteristics of a natural monopoly, the natural monopoly argument has not been an important justification for government intervention in medical care.

Although price-competitive markets may not fulfill the assumptions of a textbook model of competition, namely, many firms and a homogeneous product, workable competition can exist as long as entry is possible and the firms are prohibited by the anti-trust laws from engaging in anticompetitive behavior (e.g., boycotts, price fixing, and other forms of monopolizing the market). Competing firms are not perfect substitutes for one another; consequently each firm will have a downward-sloping demand curve (hence price will exceed marginal cost), because each provider is somewhat different, given their location, services available, and so on. In these competitive situations government intervention is not necessary, since it has not been shown that regulation can improve market performance without imposing greater economic inefficiency.

An important reason for market failure is the existence of externalities. Externalities occur when an action undertaken by an individual (or firm) has secondary effects on others, which may be favorable or unfavorable. Externalities result in a nonoptimal amount of output being produced because individuals or firms consider only their own benefits and costs when making a production or consumption decision. If costs or benefits are received by others as the result of someone's private decision, the level of output produced in the market will be based on either too small a level of benefits (i.e., positive external benefits) or too small a level of costs of production (i.e., positive external costs).

For example, as shown in Figure 16.1B, when there are external benefits (*MEB*), the result of an individual's considering only the (marginal private) benefits (*MPB*) that are expected to be derived from that purchase would be a level of output determined by the intersection of the marginal private benefit (*MPB*) schedule and the marginal private costs (*MPC*) of producing that service. (The marginal private benefit curve is the demand curve for that service.) The resulting level of output, Q_0, would be smaller than if the external benefits to others (*MEB*) were also included. If the marginal private benefits and the marginal external benefits were added together (to result in the marginal social benefits [*MSB*] curve), the resulting level of output would be Q_1, which is greater than Q_0.

One would use a similar approach for determining the optimal level of output when there are external costs, although the effect would be opposite that of external benefits. A firm deciding how much output to produce would consider only the marginal private

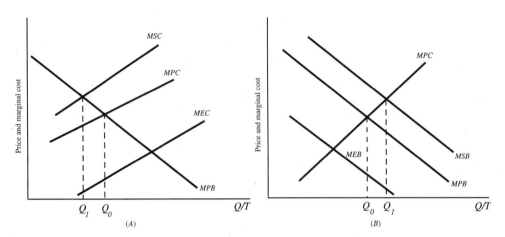

FIGURE 16.1 • Externalities in production and consumption: (A) a case of external costs, (B) a case of external benefits.

benefits and marginal private costs; it would not take into account any costs imposed on others, such as air pollution. If the marginal costs imposed on others (MEC) were added to the firm's costs of production (MPC), the resulting costs of producing that output, the marginal social cost curve (MSC), would represent the full costs of production. The level of output that would then be produced would be smaller, Q_1, than when the external costs were not considered, Q_0.

Individual consumers and producers in a competitive market do not take into consideration the external benefits or costs imposed on others as a result of their decisions. When such external costs and benefits are not incorporated into the private decision-making process, the resultant output level is not optimal. Some persons receive benefits for which they would be willing to pay but do not, whereas others bear additional costs for which they did not receive any benefits. (In the case of external costs, the persons purchasing that good or service pay a price that is less than the full cost of producing that service; they should bear the full cost of their consumption decisions.)

Externalities therefore have two effects. The first is on economic efficiency: it is only when all the marginal benefits (MSB) equal all the marginal costs (MSC) that the optimal level of output is determined. The second effect is redistribution: some persons receive an external benefit for which they do not compensate those providing it, or a cost is imposed on them for which they are not reimbursed.

The reason externalities occur is because of a lack of ownership or property rights. If someone owned the air or stream that is polluted as a result of a firm producing that product, the polluter could be charged for the pollution and that charge would become part of the cost of producing that product. Similarly, if persons who receive an external benefit could be charged for their benefit, then the appropriate level of output would occur. At times the cost of monitoring and collecting from those who impose or receive an externality exceeds the benefits of doing so, in which case it is not done.

Because of the lack of ownership rights, collective nonmarket decision making is needed to incorporate external costs and benefits into the private decision-making calculus.[3] When large numbers of persons are involved, it becomes difficult to make voluntary arrangements that are satisfactory to all concerned. Group or collective decision making, in which all persons must abide by the decision, is required to determine both the optimal level of output and to whom the compensation is to be paid (and on whom the taxes should be assessed). It is legitimate for government to serve as the group's agent in a nonmarket situation.

The existence of externalities legitimizes a role for government in health care, but of what should that role consist? It is not sufficient merely to claim that externalities exist and then justify all types of government intervention and financing of health and medical care. [4] The proper role of government is twofold. First, it must determine the exact nature and size of external benefits and costs. The measurement of externalities is a difficult task, both conceptually and empirically, as will be discussed below. Nonmarket studies, referred to as cost/benefit analysis, are important for determining the optimal level of output when externalities exist (2).

It is not appropriate, however, for the government to undertake *any* program that has 'favorable' cost/benefit ratios. For example, with respect to personal medical programs that have no external effects, the analyst may propose government subsidies based solely on a finding of a favorable cost/benefit ratio. If there are no external effects and the individuals involved do not wish to spend their own funds on the program, it is inappropriate to have the government intervene, unless one is willing to declare that the individuals making the decision are not rational. More likely, the individuals do not share the same values or perception of benefits as does the analyst.

The second appropriate role of government when externalities exist is to determine how the externalities should be financed—who will be compensated and who will be taxed. For example, air pollution is an external cost imposed on others. The government should determine the magnitude of the external costs and then place a unit tax (equivalent to the size of the external costs) on those who are producing the particular product that is causing the pollution. The per unit tax will cause an increase in the polluters' costs of production and a consequent decrease in production and pollution (as shown in Figure 16.1A). The proceeds of the tax can then be used to reimburse those who bear these external costs. Similarly, when there are external benefits, as in the case of medical re-

---

[3]When few individuals are involved, it is possible that they will reach agreement among themselves as to the proper levels of compensation, and the resulting level of output will be optimal.

[4]Not all externalities require government intervention. Externalities may exist in a market; however, they may be relatively small so that when the *MEB* is added to the *MPB* curve the sum of the two curves intersect at a point to the left of the intersection of the *MPB* and *MPC* curves. Thus the optimal rate of output is unaffected by including the *MEB*. When the market produces more than the amount demanded by the *MEB* then this is referred to as "inframarginal" externalities. This subject is discussed in Chapter 14, with reference to whether medical education should be subsidized.

search, then those receiving the external benefits should be similarly taxed and the proceeds used to subsidize an increase in medical research.

The principle underlying financing should attempt to affix the taxes and subsidies to those who generate the external costs and benefits. A system of financing based on ability to pay would be inappropriate unless such a system reflected the extent of the external benefits and costs. Further, not all nonmarket decision making should be at the federal level. For some health programs the benefits and costs are purely local in character (e.g., water fluoridation); the appropriate level of financing, therefore, should be local.

Situations involving externalities do not necessarily require government production or provision of particular services. If a particular service does not have the characteristics of a natural monopoly, there is no reason why there could not be competition in the provision of that service. Medical schools and other research institutions could compete for research grants. Research is not necessarily produced more efficiently if undertaken solely by federally employed researchers. The criterion for whether the service should be governmentally or privately provided should be efficiency; there is nothing inherent in the nature of externalities that suggests that services should be publicly provided.[5]

Several types of situations in the health and medical fields give rise to externalities. The first type may be referred to as the "consumer protection" argument, discussed previously. Given the technical nature of medical care and the patients' lack of knowledge regarding diagnosis, treatment needs, and the provider's competence, consumers might benefit from the establishment of certain minimum standards and the provision of information. If the private market did not provide minimum standards (possibly through monitoring of providers and malpractice actions) or the necessary information required by consumers, or if all consumers desired the government to ensure some minimum standards, consumer protection would become an externality and hence a legitimate role of government. The methods by which the government could fulfill this public demand for protection would be similar to those discussed previously.

Another externality with regard to personal medical services is what may be referred to as "externalities in consumption." If healthier and wealthier individuals do not want to see persons less fortunate than themselves go without necessary medical care and are willing to contribute to their medical care, an externality in consumption is said to exist. This

---

[5]Using the criterion of efficiency, is there any reason for allowing the federal government to have a monopoly on the provision of medical care for veterans? Presumably, the government could determine how much it was willing to spend on medical care for a specific class of veterans (those with a service-connected disability) and then allow them to choose whether they want to purchase care in the private medical sector or in the government's VA hospitals. Such potential competition would be threatening to the VA bureaucracy. Prohibiting competition for the provision of governmentally financed services often has less to do with efficiency and choice considerations than with the survival of an entrenched government agency. It would also reduce the size of the VA organization, since many of its beds are filled with veterans who do not have a service-connected disability. (Instead of reducing the size of its bureaucracy and budget as the number of veterans of the type for whom it was originally established to provide medical care decreases, the VA would prefer to maintain its institutions and budget by expanding the eligible class of veterans.)

is because the utility of individuals depends not only on the quantity of goods and services they themselves purchase, but also on the amount of certain goods and services (such as medical care) purchased by others. Under such circumstances, if some contribute to the medical services of the less fortunate, then other persons, who similarly would have been willing to contribute, receive an external benefit; everybody receives the benefit of seeing the less fortunate receive medical care, even though everybody did not necessarily contribute. Theoretically, each person who receives an external benefit should contribute according to the size of the external benefit. Unless there is some form of nonmarket decision making, it will not be possible to collect from all the persons who receive an external benefit.

The implications of the preceding discussion are twofold. First, government, acting as the agent for the collective desires of those wishing to contribute, should tax those persons (assuming the government knows the amount each person is willing to spend on those less fortunate than himself) and provide a subsidy to the desired recipients equivalent to the magnitude of the collected tax. Second, the form of that subsidy (e.g., medical services) and the determination of its method of distribution (possibly an income-related determination of recipients) should represent the desires of the *donors,* not those of the recipients (3). This is because some donors may be willing to contribute, and thereby receive an external benefit, only if their contributions go to a particular income group, for a particular type of service, and are distributed in a certain manner.

There are a number of ways in which subsidies could be provided to help those who are ill or who have low incomes. These persons could be given an income supplement rather than just an increase in their medical services; with an increase in their incomes, they could spend those funds on housing, nutritional foods, or medical services. If it is a lack of access to medical services that the more fortunate wish to redress, it would be inappropriate, from the donor's perspective, to allow those funds to be spent on goods and services other than medical care. Under circumstances of externalities in consumption, in-kind subsidies are efficient.

The justification for national health insurance and other forms of in-kind subsidies (to be discussed more completely in chapter 18) is presumably based on the assumption that there are externalities in consumption; otherwise, proposed in-kind subsidies would not be efficient. If the objective of the subsidies were the redistribution of income, direct cash supplements would be a more efficient means to this end. The recipients of the subsidy would always prefer cash, which can be used to satisfy their most important needs, rather than a subsidy that can be used for only one of their needs, a need that may not represent their highest priority (4).

For in-kind subsidies to be efficient, therefore, the intent must be to satisfy the preferences of the *donors* rather than the recipients. When an in-kind subsidy is called for, as in the case of externalities in consumption, the type of person the donors are willing to subsidize and the amount of subsidy to be provided to each person are most likely inversely related to the recipient's income: the lower the recipient's income, the greater will be the donor's willingness to provide a subsidy. It is unlikely that a person will receive an external benefit from seeing a person with a possibly higher income than her own receive a subsidy. These aspects of in-kind subsidies should be kept in mind when national health insurance and other in-kind subsidies are discussed.

Requiring everyone to purchase at least catastrophic health insurance can be justified on grounds of externalities. If a person decides to self-insure, then other persons are bearing part of the cost of that decision. If the person who self-insures is unfortunate enough to incur catastrophic medical expense that he is unable to pay, the community (through welfare payments) will have to reimburse the medical providers for that person's medical services. The rest of the community will have to bear part of the cost (in terms of higher taxes) of that individual's decision to self-insure (or purchase less than catastrophic insurance). It would be more equitable, therefore, if these costs were borne in full by individuals at risk, similar to an uninsured motorists' fund.

The third type of externality that occurs in the health field is usually associated with public health programs rather than with personal medical services. Vaccination programs, clean water supplies, air pollution abatement, and medical research are examples of goods that result in large, external benefits. It has generally been with respect to these types of programs that a great many cost/benefit studies have been undertaken.

REDISTRIBUTION USING IN-KIND SUBSIDIES

There are many types of in-kind subsidies in medical care. Some of these are demand subsidies, others are supply subsidies; some are indirect with regard to the beneficiary groups they hope to affect, others are direct. National health insurance would be classified as a direct demand subsidy. Before discussing national health insurance, it would be instructive to discuss the different types of in-kind subsidies in medical care, their magnitude, their probable effects, and their probable beneficiaries. With a better understanding of in-kind subsidies, their actual as compared to their stated purpose becomes clearer, and a context within which national health insurance can be analyzed is provided. If national health insurance is an efficient in-kind subsidy, then it is questionable whether other in-kind subsidies should be continued.[6]

---

[6]Regardless of their stated intent, in-kind medical care subsidies do not have as their actual objective an increase in health status. Instead, their goal appears to be an increase in use of medical services. For example, total public spending on medical services for those 65 years of age and older were $3,356 per person in 1987; for those 19 to 64 and under 19 the equivalent figures were $395 and $198. If the actual purpose of government medical care expenditures were to achieve an increase in health levels, these expenditures might well have been allocated to different population groups, disease categories, and nonmedical care programs. Even if it were agreed that the in-kind subsidy was to be provided to the aged alone, a different allocation of funds for nonmedical care services would be called for. An equivalent cash supplement to the aged to enable them to increase their consumption of food, housing, and heating would probably contribute more to their health than a subsidy restricted to medical services alone. Daniel Waldo et al., "Health Expenditures by Age Group, 1977–1987," *Health Care Financing Review,* 10(4), Summer 1989: 111–120.

The major in-kind subsidies on the demand side are Medicare, Medicaid, the tax exemption of employer-paid health insurance, and the tax deductibility of medical expenses in excess of 7.5 percent of adjusted gross income. Expenditures under Medicare and Medicaid (excluding other direct government subsidies on the demand side, such as maternal and child health care) were $317 billion in 1995 (5). The exclusion from taxes of employer-paid health insurance premiums were estimated to cost the federal government $74 billion a year in lost federal income and Social Security taxes in 1994 (excluding lost state income taxes)(6).

On the supply side there are (and have been) both direct and indirect subsidy programs. Subsidies are provided for health manpower education, graduate medical education, hospital construction, and provision of medical services through the VA and state and local government hospitals, as well as numerous indirect subsidies, such as those that grant tax-exempt status to nonprofit hospitals and state assistance in financing hospital bond issues.

The magnitude of these direct and indirect demand and supply subsidies has been and still is very large; it is clear that the role of government in the financing and provision of personal medical services has been substantial.

Given the significant role of government in personal medical services, it is important to determine who the beneficiaries of these subsidies are and the efficiency with which they are being distributed. These two issues are interrelated; as discussed previously, the argument for in-kind subsidies is based on externalities in consumption. As such, the primary recipients should be those persons with low incomes and poor health. If the subsidies are distributed in such a way as to benefit higher-income groups or provide them with a greater proportionate share of the subsidy, then the distribution of the subsidy is inefficient; that is, the desired beneficiary group (low-income persons) could receive a greater amount of the subsidy if it were provided in a different, presumably more direct, manner.[7]

It is generally easier to determine the beneficiary groups under demand rather than supply subsidies. Under the Medicaid program, for example, the designated beneficiaries are the medically indigent. Since Medicaid is a federal–state matching program, the definition of medical indigency and the benefits provided under the program vary by state. However, as shown in Table 16.1, expenditures under Medicaid go predominantly to the poor and near-poor. This relationship between income level and Medicaid expenditure holds for both per capita and total Medicaid expenditures.

When indirect demand subsidy programs are examined, it becomes less obvious that the subsidies are going to those persons with the lowest incomes and greatest medical needs. Under Medicare, because the beneficiary group is defined by age rather than income level, the subsidy is more evenly distributed across income levels. Not all aged

---

[7]This assumes that the method of distribution is not prescribed by the same externalities argument that gave rise to the subsidy in the first place.

TABLE 16.1 Major Federal Government Expenditures on Health Services, 1977

All Persons	Income Tax Savings		Medicare[a]		Medicaid		Total Federal[b]	
Per Capita Government Expenditures								
Poor and near-poor	$2		$141		$184		$327	
Other low-income	16		99		63		178	
Middle-income	43		57		16		116	
High-income	90		48		4		142	
Total Government Expenditures (Billions)								
	$	%	$	%	$	%	$	%
Poor and near-poor	0.1	1	4.3	28	5.6	62	10.0	29
Other low-income	0.5	5	3.1	20	2.0	22	5.6	16
Middle-income	3.5	34	4.7	31	1.3	14	9.5	27
High-income	6.2	60	3.3	21	0.2	2	9.7	28
Total expenditures	10.3	100	15.4	100	9.1	100	34.8	100

Source: This table is from Gail R. Wilensky, "Government and the Financing of Health Care," *American Economic Review,* 72(2), May 1982: 202–207, Table 2.

[a]Less Part B premiums.

[b]Excludes expenditures from veterans programs and small federal programs. The definition of income groups are as follows: The "poor" includes those whose family income was less than or equal to the 1977 poverty level as well as those whose income was between 101 and 125 percent of that level. "Other low-income" includes those whose income is 1.26 to 2 times the poverty level, "middle-income" is 2.01 to 4 times the poverty level, and "high-income" is 4.01 times the poverty level or more. For a family of four in 1977, these four groups distribute as follows: less than $8,000 to $9,999, $10,000 to $15,999, $16,000 to $31,999, and greater than $32,000. The percent of the population in each group is 14, 15, 39, and 32 percent, respectively.

persons have lower incomes than nonaged persons. Although per capita Medicare expenditures decrease with higher income levels (because older aged have lower incomes), the percent of total Medicare expenditures going to each income level is more evenly distributed. The poor and near-poor received 28 percent of total Medicare expenditures as compared to the high-income group, who received 21 percent.

When tax subsidy programs, such as the exclusion of employer-provided health insurance premiums from taxable income and the deduction of medical expenses are examined, higher-income groups are the major beneficiaries. Middle-income and high-income groups together receive 94 percent of those subsidy dollars.

When government expenditures for all three programs are combined, the total benefits are evenly divided across the different income groups except for the "other-low-income group," with 16 percent of total government expenditures; the incomes of this group are too high for Medicaid; thus they receive few Medicaid benefits and their incomes are too low to benefit from the tax subsidy programs. The poor and near-poor, middle-income, and high-income groups received 29, 27, and 28 percent, respectively.

Medicaid expenditures, which heavily favor the low-income groups, are offset by the tax subsidy programs. The redistributional effects of Medicare are small.

It would thus appear that the more directly the demand subsidy is aimed at a designated population group, the more likely it is that the intended recipients will receive a larger proportion of that subsidy. Direct subsidy programs of this sort would be more in accordance with the stated goals of the legislation. Indirect demand subsidy programs are a less efficient way of subsidizing a particular beneficiary group. If in-kind medical subsidies are justified on grounds of externalities, the beneficiaries should presumably be those with lower incomes and greater needs for medical care than the persons favoring such subsidies. Direct demand subsidies would be both a more obvious and a more direct means of assuring that this objective is achieved.

It is perhaps an indication of what the true, as compared to the stated, intent is of the legislation that in-kind subsidies are indirect, such as the tax subsidy programs. The legislation's real goal is not to just assist the poor, but to provide a benefit to those in the middle- and high-income groups as well.

Demand subsidies impose costs on those persons not receiving them in two ways. First, those persons must pay increased taxes to pay for the subsidy program. Second, an increase in demand by the recipients of the subsidies results in an increase in the price of medical services, which (depending on the price elasticity of demand) both increases the cost and decreases the use of medical services for those who are not being subsidized. After Medicare and Medicaid were introduced, prices in the medical sector more than doubled, as shown previously.

The demand subsidy will have secondary effects throughout the entire medical sector. A demand subsidy will cause an increase in demand in the different institutional markets: hospitals, physician services, and so on. How large the increase in demand will be in each of the separate institutional markets will depend, in part, on the type of demand subsidy (i.e., how much price is reduced to the beneficiaries) in each of the institutional settings and the elasticity of supply in that market. A more inelastic supply will result in greater price increases, which will tend to reduce demand in both the beneficiary and nonbeneficiary groups.

As demand increases in each of the institutional settings, there will be an increase in the derived demand for the inputs (different types of health manpower and nonlabor inputs) used in that setting. With increased demands for health manpower, wages and incomes in the manpower markets will increase, together with participation rates. In the long run, an increase in the incomes of health personnel will result in increased demands for a health professional education, and if the health education market responds, there will be an increase in the stock of trained health manpower.

How much of the demand subsidy ends up in higher prices rather than in increased services will depend on the elasticity of supply in the various medical markets. The greater the number of restrictions on entry into the health professions, and on the tasks that different health personnel can perform, and the greater the lack of efficiency incentives in methods of provider payment, the greater the inelasticity of supply and the higher the increases in medical prices.

Supply subsidies may also be classified according to whether they are directly targeted to a beneficiary group or whether their benefits are diffused among many population groups. An example of a direct supply subsidy to a designated beneficiary group is the provision of funds to establish a clinic in a low-income neighborhood. Even if there is no corresponding demand subsidy, the new clinic will result in an increased use of medical services by those with low incomes because it will decrease the patients' cost of travel to the facility. Most direct supply subsidies are not of this type; the major direct supply subsidies are the VA hospitals and state and local government hospitals.

The VA medical system is fairly extensive, consisting of 171 hospitals, 362 outpatient clinics, 128 nursing homes, a $16 billion (1994) budget, and 266,000 employees. Although the major stated role of the VA is to provide medical care to veterans with a service-connected disability, only 10 percent of the veterans in VA hospitals are there for that purpose. The remaining 90 percent have low incomes and receive care for illnesses unrelated to their military service (7).

State and local government hospitals account for approximately 17 percent of all admissions to short-term general hospitals and approximately 17 percent of all hospital outpatient visits. These hospitals have served as important sources of medical care for the indigent and have relieved the private hospitals and physicians of the financial risk of caring for these patients.

In view of the amount being spent on Medicare and Medicaid, which is targeted to similar population groups served by the VA and other government hospital systems, what is the likely and proper role for these government providers? If the medically indigent were to receive a demand subsidy with benefits at least as complete as those presently available to them in the VA and other government hospitals, the demand for care in these institutions is likely to decline sharply. State and local government hospitals have had a reputation for providing lower-quality or less-satisfying care to patients than that provided by community nonprofit hospitals. VA hospitals are inconveniently located in relation to their beneficiary population (there are only 171 VA general and psychiatric hospitals as opposed to more than five thousand community hospitals).

If all providers, including the VA and the other government hospitals, had to compete for patients under a demand subsidy arrangement, the VA and governmental hospitals would either have to adapt or they would not be able to survive in a competitive environment. For the VA system to compete for the 90 percent of its population who use the VA because they are medically indigent, it would have to provide ambulatory services, change its organizational and reimbursement arrangements with its physicians, increase its relative efficiency by lowering length of stay and using less costly substitutes for inpatient care, and compete on a more local basis for patients, since patient travel costs and time are likely to be significant determinants in choosing medical delivery systems. If the VA cannot survive under competitive conditions where patients are provided with a demand subsidy and are free to choose, what economic justification is there for providing additional large subsidies to enable the VA to maintain its current role?

State and local governmental hospitals in many states are being forced to compete with HMOs and other providers as more of the Medicaid population is being enrolled in capitated managed care systems. If everyone were enrolled in either private or public insurance programs, then it would not be necessary to separately subsidize local governmental hospitals. Unfortunately, not everyone is covered by private insurance or eligible for demand subsidies, such as the uninsured and illegal immigrants. Local governmental hospitals will continue to remain as the providers of last resort, requiring a supply subsidy. Under a competitive system, the existence of public hospitals would be an indication that either the size of the direct demand subsidies is insufficient for the private sector to serve these population groups or that certain groups are ineligible for subsidized medical care.

Indirect supply subsidies, the other major type of in-kind supply subsidy, are exemplified by funds for training additional health manpower and capital grants to hospitals. These indirect supply subsidies have their initial effects on a particular medical market. For the subsidy to increase medical services, its effect must eventually be transmitted through several medical markets. For example, when a subsidy is given to medical schools to increase the number of physicians, several years pass before there is an increase in the number of graduates. These graduates will then work in a number of settings, ranging from hospitals to physicians' offices.

The increase in the amount of services eventually received by the members of a particular beneficiary group (i.e., those with low incomes) will depend on their elasticity of demand for those services. (The increased supply of services is a downward shift along a patient's demand curve for that service.) If demand by members of the beneficiary group is relatively inelastic (i.e., not very responsive to changes in the price of the service), there will be relatively little increase in their use of medical services. Since indirect supply subsidies are not generally targeted to particular beneficiary groups, the beneficiaries will be everyone using the service; they will be paying a lower price than before the subsidy. Because low-income persons do not use medical services as much as those with high incomes, they may receive less benefit than high users from such subsidies; the high users may also have relatively higher incomes.

In addition to being inefficient, in that the greatest portion of the subsidy does not go to those with low incomes, general supply subsidies present further problems. When only one input into the process of producing medical care is subsidized, a manager who is attempting to use the lowest-cost combination of inputs will tend to use more of the subsidized input because its cost has been artificially reduced. For example, a subsidy to train additional registered nurses will, if it is successful, result in a greater increase in the supply of nurses and a relatively lower wage for them. Because the wage of nurses is lowered, hospitals will substitute away from other nursing personnel toward more registered nurses in providing patient care.

Subsidizing a specific input is less efficient than if the hospital were merely awarded an equivalent unrestricted subsidy. In the latter case, the hospital would use a combination of registered and nonregistered nurses and other inputs based on their relative prices and productivities. Consequently, the hospital would use fewer registered nurses than if only RN wages were artificially reduced through a subsidy. Subsidies that increase the supply of a particular input are therefore less efficient (more costly) than an equivalent dollar subsidy.

It is also often difficult to determine what additional services have been produced as a result of a supply subsidy. Although one might be able to count the number of additional persons trained as a result of the subsidy (which is not as easy as it might appear), it is more difficult to calculate the net increase in services resulting from the additional health manpower. Without additional nurses, the wage rate of existing nurses would have risen more rapidly, thereby causing an increase in the nurse participation rate. In the long run, higher wages would cause an increase in the number of persons seeking a career in nursing. Similarly, without a subsidy to increase the number of physicians, the productivity of existing physicians might be greater. To assume that the additional services provided by the subsidized manpower are the net benefits of the supply subsidy greatly overstates its benefits.

To understand exactly what impact supply subsidies have on increased use of services, and for which beneficiary groups, it is necessary to use a complex econometric model of the medical sector. For example, a subsidy to increase the number of registered nurses will have its initial impact on the nursing education market. How many additional nurses will be graduated as a result of that subsidy will depend, in part, on the objectives of the different types of nursing schools and on which schools receive the subsidies. The number of nurses will also depend on the elasticity of demand for a nursing education by prospective nurses, since the subsidy will reduce their educational costs.

The impact of additional nurses on the market for nurses will affect nurses' wages, participation rates, and nurse employment. How many additional nurses will be employed in the various institutional settings will depend on the elasticity of demand for nurses in each of the different settings and the new wage for nurses. (The determination of wages and employment will, of course, be a simultaneous process.) The greater the substitutability of registered nurses for other types of nursing personnel, the higher will be the elasticity of demand and the greater will be the decrease in demand for nonregistered nurses. Each of the institutional settings that employs registered nurses will have a slightly lower cost for its nursing personnel; the cost of care in each institutional setting will also be lower. How much lower will depend on how many registered nurses are employed and the elasticity of the demand for nurses (i.e., whether many more nurses are hired as a result of their relatively lower wage).

The effect of the nurse subsidy on cost of care will vary for each institutional setting; hospitals, which hire the majority of nurses, would receive the largest cost reduction. Since the relative cost of the different institutional settings has changed, how much the price of care will be reduced in each of the institutional settings as a result of a lowering of costs will depend on the elasticity of demand for services and the environment in which an institution competes. If there are no competitive pressures on the institution or if the institution attempts to maximize its prestige, it is less likely that the cost savings will be passed on to patients and other third-party payers.

As seen from the above discussion, it is much more difficult to determine the end result of supply subsidies compared with the impact of demand subsidies. It is equally difficult to determine which consumer or payer group receives the major benefit, if any, of the supply subsidy.

When the government has served as the supplier of medical services (e.g., state hospitals), such supply subsidies have generally had a direct impact on low-income persons. When supply subsidies have been indirect, in-kind subsidies have provided benefits to all those persons who use medical services; but as with the Hill–Burton program for hospital construction, nothing was done to help those who could not afford to use the hospital. A demand subsidy was still required for the medically indigent.

In-kind supply subsidies take longer than direct demand subsidies to provide greater access to medical services to a beneficiary group. They are also economically inefficient, either because patients have no choice as to provider, as under the VA system, or because the relative cost of inputs is distorted. Finally, the benefits of indirect supply subsidies are overstated, since employee participation rates and productivity increases are, in fact, likely to be lower than what they would otherwise have been.

Although direct demand subsidies would appear to be a more efficient method of providing an in-kind subsidy, supply subsidies are legislatively popular. The probable reason is not that legislators are necessarily unaware of which is the more efficient subsidy method, but rather that the providers of medical care and manpower education are important beneficiaries of such proposals. Such supply subsidies are generally the direct result of lobbying by these interest groups.

The intent of the preceding discussion on existing in-kind subsidies in medical care was to provide both an indication of the magnitude of such subsidies and criteria by which to judge the efficiency of alternative types of in-kind subsidies. If national health insurance were enacted, which of the many demand and supply (direct and indirect) subsidies should remain needs to be examined; any funds saved could be used to lessen the cost of national health insurance.

SUMMARY

Poor performance may occur when the assumptions of a competitive market are not fulfilled. Such market imperfections may be the result of a lack of consumer information, inadequate purchaser and supplier incentives to be efficient, and barriers to the mobility of resources. When such market imperfections exist, there may be a role for government. Unfortunately, many of these market imperfections, such as entry barriers and lack of patient and provider incentives, have been created by government itself.

The appropriate role of government when such market imperfections exist should be to eliminate them and directly address the stated purpose for which they were imposed, namely, consumer protection. That the stated goal of such restrictive practices can be achieved more directly and more efficiently and are not suggests that the intended objective is different from the stated goal.

A second justification for government intervention is the existence of externalities. Individual consumers and producers do not take into consideration the external benefits and costs imposed on others as a result of their actions. When externalities exist, the appropriate role of government is to calculate their magnitude and use a system of taxes or subsidies to achieve the optimal rate of output. One such externality, to provide medical care to the poor, is an important justification for in-kind demand and supply subsidies.

Indirect subsidies are less efficient (more costly) than direct subsidies since many who are not part of the intended beneficiary group also benefit. Direct demand subsidies are both the fastest and most efficient means for increasing the use of services by a designated beneficiary group.

Key Terms and Concepts

- Consumer sovereignty
- Economic efficiency
- Externalities
- Market failure
- Market imperfections

- Externalities in consumption
- Direct and indirect subsidies
- In-kind subsidies
- Optimal level of output with externalities

Review Questions

1. Explain the economist's definition of the correct or optimal rate of output.
2. Define externalities. Why do they occur? What are examples of externalities in the health field? Explain why the presence of externalities will, in the absence of some collective action, lead to a suboptimal rate of output. What type of collective action is called for?
3. Is there an optimal amount of pollution? What would occur if government were to mandate the elimination of all pollution?
4. If a cost/benefit analysis is "favorable," does this suggest that the government should always undertake such an expenditure? In your answer, discuss the criteria that should be used or who should undertake such projects, and how they should be financed.

5. What are the economic rationales for different types of government intervention in health care?
6. Explain the rationale for requiring everyone who can afford it to purchase, at a minimum, catastrophic health insurance.
7. What economic arguments support government financing of personal health services to certain population groups?
8. If the objective is one of redistribution, what are the welfare implications of achieving this redistribution by providing cash supplements versus medical care to the desired beneficiary group?
9. "We all benefit by having physicians available in case we need them. Therefore the government should subsidize medical education." Critique this justification of government subsidies based on an externalities argument.

REFERENCES

1. For a complete discussion of the role of government, see Richard A. Musgrave and Peggy B. Musgrave, *Public Finance in Theory and Practice* (New York: McGraw-Hill, 1989). The Musgraves categorize government programs into those that affect the allocation of resources, those that alter the distribution of incomes, and stabilization programs (i.e., those that regulate the level of economic activity).
2. For an extensive discussion of cost/benefit analysis, see Edward M. Gramlich, *A Guide to Benefit-Cost Analysis,* 2nd ed. (Englewood Cliffs, N.J.: Prentice-Hall, 1990).
3. For a more extended discussion of this proposition, see Paul Feldman, "Efficiency, Distribution, and the Role of Government in a Market Economy," *Journal of Political Economy,* 79(3), May–June 1971: 508–526.
4. A proof of this statement may be found in a number of texts on microeconomics. See, for example, Robert H. Frank, *Microeconomics and Behavior,* 2nd ed. (New York: McGraw-Hill, 1994), pp. 89–91.
5. Katherine R. Levit et al., "National Health Expenditures, 1995," *Health Care Financing Review,* 18(1), Fall 1996: Table 17, p. 212.
6. *The Tax Treatment of Employment-Based Health Insurance,* Congressional Budget Office, Congress of the United States, March 1994, p. xi.
7. Communication with the Veterans Administration, March 1, 1991, based on the fiscal year 1989 Report of The Secretary of Veterans Affairs.

CHAPTER

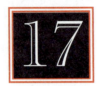

The Legislative Marketplace

THE LEGISLATIVE MARKETPLACE

There has been and continues to be extensive government intervention in the financing and delivery of medical services. For example, on the demand side of the market, there are substantial government subsidies, such as Medicare, Medicaid, and the exclusion from taxable income of employer-purchased health insurance. On the supply side, government subsidizes medical schools, nursing schools, and other health professional educational institutions; state licensing boards establish barriers to entering the various health professions and define the tasks permitted to various health professionals. Some states subject health facilities investment to state review and determine which benefits must be offered under health insurance plans. And the federal government regulates hospital and physician prices for Medicare patients. These are just some of the more significant examples of government involvement in health care.

To gain a better understanding of the reasons for extensive government intervention, which at times may seem contradictory in its effects, it is necessary to develop a framework within which to view government behavior. Different theories of legislative outcomes exist. At different ends of the theory spectrum are the "public interest" and "economic" theories.

THE PUBLIC INTEREST VIEW OF GOVERNMENT

The traditional or public interest view of government assumes that legislation is enacted to serve the public interest. To accomplish this, the public interest theory assumes that there are two basic objectives of government: to improve efficiency and to redistribute income in a more equitable manner.

The efficiency objective of government is to improve the allocation of resources. Inefficiency in resource allocation can occur, for example, when firms in a market have monopoly power or when externalities exist. A firm has monopoly power when it is able to charge a price that exceeds its cost by more than a normal profit. Monopoly is inefficient because it produces too small a level of service (output). The additional benefit to purchasers (as indicated by its price) from consuming a service is greater than the cost of producing that benefit; therefore more resources should flow into that industry until the additional benefit of consuming that service equals the additional cost of producing it.

The bases of monopoly power are several: there may be only one firm in a market, such as when there is a natural monopoly (e.g., an electric company); there may be barriers to entry in a market; firms may collude on raising their prices; or, because of a lack of information, consumers are unable to judge price, quality, and service differences among different suppliers. In each of these situations, the prices charged will exceed the costs of producing the product (which includes a normal profit). The appropriate government remedy to decrease monopoly power is to eliminate barriers to entry into a market, prevent price collusion, and improve communication of information to consumers.

The second situation where the allocation of resources can be improved is when there are "externalities"; these occur when someone undertakes an action and in so doing affects others who are not part of that transaction. The effects on others could be positive or negative. For example, a utility using high-sulfur coal to produce electricity also produces air pollution. As a result of the air pollution, residents in surrounding communities may have a higher incidence of respiratory illness. Resources are misallocated since the cost of producing electricity excludes the costs imposed on others. As a result, too much electricity is being produced. If the costs of producing electricity also included the costs imposed on others, the electricity price would be higher, and, consequently, its demand would be less. The allocation of resources would be improved if the utility's cost included both types of costs.

The appropriate role of government in such a situation is to determine the costs imposed on others and to tax the utility an equivalent amount.

Redistribution, the second objective of government, causes a change in wealth and is based on the values of society, namely, how equitable the distribution of resources should be. If society decides that medical services should be more equitably distributed, then those with lower incomes would be expected to receive net benefits (their benefits exceed their costs or taxes) and those with higher incomes should incur net costs (their taxes exceed their benefits) from the legislation. Crucial to the evaluation of redistributive legislation is which population groups are eligible for the benefits and the types of taxes imposed to finance those benefits. When eligibility is by income and income taxes are used to finance the program's benefits, it is likely that redistribution occurs from high- to low-income groups. Two large redistributive programs are Medicare for the aged and

TABLE 17.1 Determining the Redistributive Effects of Government Programs

	Low Income	High Income
Benefits	X	
Costs		X

Medicaid for the medically indigent. The benefits and costs of a redistributive medical program, such as Medicaid, are shown in Table 17.1.

These traditional objectives of government, redistribution and efficiency, can be achieved by using one or more of the following policy instruments: expenditures, taxation, or regulation. These policy objectives and instruments are shown in Table 17.2. The policy instruments can be applied to either the purchaser (demand) or the supplier side of the market (1). For example, the government has subsidized (expenditure policy) medical schools to increase the number of physicians (supply side) and has also subsidized the purchase of medical services by the aged (demand side). Tax policy has benefited employees by excluding employer-paid health insurance from taxable income (demand side) and enabled nonprofit hospitals to pay lower interest costs by issuing tax-exempt bonds (supply side). State government regulations specify which medical services and practitioners must be included in health insurance sold in that state (demand side), and some states require government approval for building a hospital facility (supply side).

AN ECONOMIC THEORY OF GOVERNMENT

Dissatisfaction with the public interest theory occurred for several reasons. Instead of just regulating natural monopolies, government has also regulated competitive industries,

TABLE 17.2 Health Policy Objectives and Interventions

Government Policy Instruments		Government Objectives	
		Redistribution	Improve Efficiency
Expenditures	{ Demand side { Supply side		
Taxation (+/−)	{ Demand side { Supply side		
Regulation	{ Demand side { Supply side		

such as airlines, trucks, taxicabs, as well as various professions. Further, nonregulated firms always want to enter regulated markets. To prevent entry into regulated industries, the government establishes entry barriers. If the government supposedly reduces prices in regulated markets, hence a firm's profitability, why should firms seek to enter a regulated industry?

To reconcile these apparent contradictions with the public interest view of government, an alternative theory of government behavior, the economic theory of regulation, was developed (2). The basic assumption underlying the economic theory is that political markets are no different from economic markets; individuals and firms seek to further their self-interest. Firms undertake investments in private markets to achieve a high rate of return. Why wouldn't the same firms invest in legislation if it also offered a high rate of return? Organized groups are willing to pay a price for legislative benefits. This price is political support, which brings together the demanders and suppliers of legislative benefits.

The suppliers of legislative benefits are legislators, and their goal is assumed to be to maximize their chances of reelection. As the late Senator Everett Dirksen said, "The first law of politics is to get elected, the second law is to be reelected." To be reelected requires political support, which consists of campaign contributions, votes, and volunteer time. Legislators are assumed to be rational, to make cost/benefit calculations when faced with demands for legislation. However, the legislator's cost/benefit calculations are not the costs and benefits to society of enacting particular legislation. Instead, the benefits are the additional political support the legislator would receive from supporting the legislation. The costs are the lost political support she would incur as a result of her action. When the benefits to the legislator exceed her costs, she will support the legislation.

Those who have a "concentrated" interest (that is, the effect of the legislation will have a large impact on their profitability, by affecting either their revenues or their costs) are more likely to be successful in the legislative marketplace. It becomes worthwhile for the group to organize, to represent their interests before legislators, and to raise political support to achieve the profits that favorable legislation can provide. It is for this reason that only those with a concentrated interest will demand legislative benefits.

Whenever legislative benefits are provided to one group, others must bear those costs. When only one group has a concentrated interest in the legislation, they are more likely to be successful if the costs to finance those benefits are not obvious and can be spread over a large number of people. When this occurs, then the costs are said to be "diffuse."

For example, assume that there are ten firms in an industry and, if they can have legislation enacted that would limit imports that compete with their products, they would be able to raise their prices and thereby receive $280 million in legislative benefits. These firms have a concentrated interest ($280 million) in trying to enact such legislation. The costs of these legislative benefits are financed by a small increase in the price of their product amounting to $1 per person. It is often not obvious to consumers that the legislation increases their costs. Further, even if consumers were aware of the legislation's effect, it would not be worthwhile for them to organize and represent their interests so as to forestall a price increase that will decrease their income by $1 a year. The costs of trying to prevent the cost increase would exceed their potential savings.

It is easier (less costly) for providers than for consumers to organize, provide political support, and impose a diffuse cost on others. It is for this reason that there has been so much legislation affecting entry into the health professions, which tasks are reserved to certain professions, how (and which) providers are paid under public medical programs, why subsidies for medical education are given to the school and not to the student (otherwise they would have to compete for students), and so on. Most health issues have been relatively technical, such as the training of health professions, certification of their quality, methods of payment, controls on hospital capital investment, and the like. The higher medical prices resulting from regulations that benefit providers have been diffuse and not visible to consumers.

The economic theory of legislation provides an explanation for the above dissatisfactions with the public interest theory. Firms in competitive markets seek regulation so as to earn higher profits than are available in competitive markets. Prices in regulated markets, such as interstate airline travel, were always higher than nonregulated markets, such as intrastate air travel, thereby enabling regulated firms to earn greater profits. These higher prices provided nonregulated firms with an incentive to try to enter regulated markets. Government, on behalf of the regulated industry, imposed entry barriers to keep out low-priced competitors. Otherwise the regulated firms could not earn more than a competitive rate of return.

Firms try to receive through legislation the monopoly profits they are unable to achieve through market competition.

When only one group has a concentrated interest in the outcome of legislation and the costs are diffuse, legislators will respond to the political support the group is willing to pay to have favorable legislation enacted. When there are opposing groups, each with a concentrated interest in the outcome, legislators are likely to reach a compromise between the competing demanders of legislative benefits. Rather than balancing the gain in political support from one group against the loss from the other, legislators prefer to receive political support from both groups and impose diffuse costs on those unable to offer political support.

When the beneficiaries are specific population groups, such as the aged, the redistributive effects of the legislation are meant to be very visible. An example of this is Medicare. By making it clear which population groups will benefit, legislators hope to receive their political support. The costs of financing such visible redistributive programs, however, are still designed to be diffuse so as not to generate political opposition from others. A small diffuse tax imposed on many people, such as a payroll tax, is the only way large sums of money can be raised, with little opposition, to finance visible redistributive programs.

Payroll taxes that include a maximum wage level to which the tax applies, such as the one used to finance Medicare, were regressive. The tax represented a greater portion of income from low-income employees. Economists have determined that payroll taxes, even when imposed on the employer, are borne mostly by the employee. However, the advantage of imposing part of the tax on the employer is that it appears that employees are paying a smaller portion of it than they really are. The remainder of the tax is shifted forward to consumers in the form of higher prices for the goods and services they purchase.

Differences in the sources of political support are important for understanding the two main redistributive programs in the United States. Medicaid is a means-tested program for the poor and is funded from general tax revenues. Since the poor (who have low voting participation rates) are unable to provide legislators with political support, the support for Medicaid comes from the middle class, who must agree to higher taxes to provide the poor with medical benefits. The inadequacy of Medicaid in every state, the conditions necessary for achieving Medicaid eligibility, the low levels of eligibility, and the poor's lack of access to medical providers are related to the generosity (or lack thereof) of the middle class. The beneficiaries of Medicare, on the other hand, are the aged who (together with their children) provide the political support for the program. As the cost of Medicare has risen, government has raised Social Security taxes and reduced payments to providers rather than reducing benefits to this politically powerful group.

Provider organizations also have a concentrated interest in redistributive programs. When Medicare and Medicaid were enacted, physician and hospital associations were concerned with how their members would be paid by the government. These provider associations were also interested in precluding competition by competitive industries, such as HMOs, nurse practitioners, psychologists, and so on. Given their concentrated interest in these issues, physician and hospital associations were important contributors of political support for the purpose of defining the regulations determining provider payment and eligibility of providers to participate in these programs

The political necessity of keeping costs diffuse explains why the financing of both Medicare and producer regulation relies on regressive taxes, either payroll taxes or higher prices for medical services. Spreading the costs over large populations keeps these costs diffuse. The net effect is that low income persons pay the costs and higher income persons, such as physicians or high-income aged, receive the benefits. Those receiving the benefits and those bearing the costs, according to the economic theory, are not based on income, as shown in Table 17.1, but instead on which groups are able to offer political support (the beneficiaries) and which groups are unable to do so (they bear the costs). Regressive taxes are typically used to finance producer regulation as well as provide benefits to specific population groups.

Health policies change over time because groups who previously bore a diffuse cost develop a concentrated interest. Until the 1960s, medical societies were the main group with a concentrated interest in the financing and delivery of medical services. Thus the delivery system was structured to benefit physicians. Increases in the physician/population ratio remained constant for fifteen years (until the mid-1960s) at 141/100,000, state restrictions were imposed on HMOs to limit their development, advertising was prohibited, and restrictions were placed on other health professionals to limit their ability to compete with physicians. Financing mechanisms also benefited physicians; until the 1980s, capitation payment for HMOs was prohibited under Medicare and Medicaid and competitors to physicians were excluded from reimbursement under public and private insurance systems.

As the costs of medical care continued to increase rapidly to government and employers, their previously diffuse costs became concentrated. Under Medicare, the government was faced with the choice of raising taxes or reducing benefits to the aged, both of which would have cost the administration political support. Successive administrations developed a concentrated interest in lowering the rate of increase in medical expenditures. Similarly, large employers were concerned that rising medical costs were making them less competitive internationally. The pressures for cost containment increased as the "costs" of an inefficient delivery and payment system grew larger. Rising medical expenditures are no longer a diffuse cost to large purchasers of medical services.

Other health professionals, such as psychologists, chiropractors, and podiatrists, saw the potentially greater revenues their members could receive if they were better able to compete with physicians. These groups developed a concentrated interest in securing payment for their members under public and private insurance systems and expanding their scope of practice. The rise in opposing concentrated interests weakened the political influence of organized medicine.

The public interest and economic theories of government provide opposing predictions of the redistributive and efficiency effects of government legislation, as shown in Table 17.3. To determine which of these contrasting theories is a more accurate description of government it is necessary to match the actual outcomes of legislation to each theory's predictions. Do the benefits of redistributive programs go to those with low incomes? Are they financed by taxes that impose a larger burden on those with higher incomes? Does the government try to improve the allocation of resources by reducing barriers to entry and, when information is limited, monitoring and publishing quality of physicians' and other medical services?

The economic theory of regulation provides greater understanding of why health poli-

TABLE 17.3 Health Policy Objectives under Different Theories of Government

Theories of Government	Objective of Government	
	Redistribution	Improve Efficiency
Public Interest Theory	Assist those with low incomes	Remove (and prevent) monopoly abuses and protect environment (externalities)
Economic Theory of Regulation	Provide benefits to those able to deliver political support and finance from those having little political support	Efficiency objective unimportant; more likely to protect industries so as to provide them with redistributive benefits

cies are enacted and why they have changed over time than alternative theories. The economic theory predicts that government is not concerned with efficiency issues. *Redistribution is the main objective of government, but it is to redistribute wealth to those who are able to offer political support from those who are unable to do so.* Thus the reason medical licensing boards are inadequately staffed, have never required reexamination for relicensure, and have failed to monitor practicing physicians is that organized medicine has been opposed to any approaches for increasing quality that would adversely affect physicians' incomes. Regressive taxes are used to finance programs such as Medicare, not because legislators are unaware of their regressive nature, but because it was in the economic interest of unions to ensure that all their members would be eligible for Medicare.

The structure and financing of medical services is rational; the participants act according to their calculation of costs and benefits. Viewed in its entirety, however, health policy is uncoordinated and seemingly contradictory. Health policies are inequitable and inefficient; low-income persons end up subsidizing those with higher incomes. These results, however, are the consequences of a rational system. The outcomes were the result of policies intended by the legislators.

THE DEMAND FOR LEGISLATION BY HEALTH ASSOCIATIONS

Producer-type regulation has affected the structure and efficiency of the health care market. While it has not been as visible as redistributive legislation, such as Medicare and Medicaid, producer regulation has influenced the costs of these programs. It has also affected the performance of each of the medical markets. The following discussion provides an analysis of the different types of producer regulation demanded together with past examples of their use. Understanding the types of regulation demanded by health associations provides insights into the types of legislation health associations will favor or oppose in the years ahead.

Although differences existed in the objectives of health associations representing health professionals, hospitals, medical and dental schools, and Blue Cross and Blue Shield plans, the members of these associations all tried to make as much money as possible. They would then retain it for themselves, as did health professionals, or spend it to achieve prestige goals, as did hospitals and medical schools; the incomes of employees of prestigious institutions are likely to exceed those of less prestigious institutions. Thus the objective underlying the demand for legislation is the same for each health association.

Each association attempts to achieve for its members through legislation what cannot be achieved through a competitive market, namely, a monopoly position. Increased monopoly power and the ability to price as a monopolist seller of services was, and is, the best way for the associations to achieve their goals.

There are five types of legislation that health associations demand on behalf of their members. As government policy shifted from increasing to decreasing health expenditures (given the concern over the budget deficit) the emphasis devoted to each of these types of legislation by health interest groups has changed over time.

Demand-Increasing Legislation

An association favors demand-increasing legislation since an increase in demand, with a given supply, will result in an increase in price, an increase in total revenue, and, consequently, an increase in incomes or net revenues.

The most obvious way to increase the demand for the services of an association's members is to have the government subsidize the purchase of insurance for the provider's services. Health providers, however, do not want the government insuring everyone. Instead, the providers' demand for insurance subsidies was always discussed in relation to specific population groups in society, that is, people with low incomes.

The reason for selective government subsidies is twofold: first, people with higher incomes presumably have private insurance coverage or can afford to purchase the provider's services. The greatest increase in demand would result from extending coverage to those unable to pay. Second, extending government subsidies to those currently able to pay for the services would greatly increase the cost of the program to the government. A greater commitment of government expenditures would result in the government developing a concentrated interest in controlling the provider's prices, utilization, and expenditures. Thus, when demand subsidies were favored by health associations, they were always in relation to specific population groups or services rather than to the population at large.

Examples of the above approach were the AMA's position on national health insurance, Medicare, and Blue Shield. The AMA successfully defeated President Truman's national health insurance proposal in 1948 because subsidies would have been provided to all regardless of income level. The AMA's opposition to Medicare was also based on the fact that all aged, regardless of income, were to be subsidized. The approach favored by the AMA was a system of tax credits for the purchase of health insurance, which would decline as a person's income rose.

In recent years, as concern with the federal deficit has increased and federal funds to subsidize those with low incomes were unlikely to be available, the AMA has favored an employer mandate, whereby employers are required to purchase health insurance on behalf of their employees. An employer mandate would increase the demand for physician services by requiring the working uninsured to have private coverage. It would also move low-income employees and their families off Medicaid onto private insurance, which also reimburses providers at a higher rate.

The American Dental Association's (ADA) major demand-increasing effort has been to expand private insurance coverage for dental services. Insurance is generally purchased for events that are very expensive, such as hospital care and in-hospital physician services, and that have a low probability of occurring. Dental expenditures, which are relatively small, expected, and not catastrophic, are therefore not insurable in the same sense as hospital or surgical services; in fact, dental prepayment is not really insurance but a form of forced savings.

If special incentives to purchase dental insurance did not exist, most people would just pay for dental care when they needed it. The use of dental services is also highly related to income. Thus, a major reason for the growth in dental insurance has been the favorable tax treatment of employer-paid health insurance premiums. Such contributions are not considered part of the employee's income; the employee does not have to pay federal, state, or Social Security taxes on employer-paid health benefits.

Eliminating or "capping" the amount of employer-paid health benefits that are excluded from taxable income has been proposed in some health care reform proposals as a means of raising revenues to finance health benefits for those with low incomes.

The ADA's major legislative strategy in the past several years has been to defeat any such tax cap. If a tax cap were passed, employees would want less comprehensive health benefits because they would have to pay for additional benefits with after-tax dollars. The ADA believes, and rightly so, that if the tax discount for purchasing dental insurance were eliminated, the incentive for employees to purchase such insurance would decline. With less dental insurance, consumers would have to pay the full price of dental care. The demand for dental care would decline and consumers would be more inclined to "shop" among dentists for the lowest price (3).

The American Nurses' Association has favored three types of demand-increasing legislation. The first are proposals that increase the demand for medical services. An example is the ANA's support of national health insurance. Increases in demand for medical services would increase the demand for institutions in which RNs are employed, thereby increasing the demand for RNs. However, since health insurance coverage for hospital care is more extensive than for any other delivery settings (and two-thirds of nurses work in hospitals), nurse associations have also favored other demand-increasing proposals. The ANA has favored requiring minimum nurse staffing ratios in hospitals, nursing homes, and home health agencies.

Second, nurse associations have opposed hospital attempts to substitute lower-paid nurse aides to perform more of the RNs' tasks, which would decrease the demand for RNs.

A third type of demand proposal favored by nurse associations is one that widens the nurse's role, that is, increases the number of tasks nurses are legally able to perform. The nurses' value to an institution increases as they are permitted to perform more, and higher-valued, tasks. The demand for their services will increase, with a consequent increase in their incomes. In attempting to increase their tasks, nurses have come in conflict with the AMA. The AMA is fearful that changing state laws that limit the scope of what nurses with advanced training can do would decrease the demand for physicians (4).

As nurses work to increase their roles, they wage a struggle in the legislative marketplace to prevent other health professionals, such as licensed practical nurses (LPNs), from performing tasks previously reserved to RNs. The ANA is also in competition with physician assistants (PAs) over which profession will be able to perform tasks previously reserved to physicians.

The health professional association that is successful in enabling its members to increase their role, while preventing other health professionals from encroaching on their own tasks, will be able to increase the demand, hence the incomes, of its members. Examples of the legislative conflict over state practice acts are the attempts by optometrists to increase their role at the expense of ophthalmologists—as well as the struggles of psychologists versus psychiatrists, obstetricians versus nurse midwives, and podiatrists versus orthopedic surgeons.

The initial approach used by hospitals to increase the demand for their services was their establishment and control of Blue Cross. When hospitals started Blue Cross, Blue Cross only paid the costs of hospital care. Even if it was less costly to perform diagnostics in an outpatient setting, for the patient with Blue Cross coverage it was less expensive to have it performed in the hospital. The patient with Blue Cross did not have to pay any additional out-of-pocket hospital payments; thus high-cost hospitals were not at a price disadvantage with low-cost hospitals, thereby precluding price competition for Blue Cross patients. Further, every Blue Cross plan had to have at least 75 percent of the hospitals in its area participate in Blue Cross. This requirement precluded Blue Cross from contracting with only a lower-cost panel of hospitals. (The 75 percent rule also meant that Blue Cross would not have to compete with another Blue Cross plan in its area.)

As the price of hospital care became free to the Blue Cross subscriber, hospital use increased. Hospitals were reimbursed generously by Blue Cross for their services.

Legislatively, the American Hospital Association (AHA) favored government subsidies to stimulate the demand for hospital services by the aged and the poor. Medicare, which provided generous hospital coverage for the aged, increased the demand for hospitals by a high user group with generally low incomes. Hospitals have been in the forefront of lobbying efforts to receive federal subsidies for "uncompensated care," that is, the provision of hospital care to the poor for which they are not reimbursed. In the 1990s debate over national health insurance, the AHA has favored an employer mandate, which would increase the demand for private health insurance by those who are uninsured and by those whose hospital bills are being paid by Medicaid.

The Association of American Medical Colleges (AAMC) has favored legislation, at both state and federal levels, that provide such schools with unrestricted operating subsidies. Such subsidies would increase the demand for medical and dental schools by enabling them to set tuition levels greatly below the actual costs of education. With artificially low tuition levels and limits on the number of students they would accept, there would be an excess demand for their spaces. As long as there is an excess demand for a medical education—and the schools do not willingly expand their spaces to satisfy this demand—then the schools can determine the type of educational curriculum that comes closest to meeting their (and the AMA's or ADA's) preferences.

Securing the Highest Method of Reimbursement

The method of reimbursement, or the method used by the provider to charge for services, has been crucial to understanding provider economic behavior.

Two basic approaches have been used by health associations to achieve the highest possible reimbursement for their members. The first has been to try and eliminate price competition. The ability to engage in price competition is more important to new practitioners or firms desiring to enter a market. New competitors must be able to let potential patients know (through advertising) they are available and new surgeons must be able to provide primary care physicians with an incentive (fee splitting) to switch their surgical referrals away from established surgeons.

To prevent price competition from occurring, health associations have termed the elements of price competition, such as advertising and fee splitting, "unethical behavior" and have prohibited such behavior in their state practice acts (5). The medical and dental professions have used strong sanctions against practitioners who engaged in unethical behavior. A physician could have her license suspended and be assessed financial penalties. Previously, medical societies were able to deny hospital privileges to physicians who advertised or engaged in price competition (6). Without hospital privileges a physician could not offer patients complete medical service. Since physicians new to an area had the greatest incentive to engage in such "unethical" behavior, they were given probationary membership in the local medical society. They were thereby placed on notice that they could lose their hospital privileges if they engaged in such behavior. (Since the application of the anti-trust laws to health care in 1982, such anticompetitive behavior by medical societies is no longer permitted.)

The second approach used by health providers to secure the highest possible payment for their services was to engage in price discrimination, which means charging different patients or payers different prices for the same service. These different prices do not result from differences in costs, but from the patients' or their payers' abilities to pay. Charging according to ability to pay results in greater revenues than a pricing system that charges everyone the same price.

The desire by organized medicine to maintain a system whereby physicians could price discriminate influenced the financing and delivery of medical services for many years. Once medical insurance was introduced, organized medicine attempted to retain the physician's ability to price discriminate. For example, when medical societies started Blue Shield plans, the physician's fee was paid in full for those subscribers whose incomes were below a certain level. Physicians were permitted to charge higher-income patients an amount in addition to the Blue Shield payment. The Blue Shield income limits were eventually eliminated as the large majority of subscribers' incomes exceeded the income limit. Blue Shield insurance was not worth as much to high-income people if they had to pay a significant amount each time they went to the physician, in addition to the annual premium. As Blue Shield organizations dropped their income limits so as to be able to enroll more high-income subscribers, some medical societies dropped their sponsorship of the Blue Shield plans.

Once the income limits were removed, physicians could still maintain some ability to price discriminate by deciding when they wanted to participate in Blue Shield and when they wanted to charge the patient directly. In the latter case, the patient would then receive payment from Blue Shield for an amount less than the physician's charge. For persons with higher incomes, physicians would charge the patient directly, which would provide them with a higher payment than if the physician participated in Blue Shield.

The physician payment system under Medicare was based on the same principle. Physicians decided whether to participate in Medicare on a case by case basis. If they thought they could make more money by charging the patient directly, they would do so. When they accepted the Medicare fee, the patient was responsible for a 20 percent co-payment. When the physician chose not to participate, the patient had to pay the physician's fee, which was greater than the Medicare fee, and the patient was responsible for the difference in the fees as well as the co-payment. By having the option of participating when they wanted to, physicians were assured of payment from low-income persons, while still being able to charge a higher price to the higher-income patient. The method of pricing and flexibility of physician participation under Blue Shield and Medicare were crucial to their acceptance of these plans.

Organized medicine's desire to maintain a physician's ability to price discriminate limited the growth of prepaid health plans. HMOs charge patients the same premium regardless of income level. When fee-for-service physicians charge higher-income patients a higher fee, then an HMO that charges all persons the same premium is a form of price competition; it limits the physician's ability to price discriminate. When physicians moved into an area with the intention of joining a prepaid plan, local medical societies prevented them from receiving hospital privileges. Unless the plan had its own hospital, which was unlikely, this effectively eliminated competition. Medical societies were subsequently successful in having restrictive legislation enacted at a state level, which effectively limited the growth of these plans.

In the mid-1980s the AMA opposed the federal government's attempt to pay HMOs an annual capitated price for each Medicare enrollee (referred to as Medicare risk contracts).

Dental societies have acted similarly with respect to advertising and price competition. Until the successful FTC suit against the AMA, dental societies included bans on advertising in their state practice acts.

An important recent legislative activity of many state medical and dental societies has been to enact "any willing provider" legislation, which seeks to ensure that all patients have free choice of any provider. Providers included in closed provider panels established by HMOs and PPOs are willing to discount their fees and practice cost-effectively in return for receiving a greater volume of patients. HMOs and PPOs are thereby able to offer their services to employers at premiums lower than those prevailing in the area. Providers who are not a part of these closed panels do not have access to the HMOs' and PPOs' patient population. Providers in closed panels are engaged in price competition with providers who are not in the closed panels.

By enacting "any willing provider" legislation, medical and dental societies remove providers' financial incentive to discount their fees in return for more patients. If providers in closed panels have to share their patients with providers who are not in closed panels, providers are unlikely to join closed panels and discount their fees.

To enable dentists to charge what the market will bear, the American Dental Association (ADA) has opposed the use of insurer fee schedules. Several years ago, the Pennsylvania Blue Shield (PBS) won an anti-trust suit against the Pennsylvania Dental Association (PDA) on grounds that the PDA boycotted PBS because the Blue Shield dental plan paid dentists according to a fee schedule. The PDA wanted dentists to be able to charge the patient an additional amount if they so desired.

Similar to the above, the ADA has also opposed the practice of insurance companies reimbursing a patient a lower amount if he goes to a nonparticipating dentist. The ADA has called for legislation prohibiting insurance companies from this payment approach. (The dentist is not prohibited from participating with the insurance company. However, the dentist would prefer not to participate, to receive the same amount as participating dentists, as well as to be able to charge the patient an additional amount.)

The American Nurses' Association has long been in favor of permitting advanced practice nurses to bill fee-for-service. Against the opposition of the AMA, registered nurses are striving to become independent practitioners, such as nurse practitioners and nurse midwives, who will then be able to bill the patient on a fee-for-service basis. Fee-for-service payment to a health professional, which in most cases is reimbursed by the government or private insurance, is the most direct way for a health professional to increase income and to work independently of physicians.

Nurse practitioners have been able to work independently and be reimbursed by many state Medicaid programs that serve low-income people and by Medicare for patients in rural areas. The numbers of independent nurse practitioners are likely to increase as a result of a decision in 1997 by the VA to formally accept nurse practitioners without links to physicians and of a new federal law (effective 1998) allowing Medicare to pay nurse practitioners who work in cities and suburbs, not just in rural areas, directly.

The American Hospital Association was, until the 1980s, successful in eliminating any incentive for hospitals to engage in price competition. When hospitals started Blue Cross, the plans were required to offer their subscribers a service benefit plan, which provides the hospitalized patient with services rather than dollars, a characteristic of an indemnity plan. By guaranteeing payment to the hospital for the services used by the patient, the service benefit policy removes any incentive the patient (or the hospital) may have regarding the cost of hospitalization. Since the patient does not have to make any out-of-pocket payments, the prospective patient has no disincentive to enter the most expensive hospital, which may or may not be the highest-quality hospital. Under a service benefit policy, hospitals cannot compete for patients on the basis of price.

When Medicare was enacted, the AHA proposed a method of hospital payment, which was adopted by the government, that paid hospitals for providing care to Medicare patients based on each hospital's costs plus 2 percent. Once patients paid a deductible, they were not assessed any co-payments. Not only did this method of payment eliminate any incentive for patients to select less costly, more efficient hospitals, but it provided hospitals with an incentive to increase their costs. (Further, hospitals were not permitted to compete for Medicare patients by offering to reduce the hospital deductible.)

Hospitals have also tried to price discriminate. When hospitals started Blue Cross, they gave Blue Cross a 20 percent discount compared to what commercial insurers were charged. This discount enabled Blue Cross to offer a more expensive policy (a service benefit) that was in the hospitals' interest. The discount was also a competitive advantage for Blue Cross and enabled them to increase their market share over the commercial companies.

Hospitals did very well financially under the initial Medicare payment policy. The government was anxious for hospitals to participate in Medicare and therefore accepted many of the AHA's payment proposals. Not only were hospitals able to negotiate a 2 percent addition to their costs of serving Medicare patients and receive favorable treatment for depreciating their assets, but the manner in which hospital costs were calculated gave hospitals additional payment. Hospitals could not separate the actual costs of serving Medicare patients from those of other patients. The method used to calculate Medicare costs was to use the ratio of what hospitals charge for Medicare patients to the charges for non-Medicare patients. That ratio was then used to determine the portion of the hospitals' total costs that should be paid by Medicare. The effect of this policy was to provide hospitals with an incentive to raise charges on those services used predominantly by the elderly, such as bed rails. By raising the proportion of their charges for the aged, a greater portion of the hospitals' total costs were paid by the government. The hospital would then be able to make a higher profit on its charges to commercial insurance companies.

Hospitals were also able to price discriminate by setting a higher price/cost ratio for those services for which there was a greater willingness to pay, that is, services that were less price elastic. Ancillary services, such as lab tests and x-rays, had higher price/cost ratios than the hospital's basic room charge. Once patients were hospitalized they had little choice on the use or price of ancillary services. Patients who paid part of the hospital bill themselves could, before they entered a particular hospital, more easily compare charges for obstetric services and room rates. The charges for these services were much closer to their costs.

The method by which public medical and dental schools are subsidized is very important. Subsidies go directly to the school, as do government funds distributed for loans and scholarships. Under this arrangement, the student receives a subsidy (tuition less than costs) only by attending a subsidized school. This method requires that students compete for medical and dental schools. If government subsidies went directly to the student, then the schools would have to compete for students. As with subsidies, medical and dental schools prefer to distribute loans and scholarships themselves rather than have students apply directly to the government for such financial assistance. If the students received the subsidies and loans directly, then they would have an incentive to shop and select a school based on its tuition rates and reputation. The current system provides a competitive advantage to schools receiving subsidies. Needless to say, private schools would prefer that the subsidies go directly to the students.

The methods used by health professionals and health institutions for pricing their services has enabled these providers to maximize their revenues. The health associations representing each provider group have had, in negotiating with the government, in establishing their own insurance organizations, and in proposing legislation, a clear appreciation for which pricing strategies are in their members' economic interest.

Legislation to Reduce the Price or Increase the Quantity of Complements

A registered nurse may be a substitute or a complement to the physician. It is difficult to determine when an input, such as a nurse, is a complement or a substitute based only on the task performed. A nurse may be as competent as a physician in performing certain tasks. If the nurse works for the physician and the physician receives the fee for the performance of that task, then the nurse has increased the physician's productivity and is a complement. If, however, the nurse performs the same task and is a nurse practitioner billing independently of the physician, then the nurse is a substitute for the physician providing that service. The essential element in determining whether an input is a complement or a substitute is who receives the payment for the services provided by that input. Whoever receives the payment controls the use of that input.

The state practice acts were the legal basis for determining which tasks each health professional can perform and under whose direction health professionals must work. A major legislative activity for each health association was to ensure that the state practice acts worked to their members' interests. Health associations that represent complements (e.g., nurses and denturists) attempt to have their members become substitutes. Health associations whose members control complements seek to retain the status quo.

In the past, almost all the health professions and health institutions were complements to the physician. That situation is now changing. The physician is no longer the sole entry point to the delivery of medical services. HMOs, for example, may use nurse practitioners to serve their enrollees. The AMA has continued to oppose the use of independent nurse practitioners and has lobbied against state laws that allow advance practice nurses to provide medical care without the supervision of a physician. The American Academy of Family Practitioners (who would be most adversely affected by independent nurse practitioners) has stated that such nurses should only be paid by insurers when they work in a "collaborative" relationship with physicians.

Providers can increase their incomes if an increase in demand for their services is met through greater productivity than through an increase in the number of competing providers. The providers' income can be increased still further if their productivity increases are subsidized and they do not have to pay the full cost of the increased productivity.

The following are several examples of legislation that has subsidized providers' productivity. The American Hospital Association lobbied for passage of the Nurse Training Act in the belief that federal educational subsidies would increase the supply of RNs available to hospitals. With a larger supply of nurses, nurses' wages would be lower than they otherwise would have been. The AHA was a strong proponent of the Hill–Burton program, which provided capital subsidies to modernize hospitals. The AHA opposed legislation that would have increased the cost of inputs to hospitals. It opposed the extension of minimum wage legislation to hospital employees and has called for a moratorium on the separate licensing of each health professional. (Separate licensing limits the hospital's ability to substitute different health professionals in the tasks they perform and to use such personnel in a more flexible manner.) Conversely, separate licensing is demanded by each health professional association so as to increase the demand for its members' services by restricting the tasks that other professions can perform.

The AMA has favored internship and residency programs in hospitals. Interns and residents are excellent complements for physicians; they can take care of the physician's hospitalized patients and relieve the physician from serving in the hospital emergency room and from being on call. The more advanced the resident is, the closer the resident is to being a potential substitute for the physician. Residents, however, are complements since it is the physician who bills for the service. For this reason the AMA has favored the use of foreign medical graduates to serve as interns and residents. Once they graduate, however, they become substitutes to existing practitioners. The AMA has, therefore, favored the return of foreign medical graduates to their home country once their residencies are completed. (The AMA advocated a time limit on how long foreign medical graduates can remain in the United States, as well as the requirement that they be out of the country two years before returning.)

The main concern of the AMA toward emerging health professionals, such as physician assistants, was to ensure that these types of personnel become complements to, not substitutes for, the physician. Thus, whether there is direct or indirect supervision of the PA by the physician is less important to the AMA's political position than who gets the fee for the PA's service.

The legislative attempt by physicians and dentists to lower the cost of their inputs has been action at both the federal and state levels to limit increases in malpractice premiums. There are many reasons why malpractice premiums have risen (7). Professional associations have been more willing to seek legislation to place limits on the size of malpractice awards than to make a concerted effort to eliminate unqualified practitioners.

Up until the mid-1980s (at which time large employers placed pressure on insurance companies to reduce their premiums), the Blue Cross premium consisted almost entirely of the costs of hospital care. Its main cost therefore has been the cost and quantity of hospital care used by its subscribers. Commercial insurance companies had broader coverage (although it included deductibles and cost sharing), and therefore hospital care was a smaller portion of the total premium. Thus to remain competitive against commercial insurance companies, Blue Cross had to keep the cost of hospital care (both hospital use and cost per unit) from rising so rapidly. Under the service benefit policy, however, patients, their physicians, and the hospital had no incentive to be concerned with cost or use. In fact, it was in the hospital's interest to add facilities and services and pass the costs on to Blue Cross. As more hospitals added facilities and services in a race to determine who could be more prestigious, there was a great deal of duplication of costly facilities and services and, consequently, low use. Blue Cross, however, was committed to pay. To limit the increase in these costly facilities, Blue Cross favored legislative restrictions on hospital investment.

Given the control hospitals had over Blue Cross, Blue Cross was not aggressive in trying to limit the rapid rise in hospital costs, such as by limiting what they would pay hospitals. Blue Cross and large hospitals favored an indirect approach that prevented smaller hospitals from expanding their beds and facilities and the entry of new hospitals. To receive Blue Cross (and Medicare) reimbursement for capital expenditures, a hospital had to receive the approval of a planning agency for its investment. Existing large hospitals either had the latest facilities or were the likeliest candidates to receive approval from the planning agency, whose criteria favored large, full-service hospitals. These large institutions also favored the development and strengthening of planning agencies because it limited competition.

Blue Cross relied on controls to hold down hospital investment and rising Blue Cross premiums. All studies have shown that controls on capital investment were not effective in holding down either hospital investment or the rise in hospital costs (8). It was not until Blue Cross began to experience strong competitive pressures, sufficient to affect its survival, that it finally undertook more direct means of lowering the costs of its major input. Blue Cross began including lower-cost substitutes to hospitals as part of its benefits, instituting utilization control programs, and changing the method by which it pays hospitals.

Legislation to Decrease the Availability or Increase the Price of Substitutes

All health associations try to increase the price of services that are substitutes to those provided by their members. (Similar to increasing the price of a substitute is decreasing its availability.) If the health association is successful in achieving this, then the demand for its members' services will be increased.

Health associations use three general approaches to accomplish this. The first is to simply have the substitute declared illegal. If substitute health professionals are not permitted to practice, or if substitutes are severely restricted in the tasks they are legally permitted to perform, then there will be a shift in demand away from the substitute service.

The second approach, used when the first approach is unsuccessful, is to exclude the substitute service from payment by any third party, including government health programs. This approach raises the price of the substitute. The third approach is to try and raise the costs of the substitutes, who must then raise their own prices if they are to remain in business. The following examples illustrate the behavior of health associations for each of these approaches.

For many years the AMA regarded osteopaths as "cultists." It was considered "unethical" for physicians to teach in schools of osteopathy. Unable to prevent their licensure at a state level, the AMA tried to deny osteopaths hospital privileges. (A physician substitute is less than adequate if that substitute cannot provide a complete range of treatment.) As osteopaths developed their own hospitals and educational institutions, medical societies decided the best approach to controlling the increase in supply of these physician substitutes was to merge with the osteopaths, make them physicians, and then eliminate any future increases in their supply. An example of this approach, which was used in California until it was overturned by the state Supreme Court, was to allow osteopaths to convert their D.O. degree to an M.D. on the basis of twelve Saturday refresher courses. After the merger between the two societies occurred in California, the Osteopathic Board of Examiners was no longer permitted to license osteopaths.

Medicare has been the vehicle for much legislative competition. The AMA has lobbied for covering only physician services under Medicare Part B while excluding nonphysician services. By including only physician services the prices of substitute providers to the aged are effectively increased relative to those of physicians. For example, optometrists and chiropractors are potential substitutes for ophthalmologists and family physicians. By including physician services under Medicare, but excluding payment for nonphysicians, the price of nonphysicians is increased relative to physicians. An aged person with Medicare Part B pays less for a physician's services, since the out-of-pocket price to the aged of physician services has been lowered. The AMA has similarly opposed direct payment of nurse anesthetists and nurse practitioners under Medicare.

In one case, the intervention of the courts prevented physicians from artificially raising the price of a substitute. In Virginia, Blue Shield did not reimburse psychologists as providers of psychotherapy. Psychiatrists' services were therefore less expensive than psychologists' to a patient with Blue Shield. The psychologists brought a successful anti-trust case against Blue Shield in 1980, claiming discrimination of nonphysician providers.

An example of the legislative behavior of dental societies toward substitute providers is illustrated by dentistry's actions toward denturists. Denturism is the term applied to the fitting and dispensing of dentures directly to patients by people not licensed as dentists. Independently practicing denturists are a threat to dentists' incomes since they provide dentures at lower prices. Denturists are legal in most of Canada. As a result of their political success in Canada, denturists in the United States became bolder, forcing referendums on the issue and lobbying for changes in the state practice acts. Several states have passed laws legalizing denturism.

Occasionally denturists have sold dentures directly to patients illegally. To eliminate this competition and to prevent its increase, local dental societies, such as in Texas, responded in two ways: first, they offered to provide low-cost dentures to low-income persons; second, they pressured state officials to enforce the state laws against illegal denturists.

It was only the threat of competition that resulted in the dental profession's offer to provide low-cost dentures to the indigent or near-indigent. If the denturists' competitive threat is eliminated through dentistry's successful use of the state's legal authority, the net effect will be to cause the public, particularly the poor, to pay higher prices for dentures.

The ADA is also concerned that dental hygienists remain complements to, not become substitutes for, dentists. Several state dental hygienist associations have attempted to change the state practice act to permit hygienists to practice without a dentist's supervision and to become independent practitioners. In 1986, although opposed by the ADA, the hygienists were successful in achieving this goal in Colorado.

One of the most important substitutes for registered nurses is foreign-trained registered nurses. Nurses' salaries are considerably higher in the United States than in other countries, providing a financial incentive for foreign nurses to enter the country. The ANA has tried to decrease the availability of a low-cost substitute for U.S. registered nurses by making it more difficult for foreign-trained RNs to enter the country. For example, the ANA has proposed that foreign RNs desiring to enter the United States be screened by examination in their home country before being allowed to immigrate. If the screening exam were administered only in the United States, then foreign-trained RNs could still work in some nursing capacity in this country even if they did not pass the exam. The foreign-trained nurse could then retake the exam in the future. As it is, the screening exam is an additional barrier for foreign nurses to pass before they can enter the United States; if they do not pass the exam, they are unlikely to emigrate.

An additional legislative approach used by the ANA is to prevent other personnel from performing tasks performed by the RN. The ANA has opposed permitting physicians to decide which personnel can perform nursing tasks; the ANA has opposed permitting LPNs to be in charge of skilled nursing homes, otherwise there would be substitution away from RNs (who receive higher wages) currently performing such functions. The California Nurses Association opposed a bill that would have authorized firefighters with paramedic training to give medical and nursing care in hospital emergency departments. As a means of preventing physician assistants from assuming a role that the RN would like, the ANA has favored a licensing moratorium. A moratorium would prevent any new health personnel from being licensed to perform tasks that RNs do or would like to perform.

The American Hospital Association opposed the growth of freestanding ambulatory surgicenters. Surgicenters are low-cost substitutes for hospitals; performing surgical procedures in a surgicenter decreases the use of the hospital, and its revenues. To limit the availability of these low-cost substitutes, hospital associations have argued that surgicenters should be permitted only when they are developed in association with a hospital.

Denying Blue Cross reimbursement to freestanding surgicenters and including surgicenters under CON legislation were approaches favored by hospital associations. Health maintenance organizations were also included in state CON legislation for the same reason, since they decrease the use and revenues of hospitals.

Hospital associations have used several approaches to raise the price of their competitors, for-profit hospitals. For example, hospitals opposed granting for-profit hospitals Blue Cross eligibility. Being ineligible for Blue Cross payment precludes the use of the hospital by patients with Blue Cross coverage.

Substitutes for American medical and dental schools are foreign schools whose graduates (who may be U.S. citizens) want to practice in the United States. To reduce the likelihood that foreign medical schools will substitute for U.S. medical schools, the AAMC has been a strong proponent for eliminating Medicare graduate medical education payments for residents trained in foreign medical schools. This reduction to teaching hospitals would be a strong incentive for these hospitals not to accept foreign-trained graduates.

The American Dental Association and the Association of American Dental Schools have been more successful in reducing the attractiveness of a foreign dental education. Practicing dentists do not use residents as do physicians. Therefore their interest is solely with decreasing the supply of dentists. There are increased time requirements for a foreign-trained dentist wishing to practice in the United States. A minimum number of years of training in the foreign country is required, as well as a license to practice in that country. (For a U.S. citizen, this would mean learning a different language.) And once foreign-trained dentists enter the country, additional requirements are then imposed on them. They are required to take the last two years of dental school in an accredited U.S. dental school. They may also be required to take additional examinations before the licensing exam. To date, such restrictive practices have raised the cost of a U.S. dental license for foreign-trained dentists (both U.S. and non-U.S. citizens). The consequence has been a decreased demand for a foreign dental education as a substitute for a U.S. dental education. The measure of how successful the dental profession and the dental schools have been is that less than 5 percent of all practicing dentists in the United States are foreign-trained.

Legislation to Limit Increases in Supply

Essential to the creation of a monopoly are limits on the number of providers of a service. Health associations, however, have justified supply control policies on grounds of quality. Restrictions on entry, they maintain, ensure high quality of care to the public. These same health associations, however, oppose quality measures that would have an adverse economic effect on existing providers (their members). This apparent anomaly—stringent entry requirements and then virtually no quality assurance programs directed at existing providers—is only consistent with a policy that seeks to establish a monopoly for existing providers.

If health associations were consistent in their desire to improve and maintain high quality standards, then they should favor all policies that ensure quality of care, regardless of the effect on their members. Quality control measures directed at existing providers, such as reexamination, relicensure, and monitoring of the care actually provided, would adversely affect the incomes of some providers. More important, such "outcome" measures of quality assurance would make entry or "process" measures less necessary, thereby permitting entry of a larger number of providers.

As previously discussed in the chapter on physician manpower, a test of the hypothesis that entry barriers are primarily directed toward developing a monopoly position rather than improving quality of care would be as follows: Does the health association favor quality measures, regardless of the effect on its members' incomes, or does it only favor those quality measures that enhance members' incomes? If the health association only favors those quality measures that have a favorable impact on its members' economic position, then it can be concluded that the real intent of those quality measures is the improvement of its members' competitive position rather than the assurance of quality care in the most efficient manner.

In recent years there has been a growing concern among dentists (as well as among other health professions) that there are too many practitioners. As would be expected, rather than relying on market forces to determine the number of dentists, the ADA approach is to reduce the number of dental school spaces. Indicative of this approach is the ADA's statement, "Resolved, that public statements made by the American Dental Association . . . include the recognition that a surplus of dentists does exist to meet the current demand for dental services, . . . [and that] the ADA encourage and assist constituent societies in preparing legislation that may be used to petition state legislatures and governmental bodies with respect to private schools to adjust enrollment in dental schools" (9).

Optometrists have followed the same supply control policies as previously discussed for medicine and dentistry. Similarly, as educational requirements were increased, existing members of the profession were grandfathered in. By the early 1900s, optometrists were able to secure licensure in all states. However, there were many private schools for training optometrists. By the 1920s, the American Optometric Association was successful in disqualifying twenty of the thirty optometric schools and in raising educational requirements. Optometry requires six years of education in an approved optometric school and at least three years (most applicants have completed four years) of traditional undergraduate college education (10). Increasing educational requirements for a profession involves not just increasing the number of years of professional training but also requiring more years of undergraduate training.

Nursing also tried to impose stringent educational requirements. The ANA has proposed and has lobbied state legislatures that nursing education take place only in colleges that offer a BA (11). Only four-year nurse graduates would be referred to as professional nurses, otherwise the nurse would be a "technical nurse." By proposing an increase in the educational requirement of two-thirds of the nurse graduates, the ANA must be well aware that the result will be a decrease in the number of nurse graduates. The effect of increased education and an increase in nursing tasks would be an increase in the incomes of existing nurses, who would be grandfathered in as professional nurses.

It is unlikely one would ever observe a health association proposing increased educational requirements that are then applied to its existing members. Only to forestall more stringent requirements proposed by others would a health association favor additional training requirements for its existing members. Health associations do not favor relicensure or reexamination requirements for their current members, even though increased knowledge is the basis for requiring additional training for those entering the profession. Reexamination and relicensure would lower the incomes of their members, since they would have to take the time to study for the exam. Current practitioners also may not be able to pass the exam. No health association proposes that the time required to prepare a person to enter their profession be reduced.

As knowledge increases and educational requirements for new graduates in the health professions lengthen, the public is led to believe that all persons in a profession are equally (or at least minimally) qualified. This is unlikely to be the case, particularly for those practitioners who were trained thirty years ago and have not kept up with current information.

At times the profession has imposed requirements on new entrants that are blatant barriers. For example, foreign medical and dental graduates were required to be U.S. citizens before they were allowed to practice in some states (12). Further, a dentist desiring to practice in Hawaii, for example, no matter how well-trained or how long in practice in another state, is required to complete a one-year residency requirement before being allowed to practice (13). Such requirements cannot be remotely related to the profession's concern with quality.

If the members of a profession are concerned with quality, then they should favor monitoring quality among themselves. Yet associations have opposed any attempts by others to review the quality of care practiced by their members. Health associations that have proposed continuing education for their members have done so in response to demands by those outside the profession. These requirements are made easy to achieve and at low cost to the members of the profession.

SUMMARY

Health professionals and health institutions do not exhibit characteristics of a natural monopoly, that is, large economies of scale for a given size of market sufficient to preclude entry of competitors. Because these professionals and institutions cannot achieve a monopoly position through the normal competitive process, they seek to achieve it through legislation. The first step toward increasing their monopoly power is to erect barriers to entry. The next is to limit competition among their members. They then attempt to improve their monopoly position by further demanding legislation that will increase the demand for their services, permit them to price as would a price-discriminating monopolist, lower their costs of doing business, and disadvantage their competitors either by causing them to become illegal providers or by forcing them to raise their prices.

Health professionals, particularly physicians and dentists, have been successful in the legislative marketplace, as evidenced by the design of public programs to pay for their services and by their relatively high incomes. However, three types of "costs" are imposed on the rest of society as a result of the restrictions that cause a redistribution of wealth to members of health associations that have achieved legislative success.

The first is higher prices. The more successful a health association is in achieving their members' goals, the higher will be the price of their members' services. However, once price competition occurs between members of different health associations, the lower will be the prices of both groups' services. Allowing freestanding surgicenters to compete with hospitals lowered the cost to the patient for surgical procedures (through reduced insurance premiums). Other tactics used by health associations to prevent price competition among their members included prohibitions against advertising, limiting productivity increases to prevent excess capacity, preventing physicians in HMOs from having hospital privileges, and requiring free choice of provider under both public and private insurance plans. These restrictions have resulted in health care prices being higher than they would be otherwise.

The second implication of successful legislative behavior by health associations is that the public is provided with a false assurance with respect to the quality of the medical care it receives. The state delegated its responsibility for protecting the public to the individual licensing boards, which in turn have been controlled and operated in the interests of the providers themselves. The approach toward quality assurance used by both the profession and licensing boards is needlessly costly and inefficient. It has been more concerned with the process of becoming a health professional, such as entry into the profession, than with monitoring the care provided. As such, state licensing boards have devoted too few resources to investigating complaints against and removing incompetent or unethical providers. Too rarely do state licensing boards take disciplinary action against their members.

The movement toward a competitive market in medical services has resulted in a new emphasis on quality of care. Large employers are pressuring HMOs to provide information on their enrollees' medical outcomes, preventive measures undertaken, and health status indicators of their subscriber population. It is through actions by such large purchasers that HMOs are developing "report cards." Employer emphasis on "outcome" measures is forcing HMOs and medical groups to reexamine how medical care is provided. It is doubtful that this new approach toward quality would have occurred had market competition not developed (14).

The third effect of legislative success by a health association is that innovation in the delivery of medical care was inhibited. Innovation provides benefits to consumers; they have greater choice, higher quality, and lower costs. Innovation, however, threatens the monopoly power of a protected provider group, and is therefore opposed. Medical and dental societies have been protectors of the fee-for-service delivery system. These organizations have delayed the introduction of alternative delivery systems, such as HMOs and PPOs.

Rather than being procompetitive, "any willing provider" laws and "free choice of provider" have been used by the professions to eliminate competition from "closed" provider panels. HMOs and PPOs cannot negotiate volume discounts with closed panels of providers if they have to offer their subscribers free choice of any provider. HMOs and managed care organizations are able to offer lower premiums than traditional insurance because they are able to impose restrictions on the types of participating providers and institute medical management programs. Legislative restrictions against closed panels, such as by requiring free choice of provider, have prevented managed care organizations from successfully competing against traditional insurance plans.

Medical and dental societies have inhibited the development of new types of health personnel, such as nurse midwives, nurse practitioners, and expanded function dental auxiliaries, because they might become substitutes. The determination of which tasks a health professional is able to perform is related more to their economic effects on another health profession than to the professional's qualifications and training.

Hospital associations have sought, through certificate-of-need legislation, to stifle innovations such as the growth of freestanding surgicenters. It was the commercial insurance companies that introduced major medical insurance, a distinct innovation that also increased their share of the health insurance market. The process of receiving a professional education (medical, dental, and optometric) has changed little over time (except for an increase in years required) because it has remained under the auspices of accredited schools and their professions. It is highly likely that the necessary knowledge could be provided to students in a shorter period of time, thereby decreasing the total cost of such an education.

Innovation offers the hope of greater productivity, lower costs, and increase in quality. The political activities of health associations should be viewed in their proper perspective, namely, to benefit their members while imposing a cost on the rest of society. Past reliance on professional regulation to protect the patient has reduced incentives for innovation.

The usefulness of the different theories of government should be judged by their predictive ability. While it is unlikely that any one theory will be able to explain all or even a very high percentage of all legislation, a theory is necessary for trying to understand why certain types of legislation were passed and why others were not, unless one believes that all legislation is ad hoc. It is natural to try to organize what we observe in some meaningful manner. The criteria for selecting one theory over another should be based on pragmatic grounds: Which approach is better at explaining events under a broad range of circumstances? To reject a theory it is necessary to have a better theory.

The economic theory of government assumes that human behavior is no different in political than in private markets. Individuals, groups, firms, and legislators seek to enhance their self-interests. They are assumed to be rational in assessing the benefits and the costs to themselves of their actions. This behavioral assumption enables us to predict that firms in private markets will try to produce their products and services as efficiently as possible to keep their costs down and that they will set their prices so as to make as much profit as possible. They will be motivated to enter markets where the profit potential is greatest and, similarly, to leave markets where the profit potential is low.

It is merely an extension of the above discussion to include political markets. Individuals and firms use the power of the state to further their own interests. Firms try to gain competitive advantages in private markets by investing in technology and advertising. Why shouldn't firms also make political investments to be able to use the powers of government to increase or maintain profit?

The actions of organizations representing individuals are no different from those representing firms. Many people would like to use the power of the state to assist them in what they cannot otherwise achieve. For some, this may mean using the state to help them impose their religious or social preferences on others. Still other groups would like to use the state to provide them with monetary benefits that they could not earn in the market and that others would not voluntarily provide to them, such as low-cost education for their children, pension payments in excess of their contributions, and subsidized medical benefits.

It is usually with regard to our public "servants" that the assumption of acting in one's self-interest becomes difficult to accept. After all, why would a person run for office if not to serve the public interest? However, to be successful in the electoral process requires legislators to behave in a manner that enhances their reelection prospects. Political support, votes, and contributions are the bases for reelection. Legislators must therefore be able to understand the sources of such support and the requirements for receiving it. A hungry man quickly realizes that if money buys food then he must have money to eat. Legislators act no differently than others.

Political markets have several characteristics that differentiate them from economic markets. These differences make it possible for organized interests to benefit at the expense of majorities. First, individuals are not as informed about political issues as they are about the goods and services on which they spend their own funds.

Second, in private markets individuals make separate decisions on each item they purchase. They do not have to choose between sets of purchases, such as between one package that may include a particular brand of car, a certain size house in a particular neighborhood, several suits, and a certain quantity of food. Yet in political markets their choices are between two sets of votes by competing legislators on a wide variety of issues.

Third, voting participation rates differ by age group. The young and future generations do not vote, and yet policies are enacted that impose costs on them. Future generations depend on current generations and voters to protect their interests. However, as has been the case many times, such as with respect to the federal deficit, Social Security, and Medicare, their interests have been sacrificed to current voters.

Fourth, legislators use different decision criteria from those used in the private sector.

A firm or an individual making an investment considers both the benefits and the costs of that investment. Legislators, however, have a different time horizon, which not only affects the emphasis they place on costs and benefits but also on when each is incurred. Since members of the House of Representatives run for reelection every two years, they are likely to favor programs that provide immediate benefits (presumably just before the election) while delaying the costs until after the election or years later.

Further, from the legislator's perspective, the program does not even have to meet the criterion that the benefits exceed its costs—the immediate benefits only need to exceed any immediate costs. Future legislators can worry about future costs.

It is for these reasons that organized groups are able to receive legislative benefits while imposing the costs of those benefits on the remainder of the population. For those bearing the costs of legislative benefits that others receive, it may be perfectly rational not to oppose such legislation. As long as the cost of changing political outcomes exceeds the lost wealth imposed by legislation, it is rational for voters to lose some wealth rather than to organize and bear the cost of changing the legislative outcome.

At times self-interest legislation may be in the "public interest." When this occurs, however, it is because it is a byproduct of the outcome rather than its intended effect.

Key Terms and Concepts

- Concentrated interests
- Diffuse costs
- Government policy instruments
- Government policy objectives
- Price of legislation
- Regressive taxes

- Economic theory of government
- Five types of producer legislation
- Public interest theory of government
- Visibility of legislation's effects

Review Questions

1. Describe the economic theory of regulation. Contrast its predictions to the public interest theory of regulation with respect to certificate-of-need legislation. What evidence leads you to select one theory over the other?
2. Predict which organizations would oppose and support:
   a. Subsidies for the training of nurse midwives

    b. state mandates requiring all health insurers include chiropractic services in their benefits

    c. inclusion of psychologists as covered providers in a health insurance plan.

3. Why are concentrated interests and diffuse costs important to predicting legislative outcomes?

4. Contrast the cost/benefit calculations of legislators under both the public interest and economic theories of government.

5. Evaluate the following policies according to the public interest and economic theories:
    a. The performance of state licensing boards in monitoring physician quality
    b. Medicare reform

6. There are a number of restrictions in the methods by which medical care is organized and provided. With regard to restrictions on entry, on tasks performed, and (previously) on information, contrast the reasons for such restrictions in terms of improved quality versus enhancement of provider incomes.

7. Apply the theoretical model of the demand for legislation to predict legislation demanded by the AMA or the ADA. Be explicit regarding the objective of the AMA or ADA, and justify the choice of that objective.

8. What are some practices in medical care that are purported to result in higher standards of quality that are in effect restrictive devices intended to confer monopoly power on the practitioners of the profession? What are alternative ways of achieving the goal of higher quality without the restrictive element?

REFERENCES

1. In his review article, Barr uses a different classification of government interventions, regulation, which can apply to quality, quantity, or price of a product or service; a price subsidy, which can be direct or through the tax system; public production, such as when the government is the supplier of the service; and income transfers, which can be tied to specific products, such as food stamps or general, as with Social Security. Nicholas Barr, "Economic Theory and the Welfare State: A Survey and Interpretation," *Journal of Economic Literature,* 30, June 1992: 741–803.

2. The economic theory of regulation was first proposed by G. J. Stigler, "The Economic Theory of Regulation," *The Bell Journal of Economics,* Spring 1971: 3–21. For additional references and a more complete discussion of this theory and its applicability to the health field, see P. J. Feldstein, *The Politics of Health Legislation: An Economic Perspective,* 2nd ed. (Chicago: Health Administration Press, 1996).

3 One demand-increasing proposal is reputed to have had an adverse effect on patients' oral health. In 1974 the Federal Social Court in Germany ruled that false teeth should be included in the country's compulsory health insurance programs. "Fillings went out of fashion and prevention was ignored as vast quantities of teeth were pulled and replaced. By 1980, German

dentists were using 28 tons of tooth gold a year, one third of the world total." Dentists' incomes soared, exceeding those of physicians by 30 percent. The sickness funds reported a huge deficit, forcing them to raise the level of compulsory contributions. "Dentists Gnashing Teeth in West Germany," *The Wall Street Journal,* December 26, 1985, p. 11.

4. "Doctors Group Denounces Nurses' Demand for Power," *The Washington Post,* December 7, 1993, p. A3.

5. Fee splitting occurred when a physician referred a patient to a surgeon and in return received part of the surgeon's fee. Fee splitting is an indication that the surgeon's fee is in excess of her cost; the surgeon can still make a profit though rebating part of the fee. If the fee was not in excess of the costs (including the opportunity cost of the surgeon's time), the surgeon would be unwilling to split the fee. The state practice acts permitted surgeons to act as a cartel by preventing any one surgeon from engaging in this form of price competition. Fee splitting was a way of eroding the surgeons' monopoly power. Surgeons opposed to fee splitting consider it unethical because the referring physician has a monetary incentive to select the surgeon. Any concern the medical profession had with the quality of surgeons or with the ethical behavior of physicians should have been addressed directly through examination and monitoring procedures and not by prohibiting price competition. Unfortunately, the medical profession has opposed reexamination and monitoring. For a more complete discussion of fee splitting, see Mark V. Pauly, "The Ethics and Economics of Kickbacks and Fee Splitting," *The Bell Journal of Economics,* 10(1), Spring 1979: 344–52.

6. Reuben Kessel, "Price Discrimination in Medicine," *Journal of Law and Economics,* 1, October 1958: 20–53.

7. Patricia M. Danzon, *Medical Malpractice: Theory, Evidence and Public Policy* (Cambridge, Mass.: Harvard University Press, 1985).

8. David S. Salkever and Thomas W. Bice, *Hospital Certificate-of-Need Controls: Impact on Investment, Costs, and Use* (Washington, D.C.: American Enterprise Institute, 1979).

9. 1984 House of Delegates Resolutions, October 25, p. 537. This resolution follows a previous one (124H-1981), where the ADA was to encourage their "constituent dental societies to utilize these reports (on dentist supply) in petitioning their legislative bodies to consider by lawful means the number of dentists that should be trained." *Transactions,* 125th Annual Session, October 20–25, 1984 (Chicago: American Dental Association, 1984).

10. James W. Begun, *Professionalism and the Public Interest: Price and Quality in Optometry* (Cambridge, Mass.: MIT, 1981). Also see James W. Begun and Ronald C. Lippincott, "A Case Study in the Politics of Free-Market Health Care," *Journal of Health Politics, Policy and Law,* 7(3), Fall 1982: 667–85.

11. For a more complete discussion of this proposal, see Andrew K. Dolan, "The New York State Nurses Association 1985 Proposal: Who Needs It?" *Journal of Health Politics, Policy and Law,* 2(4), Winter 1978: 508–30.

12. Many states adopted the citizenship requirement for foreign medical graduates after the AMA's House of Delegates passed such a resolution in 1938. Five states continued such a requirement as late as 1975. Citizenship is no longer required in any state.

13. Another entry barrier used in dentistry is restrictions on interstate mobility. Various studies have shown that dentists graduating from a dental school within a state have a greater chance of passing that state's licensing exam than dentists from other states. Unlike medicine, most

states do not permit reciprocal licensing for dentists. See, for example, Lawrence Shepard, "Licensing Restrictions and the Cost of Dental Care," *Journal of Law and Economics,* 21, April 1978: 187–201. See also B. Friedland and R. Valachovic, "The Regulation of Dental Licensing—The Dark Ages," *American Journal of Law and Medicine,* 17(3), 1991: 249–270.

14. For an excellent discussion of licensure, quality, and the production of information concerning comparative performance of physicians and hospitals, see Lee Benham, "Licensure and Competition in Medical Markets," in H. E. Frech, *Regulating Doctors' Fees* (Washington, D.C.: American Enterprise Institute, 1991).

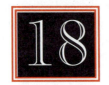

CHAPTER
18

National Health Insurance: An Approach to the Redistribution of Medical Care

THE ECONOMIC AND POLITICAL FRAMEWORKS

National health insurance (NHI) has been a highly visible political issue many times, most recently with the Clinton administration. Each time its proponents have been disappointed. It is an issue that is unlikely to go away. To understand the issues surrounding NHI requires both an economic and a political framework. The latter explains why efficiency and equity criteria are unlikely to be the basis of any enacted NHI plan.

This chapter begins with a theoretical framework that can be used to analyze various NHI proposals in terms of the efficiency with which they achieve the different values that underlie proposals for NHI. No attempt will be made to select one set of values over another; instead, the analysis will be concerned with the most efficient means for achieving a given set of values. Some empirical evidence based on Medicare will be used to support the theoretical conclusions. This theoretical discussion will then be used as a basis for developing a set of criteria for evaluating alternative health insurance proposals. The current system of financing medical care and several suggested proposals for NHI will then be discussed according to the criteria developed. No attempt will be made to provide a detailed discussion of various legislative proposals. Since new legislative proposals are constantly being introduced, a basic understanding of the concepts underlying such proposals would be more useful for understanding both current and future proposals (1). The chapter concludes with a discussion of why the United States has not enacted NHI.

ACHIEVING EFFICIENCY FOR DIFFERENT VALUES UNDERLYING NATIONAL HEALTH INSURANCE

A Theoretical Discussion

NHI may be viewed as an in-kind demand subsidy based on the argument that there are externalities in consumption. Assuming the nonpoor wish to subsidize the poor, this will result in a demand for government subsidies. The nonpoor benefit by knowing that the poor receive medical services when ill. Unless the government were to tax the nonpoor for this benefit, some nonpoor would "free ride," that is, receive the benefit without contributing to assist the poor with their medical care.

The extent of government subsidization will differ depending on the values held by the nonpoor with respect to redistribution of medical care services. One set of values may be termed "minimum provision," meaning that no person in society, when ill, should receive less than a certain quantity of medical care. A second set of values might be called "equal financial access to medical care." If these values were the basis for the externalities in consumption, they would suggest an NHI plan that would equalize the financial barriers to all persons. The third set of values that people may share with respect to redistribution of medical care services goes beyond equal financial access to require equal treatment for equal needs—in other words, equal consumption of medical services regardless of economic or other factors affecting utilization. The different demands for government subsidies reflect varying sets of values that are believed to exist in the population. The first set of values would require the smallest level of subsidization; the third set of values would be the most expensive to achieve.

It is not possible for an economist to state which set of values is most appropriate; whichever set of values the population selects would be the proper basis for the level of government subsidies under NHI. Although it is not possible to determine a priori the set of values that is likely to be chosen by the population, it is possible to determine the most efficient approach for achieving each of the three sets of values. It should be possible to state which types of national health insurance are likely to be more efficient than others, regardless of the set of values one selects.

Minimum provision may be achieved in one of two ways: those persons whose consumption of medical care is below the minimum may be subsidized to bring their consumption up to the minimum, or, alternatively, a subsidy can be provided to *everyone* so that at the resulting new, lower price, no one person's consumption would be below the minimum specified by society. These two alternatives are shown in Figure 18.1. Assuming that there are three different income groups—high incomes (HY), middle incomes (MY), and low incomes (LY)—their demands for medical care would be shown by the three demand curves, *HY, MY,* and *LY,* respectively. The aggregate demand curve of all three income groups is shown by *HYMLY.*

The reason the three demand curves do not result in the same consumption of medical care at zero price is that there are factors, other than financial ones, that result in differences in demand between different income groups. For example, low-income groups may incur greater costs in traveling to providers than do higher-income groups; differences in attitudes may also affect their utilization. Provider preferences in dealing with different income groups may also play a role. If the current price of medical care is P_{mc} the utilization of the three income groups would be Q_1, Q_2, and Q_3, and their aggregate utilization would be Q_0, which is the intersection of the aggregate demand curve and the supply of medical care (assuming, for simplicity, perfect elasticity).

If society wanted to assure that no one received less than a minimum amount of medical care, Q_m, a national health insurance system could use one of two approaches to achieve this goal. A system of subsidies that lowered the price of medical care just for those whose consumption is less than the minimum would be one approach. Alternatively, a "universal" program that reduced the price of medical care for everyone (or set to zero for everyone) would also achieve this goal. If medical care were free, everyone's consumption would increase, with the total going from Q_0 to Q_4. If, instead, a subsidy were provided to just those persons whose consumption was below the minimum (i.e., by low-

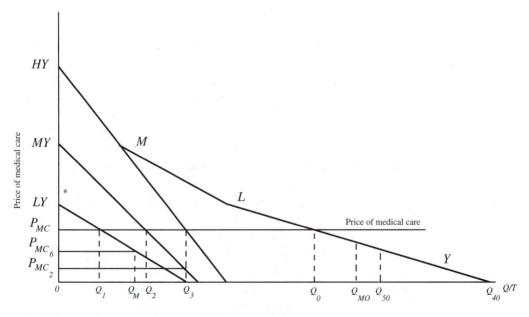

FIGURE 18.1 • Demand curves of different income groups.

ering the price to lower-income persons to P_{mc1}), the aggregate increase in use of medical care would be from Q_0 to Q_{m0}.

The cost to society of this approach to achieving minimum provision would be the subsidy required to increase the low-income group's utilization, which is $P_{mc} - P_{mc1}$, multiplied by that group's utilization, Q_m. The cost of making medical care free to all persons would be the price of medical care multiplied by the new and greater quantity that would result when the price was reduced to everyone, which is P_{mc} multiplied by Q_{40}. Both approaches would achieve the goal of minimum provision; however, the approach that provided a subsidy to the lower-income group only would be less costly, hence more efficient, than a scheme that reduced the price for everyone.

The second value with respect to redistribution of medical care is that all persons should have equal financial access to medical care. This value could again be achieved by establishing a universal program, that is, a free medical care system (or a low price to all persons), as in the previous illustration, which would equalize financial barriers among different income groups. Alternatively, a system of subsidies that varied according to income could be used. Subsidizing the price of medical care to low-income persons so that it is reduced to zero would increase their consumption to Q_3. A subsidy to middle-income groups equal to $P_{mc} - P_{mc2}$ would also increase their consumption to Q_3. At consumption level Q_3, the utilization of medical care for the three income groups would be equal. The aggregate increase in medical care use would go from Q_0 to $Q_{50.}$

Equal financial access requires a more expensive subsidy than would be required for achieving minimum provision. However, providing this subsidy according to income ($Q_3 \times P_{mc}$) for the low-income group, plus $Q_3 \times [P_{mc} - P_{mc2}]$ for the middle-income group), would still be less costly than a medical care system that eliminated all financial barriers for everyone (a universal program).

It is unlikely that the external demand for subsidization, based on the value that there should be equal financial access, would include the value judgment that the demands of higher-income persons should be increased beyond levels that they currently spend, and that this increase should be financed through higher taxes. If such persons are currently purchasing Q_3 amount of medical care, then the value to them of additional units of care is less than the price they would have to pay to consume it. It would be illogical for people to vote for an additional tax on themselves to purchase additional units of medical care when they were previously not willing to pay the equivalent amount of money to purchase those same units.

Equal treatment for equal needs expresses the third set of values that give rise to a demand for medical care subsidies. Since demands for medical care vary for more reasons than just financial ones, merely making the price of medical care free to all will not result in equal consumption. As shown in Figure 18.1, high-income groups would still consume more medical care at zero price than would those with middle and lower incomes. Thus a free medical care system would not be able to achieve that set of values defined as equal treatment for equal needs.

The value likely to be achieved through a free medical care system would be equal financial access, which, as we have shown, could be achieved at lower cost by a system of subsidies that varied by income.

The only way in which equal treatment for equal needs could be achieved would be by differential subsidies, varying according to income level. For example, as shown in Figure 18.2, lowering the price of medical care to zero for both low- and middle-income groups would still not increase their utilization to where it equaled that of the high-income group. Only if the low- and middle-income groups were subsidized further, through a system of negative prices, could their utilization be equal. (Negative prices mean that such groups are paid to increase their use.) How large the negative prices would have to be would depend, in part, on the consumption levels of the high-income groups.

Legislation would not be enacted that would actually pay people to increase their use

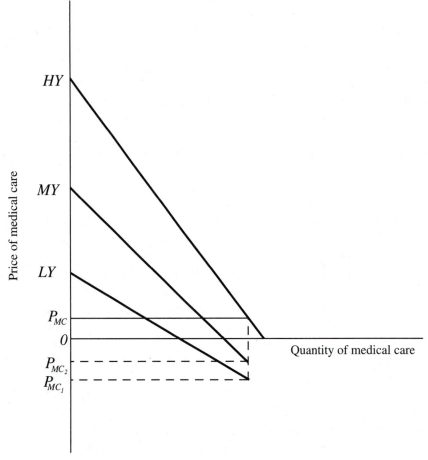

FIGURE 18.2 • Equal treatment for equal needs through a system of negative prices.

of medical care. Instead, a negative price would be paid by means of a direct in-kind supply subsidy to low-income groups. For example, although the price of medical care to a low-income person would be zero, substantial travel and access costs might deter that person from using more medical services. Establishing clinics and neighborhood health centers in low-income areas and providing incentives for health personnel to practice there would increase access and decrease travel costs, thereby increasing use.

The cost in resources and the consequent increase in taxes required to achieve each of the three sets of values are even greater when the more realistic assumption is made that supply is not perfectly elastic but is, instead, relatively inelastic. Figure 18.3 is similar to Figure 18.1, except that the supply of medical care is less elastic. The consequence of a rising supply curve is that as demand is subsidized, the cost of a subsidy will be greater than if supply were more elastic. The cost of the subsidy necessary to achieve minimum provision is the utilization of the low-income group multiplied by the higher price of medical care (point *A* on the supply curve). This higher price will also be borne by those persons in society who favor medical care subsidies to low-income groups.[1] The taxes required to fund equal financial access will be greater than those required to achieve minimum provision.

As might be expected, as the price to those who are not being subsidized rises, and the cost of achieving a given set of values increases, the amount that they are willing to pay to subsidize others will decline.

For national health insurance to have the redistributive effects that are desired by society, increased utilization must occur; it will most readily occur when there is a high price elasticity of demand for medical services by those persons receiving subsidies. However, the greater the price elasticity of demand, the greater will be the increase in demand along an inelastic supply; the consequence will be rapidly increasing prices and total expenditures.

It is precisely because of these expected higher costs that proposals for national health insurance have also included approaches for changing the delivery system. In evaluating alternative national health insurance proposals, demand proposals should be analyzed separately from supply proposals. Presumably, proposals to enhance efficiency on the supply side, which were discussed in a previous chapter, can be incorporated into any NHI plan. A supply proposal becomes an integral part of the demand proposal only when its proponents are not willing to accept the criterion of economic efficiency in supply.

Under one NHI approach, a Canadian-type system that would make medical care free to all, a great deal of emphasis is placed on how the supply side will be financed and organized. Expenditure limits by region and by type of provider would be established. As shown in Figure 18.3, total expenditures and prices would increase sharply under a free

---

[1]Because the supply of medical care is not elastic, it is necessary to think in terms of the postsubsidy market price that an income group will face when the price of medical care is subsidized. National health insurance based on a tax credit is one way of achieving this.

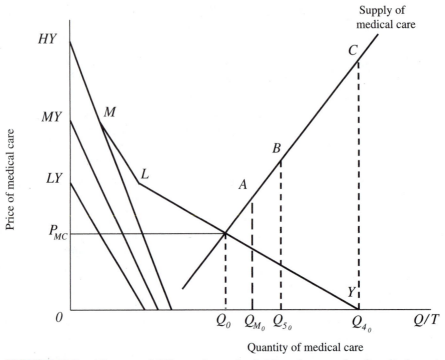

FIGURE 18.3 • The cost of different demand subsidies when supply of medical care is relatively inelastic.

medical care system. Arbitrary establishment of dollar limits is an outgrowth of a political process and is unrelated to underlying supply and demand conditions. Expenditure limits would serve as a cost control mechanism, but if cost control is the consequence of this approach, either intended or otherwise, the proponents of a free medical care system should be more explicit in defining the set of values that underlie this approach. They should also demonstrate how arbitrarily determined expenditure limits on the supply side would achieve these values.

The advocates of a free medical system might argue that it would still be possible to achieve, through greater efficiency, the program's stated goals at a lower expenditure level than indicated by the supply curve in Figure 18.3. Since the advocates of a free medical system are opposed to competition as a way of determining the most efficient system and set of providers, reliance would have to be placed on government to manage the medical system and to bring about greater efficiency in supply. Previous attempts by government to regulate or manage the supply of a good or service, both outside and within the medical care field, lend little credibility to the belief that the government will become an efficient and innovative manager in the near future.

It is more likely that under a free medical system the system would be frozen in existing patterns. The government has not been able to close VA, Public Health Service, or any municipal hospitals, when it wanted to do so on grounds of efficiency because of political pressure from employee groups and the constituencies of these facilities. It is likely that each provider group within each region would attempt to protect its expenditure allocation each year; such actions would prevent changes in methods of delivery when dollar allocations to providers are affected.

The ability of government to bring about greater efficiency is not borne out by the evidence, even in the health field. Lengths of stay in VA hospitals are much longer than in nongovernment hospitals (for similar diagnoses), and there has been little substitution away from hospitals, when medically possible, to less expensive services, such as ambulatory care. The use of HMOs, PPOs, and managed care techniques used so widely in the private sector have not been adopted in the Canadian health system. It is unlikely that the quality of managers in a medical system controlled by government would be improved. It is more likely that the quality of management would decline because such an all-inclusive system would preclude a point of reference outside itself by which managers could be evaluated.

There also would be no incentives for managers to seek to change the system; the financial rewards to good management would be greater in nongovernment-controlled sectors. Evidence to support this contention may be found not only in VA hospitals, but also in the postal service. In the medical system, too, unions would become more powerful in the decision-making process, and as in the postal service, might inhibit the introduction of labor-saving innovations and flexibility in use of personnel.

For each set of values examined—minimum provision, equal financial access, and equal treatment for equal needs—it was shown that these values can be achieved more efficiently when the subsidy varies by income level rather than through a universal system that either provides an equal price reduction to all or makes medical care free to everyone, regardless of income level. Although this analysis was theoretical, empirical data support these conclusions.

Some Empirical Evidence from the Medicare Program

Medicare is an existing in-kind demand subsidy to the aged. (Part A of Medicare provides hospital coverage, while Part B is a voluntary program primarily for physician services, with 75 percent of the premium being subsidized by the government.) The benefits available to all the aged under Medicare are similar, as is the reduced price they must pay for the use of medical care. To use physician services (Part B of Medicare), an aged person was initially required to pay a $50 deductible and a 20 percent co-payment.

It would appear that the pricing mechanism was designed to ensure either equal financial access to medical care or equal treatment for equal medical needs for the aged.

As long as demand for medical care among the aged differs according to income and accessibility, then, as shown in Figure 18.1, a similar price for all persons, such as the aged under Medicare, would result in differences in utilization. Setting the same price for the aged of all incomes will result in higher utilization for higher, rather than lower-income aged. The reduced price would represent a smaller financial burden to higher-income aged. Also higher-income aged are likely to have lower travel costs, since they are likely to live in areas that are closer to medical providers.

According to data shown in Table 18.1, in 1968, higher-income aged were more likely to pay the deductible and use the Part B supplementary coverage under Medicare: 552.3 persons per 1,000 Medicare enrollees with incomes in excess of $15,000, 431.7 persons per 1,000 among those aged with incomes less than $5,000. Services used by the higher-income aged also cost the government more: $10.40 compared with $7.02 per reimbursable service. (These higher prices represent higher prices for the same services as well as possibly higher-quality services, as when specialists are used.) Medicare reimbursement per person enrolled was more than twice as high for the higher-income aged, $160.30 compared with $78.77.

When Medicare utilization in 1968 was examined for differences according to race, there were large disparities, as shown in Table 18.2. Whites were more likely than non-whites to use physician services; one reason is that nonwhites received more ambulatory services from hospital outpatient departments than did whites. Medicare reimbursement was also on average higher for whites than for nonwhites.

If Medicare were based on the assumption that there should be equal treatment for equal needs, one would expect to observe an equal number of physician visits according

TABLE 18.1 Medicare Reimbursements for Covered Services under the Supplementary Medical Insurance Program and Persons Served, by Income, 1968 and 1977

Income Group	Persons Receiving Reimbursable Services per Thousand Medicare Enrollees	Medicare Reimbursement per Reimbursable Service	Medicare Reimbursement per Person Enrolled
	_1968_		
Under $5,000	431.7	$7.02	$78.77
Over $15,000	552.3	10.40	160.30
Ratio, over $15,000 to under $5,000 incomes	1.28	1.48	2.04
	_1977_		
At or near poverty line	773.4	6.43	60.32
High-income	801.7	5.82	57.72
Ratio, high income to at or near poverty line	1.04	0.91	0.96

Source: For 1968 data: Karen Davis, "Equal Treatment and Unequal Benefits: The Medicare Program," _Milbank Memorial Fund Quarterly/Health and Society,_ 53(4), 457, Table 1, Copyright Milbank Memorial Fund. For 1977 data: G. Wilensky, L. Rossiter, and L. Finney, "The Medicare Subsidy of Private Health Insurance," Rockville, Md.: National Center for Health Services Research, _National Health Care Expenditure Survey,_ 1983.

TABLE 18.2 Persons Served and Medicare Reimbursement per Person Served, by Race, 1968 and 1977

	Persons Served per Thousand Enrollees		Reimbursement Per Person Served		
	Physician Services	Hospital Outpatient Services	Physician Services	Hospital Outpatient Services	Medicare (Part B) Reimbursement per Person Enrolled
			1968		
White (age 65+)	394.9	71.6	$199.44	$39.02	$82.70
Other races (age 65+)	279.4	89.9	173.37	50.43	54.20
Ratio, white to other	1.413	0.796	1.150	0.774	1.526
			1977		
White (age 65+)	770.0	227.0	60.01	70.46	62.23
Other races (age 65+)	652.0	315.0	42.99	47.57	43.04
Ratio, white to other	1.18	0.72	1.40	1.48	1.45

Sources: Karen Davis, "Equal Treatment and Unequal Benefits: The Medicare Program," *Milbank Memorial Fund Quarterly/Health and Society,* 53, 1995: 468, 469. The 1977 data are from G. Wilensky, L. Rossiter, and L. Finney, "The Medicare Subsidy of Private Health Insurance," National Center for Health Services Research, *National Health Care Expenditure Survey*, 1983.

to level of medical need. This is unlikely to occur when all aged recipients face the same price but differ according to income, race, and accessibility, as shown in Table 18.3. Regardless of health status, aged persons with higher incomes had more physician visits than did aged with lesser incomes. Of those aged who are classified as being in poor health, in 1969 the low-income aged (less than $5,000 in income) had 10.47 physician visits per year compared to 16.98 visits per aged person with a high income (greater than $15,000 per year).

By 1977 differences in visit rates among the aged in different income groups were less and visit rates among the high-income aged decreased. Between 1969 and 1977 the "real" price (adjusted for inflation) declined for the low-income aged, hence increasing their visit rates, while the "real" price faced by the high-income aged increased, thereby decreasing their visit rates. Physicians serving low-income aged were likely to accept Medicare assignment; that is, they were willing to accept the Medicare fee as the price for their services. Medicare fee increases were limited by the Medicare economic index, which increased much more slowly than the rate of inflation. Thus, to low-income aged, the "real" price of a physician visit (the 20 percent co-payment of a physician's fee, which was not permitted to rise rapidly) declined. The physician assignment rate, those physicians participating in Medicare, declined after Medicare started, reaching a low of 50.5 percent in 1977.

Physicians were also less likely to take assignment for those aged who had higher incomes. All aged were required to pay a deductible and a co-payment. However, a high-

TABLE 18.3 Average Physician Visits for the Elderly, by Health Status and Family Income, Adjusted for Other Determinants, 1969 and 1977

| | Health Status[a] | | |
	Good	Average	Poor
	1969		
Family Income: Under $5,000			
No aid[b]	2.78	5.64	10.47
Aid	3.86	7.52	13.42
$5,000–9,999	3.14	6.60	11.70
$10,000–14,999	3.75	7.27	12.98
$15,000 and over	5.35	9.53	16.98
	1977[c]		
At or near poverty line			
No Medicaid	3.72	6.56	9.06
Medicaid	5.89	7.36	10.46
Middle-income	4.21	7.31	10.66
High-income	4.34	7.30	—[d]

Source: 1969 data are from Karen Davis, *National Health Insurance: Benefits, Costs, and Consequences* (Washington, D.C.: Brookings Institute, 1975), p. 85. The 1977 data are from G. Wilensky, L. Rossiter, and L. Finney, "The Medicare Subsidy of Private Health Insurance," National Center for Health Services Research, *National Health Care Expenditure Survey,* 1983.

[a]Good health status is defined as absence of any chronic conditions, limitations of activity, or restricted activity days. Average and poor health are defined at the mean and twice the mean level, respectively, of the three morbidity indicators used.

[b]Aid indicates public assistant recipients.

[c]For 1977 data, respondents are asked to characterize their own health status relative to people of the same age.

income aged person going to a nonparticipating physician also had to pay the full difference between what Medicare reimbursed as the physician's fee and the physician's actual fee. Physicians not accepting assignment were also able to raise their fees more rapidly than the increases permitted under the Medicare economic index. Thus high-income aged, using nonparticipating physicians, experienced an increase in the "real" prices they paid for physician visits.

The 1969 data are therefore consistent with the expectation that visit rates will differ when different income groups face the *same* price. The 1977 data (and the change from 1969) are also consistent with what would be expected when different income groups pay *different* prices for physician visits. (Since the early 1990s physicians must either participate for all Medicare patients or for none. Thus once again both high- and low-income patients pay the same physician fees.)

Based on the Medicare experience, it is obvious that a reduced but similar price to all aged persons will achieve neither equal financial access nor equal treatment for equal needs. As could have been hypothesized based on the earlier theoretical discussion, Medicare is an inefficient approach for achieving either of the foregoing sets of values, because higher-income persons use a greater number of services than do lower-income persons, and the services they use are more costly.

If the Medicare subsidy varied according to income level, the same services could have been provided to lower-income aged at a lower total cost. Not only would the overall level of utilization under Medicare be less with a subsidy that varied by income, but with a smaller overall increase in demand, the rise in medical prices would also have been less. The record of the Medicare program should be kept in mind when specific proposals for national health insurance are analyzed.

SPECIFIC CRITERIA FOR EVALUATING NATIONAL HEALTH INSURANCE PLANS

Before discussing specific proposals for national health insurance, it would be useful to have a common set of criteria by which these alternative plans may be evaluated.

The Beneficiaries

Based on the previous discussion of the different sets of values held by society regarding redistribution of medical care, the primary recipients of national health insurance should be those who are or might become medically indigent. The medically indigent are those persons who have low incomes and cannot buy as much medical care as society would prefer them to have. Another category of beneficiaries are those persons who are potentially medically indigent; their medical expenses are large in relation to their incomes. Even persons with middle incomes may be hard-pressed to pay their medical bills if they have a chronic or preexisting medical condition requiring large expenditures.

Subsidies under national health insurance, therefore, should vary according to income (decline as income increases). An upper limit on liability for medical expenses should be available to protect even higher-income persons from suffering an undue financial hardship. Everyone should, therefore, be required to have, at a minimum, catastrophic insurance coverage.

The primary beneficiary groups included under national health insurance should be categorized according to both income and the size of the medical bill in relation to income. Categorizing population groups by age is a less direct approach for determining current medical need and potential financial hardship. Although many of the aged are low-income, not all of them require the same degree of financial subsidy; many younger persons have greater medical and financial needs than do some of the aged.

The size of the medical subsidy for low-income persons is basically a value judgment. Some persons would prefer that the poor receive all their medical care, including preventive care, without any charge; others would prefer a less generous subsidy. Any plan for national health insurance should be able to incorporate either of these conflicting values by varying the degree of subsidization in relation to income levels.

Incentives for Efficiency

A second criterion by which alternative health insurance plans should be judged is whether there are incentives to encourage the efficient use of medical resources by both demanders and suppliers. This may be accomplished in several ways. First, coverage should be sufficiently broad so that the combination of medical services that is least costly for providing a medical treatment should be used. For example, when Medicare previously excluded ambulatory and other nonhospital services, more of the care was provided in the hospital even though it is less costly to substitute ambulatory, nursing home, and home care services.

Second, consumers should be provided with incentives to seek out less costly providers and not to overutilize. When consumers have a choice of managed care plans and must pay the additional cost of more expensive plans they have an incentive to weigh the benefits and the costs of the competing health plans. Similarly, including deductibles and co-payments in indemnity plans provides consumers with an incentive to select providers on the basis of price, as well as other attributes.

Third, providers of medical services should also be provided with efficiency incentives. For example, if consumers choose among competing health plans based on premiums and other attributes of the plan, then providers would have to similarly compete on price and those other attributes to be included in those plans. Physicians would be fiscally responsible for their use of medical resources when their incomes and employment are affected by the market success of the health plan with which they are associated.

Equitable Financing

A third criterion for evaluating alternative NHI plans is the equitability of their financing. Any one or combination of the following taxes could be used (and have been suggested) to finance NHI. An income tax, which would place the greater cost burden on those with higher incomes, would be the most equitable method of financing a redistributive program. (While income tax financing is generally regarded as being more equitable, it is a tax on work effort and may therefore cause a decrease in the supply of such effort.) Deficit financing, whereby the government borrows the money to subsidize different population groups, would shift the cost burden to future generations. (Future generations do not vote on current policies, thereby enabling politicians to provide benefits without imposing costs on current recipients. Therein lies both its political advantage and its inequity.)

A sales tax, particularly if it does not exclude such expenditures as food, could be regressive in that those with lower incomes contribute a higher percent of their incomes than those with higher incomes. "Sin" taxes, such as taxes on alcohol and cigarettes, are also regressive, but are economically efficient when the beneficiaries of such goods are required to pay the full costs of their consumption. And lastly, a payroll tax, which will be discussed more completely, is also regressive.

The two major approaches used in the past have been an income tax, which funds Medicaid and Medicare Part B (physician and nonhospital services), and a separate Medicare payroll tax, which pays for Medicare Part A (hospital services). Medicare Part A was initially financed by an increase in the Social Security tax. In 1965 the Social Security tax paid by both employee and employer was 3.625 percent (for a total of 7.25 percent) of the employee's wage up to a maximum annual wage of $4,800. To finance Medicare, the Social Security tax was increased to 4.2 percent (a total of 8.4 percent) on an increased wage base of $6,600. By 1998 the Social Security tax on both the employee and employer had risen to 7.65 percent (a total of 15.3) up to a maximum wage base of $68,400. However, to prevent Medicare from going bankrupt, the Medicare portion of the Social Security tax and the wage base to which it applied kept increasing. It is currently 1.45 percent (a total of 2.9 percent) and imposed on all wages (other income is excluded from the tax). Thus, Medicare is now financed by an almost proportional tax rather than the regressive tax with which it started and which still funds Social Security.

While part of the funding for any NHI plan might come from "sin" taxes, the large amount of funds required would necessitate an increase in either income or payroll taxes. Although the most equitable method of financing a redistributive program would be an income tax, it would be obvious who is bearing the cost burden to assist those with low incomes. Although proposals to use a payroll tax to fund NHI (given the way they are structured) are regressive, it has had many proponents. Unlike the income tax, a payroll tax would not affect the budget deficit and it would not place a large burden on those with the highest incomes, who are also more politically active.

If all or part of the payroll tax is imposed on the employer, as has been proposed, then the burden of the tax is less visible, since it is believed by many to be borne by the employer, not the employee.

In actuality, the incidence of the tax is determined by the elasticity of the demand and supply curves for labor. Assume that the initial wage rate is $10 an hour, as shown in Figure 18.4A. If the government were to impose a $2 an hour tax on the employee, the new labor supply curve would be *ST*, which is equal to the initial labor supply curve, *S*, plus the tax of $2 an hour. The new equilibrium wage will rise to $11 an hour. However, the employee would have to pay $2 of the $11 an hour to the government. The employees' net wage is $9 an hour, $1 less per hour than their previous earnings. The employer pays $1 an hour more than previously. Thus in the above example the employee pays 50 percent of the $2 an hour tax, while the employer pays 50 percent.

Assume that instead of placing the tax on the employee, the $2 an hour tax is placed

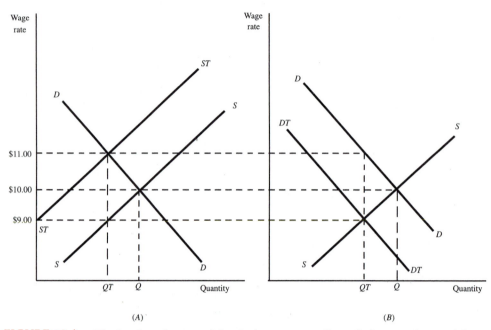

FIGURE 18.4 • The burden of a tax on labor is the same regardless of who pays the tax: (A) employees pay the tax, (B) employers pay the tax.

on the employer. As shown in Figure 18.4B, the size of the tax is indicated by the vertical distance between the two equilibrium points. (The employer's demand for labor shifts down with a per unit tax because the initial demand represents the maximum amount of labor the firm will hire at any given wage.) The burden of the tax when it is imposed on the employer is the same as when it was imposed on the employee. The employee receives $9 an hour, the employer pays the government $2 per hour, and the employer ends up paying $11 an hour, $1 an hour more than previously. In both cases less labor is hired.

Thus it does not matter who pays the tax or on whom the tax is imposed, the employee or the employer, the effect is the same.

Figure 18.5 shows who bears the burden of a tax on labor when the demand for labor is less elastic (Figure 18.5A) and more elastic (Figure 18.5B). The elasticity of labor supply is the same in both cases.

When the demand for labor is less elastic (Figure 18.5A), a greater portion of the tax is borne by the employer. The greater the elasticity of demand for labor (Figure 18.5B), the greater the burden of the tax on the employee. The demand for unskilled labor is believed to be more elastic than the demand for skilled labor.

Figure 18.6 depicts the situation under different elasticities of labor supply. When the tax is imposed on business, as shown by a downward shift of $2 an hour in the demand for labor, and the labor supply is completely inelastic with regard to the wage (Figure 18.6A), a tax on labor is shifted entirely onto labor. As the labor supply becomes more elastic (Figure 18.6B), the employer pays a portion of the tax.

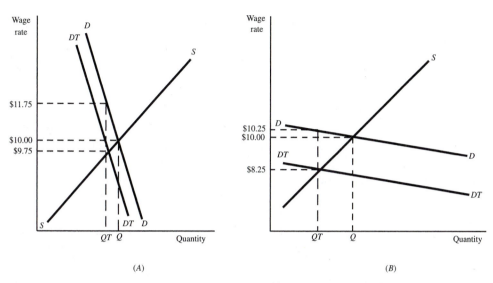

FIGURE 18.5 • The burden of a tax on labor according to different elasticities of demand for labor: (A) less elastic demand for labor, (B) more elastic demand for labor.

As shown above, the burden of the Social Security tax is determined by the elasticity of the demand and supply for labor and not on who is obligated by the government to pay the tax. (Although the net wage received by labor is shown to decrease as a result of the tax, in a dynamic economy increases in the Social Security tax may result in wages not rising as much as they would have otherwise.)

A crucial issue, therefore, for determining the burden of a payroll tax is the wage elasticity of the supply of labor. Economists believe that the supply of labor facing any one industry is relatively elastic since labor can move to other industries. The aggregate sup-

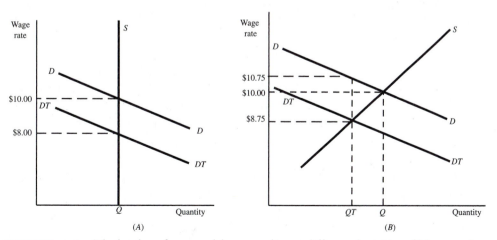

FIGURE 18.6 • The burden of a tax on labor according to different elasticities of labor supply: (A) inelastic supply of labor, (B) more elastic supply of labor.

ply of labor to the economy, however, is believed to be relatively inelastic, similar to that shown in Figure 18.6A.

Most people believe that only half of the Social Security tax is imposed on labor. Thus the size of the tax on labor appears smaller than it is. The main advantage of placing half of the Social Security tax on the employer is political. It is not obvious to the employee who bears the true burden of the entire tax.

There are two additional effects of the Social Security tax that should be considered. When business bears a portion of the tax, as shown in Figure 18.4, the prices of the firm's goods and services are increased. (An increase in the wage results in an increase in the firm's marginal and average total cost curves.) Those industries most adversely affected by the tax on labor are those that are more labor-intensive and those that face increased price competition from foreign competitors. Second, when the price of labor is increased, employers will hire fewer employees. The decline in the demand for labor is greater, the greater is the employer's elasticity of demand for labor; this is shown in Figure 18.5. The lower the skill level of labor, the greater the elasticity of demand.

An increase in the income tax (to raise an equivalent amount of money as a Social Security tax) will not cause the firm to raise its prices or decrease its demand for labor. This is because the firm's cost of labor is not affected by an income tax.

One other issue to be considered in evaluating the Social Security tax as a method of financing medical services is which income groups will bear the greatest burden of the tax. If all employees must pay 7.65 percent of their wages, up to a maximum of $68,400, then a person with $68,400 of income as well as a person with $100,000 of income each pays $5,233 a year (plus the employer's contribution of $5,233). The $5,233 payment represents a greater proportionate tax on a low-income than on a high-income employee. For this reason the Social Security tax is referred to as a "regressive" tax. As the Social Security wage base has increased over time, the Social Security tax has become more of a proportionate tax. While low-income individuals may have too low an income to pay any income taxes, they still have to pay Social Security taxes on their earnings.

To the extent that not all of the tax is shifted and employers must pay part of it, the prices of goods and services will increase. These price increases are also regressive in their effects, representing a greater portion of income for low-income persons.

An analysis of the Social Security tax is important not only for understanding the financing of the original Medicare legislation but also for determining who bears the burden of NHI proposals to mandate employer coverage of employees' health benefits.

In addition to these three criteria—the population group to be covered, incentives for efficiency, and the method of financing—two other supplementary goals are usually mentioned. First, the national health insurance plan should not be very costly to administer, so that as much of the money as possible goes to pay medical rather than administrative expenses. Second, it should be politically acceptable to the public, the providers, and the government. Political acceptability includes such issues as methods of reimbursing providers, whether there is a role for insurance companies, how large a tax increase would be necessitated by the program, and the impact on the federal budget.

THE CURRENT SYSTEM
FOR FINANCING MEDICAL SERVICES

Using the criteria that have been presented, we will present a brief evaluation of the current system for financing care, some suggestions for improvements in the current system, and then a discussion of several generic types of NHI proposals.

There are a myriad of government subsidies, direct and indirect, to decrease the price of medical services to various population groups. For example, there is the Veterans Administration, CHAMPUS (Civilian Health and Medical Program for Uniformed Services), the Indian Health Services, state and county health services, as well as Medicare, Medicaid, and the exclusion from the employees' taxable income of employer-paid health insurance (to be referred to as employer-paid health insurance). Since these last three programs comprise the vast majority of demand subsidies, each will be briefly discussed.

Medicare

Medicare, a federal program to cover the medical expenses of the aged, started in 1966. It was extended in 1974 to cover all persons with chronic renal disease. All aged, regardless of their income levels, are presently included. The benefits and the prices the aged must pay, including the monthly premium for Part B (physician services), and the deductibles and co-payments for both hospital and physician services, are the same for each aged person, regardless of income. Those aged with higher incomes can afford to purchase more medical services and to buy supplementary coverage for those gaps not covered by Medicare. Catastrophic coverage under Medicare is incomplete and the services covered are not comprehensive. There are limited benefits for posthospital care, particularly for outpatient prescription drugs.

Because Medicare benefits are not income-related, many aged find it difficult to pay the necessary out-of-pocket expenses. The consequence of these large expenses and gaps in benefit coverage is that approximately 20 percent of the aged must rely on Medicaid.

Medicare can also be improved with regard to the efficiency with which services are delivered. Medicare expenditures have risen almost 11 percent per year between 1990 and 1995, reaching $187 billion in 1995 (2). Medicare expenditures have risen more than 8 percentage points a year faster than the private sector. These differences in annual rates of increase between Medicare and the private sector are believed to be the result of growth in managed care in the private sector. Medicare has had much lower rates of managed care growth.

The method used to finance Medicare is inequitable and results in large intergenerational transfers to the aged (3). A couple who turned 65 in 1980 could expect Medicare to spend $114,000 on them during their lifetime. The total lifetime estimate climbs to $232,000 for a couple turning 65 in 1995. By the year 2020, the estimate increases to $428,000. These couples will have contributed much less than the costs of those benefits.

Also, higher-income aged tend to live longer and therefore receive several times the lifetime benefits that those with low incomes receive.

Once again this special Medicare trust fund is expected to be bankrupt in the year 2007. When the trust fund was expected to go bankrupt previously, changes in payroll taxes and provider payments were instituted to forestall bankruptcy. Few, if any, burdens were placed on the aged. It is likely similar types of changes will be made by Congress in the next several years.

Medicare Part B (generally nonhospital services) is financed by a monthly premium by the aged, covering only about 25 percent of the program's cost. The remainder is funded from general tax revenues, a large portion of which comes from income taxes. Part A expenditures reached $70 billion in 1996, a large increase over 1990, when it was $42 billion. Since Part B is not funded by an earmarked tax, these federal subsidies contribute directly to the budget deficit.

Medicare faces two types of problems. In the short run, the Medicare trust fund will go bankrupt around 2010 if no changes are made. In the long run, as the baby boomer generation becomes eligible for Medicare around 2010, there will be huge needs for additional funds to keep the program solvent. Proposals to solve the short-run problem, such a decreasing hospital and physician payments, will not be sufficient to provide a solution to the long-run problem. The short-run solutions merely keep the trust fund solvent until about 2010. The longer the delay before long-run solutions are implemented, the more costly will be each of the options, the more taxes required, the larger the benefit reductions, and the steeper the reductions in provider payments.

The long-run problem of Medicare arises because of unlimited access to medical services and to new, expensive, technology, an aging population, longer life expectancy, and lower birth rates. In 1900 for every person over 65 years of age there were 10 children under the age of 10. By 1990 that ratio has fallen to 2 children per aged person. The ratio is continuing to fall, leading to a huge financial burden on future generations. The working population will begin to experience that burden when the baby boomers begin to retire, starting in 2010.

As the very large number of baby boomers (born between 1946 and 1964) start becoming eligible for Medicare, it will become increasingly difficult to make drastic reductions in their benefits on the eve of their retirement. Given the timing of presidential elections, particularly the election in 2004, unless changes occur before then, it is unlikely that a presidential candidate will run on a platform of promising to decrease benefits to those population groups (who have the highest voting participation rates) and would be most adversely affected. Thus long-run solutions must be gradually phased in, otherwise the political opposition by the various groups adversely affected will make an equitable solution more difficult to achieve.

A number of long-term proposals have been made to maintain Medicare; the following are several such options, which are not mutually exclusive. The first is to phase in an increase in the eligibility age so that it will be the same as the higher Social Security eligibility age, which will be sixty-seven.

Second, the financial burden on the working population can be sharply increased by raising payroll taxes. This approach has been used in the past. However, as the number of aged beneficiaries per employed person increases, many believe that the tax burden will become too great; the employed population will oppose such large taxes to pay for the medical services of the many aged who are well to do.

A third option is to make Medicare an income-related program. This can be achieved is several ways. Higher-income aged can be required to pay a larger premium than lower-income aged or the value of the benefits could decline with increased income, similar to a fixed and refundable tax credit (discussed below).

A fourth approach would be to change Medicare from a defined benefit program, where the government pays the cost of providing those benefits, to a fixed contribution program, where the government pays a fixed dollar amount toward a health plan (perhaps equal to the lowest cost health plan). (This proposal could also be income-related and combined with medical savings accounts.)

Fifth, to reduce medical expenditure increases could be reduced through changes on the supply side, such as decreasing payment to hospitals and physicians. Also, under Medicare risk contracts paying HMOs less than 95 percent of the average area per capita cost (AAPCC). Further changes on the supply side could involve providing Medicare beneficiaries with a choice of health plans so that the plans must compete. (Coupled with this last approach could be a voucher for a low-cost health plan with the aged person paying the additional cost of more expensive plans.)

Merely making the health care system more efficient will not solve the long-run financial burden of maintaining Medicare. Further, reducing benefits for all the aged, such as increasing deductibles, co-payments, premium increases, and increases in the eligibility age will adversely affect low-income aged. Instead, to make the Medicare system more efficient and more equitable (both across generations as well as redistributing toward low-income aged away from high-income aged) the Medicare system should include two principles: income-related subsidies (or declining voucher amounts as income rises) and allowing Medicare beneficiaries a choice of health plans.

These principles of equitable financing and efficient provision of services raise the question, "Why should Medicare and Medicaid be maintained as a separate systems?" Why should there not be just one system for those over and under sixty-five years of age based on income-related subsidies and choice of competing health plans?

Medicaid

Medicaid, which also began in 1966, is a federal–state matching program whose designated beneficiary group is the poor. There are three main beneficiary groups under Medicaid: the elderly, the blind and disabled, and low-income women and children. The role of the federal government is primarily one of sharing the costs of the program with the states, who are responsible for defining the eligibility requirements and determining the benefit coverage. The states were required to cover those who are eligible for cash assistance, such as those receiving Aid for Dependent Children (these are referred to as the "categorically needy"). Previously this meant single women with children having incomes below the federal poverty level. The states determine the income levels for those who are medically needy (unable to pay their medical expenses but not poor enough to qualify as categorically needy). Income eligibility for the medically needy category varies greatly among the states; in some states it is as low as 25 percent of the federal poverty level.

As in the case with Medicare, although the direct beneficiaries of Medicaid have been helped, there are equity and efficiency concerns with the current program.

Because Medicaid is administered by each state, there are wide variations in eligibility requirements and in services covered. In some states, people may lose all of their eligibility if their income rises so that it is slightly above the cutoff level; in other words, eligibility is not graduated according to income level. Although the beneficiary group is the poor, about half of the population below poverty level is eligible for Medicaid benefits. No state covers all those whose incomes are below the federal poverty level. Even within a state there are variations in access and use of services between white and nonwhite persons and between urban and rural dwellers.

Medicaid is financed through a state's general tax revenues and from federal income taxes. This is a more equitable method of financing than is a Social Security tax.

Congressionally mandated benefit and eligibility expansions, along with an increase in the number of uninsured, have caused Medicaid expenditures to sharply increase. Beginning in 1987, Congress expanded Medicaid eligibility by increasing the percent of the poverty level that pregnant women and children could qualify. States could also expand eligibility to as high as 185 percent of the federal poverty level and still receive federal matching funds.

An important policy concern with regard to increased Medicaid eligibility is whether the new beneficiaries dropped their private insurance because Medicaid became available as a lower-cost substitute. During the period since 1987, the nonelderly population on Medicaid greatly increased as private insurance for that population decreased. In addition to greatly increasing Medicaid expenditures, the Medicaid eligibility expansions also had an adverse effect of private coverage. Thus the cost to the government of decreasing the number of uninsured became more costly since some of the increased Medicaid spending is for individuals who dropped their private coverage. Cutler and Gruber estimate the magnitude of this effect and propose that a preferable approach would be to subsidize the purchase of private insurance by those with low incomes with a subsidy that decreases as income increases (4).

States have found themselves under pressure to reduce their share of rising Medicaid costs; it has been the states' fastest-increasing expenditure. States have attempted to reduce these expenditure increases by limiting eligibility of other groups, reducing benefits, and paying medical providers less. This latter approach has reduced the poor's access to medical care; lower reimbursement levels have limited the willingness of many providers to serve Medicaid patients. With the difficulties that states have in meeting projected increases in Medicaid expenditures, the gaps in Medicaid are unlikely to be resolved and are likely to worsen.

Various proposals have been made to improve both the efficiency and equity of the Medicaid program. One approach is to have uniform eligibility standards across states. Second, as mentioned above, subsidies could be provided to low-income people on a decreasing scale, phasing out at a certain percent of the poverty level. Alternatively, it has been suggested that low-income persons above a certain poverty level should be able to buy in to Medicaid eligibility by paying a premium that is less than its actuarial value. The size of the premium subsidy would decline with higher income levels.

There are a number of advantages to this approach. The benefits are directed to those with lowest incomes; there is a gradual decline in benefits as income rises so as to provide an incentive to earn more income; the financing is based on general tax revenues, which raises more funds from those with higher incomes; the eligibility and benefits are uniform across the states, thereby eliminating any incentive for those with low incomes to move to states with higher eligibility criteria.

There are, however, a number of problems with this approach. The first is political. Constituencies of the Medicaid program are those with low incomes, both the young and those aged who are in nursing homes; thus, their voting participation rates have been lower than those of other population groups. It is for these reasons that states have been reluctant to raise taxes on the middle class to adequately fund Medicaid.

Second, under the proposed approach, states could still reduce their Medicaid expenditures by reducing payments to providers. Inadequate hospital and physician payments have decreased provider participation and thereby decreased access to care by the poor. Unless payments to providers were competitive, providers would be unwilling to serve the larger eligible populations. There would also be a reluctance for those with low incomes to buy in to Medicaid if they had limited access to medical providers.

To improve provider participation with Medicaid patients and to increase the efficiency of Medicaid expenditures, many states are beginning to contract on a capitation basis with managed care organizations, using a bidding process. In contrast to past practices, patients will no longer be able to go to an emergency room for nonemergent services and providers will have to respond to the Medicaid patient's needs for service. The current excess capacity among hospitals and physicians has increased their willingness to participate in Medicaid managed care programs. Crucial to its success is the state's willingness to monitor the quality, outcomes, and patient satisfaction of the care provided by managed care organizations. Access to care and the quality of those services are more easily monitored in a managed care system than in a fee-for-service system. Provider efficiency incentives are also greater.

The Tax Treatment of Employment-Based Health Insurance

The major approach used by the federal government to subsidize the purchase of medical care and insurance by the nonpoor is through employer contributions to their employees' health insurance plans, which are not considered part of an employee's taxable income. This exclusion is equivalent to a discount or a subsidy on the purchase of insurance equal to the employee's marginal tax rate. The effect of tax-free employer-purchased insurance is to have a greater demand for insurance than if the employee had to pay for such coverage with after-tax dollars; more comprehensive insurance, as well as coverage for additional benefits, is purchased. It has been estimated that the cost of these subsidies, in terms of lost federal income and Social Security taxes (excluding state income taxes), was approximately $74 billion in 1994 (5).

The beneficiaries of these subsidies are those who are employed and who file tax returns, but the major beneficiaries are those in higher-income groups. A deduction from income is worth more to a person in a higher-income bracket than to a person with a lower income. For example, the after-tax cash equivalent of an employer-paid premium for health insurance totaling $1,000 would be $850 for a person in a 15 percent tax bracket, whereas it would be $666 for a person in the 33 percent bracket. (It would be even less than $666 since employer-purchased health insurance is not subject to either Social Security or state taxes.) If the true actuarial value of that premium is $900 (the remaining $100 going for administrative cost), the person in the 33 percent bracket will demand more insurance because it costs much *less* than the actuarial value of that insurance.

As shown in Table 18.4, both the percentage of households receiving employer contributions and the average employer contribution increase with higher household incomes.

Up until the 1980s, tax brackets were much higher, up to 70 percent (plus state and

TABLE 18.4 Employer Contributions to Health Benefit Plans and Employee Tax Benefits, 1994

	Families Receiving Contributions		
Family Income[a]	Percentage Receiving Employer Contribution	Average Employer Contribution	Average Subsidy
$ 1–9,999	8	$1,519	$ 190
$ 10,000–19,999	34	1,896	450
$ 20,000–29,999	62	2,587	800
$ 30,000–39,999	78	3,066	900
$ 40,000–49,999	85	3,758	1090
$ 50,000–74,999	89	4,420	1320
$ 75,000–99,999	91	5,229	1740
$100,000–199,999	89	5,641	1910
Over $200,000	76	4,922	1830

Source: The Tax Treatment of Employment-Based Health Insurance (Washington, D.C.: Congressional Budget Office, 1994), p. 30, Table 4.

Note: The table excludes families in which all members are covered by Medicare or Medicaid.

[a]Adjusted gross income reported on tax returns plus certain nontaxable forms of income, including employers' contributions to the cost of health insurance premiums and tax-exempt interest.

Social Security taxes). At that time, the incentive for high-income persons to have their employers purchase their health insurance was even greater.

The consequences of these tax subsidies were (and are) that higher-income persons receive greater benefits than do lower-income persons and that "too much" health insurance coverage is purchased by the higher-income person. It becomes worthwhile for higher-income persons to insure (through their employer) against small, routine medical expenses. This is because the cost of the insurance is less than the cost of those services if high-income persons were to pay for it with after-tax dollars.

Economists have often proposed that employers' contributions toward their employees' insurance become completely taxable or, to make it more politically acceptable, that a "cap" or dollar limit be established, above which employer contributions become taxable. Depending on where the cap was set, it could increase federal tax revenues by $30 billion a year. Equity would be improved; those with the highest incomes would receive less of a tax subsidy for the purchase of health insurance. Importantly, a cap would make employees more price-sensitive to alternative health plans; they would either join managed care plans or purchase less health insurance, namely, policies with more deductibles and co-payments. Greater competition among managed care plans and increased patient sensitivity to medical prices would lead to greater efficiency in the provision of medical services.

There are, however, political difficulties in placing a limit on the employer's contribution. Unions that have bargained for and received generous health benefits have opposed making such contributions taxable; their members' taxes would be increased. Health insurance companies have also opposed such proposals since they would raise the after-tax price of insurance, thereby decreasing the demand for such insurance. Provider interest groups, such as the American Dental Association, have also opposed eliminating the tax subsidy or even placing a limit on the amount that is nontaxable, since it would reduce, if not eliminate, insurance coverage for their members' services, which are highly income elastic.

Placing a limit on the tax exclusion has desirable consequences, but it is not NHI. It would improve equity as the tax subsidy for those with high incomes is reduced; greater efficiency would also be introduced into the system as employees make choices of health plans and use of services according to their relative premiums and medical prices. Thus this proposal is worthwhile in and of itself. However, such a proposal must be combined with another proposal if NHI is to be a universal program and also cover those with low incomes and the unemployed. Limiting or ending the tax exclusion would generate additional tax revenues that could be used to finance medical services and insurance to those with low incomes.

NATIONAL HEALTH INSURANCE PROPOSALS

Many proposals have been made to increase access to care by those with low incomes. In what follows, each of the major types of proposals are described together with an evaluation of their redistributive and efficiency effects.

A Canadian-Type Health System

The most far-reaching of all the proposals for NHI is to introduce a system similar to the Canadian health system (referred to as "single payer") (6). Under such a system the entire population would be covered, the benefits would be uniform for all, and there would be no out-of-pocket expenses ("zero" price) for basic medical services. An important characteristic of this plan is that private insurance for hospital and medical services is not permitted. In other words, it is not possible to "buy out" of the system. Access to care by those with low incomes and the uninsured is likely to be improved under this proposal.

The proposed method of financing is a combination of employer taxes, Medicare and Medicaid expenditures, private insurance payments, and a tax to raise the equivalent amount consumers currently spend out of pocket and on health insurance premiums.

To prevent expenditures from rising rapidly, since there are no cost constraints on either consumers or suppliers, regional expenditure limits would be imposed on hospitals and physicians. Single-payer proponents claim that administrative costs will be greatly reduced since insurance companies would no longer be necessary.

The simplicity of the Canadian approach (everyone receives the same health benefits at no out-of-pocket cost and the government controls cost by limiting the growth in health expenditures) is deceptively appealing (7). First, there is the issue of choice. While eliminating choice reduces administrative cost, it makes many people worse off since the nonpoor are required to purchase (through payment of taxes) benefits they previously chose not to when they had a choice. Comprehensive, first-dollar coverage is expensive and when offered the choice many would prefer to self-insure for these expenditures.

Second, gross comparisons of administrative costs between the Canadian and U.S. health system are inappropriate as a measure of relative efficiency. One reason is that in the United States there are a great variety of insurance plans, necessitating marketing and administrative costs. This competition among health plans offers consumers greater choice at different premiums. Some people are willing to pay to have a choice between more restrictive and less restrictive plans. Choice is costly. However, without it, there would be less innovation in benefit design, patient satisfaction, and health plan premiums. Further, part of the administrative cost involves utilization management, which, if it did not reduce medical expenses and overutilization, would not be undertaken by the health plan.

For example, Medicare, which has a similar design as the Canadian system, has much lower administrative costs than private health plans. However, the Government Accounting Office has criticized Medicare for having "too low" administrative costs; billions of dollars could be saved "by adopting the health care management approach of private payers to Medicare's public payer role" (8). Examples of the types of cost containment programs Medicare has been criticized for not undertaking are: paying competitively determined market prices, verifying eligibility of providers, using advanced technology to avoid paying excessive bills and inappropriate claims, and utilization review and case management of catastrophic care, all of which are performed by private health plans. Nor does Medicare offer the choice of health plans that are offered in the private sector. Cost containment programs that reduce medically unnecessary services are a benefit that more than offset their higher administrative costs.

Third, there are no incentives in the Canadian system on the part of either patients or providers to use the least costly mix of medical services or to produce them efficiently. Patients instead have an incentive to "overuse" services to the point where the benefits of additional services equal the cost to them of those services (which is zero). At that point the actual resource costs of those services exceed its additional benefits. Since providers are not rewarded for risk taking, there is little incentive to innovate in developing new delivery systems. Capital is also required for developing new methods of delivery; however, capital is allocated centrally and is less available than under a private system. The United States has been much more innovative in delivery systems, developing such models as HMOs, PPOs, and managed care techniques, than has Canada. The U.S. system has also been able to raise the necessary capital to take the risks in developing these innovations.

Further, health expenditures should not be limited to a certain percent of GNP. Changes in the rate of growth in GNP itself would arbitrarily limit the growth in health expenditures. (One reason for the smaller percent of GNP spent on health care in Canada in previous years was the more rapid rate of GNP growth in Canada.) The appropriate rate of growth in medical expenditures should be determined by the amount people are willing to pay (directly and through taxes) in an efficient medical system. There are legitimate reasons for increased health expenditures, such as an aging population, increased technology, new diseases (AIDS), shortages of personnel (thereby requiring wage increases), and so on. If expenditure growth is held below what would otherwise occur, the consequences will be shortages of services and technology and reduced access to care. This has occurred in Canada. Since there are no constraints on patient demand nor incentives for physicians to reduce use, arbitrary expenditure limits are imposed. These expenditure limits are unrelated to changes in consumer demands or to economy-wide input price increases.

The consequence of providing fewer resources than what consumers demand is that some form of nonprice rationing must occur. Resources are allocated away from prevention toward acute care services; the rate of mammograms among women aged fifty years and older were lower in Ontario, Canada, than in comparable areas of the United States (9). There are increased waiting times to receive services, there is less access to technologies, persons above a specified age are denied certain procedures, and patients travel to the United States to receive services. These forms of nonprice rationing are inefficient.

Those who have lower time costs, although their medical needs may not be greater, can afford to wait; the value of time spent in waiting is lost; there is also the discomfort involved in waiting for procedures, such as hip replacements; elderly patients must forgo driving while they wait months for cataract surgery; further, some patients will die while waiting for heart operations. These implicit costs are ignored by the proponents of the

Canadian system. These patients are clearly worse off if the system does not permit them to pay a monetary price that would enable them to have access to the latest technology, to forgo their waiting, their pain, and possible death. Canadians face increasing limits on access to technology and services.

A competitive health care market is more likely than is a government-controlled system to achieve a rate of growth in expenditures that is appropriate, that is, where the benefits are equal to the amount consumers are willing to spend to receive those benefits.

What is the goal of such a health system? If the purpose is equal financial access, then this could be achieved more efficiently by a system of subsidies that varies inversely with incomes. A Canadian-type system cannot achieve equal treatment for equal needs, even though the price of medical care is the same for all income groups (zero). Differences in use of services will still exist, owing to the value of waiting time, the location of the provider, attitudes toward seeking care, and the race of the patient. For example, as Katz and Hofer state, "Despite the long-term presence of universal insurance coverage in Ontario, the disparities in the use of cancer screening procedures by the poor were similar to the United States. Universal coverage is not sufficient to overcome the large disparities in . . . socioeconomic status" (10). As discussed previously, to increase the use of services by the poor requires "negative" prices, although these are rarely included or implemented.

Mandating Employer-Paid National Health Insurance

Requiring employers to provide health insurance benefits to their employees and families was proposed by Presidents Nixon and Carter, the Pepper Commission, and, more recently, President Clinton. There are a number of variations as to how an employer mandate would be implemented. Typically, such a plan requires that all employers offer a specified minimum health insurance plan to their employees or else pay a specified tax per employee to the state, referred to as "pay or play." (According to several of the plans proposed, it is less expensive for the employer to pay than play.) The portion of the premium to be paid by the employer, in some plans, is specified as 80 percent with the employee responsible for the remaining 20 percent of the premium. For small firms, generally with low-wage employees, there is provision for a tax credit to help the employer and employee defray part of the costs of the mandated insurance.

The employer mandate would cover all those employees who work more than half-time and firms with more than a minimum number of employees, such as five to twenty-five employees. (The minimum number of employees is very controversial; the Pepper Commission suggested that one hundred employees be the minimum number.) Large firms and unions are typically unaffected by mandated insurance since they already have employment-based health insurance and their coverage exceeds the specified minimums.

Important to any analysis of a mandated employer proposal is a determination of who are the uninsured and the characteristics of employees and firms that would be most affected by this approach.

As shown in Table 18.5, for those under 65 years of age almost 69 percent have private health insurance; 64 percent have employment-related insurance. The government covers 12.1 percent of the under 65 population through such programs as Medicaid. Approximately 19 percent of the under 65 population, about 44 million, do not have any health insurance. Persons in a family with a working adult are more likely to have insurance (73.6 percent) than persons in a family without a working adult (24.9 percent). However, because there are so many more working than nonworking adults, most of the uninsured (87 percent) are in families with working adults. Another characteristic of the uninsured is that 50 percent of the uninsured are working adults and 22 percent are children of working adults. Thus almost 75 percent of the total number of uninsured are employed or dependents of someone employed.

Selected characteristics of the uninsured are shown in Table 18.6. Those more likely to be uninsured are young adults, nineteen to twenty-four years of age (35.5 percent); persons in this age group are usually excluded from their parents' employment-related coverage and unless they are full-time students are likely to have jobs that do not provide insurance. A higher percentage of blacks (25.7 percent) and Hispanics (37.9 percent) are

TABLE 18.5 Health Insurance Coverage and Employment Status of the Civilian Noninstitutionalized Population under Age Sixty-Five, 1996

Employment status of adults in family	Total population in thousands	Private		Public only	Uninsured	Percent distribution of uninsured
		Total private	Employment-related			
		Percent distribution				
Total	231,676	68.7	64.1	12.1	19.2	100.0
Persons in families with a working adult[a]	208,574	73.6	69.0	7.9	18.5	86.9
Working adult	121,882	78.4	73.7	3.2	18.4	50.4
Nonworking adult	22,669	57.4	51.6	14.4	28.2	14.4
Child	64,022	70.2	66.3	14.4	15.4	22.1
Persons in families without a working adult[a]	23,103	24.9	20.3	49.9	25.2	13.1
Nonworking adult	15,704	32.5	26.3	37.7	29.9	10.5
Child	7,399	9.0	7.4	75.8	15.2	2.5

Source: Center for Cost and Financing Studies, Agency for Health Care Policy and Research: Medical Expenditure Panel Survey Household Component, 1996 (Round 1).

Note: Percents may not add to 100 due to rounding.

[a]Age 18–64.

TABLE 18.6 Total Population of Workers Ages Sixteen to Sixty-Four and Uninsured Workers: Percent Distribution by Selected Characteristics, United States, 1996

Characteristic	Working population in thousands	Percent distribution of workers	Percent uninsured	Percent distribution of uninsured workers
Total[a]	124,218	100.0	18.4	100.0
Age in years				
16–18	3,931	3.2	19.2	3.3
19–24	14,728	11.9	35.5	22.9
25–29	14,957	12.0	23.3	15.3
30–34	17,372	14.0	17.1	13.0
35–44	35,614	28.7	15.3	23.8
45–54	26,034	21.0	12.9	14.7
55–64	11,582	9.3	13.8	7.0
Race/ethnicity				
Total Hispanic	11,548	9.3	37.9	19.2
Total black	13,254	10.7	25.7	14.9
Total white	94,100	75.8	14.7	60.4
Total other	5,316	4.3	23.8	5.5
Self-employed	15,781	12.7	30.0	20.8
Size of establishment[b]				
Less than 10 workers	19,066	15.4	30.4	25.4
10–24 workers	15,991	12.9	22.4	15.7
25–49 workers	13,126	10.6	16.4	9.5
50–99 workers	14,328	11.5	12.1	7.6
100–499 workers	24,004	19.3	9.0	9.4
500 or more workers	17,329	14.0	6.7	5.1
Hours of work				
Less than 20 hours	8,453	7.0	23.5	9.0
20–34 hours	16,933	14.0	27.5	21.1
35 or more hours	95,536	79.0	16.1	69.8
Hourly wages[b]				
Less than $5.00	7,042	5.7	37.8	11.7
$5.00–$9.99	37,308	30.1	27.7	45.3
$10.00–$14.99	29,645	23.9	9.8	12.8
$15.00–$19.99	13,091	10.5	2.9	1.7
$20.00 or more	15,559	12.5	2.9	2.0

Source: Center for Cost and Financing Studies, Agency for Health Care Policy and Research: Medical Expenditure Panel Survey Household Component, 1996 (Round 1).

Note: Restricted to civilian noninstitutionalized population. Percents may not add to 100 due to rounding.

[a]Includes persons with unknown self-employment status, hourly wages, and size of establishment.

[b]For wage earners only.

likely to be uninsured than whites (14.7 percent). However, due to the greater size of the white population, the majority of the uninsured (60.4 percent) are white.

Examining the insurance status of the employed population, one finds that 30 percent of the self-employed are uninsured. Further, the smaller the size of firm, the greater the likelihood of the employee being uninsured; 30.4 percent of employees in firms with less than 10 employees are uninsured. In firms having between 10 and 24 employees, 22.4 percent are uninsured. Forty-one percent of all uninsured employees are working in firms with fewer than 25 employees. Proposals for mandated coverage that exclude small firms also exclude an important segment of the working uninsured. Thus the Pepper Commission's proposal to mandate coverage for firms with more than 100 employees would only affect a small portion of the uninsured.

Those who are uninsured are also low-wage employees, most likely because they are also young (19–24 years) with low skill levels. As of 1996, 57 percent of the uninsured workers were earning less than $10 an hour. Further, those working less than full-time are more likely to be uninsured.

Proponents of employer-mandated coverage point out that 87 percent of the uninsured are employed or dependents of an employee. Requiring employer coverage for all employees and their dependents would eliminate 87 percent of the uninsured, without increased federal or state spending. However, a large portion of the working uninsured are low-wage employees who cannot afford to buy insurance for themselves or for their family. Further, mandated coverage, by itself, would not achieve universal coverage since it would still leave 13 percent of the uninsured population without insurance.

Several important interest groups favor an employer mandated national health plan. For example, Congress would not have to pass a special tax to raise revenues for a mandated NHI program. Thus it offers the illusion that federal expenditures are unaffected or even reduced. State governments favor this approach since it would shift medical costs off the Medicaid budget onto small employers and their low-wage employees. Hospital and physician associations also favor this approach since it would increase the demand for their services without disrupting the current practice of medicine or payment systems. Nor does this approach change the role of private insurance companies; instead, a mandated program would have the effect of increasing the demand for insurance and, consequently, for medical services. Medical services for low-income employees and their dependents would be paid by private insurance rather than Medicaid or through bad debts.

Important interest groups, such as the health insurance companies, hospitals, physicians, and dentists would benefit from an employer-mandated plan, which was therefore favored by these organizations as their national health plan. Further, mandating a minimum set of insurance benefits does not affect large employers and their employees and permits unions and higher-income employees to retain their current negotiated benefits, which are generally greater than the mandated benefits. In fact, many large employers view a mandated plan as benefiting them because it would increase the labor costs of low-cost competitors. As Robert Crandall, chairman and chief executive of American Airlines, stated:

At American, we spend about $1,666 per employee per year—that's more than $80 million this year alone—on medical benefits for active employees and dependents. And we're spending $16 million a year for medical benefits for retirees.

Yet Continental doesn't provide any medical benefits for retirees at all—and its active employees pay for most of their own health insurance. As a result, Continental's unit cost advantage vs. American's is enormous—and worse yet, is growing!

. . . which is why we're supporting Sen. Edward Kennedy's legislation mandating minimum benefit levels for all employees. (11)

Although an employer-mandated NHI has political support from important groups, the main opposition has come from small employers who employ low wage labor and who would be most affected by this approach. The trade association of small employers (National Federation of Independent Business) played an important role in defeating President Clinton's health care reform proposal, which relied on an employer mandate.

Relying on an employer mandate as a vehicle for NHI has several problems. First, the federal government will lose revenue as taxable income is used to purchase health benefits for those employees whose benefits are below the mandated level. Employer-purchased health insurance is not considered as taxable income to the employee; instead, it is a business expense, which reduces the firm's taxable revenues. Second, requiring firms to purchase insurance for each employee is equivalent to placing a tax on each employee. The employees most affected by this tax are those working for small firms who are earning low wages. Higher-income employees already have insurance and are therefore unaffected by this tax. As the cost of labor is increased, the firm is likely to try and shift this cost to the employee, by lowering wages. (See the earlier discussion on who bears the burden of an increase in the Social Security tax). To the extent that the cost of the insurance is shifted to the employee, low-wage employees will receive reduced wages. It is equivalent to requiring workers to trade some of their taxable income for nontaxable health insurance coverage.

For those employees who are at or near the minimum wage, it will not be possible for the firm to shift the cost to them and these employees are likely to be laid off.

Third, firms will also increase overtime work and use fewer employees on whom they have to pay a tax. Further, to the extent that it takes time for the firm to shift these costs to their employees, the effect will be increased costs to the employer and, consequently, lower profits. Facing higher marginal costs, the firm will increase the prices of their goods and services. Consumers will thus bear part of the costs of mandated insurance since the increased prices are equivalent to a regressive tax on consumers.

As the firm's prices increase, there will be a decrease in demand for those goods and services, and, consequently, a decrease in the demand for labor. With an increase in prices, firms located outside the United States will be able to increase their market share. U.S. firms would have an incentive to shift their production to other countries. The decrease in demand for labor should be greater among unskilled workers, whose wages may be close to the minimum wage. Skilled labor is unlikely to be affected since their benefits are typically greater than those mandated. As their relative wages change, substitution toward skilled labor and capital, away from unskilled labor, is likely to occur. Unemployment among unskilled labor will increase. (Thus, while states will benefit by a decrease in their Medicaid expenditures, they will experience an increase in unemployment compensation and welfare payments.)

Typically, the benefits and financing mechanisms of a mandated employer program are not income-related.[2] As part of such a mandate, some form of assistance is usually proposed for small employers. However, unless such subsidies are income-related, small law firms may end up receiving subsidies.

Mandated employer insurance, if it is to achieve universal coverage, must be combined with government subsidies to individuals. There are those who would not be eligible, such as part-time employees and those who do not work; these groups, unless subsidized, would still have to rely on Medicaid.

The middle class is unlikely to oppose an employer mandate since it is a means of providing medical care to those with low incomes without having to tax the middle class to do so. It would appear to be a means of shifting the cost onto employers, even though, in actuality, the low-wage employee is being taxed to bear most of the burden of his own insurance.

Mandated employer health insurance, while politically attractive to many groups with a concentrated interest, is, however, not NHI. Most important, it does not provide the middle class with any visible net benefits. It was for this reason that President Clinton combined an employer mandate with regulatory controls on increases in medical expenditures. Under the Clinton proposal, health insurance premiums and out-of-pocket expenses of the middle class would have risen less rapidly; part of the costs of their care would be borne by the providers, who would be paid less. In this manner the middle class would have received the visible benefits of being assured of their choice of provider at lower prices; they would not be required to make any sacrifices.

The Clinton health plan was not enacted for a variety of reasons. Important among those reasons was the lack of political support by the middle class. As more information became available on the Clinton health plan and on its cost, its complexity, and the higher premiums that were to be required, the interest by the middle class in having such a radical change implemented diminished.

The structure and financing of the Clinton health plan and of national health insurance proposals generally is a *consequence* of the economic interests of politically powerful groups. The proposed financing methods and structure of the delivery system was not based on an understanding of which methods of taxation are more equitable, what their effects are on employment, which delivery systems are more efficient, and so on. Instead, it is more important to understand the political feasibility of different alternatives. It is not surprising that it is difficult to devise a politically acceptable NHI plan.

---

[2]President Clinton's health care reform plan proposed a proportional tax on wages, 12 percent. This would have greatly benefited unions, such as the United Auto Workers, whose benefits were costing about 15 to 18 percent of payroll.

546 • CHAPTER 18

Medical Savings Accounts

A new approach to financing medical care is the use of medical savings accounts (MSAs) in conjunction with catastrophic health insurance. Federal legislation enacted in 1996 provided for a pilot MSA program with the same favorable tax treatment as employer-paid health insurance. MSAs have been proposed as part of Medicare reform as well as for those under sixty-five years of age. However, MSAs were approved on an experimental basis for the self employed and for employees of small firms.

The MSA experimental plan works as follows: a person can annually contribute, tax free, an amount into her MSA equal to 75 percent of the deductible. Thus for a family policy with a high deductible between $3,000 and $4,500 and a total limit on out-of-pocket expenses of $5,500, the person can contribute a maximum of $3,375 ($4,500 180 75 percent) into her tax-free MSA. The person is at risk for the difference between the amount deposited in the MSA and the out-of-pocket limit. The contribution may be made by either the employee or the employer. The money invested in the MSA can be spent on medical services or it can be allowed to grow so the money will be there for re-tirement purposes. If it is spent on nonmedical services before retirement, the funds taken out are taxed plus a 15 percent penalty.

The advocates of MSAs claim that a fundamental problem with current health plans is their favorable tax treatment leading to comprehensive policies, which limits patients' concerns over the cost of such services. Instead, an MSA provides individuals with a fi-nancial incentive to be concerned with the costs of medical care, the prices they pay for services, and their use of services. (A high-deductible catastrophic policy has a much lower premium than a more comprehensive health insurance policy.) The result of MSAs, according to its advocates will be a lower rate of increase in medical expenditures.

Opponents of MSAs criticize this approach on several grounds. First, they claim that savings resulting from a high deductible plan would not be as large as the proponents ex-pect. After the deductible and stop loss are reached, additional expenditures are typically for inpatient care, which is not as responsive as outpatient care to patient price sensitiv-ity. Further, these expenditures are protected by insurance, so patient incentives would not be effective. Second, any savings due to switching to high-deductible catastrophic plans (which have much lower premiums) are only one-time savings and would not af-fect the rate of growth in expenditures. It is the adoption and availability of new tech-nology, typically used in an inpatient setting, that determines expenditure increases.

Perhaps the most controversial issue regarding MSAs is the issue of risk selection. MSA critics believe that MSAs will split the risk pools, with the healthier risks choosing MSAs (thereby gaining financially) while the higher risks remain with the more comprehensive health plan. The consequence of this adverse selection, if it occurred, would be that pre-miums for the traditional plan would sharply increase. To eliminate risk selection, em-ployers are likely to offer only one plan to their employees. In the individual insurance market, MSAs would also effectively segment the market, with higher-risk individuals paying much higher premiums than if the low- and high-risk groups were combined.

MSA proponents disagree that MSAs would split the insurance market according to low and high risks. They believe that high-risk groups would also choose MSAs since there would be a limit on their total out-of-pocket expenses. Those with chronic conditions or the aged, for example, would spend less on prescription drugs and other medical expenses under an MSA because of the stop-loss limit.

There is limited empirical evidence regarding the expected performance of MSAs. Several employers have adopted MSAs for their employees and report large reductions in annual rates of increase in employees' medical expenditures. However, there have been no control groups to match with these companies; thus their performance may have been affected by factors other than the adoption of MSAs. For example, annual rates of increase in medical expenditures were declining for many companies during this same period.

Two recent studies have estimated the effect of adoption of MSAs. Keeler et al. simulated the effects of several scenarios regarding MSAs. The authors conclude that while the MSA approach is unlikely to produce the large reduction in health care costs its advocates anticipate, neither is it likely to result in the adverse selection problem expected by its critics (12). The second study investigated whether those who are sick in one year also tend to be sicker on average throughout their lives. If this were the case, then MSAs would only benefit the healthy while those who are sick would not accumulate any assets in their MSAs. The authors find that health care spending of employees with the sickest families tends to diminish over time; thus, even the sickest may accumulate some savings in their MSAs (13). It is estimated that only about 20 percent of the employees would have saved less than half of their contributions while fully 50 percent of employees would have kept more than 70 percent of their contributions. This conclusion is based on the very restrictive assumption that spending one's own money would have no effect on a person's spending for medical services. If people do in fact spend less, then the accumulated savings would be much greater.

MSAs are viewed by proponents as an alternative to the current system, which relies on employer-paid health insurance. It would place much greater responsibility for medical expenses on the individual with an MSA account. MSAs, by themselves, however, will not assist those with low incomes who cannot currently afford health insurance. If the MSA concept is to be expanded to assist those with low incomes, then government subsidies to enable such persons to establish an MSA account would be needed.

An Income-Related NHI Proposal: A Refundable Tax Credit

Various tax credit proposals have been proposed over the years. The following proposal attempts to achieve universal coverage in an equitable manner, while providing incentives for efficiency in the use and delivery of medical services (14).

To achieve universal coverage, everyone would be required to have a basic level of health insurance, which, for higher-income persons would be a catastrophic policy. Mandatory catastrophic coverage is justified on the basis of externalities. If someone who can afford insurance does not have catastrophic coverage and suffers a large medical expense that has to be subsidized by the community, that person is shifting the risk, hence the cost of catastrophic coverage, to the rest of the community.

Several different definitions of catastrophic could be used. One example is a $3,000 deductible. Catastrophic proposals that rely solely on dollar limits would not be as equitable as those that are income-related. What might be considered catastrophic to low-income families is unlikely to be so to high-income groups. Alternatively, the deductible could vary according to family income, in which case, higher-income families would have higher deductibles than lower-income families. The deductible could also be a certain percentage (e.g., 10 percent) of the individual's or family's income.

Proof of insurance would be attached to the person's federal income tax forms. Lack of such evidence would result in the government collecting the appropriate premium as it would if the person paid insufficient income taxes. The government would then assign the person to a health plan, which the person could then change. (Employers could include on the individual's annual W-4 tax statement whether an amount has been deducted for health insurance.) Thus everyone who can afford health insurance will not become a burden to others if they incur a serious illness.

The refundable tax credit would work as follows: Taxpayers would be allowed to subtract from their income tax a given dollar amount that is used to purchase the mandatory health insurance. (The tax credit could be an equal dollar amount for all families [e.g., $4,000], or it could vary by income, declining with higher incomes.) Providing a tax credit of an absolute dollar amount would be politically more acceptable in that those with middle and high incomes would also receive some benefit.

Individuals whose tax credit exceeded their tax liabilities would receive a refund for the difference (a "refundable" tax credit). Thus, if a person's income were too low to pay taxes, she would receive a credit that she can use to choose a health plan. The size of the tax credit would be equal to the premium for a comprehensive set of benefits (the minimum benefits without a deductible). For those with low incomes, the tax credit would be sufficient to pay the entire insurance premium, since any sizable medical expense might be considered catastrophic in relation to their limited income. As a person's income increased the size of the tax credit would decrease, becoming zero at some level of income. At which income levels the tax credit became zero is a political decision to be determined by Congress. The government subsidy would therefore go to those with the lowest incomes. These refundable tax credits are essentially vouchers for a health plan for persons with little or no tax liability.

The current exclusion from the employee's taxable income of employer-purchased health insurance would be removed as the tax credit is substituted in its place. The lost tax revenues from this open-ended subsidy would be an important revenue source to offset the new tax credit to those with low incomes. No longer would there be the horizontal inequity of two persons with the same level of income receiving different size subsidies because one person is self-employed while the other is an employee of a large firm whose employer purchases insurance.

The financing of a tax credit proposal would be from general income taxes and would thus be financed in an equitable manner for a redistributive policy.

The obligation to purchase insurance under the above refundable tax credit proposal is placed on the individual and not on the employer ("mandated individual health insurance"). The effects on the demand for labor and the unemployment effects discussed above with respect to mandated employer insurance would therefore not occur. It is likely, however, that most employers would continue to purchase health insurance for their employees because group insurance is less expensive than if each employee did so on his own. Further, benefit managers could act as efficient agents in screening health plans and in providing information to the employees. Individuals could work for firms that did not provide health insurance as long as they purchased coverage themselves.

The premium for a minimum set of benefits that contained a deductible equal to 10 percent of income for a high-income person would be lower than the premium for the same benefits when a smaller deductible was used. Thus the premium for more comprehensive coverage (same benefits but with a small deductible) would be higher for those with low incomes.

With a large deductible-type insurance program, there may be a demand for supplementary insurance to cover all or part of what the consumer would have to pay. Consumers should be able to purchase such supplementary insurance. It would be a necessary part of this and other income-related insurance plans to take away current tax subsidies for the purchase of health insurance and for payment of medical expenses, to prevent a situation wherein "too much" health insurance would be purchased.[3]

The refundable tax credit could also replace Medicaid, using expenditures currently spent on Medicaid to partially offset the costs of the tax credit. Those eligible for Medicaid would be entitled to receive a voucher equal to the cost of a comprehensive set of benefits. Since the tax credit declines with increased incomes, there would no longer be a sharp cutoff of Medicaid benefits (the "notch" effect) with the previous disincentive to work. Since those eligible for Medicaid and others with low incomes may not file tax returns, they would register at their local welfare office to receive their insurance voucher.

Medicare could also be included in the tax credit proposal or, for political feasibility, it could be phased in for those not yet eligible for Medicare. It would be politically difficult to apply the proposed system to current Medicare beneficiaries. Thus the system could be phased in for those who are fifty-five years of age; they could receive the value of their Medicare benefits in the form of a tax credit toward their insurance premium. If Medicare and Medicaid are to be retained separately from the tax credit system, then the gaps and problems in these programs would have to be remedied.

---

[3]It has been argued that under NHI plans containing a deductible, the demand for supplementary insurance would be negligible if the favorable tax treatment of supplementary insurance were removed. It is unlikely that there would be any demand for supplementary insurance if the NHI plan covered only unreimbursed expenditures. See Emmett B. Keeler, Daniel T. Morrow, and Joseph P. Newhouse, "The Demand for Supplementary Health Insurance, or Do Deductibles Matter?" *Journal of Political Economy,* 85(4), August 1977.

An important difference from the current system will be the availability of insurance for those who do not purchase insurance through the workplace, such as the self-employed, small firms, and those on Medicaid. Such individuals and small groups will be free to purchase their own insurance, as currently occurs. The government, however, would also negotiate a "fallback" insurance plan with one or more insurers in each area. These insurers would bid for providing insurance for the minimum standard benefit coverage; there would be different premiums for the standard coverage according to the deductible percentage and for risk categories, such as age. Unless the government was willing to pay a sufficiently high premium, insurers would not be willing to become the fallback insurer. The fallback insurer would be available for those who, for various reasons, do not purchase coverage from other insurers.

No one would be required to join the fallback plan. Those joining the fallback insurer would likely be low-income persons whose premium is paid wholly or in part by the government's tax credit, those who failed to purchase insurance and were assigned by the government to the fallback plan (their premium would be collected through the income tax system), and those who chose to purchase their insurance from the fallback insurer. Each year the government would negotiate rates or take bids for the standard benefit package and each year people would be eligible to retain their coverage as long as they paid the premiums for their risk class. No one could be denied renewability of coverage from the fallback plan.

Those individuals who have specified preexisting conditions that would otherwise make them uninsurable would be eligible to join a state high-risk pool. The government would subsidize the premiums for the high-risk pool so that no individual has to pay a premium that is more than 125 to 150 percent of the standard premium for their risk class. The government would contract with an insurer to manage the risk pool. Over time there would be no need for a high-risk pool as individuals and small groups would be guaranteed renewability of insurance at standard rates.

There are a number of advantages to an income-related refundable tax credit as described above. First, those who receive the largest subsidies would be those with the lowest incomes and those whose medical bills represent the greatest financial hardship. In addition, the removal of the tax subsidy for employer-purchased health insurance would be an important source of funding for the new subsidy to those with low incomes. Other revenue sources that would be used to finance the new tax credit would also be income-related, such as Medicaid funds (which would no longer be needed) and general tax revenues. Thus the benefits would go to those with low incomes while the costs would be borne by those with higher incomes.

Second, the requirement of compulsory insurance, a competitive insurance market, and the existence of a fallback insurer would enable all persons to purchase insurance, with guaranteed renewability.

Third, consumer choice should be improved since they will have to select an approved minimum standard benefit among competing health plans. Consumers should find it easier to evaluate competing health plans and differences in their premiums when the product, the benefit, is more standardized.

Fourth, there would be greater incentives for demand efficiency. With the removal of the tax subsidy, persons desiring to spend more than the tax credit would be able to do so, but only with after-tax dollars. Those with high incomes would purchase less comprehensive insurance and have a greater incentive to be concerned with the prices and premiums they pay and the health plans they select.

Fifth, a refundable tax credit provides an incentive for increased efficiency in the provision of medical services. Competing managed care organizations would have an incentive to be concerned with the providers they use, the fees paid to providers, physician practice patterns, medical outcomes, as well as patient satisfaction.

A national health insurance system based on income-related vouchers through a refundable tax credit would achieve both increased equity and economic efficiency in the use of medical services.

WHY THE UNITED STATES HAS NOT HAD NATIONAL HEALTH INSURANCE

To understand why the United States has not had NHI, it is necessary first to understand the actual rather than the stated goal of NHI. Further, the debate over the structure and financing of NHI actually represents the controversy over the underlying objective that is to be achieved by NHI. Discussing the possible goals of NHI therefore clarifies the design features of different NHI proposals as well as providing insights as to why this country has not had NHI.

The Conflicting Goals of National Health Insurance

Increase Medical Services to Those with Low Incomes

While many individuals support increased services to the poor, this is not, nor has it ever been, the driving force behind NHI. *Medicaid is NHI for the poor.* To use the power of government to achieve one's objectives requires political power. The structure and funding of Medicaid are indicative of the limited political power of the poor and of their advocates. Medicaid's extensive inadequacies are not the actions of a few miserly bureaucrats or legislators but is instead reflective of the resources that society—the middle class—is willing to devote to the poor. The states vary in their generosity and in the criteria they use for determining eligibility for Medicaid. No state reaches the federal poverty level in determining Medicaid eligibility; and some states are only at 25 percent of the federal poverty level. How much the nonpoor are willing to spend on charity depends on how much the nonpoor themselves have, on how culturally similar the poor are to the nonpoor, and on how much it costs to provide for the poor.

Since it is the nonpoor who have the political power to determine the allocation of resources to the poor, one must assume that the inadequacies of Medicaid reflect insufficient interest or desire among the nonpoor to improve Medicaid and increase funding for the poor. *If society is unwilling to improve Medicaid, why would they be willing to tax themselves to enact NHI for the poor?*

The Use of Government to Benefit Politically Powerful Groups

Another view of NHI is that since legislators respond to politically powerful groups, these groups seek to use the power of government to provide themselves with net benefits they would not otherwise receive from the marketplace.

Politically influential groups are those who have a "concentrated" interest in a particular issue and who are able to organize themselves so as to provide legislators with political support (i.e., campaign contributions, votes, or volunteer time). A group is said to have a concentrated interest when some regulation or legislation has a sufficiently large effect on that group to make it worthwhile for them to invest resources to either forestall or promote that effect. The potential legislative benefits are greater than the group's costs of organizing and providing political support to achieve their legislative objectives.

Implicit in this discussion of concentrated interests is the assumption that legislators respond to political support, since their objective is to be reelected. Legislators, similar to the other participants in the policy process, are assumed to be rational; they undertake cost/benefit calculations of their actions. The costs and benefits of their legislative decisions, however, are not the legislation's effect on society but instead are the political support gained and lost by the legislators' actions.

In the health field, physicians and hospitals were initially the major groups with a concentrated interest in health legislation. Payment systems under both public and private insurance systems had a large effect on their revenues. Subsidies to increase the demand by those with low incomes also increased hospital and physician revenues. The availability of competitors, such as HMOs, PPOs, outpatient surgery centers, foreign-trained physicians, and so on, also affected hospital and physician revenues. Given their financial interest in issues affecting their demand for services, methods of pricing, the availability of substitutes to their services, and their overall supply, physician and hospital associations represented their concentrated interests before both state and federal legislatures. The defeat of President Truman's proposed NHI plan by the AMA was a demonstration of the AMA's political power and showed those legislators that were opposed to its economic interests that the AMA was a force to be reckoned with at election time.

The consequences of these legislative actions by physician and hospital associations were neither very obvious nor initially very costly to consumers of medical services. Medical prices were higher than they would otherwise have been and fewer alternatives, such as managed care, were available to the fee-for-service system. These costs were not sufficiently large to make it worthwhile for consumers to organize, represent their interests before legislatures, and offer political support to legislators.

The concentrated interests of medical providers and the consequent diffuse (small) costs imposed on consumers explain much of the legislative history of the financing and delivery of medical services until the early 1960s. Payment systems for physicians and hospitals and the structure of the medical services delivery system were economic benefits medical providers received as a result of government legislation.

The AFL-CIO unions had a concentrated interest in their retirees' medical costs that placed them in opposition to the AMA throughout the 1950s and early 1960s. Employers that paid for union retirees' medical costs had not prefunded these liabilities; instead they were paid as part of current labor expenses. If union retirees' medical expenses could be shifted away from the employer, then those same funds would be available to be paid as higher wages to union employees. The union's attempt to shift these costs onto others became the basis of the debate over Medicare.

To ensure that their union retirees would be eligible for Medicare, the unions insisted on Social Security financing. The AMA was willing to have government assistance go only to those unable to afford medical services, which would have increased the demand for physicians. Thus the AMA favored a means-tested program funded by general tax revenues. The AMA was concerned that subsidies to the nonpoor would merely substitute government payment for private payment. Such a program would cost too much, leading to controls on physicians' fees.

Thus the real fight over Medicare was over Social Security financing, which determined eligibility.

With the landslide victory of President Johnson in 1964, the unions were able to achieve their objective of Social Security financing. Once eligibility for Medicare was determined by Social Security financing, Part B was added, which was financed by general tax revenues.

Although the unions won on the financing mechanism, Congress acceded to the demands of the medical and hospital associations on all other aspects of the legislation. A payment system to hospitals and physicians was implemented that promoted inefficiency (cost-plus payments to hospitals) and restrictions were placed on alternative delivery systems that limited competition.

The outcome of this historic conflict in medical care between opposing concentrated interests left them both victorious. The power of government was used to benefit politically important groups.

As a result of Medicare, a massive redistribution of wealth occurred in society. The beneficiaries were the aged and medical providers; it was financed by a diffuse tax (Social Security) over a large group, the working population, who also paid higher prices for their medical services.

Medicare and Medicaid were designed to be both inefficient and inequitable because it was in the economic interests of those with concentrated interests.

This brief discussion of Medicare illustrates the real purpose of NHI. It is to redistribute wealth, that is, to increase benefits to politically powerful groups without them having to pay the full costs of those benefits or, similarly, to shift costs from the politically powerful to those who are less so.

Groups Having a Concentrated Interest in Change

An important reason why health policies change is that groups that previously had a diffuse interest develop a concentrated interest in the policy's outcome. For example, the potential benefits to unions of having their retirees' health benefits shifted from the employer to the government (via the taxpayer) under Medicare became sufficiently great as to provide them with a concentrated interest in this issue. Thus groups with a diffuse interest may develop a concentrated interest as the potential benefits or costs to their members increase. As diffuse costs become "concentrated" there is greater incentive for a group to organize and represent its interests.

There are many more groups today with a concentrated interest in health legislation. To understand the conflicting forces pressuring for change and NHI, however, one has to examine the objectives of several of the more important groups having a concentrated interest.

The Federal Government

Since Medicare and Medicaid were enacted in 1965, every administration has been faced with the problem of rapidly rising Medicare and Medicaid expenditures. As expenditures greatly exceeded projections, an initial diffuse cost became a concentrated cost to successive administrations. Each administration faced choices that were politically costly. To prevent the Medicare trust fund from going bankrupt, the administration could reduce benefits (or increase costs) to the aged, increase Social Security taxes, or pay hospitals less. All three choices were politically costly. However, it was less politically costly to increase Social Security taxes and to place limits on how much hospitals were to be paid than reduce benefits to the aged.

To limit rapidly rising Medicaid expenditures, which are funded from general tax revenues, the states chose to restrict Medicaid eligibility and reduce their payments to health providers, rather than reduce other politically popular programs or increase taxes. The percent of the poor served by Medicaid declined as did the participation of physicians and hospitals.

Medicare Part B, funded by general tax revenues, contributes to the federal budget deficit. As these expenditures began to increase, each administration's choices were limited; an increase in taxes or a larger deficit are both politically costly to the administration; increasing the aged's contribution (they currently pay 25 percent of the premium) is also politically costly; the only alternative was to pay physicians less and (as of 1993) place them under an expenditure limit.

State and federal administrations developed a concentrated interest in holding down the rise in government expenditures, which placed them in conflict with hospital and physician organizations. Currently, federal and state health policy appears to be primarily concerned with limiting the rise in Medicare and Medicaid expenditures. And the least politically costly approach is to pay providers less. Only under Medicaid are the politically weak beneficiaries also adversely affected.

Employers

Employers and their employees are interested in reducing the rise in the cost of employees' medical benefits. Rising employee medical expenses became a concern to employers in the 1980s because of more intense import competition. Many employers believe that they bear part of the cost of rising insurance premiums. More important, the stimulus for several large corporations, such as Chrysler, promoting national health insurance was a ruling by the Financial Accounting Standards Board (FASB) requiring employers who provide their retirees with medical benefits to add that liability to their balance sheet starting in 1993. This estimated liability had to include their retirees' future medical expenses, as well as the retiree benefit liability for their current employees. Retiree medical benefits have been an unfunded liability to those large corporations that provide such benefits. Previously, the employer paid retiree medical costs as they occurred; they were treated as a current expense. To place this entire liability on the balance sheet reduced the net worth and equity per share of many major corporations by a significant amount. In addition, corporate earnings will decline, since a portion of this retiree liability for medical benefits (for both retirees as well as current employees) has to be expensed annually.

Any NHI plan that restricts the growth of medical expenditures will provide a direct economic benefit to large corporations by limiting the size of their retirees' unfunded medical liabilities and by limiting the rise in their employees' medical costs, thereby improving their international competitiveness.

Unions

The percent of the working population that is unionized has been declining. Only about 15 percent of employees are unionized—down from 25 percent in 1972. The wages earned and medical benefits received by union members vary widely, from those engaged in manufacturing to those employed in the retail and construction businesses. Because unions are organized, several of the larger unions have been able to provide legislators with sufficient political support to exercise political influence greatly in excess of their proportion to the total working population.

The economic interests of the major unions, such as the UAW, have not changed since the enactment of Medicare. At that time they were successful in shifting part of the cost of their retirees onto the general working population. Since that time they have been trying to reduce the costs of their employees' medical benefits, which are among the most expensive of all employees, by limiting provider price increases. If the unions can limit cost increases for their benefits, without increasing their members' cost sharing, the savings could go toward increased wages.

Physicians and Hospitals

As other groups with a concentrated interest in limiting medical expenditures (particularly the federal and state governments) developed, the influence of physician and hospital associations declined. Also adding to their loss of political influence was the inability of their national organizations to represent the interests of their diverse constituencies under "budget-neutral" federal programs. When expenditure choices under public programs had to be made between these constituencies (urban versus rural hospitals, teaching versus nonteaching hospitals, surgical specialties versus primary care physicians, etc.), these provider coalitions split apart, each trying to gain at the expense of the other. And as these separate associations provide political support to further their own interests, the political influence of their national associations declined.

The years of excessive provider payments are over. Hospitals and physicians are striving to limit further deterioration in their financial well-being. Their objective, as opposed to that of other groups with a concentrated interest, is increased medical expenditures. The strongest lobbyists for financing medical care to the poor today are hospitals since it is in their own economic interests; they stand to gain additional revenues.

The Aged

The aged have NHI for acute care (Medicare). While the middle- and high-income aged would like lower out-of-pocket payments for their medical expenses, particularly for prescription drugs, their most pressing concern is for protection from the costs of long-term care. An extended stay in a nursing home will deplete the assets of many of the aged. Medicare does not cover long-term care or nursing home care unrelated to an acute illness. Those aged with low incomes have to rely on Medicaid for their long-term care. If an aged person's assets exceed the Medicaid limit, she must "spend down" those assets to qualify for Medicaid. Government-subsidized long-term care insurance is a means whereby the aged can protect their assets. Rather than purchasing such asset protection in the marketplace, the aged prefer government legislation, whereby they can shift part of their costs to other population groups.

To date, long-term care has not been enacted because of the reluctance of legislators to impose additional large taxes on the working population.

The Middle Class

The middle class (those in the middle income group) have a disproportionate amount of political power since they are the median voters; it is difficult to form a majority of voters without those in the middle. If national health insurance were a highly visible issue and strongly supported by the middle class, legislators would respond to the political support that would be forthcoming from the middle class. It is instructive, therefore, to consider why the middle class has not been a strong supporter of NHI.

Rapidly rising medical costs have, until recently, been a diffuse cost to the middle class. Tax-free employer-paid health insurance insulated employees and their families from the rising costs of medical care. Until the past several years, employees have had unlimited choice of providers, limited cost sharing, and small, if any, co-premiums. *Tax-free employer-paid health insurance has been a form of NHI for middle- and high-income groups.* The value of this tax subsidy is approaching $100 billion in forgone federal, Social Security, and state taxes. Given the significant tax advantages of employer-paid premiums and the fact that increased employer-paid premiums has not visibly lowered their wages, middle- and high-income employees have been insulated from rising medical costs; NHI has not been an important financial issue. Employees have probably been at greater financial risk for the long-term care needs of their aged parents than for their own acute care needs.

The middle class's dissatisfaction with the current system is increasing because they are being forced into more restrictive health plans and cannot have the free access to specialists they once had. However, they are also unwilling to pay more for less restrictive health plans or higher taxes for NHI. Basically, the public would like unrestricted access and have someone else, either government or employers, pay for their health care.

There are also other groups with a concentrated interest in any NHI plan, such as insurance companies, who do not want to be displaced by a government agency.

When one examines those groups having a concentrated interest in health policy, it becomes clear why there has not been (nor is there currently) consensus on national health insurance. The federal and state governments, as well as large employers, want to limit the rate of increase in medical expenditures. The previously politically powerful physician and hospital associations want increased medical expenditures. The aged, who have national health insurance, want a new long-term care program whose costs would be borne by the working population. The unions and the middle class want unrestricted access and at a lower cost, presumably by shifting those costs to others, either different population groups or to the providers by paying them less.

It is these conflicting objectives by powerful interest groups that explains why there is no consensus as to what NHI should attempt to achieve.

Recent Legislative Developments in Lieu of NHI

In the past several years the middle class's concern with rapidly rising medical expenses has declined as managed care competition and low inflation rates have moderated medical price increases. Instead, with the rise of managed care concern has shifted to one of access. As a result of anecdotal stories of HMO enrollees being denied access to specialists and to experimental treatments, of not being permitted to have an overnight stay for normal deliveries, "drive-through" mastectomies, HMO "gag" orders on physician communication with their patients, state legislatures and Congress have responded by enacting legislation.

The use of regulation in response to the media attention given to these instances of inadequate care is a new role for government. Regulation prescribing the practice of medicine has the potential for increasing the cost of medical services and, consequently, decreasing the demand for insurance. Managed care has been able to decrease medical costs by providing hospitals and physicians with incentives to become more efficient and to reexamine how they provide care. By specifying minimum hospital stays, ratios of nursing personnel to patients, access to a wide range of physicians, and few or no limitations on the use of specialists, managed care organizations become limited in how they may reduce their enrollees' medical costs. As government specifies certain types of practice, managed care organizations are likely to resort to more traditional indemnity approaches to limit use of services, such as increased use of deductibles and co-payments. More important, it becomes difficult for physician groups to reduce medical costs by developing innovative approaches to care for patients.

From a legislator's perspective, responding to enrollees' desire to have unlimited access to physicians and to medical services cost the legislator and the government very little, since they do not have to vote to increase taxes. Instead, a less visible cost is imposed on enrollees in terms of higher insurance premiums. The legislator receives the "benefit" of seeming to respond to the public's dissatisfaction with managed care while not incurring any cost.

Regulating the practice of medicine is a new approach for legislators to use in responding to middle-class concerns. Instead, it would be more appropriate for government to move in the direction of having health plans provide more information to the public to enable enrollees to make more informed choices when selecting a health plan. This is the approach being used by large business coalitions and nonprofit organizations that collect data on health plan performance. Incremental regulation of medical practice by Congress can have far-reaching effects on both the structure and financing of medical services. Unfortunately, these long-run effects are rarely considered.

It is unlikely that universal health insurance will be enacted in the near term. Although the number and percent of the uninsured are increasing, there seems to be little interest by the middle class, and consequently by Congress, to increase their tax burden to assist those who can offer little political support to enact such a program. Instead, it is likely that various regulatory approaches will be used to require health plans to provide more individual coverage. State and federal Medicaid expenditures will be reduced if high-risk individuals can be shifted to private health plans. However, expanding the individual insurance pool is likely to result in higher premiums, with low-risk individuals dropping their coverage.

Until NHI becomes a visible political issue for which the middle class would be willing to provide its political support, NHI is unlikely to be enacted.

Economic analysis can be a powerful tool in the analysis of alternative proposals for national health insurance in that it can sharpen the debate by providing information as to the redistributive and efficiency consequences of alternative proposals. If economists can clarify the issues by separating those that involve differences in the values underlying various goals of NHI from issues of efficiency with regard to achieving a given set of NHI goals, they will have served an important policy role.

SUMMARY

Different values underlie the extent to which government would subsidize care for the poor under any national health insurance plan. These values range from Minimum Provision to Equal Treatment for Equal Needs. Each set of values can be achieved more efficiently (at lower cost) when the subsidy varies (inversely) with income. The Medicare program was used to illustrate these theoretical conclusions.

Several criteria were specified for evaluating all NHI plans. These included defining the beneficiaries by income, providing beneficiaries and suppliers with incentives for the efficient use of resources, and that an equitable method of financing be used, namely, a greater cost burden should be placed on those with higher incomes.

Current subsidies for financing medical services were evaluated according to the above criteria, together with proposals for improving each of these programs. Several proposals for NHI, such as Canadian-type system, an employer mandate, medical savings accounts, and a refundable tax credit were also evaluated.

Rather than assuming that the intended goal of NHI is to assist those with low incomes, an alternative assumption, benefiting politically powerful constituencies, was used to explain why this country has not had NHI. This alternative hypothesis provides a more useful explanation for why many health programs are inefficiently designed and inequitably financed.

Key Terms and Concepts

- Equal financial access
- Medical savings accounts
- Negative prices
- NHI evaluation criteria

- Canadian-type health system
- Concentrated interests in health reform
- Equal treatment for equal needs
- Equity and efficiency of employer-paid health insurance
- Incidence of the payroll tax

- Medicare's redistributive effects
- Mandated employer health insurance
- Refundable tax credits
- Value judgment of minimum provision

Review Questions

1. What criteria are most appropriate for evaluating a government's health insurance scheme?

2. Describe the characteristics of the uninsured.

3. The Social Security tax is imposed on both the employer and the employee. Using supply and demand diagrams for labor, show how the elasticity of demand for labor determines who (either the employer or the employee) actually bears the burden of the Social Security tax.

4. If society were to establish as a principle for national health insurance that everyone should have equal consumption of medical care for equal needs, explain why a policy that established the same price to everyone for medical care (or makes medical care free to all, i.e., zero price) will not achieve society's goal.

5. Assume that in country X, where medical care was privately paid for, a new government was elected, with one of its policies being free medical care for all. As the new minister of health, what are the various actions you would have to undertake to ensure that at a zero price for all medical care services, an adequate supply will be available in the future?

6. Assume that an income-related tax credit NHI plan was enacted and that this replaced the current tax-exempt employer-purchased health insurance. Trace the effects of this action on the medical care system. Consider demand and supply in each of the different medical care markets (e.g., institutional, manpower, and educational markets, prices, quantities, wages, employment, and total expenditures). What assumptions become crucial to your analysis?

7. One approach that has been proposed for national health insurance system is a system whereby all employers would be required to provide their employees with a minimum set of health insurance benefits. Evaluate this proposal in terms of the demand for different types of labor, the effects on federal revenues, the effects on the prices of goods and services produced by different types of industries, and the effect on imported goods. How equitable do you believe such a proposal to be? Be explicit regarding any assumptions you make.

8. Which groups would be expected to favor and oppose an employer-mandated health insurance plan?

9. National health insurance can be financed by either a payroll or an income tax. Compare the effects on economic efficiency and equity of each of these methods of financing.

REFERENCES

1. The May 15, 1991 issue of the *Journal of the American Medical Association,* 265(19), which is devoted to issues of the uninsured, contains a number of proposals for national health insurance.

2. *Medicare and the American Health Care System: Report to the Congress* (Washington, D.C.: Prospective Payment Assessment Commission, June 1997), p.18.

3. For an excellent and comprehensive discussion of this issue, together with estimates of the intergenerational transfer, see Ronald J. Vogel, "An Analysis of the Welfare Component and Intergenerational Transfers under the Medicare Program," in Mark Pauly and William Kissick, eds., *Lessons from the First Twenty Years of Medicare* (Philadelphia: University of Pennsylvania Press, 1988). Also see Ronald J. Vogel, *The Political Economy of Medicare* (unpublished book manuscript) April 1, 1997.

4. David Cutler and Jonathan Gruber, "The Effect of Medicaid Expansions on Public Insurance, Private Insurance, and Redistribution," *American Economic Review,* 86(2), May 1996: 378–383.

5. For a more complete discussion of this and related proposals, see *The Tax Treatment of Employment-Based Health Insurance* (Washington, D.C.: Congressional Budget Office, Congress of the United States, March 1994).

6. David Himmlestein, Steffie Woolhandler, et al., "A National Health Program for the United States: A Physician's Proposal," *New England Journal of Medicine,* 320(2), January 12, 1989: 102–108.

7. The following monograph presents a critical view of the Canadian health care system; it is published by a trade association opposed to the Canadian system. Edward Neuschler, *Canadian Health Care: The Implications of Public Insurance* (Washington, D.C.: Health Insurance Association of America, June 1990).

8. *Medicare: Rapid Spending Growth Calls for More Prudent Purchasing* (Washington, D.C.: United States Government Accounting Office, GAO/T-HEHS-95-193, June 28, 1995).

9. Steven J. Katz and Timothy P. Hofer, "Socioeconomic Disparities in Preventive Care Persist Despite Universal Coverage: Breast and Cervical Cancer Screening in Ontario and the United States," *Journal of the American Medical Association,* 272(7), August 17, 1994: 530–535.

10. *Ibid.*

11. As quoted in "Notable & Quotable," *Wall Street Journal,* August 8, 1987, p. 16.

12. Emmett B. Keeler et al., "Can Medical Savings Accounts for the Nonelderly Reduce Health Care Costs?" *Journal of the American Medical Association,* 275(21), June 5, 1997: 1666–1671.

13. Mathew Eichner, Mark McClellan, and David Wise, "Insurance or Self-Insurance? Variation, Persistence, and Individual Health Accounts" (Cambridge, Mass.: National Bureau of Economic Research, NBER Working Paper 5640, 1996).

14. The following is an example of a proposal for national health insurance based on tax credits and catastrophic coverage. Mark Pauly, Patricia Danzon, Paul Feldstein, and John Hoff, "A Plan for 'Responsible National Health Insurance,'" *Health Affairs,* 10(1), Spring 1991: 5–25.

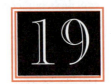

CHAPTER

19

The Market for Long-Term Care Services

DEMOGRAPHIC TRENDS AND LONG-TERM CARE

The population of this country is becoming older. This demographic trend has profound implications for society. As the proportion of retirees to the working age population increases, there are concerns regarding the fiscal burden of an aging population. Political conflict between age groups also becomes more likely as public financing of services to the aged impose greater per capita burdens on the working population.

The two largest redistribution programs for the aged are Social Security and Medicare. These programs are entitlements, which means that all aged are eligible, the benefits are adjusted for inflation, as well as for higher earnings of retirees in the case of Social Security, and legislative changes over the years have made these programs increasingly more generous. The increasing dependency ratio between the number of retired persons and the working population suggests that it will become even more difficult to provide additional benefits to the aged. Yet demographic trends will increase pressures for government to subsidize the long-term care needs of the aged. How this issue is resolved affects not only the aged with such needs, but whether additional burdens will be placed on the working-age population to finance these additional benefits.

This chapter discusses a number of long-term care issues: the growing needs and demands for long-term care, the provision of long-term care services, the financing of such services, and current government policies with respect to long-term care. To achieve an increased understanding of the public policy implications of this emerging market, the concept of economic efficiency is used for evaluating the performance of this market. Since public policy also results in redistributional consequences, the equity aspects of the financing and provision of long-term care services are also discussed.

THE DEMAND FOR LONG-TERM CARE SERVICES

Long-term care is generally not the result of a specific medical problem but is the care required to assist those whose physical and mental disabilities impair their functioning in those activities necessary for daily living. Thus long-term care refers broadly to the medical, residential, and social services that are provided to chronically disabled persons over an extended period of time, either in their own home or in a separate facility. Long-term care is more than nursing home services. The nursing home is the end of a continuum of services to assist an impaired person to function in activities necessary for daily living. When viewed in this manner, nursing homes are substitutes for independent living. The nursing home provides a limited amount of medically related services, as well as housing, food, and socialization services. Long-term care services include housing, socialization, food, in-home chore and personal care, transportation, and medical care—services that are all found in nursing homes.

The demand for long-term care services is related to the need in the population for such services, as indicated by the aging of the population, as well as economic factors. Important economic factors are the prices of institutional and noninstitutional services, government and private insurance programs, income and assets of the recipients, and "nonmarket" caregiving by family members and relatives. The extent of consumer knowledge (or lack thereof) also has an important effect on demands for long-term care services. Each of these will be briefly discussed.

Demographic Profile of the Population

About 12.6 million people require long-term care services (LTC), when LTC is defined as needing assistance in activities of daily living (ADL). Of those needing LTC, 0.5 million are children, 4.8 million are nonelderly disabled adults, and 7.3 million are over 65 years of age. Most individuals who need LTC live in the community (10.3 million) as opposed to an institution (2.3 million).

The aged number 32 million, or 12.5 percent of the population. LTC services include the need for some household tasks, such as cooking and shopping, and personal care needs, such as bathing, dressing, and eating. Of the approximately 24 percent of the elderly (7.3 million) requiring some form of assistance, only 30 percent (2 million) have limited dependencies while 20 percent (1.4 million) are completely dependent, requiring assistance in all of their activities (1). The need for long-term care services increases with age. As shown in Table 19.1, only 8.4 percent of those aged 65 to 69 years require

TABLE 19.1 Percent of the Aged Requiring Long-Term Care Services, 1987

Age	Population (thousands)	Percentage Needing Help with at Least One Personal Care or Home Management Activity	Percentage Needing Assistance, by Number of Personal Care Activities				
			At Least One	One	Two	Three	Four or Five
		Household					
65 or Older	26,517	17.1	8.1	3.6	1.6	1.0	1.9
65–69	9,048	8.4	4.2	1.6	1.0	0.5	1.0
70–74	7,327	11.7	5.0	1.7	1.2	0.8	1.2
75–79	5,096	17.5	8.2	4.7	1.2	0.8	1.5
80–84	3,015	30.9	13.4	5.4	3.3	1.7	3.0
85 or older	2,032	54.8	28.8	13.5	4.3	3.5	7.5

Source: Policy Choices for Long-Term Care, Congress of the United States (Washington, D.C.: Congressional Budget Office, June 1991), 6.

some long-term care service. For those 75 to 79 years the percentage increases to 17.5 percent; while for those 85 years and above, 54.8 percent require one or more long-term care services.

Just as personal care dependency increases with age, so does the proportion of older persons institutionalized at any point in time. Only 0.1 percent of the population under age 65 was institutionalized compared to 4 percent of the population 65 and over; this varied from 1.3 percent of those 65 to 74, 5.8 percent of those 75 to 84, and 22 percent of those over 85 years of age. The major characteristics of those institutionalized are mental disorders, severe functional dependencies, and weak social support systems (2).

Since older people have the highest dependency and institutionalization rates, and since nursing home expenditures are by far the largest commonly accepted long-term care expense, analysts examining the use of long-term care services have tended to focus on those 65 and over.

The major sources of long-term care for the dependent elderly are: with a spouse (32.7 percent), with others (20.7 percent), in a nursing home (19.4 percent), in board and care homes (3.7 percent), and living alone (23.5 percent) (3). While the dependent elderly in nursing homes are generally more disabled than those in the community, it has been estimated that for every aged person in a nursing home, there are twice as many aged in the community requiring a similar level of care.

In addition to differences in need for long-term care services by age, there are differences according to gender. Women live longer and have a higher disability rate than do men of the same age. This has important implications for substitute sources of care. Disabled males are more likely than females to have a spouse to assist them and to remain in their own homes rather than be institutionalized.

The lifetime risk of an aged person entering a nursing home and having to spend down his assets is shown in Figure 19.1. Most of the aged (59.2 percent) entering a nursing home were private-pay patients (the remainder were those already eligible for Medicaid [17.3 percent] and Medicare or other payers [23.5 percent]). Of those private-pay aged who used less than 3 months of nursing home care, 2.7 percent had to spend down their assets to qualify for Medicaid eligibility. For a stay up to 6 months, a total of 10.5 percent had to spend down. As the stay increased, up to 2 years, 18.2 percent had to spend down. For those private-pay aged who stayed 5 or more years, a total of 28.7 percent had to spend down, while 25.7 percent remained private-pay.

On average, 44.3 percent of the aged who used nursing homes were able to remain private-pay throughout their stay, while 14.3 percent had to spend down. When these data are updated for increased life expectancy, then a person turning 65 in 1995 had a 39 percent chance of entering a nursing home. The risk of a person entering the nursing home as a private pay patient and having to spend down their assets was only 6.3 percent. (These probabilities vary according to race and gender.)

Thus, based on these data, the lifetime risk of a person entering a nursing home and having to spend down her assets is relatively low. However, it is the fear of incurring this financial burden that is the basis of the demand for long-term care insurance and government subsidies.

Demographic trends will cause a huge expansion in the long-term care population and in the demand for long-term care services. In 1950, there were 12.4 million aged, representing 8.1 percent of the population. By 1990, the number of aged had increased to 32

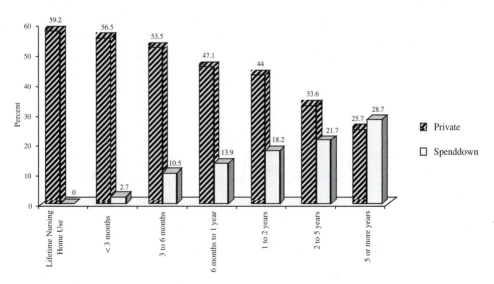

FIGURE 19.1 • Distribution of elderly decedents who used nursing homes.
Source: Brenda C. Spillman and Peter Kemper, "Lifetime Patterns of Payment for Nursing Home Care," *Medical Care,* 33 (3), March 1995: 288, Table 2.

million and constituted 12.5 percent of the population. The aged are expected to become an increasing portion of the population, reaching 17.7 percent, or 52 million, by the year 2020. (The aging of the baby boomers starting in 2010 will place major financial burdens on both Social Security and Medicare.)

The fastest-growing portion of the aged are those over 85 years of age. As shown in Table 19.2, the age group 85 and over increased by 59.1 percent between 1970 and 1980, while those aged 65 to 74 increased by 25.2 percent. Between 1990 and 2000, those 85 years and older are expected to increase by 41 percent compared to 0.5 percent for those 65 to 74 and 23 percent for those 75 to 84.

The implication of this changing age structure is clear. Studies show a greater likelihood of nursing home use is associated with advancing age, living alone, disabilities, personal care dependencies, and mental disorders (4). Demographic trends will cause a steady increase in the numbers of very dependent older persons needing long-term care services. Assuming the same dependency and institutionalization rates in the year 2000 as in 1980, the number of dependent older persons would grow by 56 percent in the two decades, while the number of institutionalized persons would grow by 73 percent. Again the fastest rate of growth is in the oldest age groups, which are more likely to require long-term care.

Economic Factors Affecting Demand

Price

The out-of-pocket price to a patient without any insurance coverage is highest for nursing home care. Nursing home prices vary, reflecting different levels of services, quality of care, levels of efficiency, and profitability. Prices are generally higher for skilled nursing facilities (SNFs), which provide a higher level of care than intermediate facilities. About 50 percent of the elderly in nursing homes receive each type of service. (The average price for a private-pay patient in a nursing home exceeds $40,000 per year in many places.)

TABLE 19.2 Percent Increase in U.S. Population for Ten-Year Intervals by Age Groups: Selected Years and Projections, 1970–2020

Year	65–74 Years	75–84 Years	85 Years or Over
1970–80	25.2	26.2	59.10
1980–90	15.8	29.5	34.90
1990–2000	0.5	23.0	41.0
2000–10	16.1	3.0	33.10
2010–20	49.0	21.2	13.90

Source: U.S. Bureau of the Census, *Current Population Report*, P-25, various issues.

The price for home health care services (HHC) also varies according to the type of service provided. A visit by a skilled nurse may be $90, while that of an unskilled personal care attendant is much less per hour ($40 in 1994) and would depend on whether the consumer purchases the service directly from the worker or contracts for the service through an agency. It is difficult to compare prices for LTC services in an institutional and a home setting since the quantity of services needed in the home can vary greatly.

It is important to estimate the price elasticity of demand by private-pay patients only, since the state pays for Medicaid patients. Scanlon, analyzing the private demand for nursing home care, found that the private-pay price had a sizable and negative effect on demand by private-pay patients—the price elasticity of demand was approximately −1.0, suggesting that there were good community substitutes for institutionalization (5). Nyman estimated the effect that price has on choice of nursing homes by private-pay patients rather than on the overall market demand for nursing homes. His price elasticity estimate of −1.7 suggests that private patients (and/or their agents) are sensitive to price differences among nursing homes (6).

The demand for marketed long-term care services depends on the supply of nonmarket or "informal" long-term care services. Everything else held constant, the higher the level of nonmarket caregiving, the lower the demand for marketed long-term care services. As shown in Table 19.3, family members provide most of the long-term care services outside of the marketplace. For all persons 65 years and over requiring personal care services, the spouse provides 53 percent of the care days to the husband; children provide 19 percent and relatives provide 18 percent of the care days. Only 11 percent of the care days are provided through a formal arrangement, although this increases for those, particularly women, over 85 years of age. As shown in Table 19.3, when the recipient is female, male spouses (who are less likely to be alive) provide only 17 percent of the care days and the largest burden falls on the children and relatives (37 and 30 percent, respectively).

The cost of nonmarket long-term care services is not easily measured. For example, the burden of an older woman caring for a still-older dependent husband can have significant emotional, physical health, and economic consequences on the caregiver. There is also the time lost from work, jobs that are given up by children of the dependent adult, lost efforts in their own homes, as well as foregone leisure to perform their caregiving tasks.

Although there are important noneconomic motivations for nonmarket caregiving, there are also powerful economic incentives to do so. Nursing homes and private insurance coverage are very expensive, and relying on Medicaid requires impoverishment. As a result, a long stay in a nursing home for a husband can mean financial ruin for a wife. It can also mean the depletion of assets that can be bequeathed to children or to relatives.

Empirical studies indicate that availability of informal care reduces the demand for nursing homes. Similarly, the higher the opportunity cost of informal support care to the providers of that care (as indicated by the labor force participation rate of adult married women), the greater the demand for institutional care. It has also been shown that Medicaid subsidies for home health services reduces the probability of nursing home use

TABLE 19.3 Percent Distribution of Helper Days, by Sex and Relationship to Individuals Sixty-Five Years of Age or over with Limitations to Activities of Daily Living, 1982

	Helper Days	
Age and Relationship	Male	Female
All persons 65 years or over		
Spouse	53	17
Offspring	19	37
Other relative	18	30
Formal	11	16
65–74 years		
Spouse	61	31
Offspring	15	27
Other relative	15	28
Formal	9	14
75–84 years		
Spouse	31	3
Offspring	18	38
Other relative	18	32
Formal	11	15
85 years or over		
Spouse	31	3
Offspring	31	47
Other relative	22	30
Formal	16	19

Source: Preliminary data from the 1982 *National Long-Term Care Survey,* Department of Health and Human Services, 1982, and published in Pamela Doty, Korfin Liu, and Joshua Weiner, "Special Report: An Overview of Long-Term Care," *Health Care Financing Review,* 6(3), Spring 1985: 70.

among at-risk elderly using formal home care. Such a subsidy also increased the use of formal home care services (7).

Incomes of the Elderly

The largest consumers of LTC services are the elderly, who pay a large portion of their expenses out of pocket. As shown in Table 19.4, the elderly pay only 4.0 percent and 28.7 percent, respectively, of hospital and physician expenditures themselves, since the remainder is in large part paid for by Medicare. For nonacute care, however, the aged pay most of it themselves. The aged pay out of pocket 56.4 percent of nursing home expenditures (Medicaid pays 36.4 percent) and 64.2 percent of other care, which consists primarily of services in the home. Medicare and Medicaid also pay for some home health care, but the total from all government sources was less than 35 percent. Examining the

TABLE 19.4 Percent Distribution of Personal Health Care Expenditures per Capita for People Sixty-Five Years of Age or over, by Source of Funds and Type of Service: United States, 1987

Total Source of Funds		Type of Service			
	Care	Hospital	Physician	Nursing Home	Other Care
Total per capita amount	$5,360	2,248	1,107	1,085	920
Percent distribution	100.0%	100.0	100.0	100.0	100.0
Private	37.4	14.8	35.5	58.4	70.0
Consumer[a]	36.9	14.2	35.5	57.7	69.4
Out-of-pocket[a]	28.7	4.0	23.4	56.4	64.2
Insurance[a]	8.2	10.2	12.1	1.3	5.2
Other private[a]	0.4	0.5	0	0.7	0.5
Government	62.6	85.2	64.5	41.6	30.0
Medicare	44.6	69.7	60.6	1.7	14.7
Medicaid	12.0	4.9	1.5	36.4	13.3
Other	6.0	10.6	2.4	3.5	2.0

Source: Daniel R. Waldo, Sally T. Sonnefeld, David R. McKusick, and Ross H. Arnett III, "Health Expenditures by Age Groups, 1977 and 1987," *Health Care Financing Review,* 10(4), Summer 1989: 111–120.

[a] These categories have been estimated based on 1984 data from: Daniel Waldo and Helen Lazenby, "Demographic Characteristics and Health Care Use and Expenditures by the Aged in the U.S., 1977–1984," *Health Care Financing Review,* 6(1), Fall 1984: 10–11.

income of the elderly therefore can shed light on their current and potential demand for marketed long-term care services and for insurance against those expenses.

The income of the elderly relative to the nonelderly has been generally underestimated. The aged pay, on average, only 13 percent of their income in taxes, compared to 23 percent for all ages (8). Over 75 percent of the aged own their homes and about three-fourths of those do not owe any mortgage (9); some form of imputed rent on these homes would substantially increase the incomes of the elderly, on average. The elderly receive many in-kind subsidies, such as Medicare, Medicaid, housing, food stamps, social services, and subsidized meal programs, the value of which is not shown as part of their reported income on surveys. The aged also earn a disproportionate share of the types of income, such as pensions, interest, and dividends, that are the most systematically underreported in income surveys (10). It has been estimated that adjusting the income of the elderly for differential tax rates, differences in household size, the value of in-kind subsidies, and imputed rent would place the average income of the elderly above that of the nonelderly population.

There has been a closing of the income gap between the elderly and nonelderly, as shown in Table 19.5. The distributions of incomes for both families and individuals are

TABLE 19.5 Estimates of Total Money Income for Those over and under Sixty-Five Years of Age, 1995

	Quintile					
	Bottom	Second	Third	Fourth	Top	Mean
Individuals Over 65 Years of Age						
1995 average income for quintile	$4,994	$7,500	$12,161	$19,242	$40,828	$17,604
Income distribution	6.0%	8.5%	13.8%	21.9%	46.4%	
Individuals Under 65 Years of Age						
1995 average income for quintile	$3,110	$9,853	$19,152	$31,081	$56,540	$25,519
Income distribution	2.4%	7.7%	15.0%	24.4%	44.3%	
Families Over 65 Years of Age						
1995 average income for quintile	$12,021	$20,000	$28,788	$42,174	$77,570	$38,675
Income distribution	6.2%	10.3%	14.9%	21.8%	40.1%	
Families Under 65 Years of Age						
1995 average income for quintile	$12,246	$27,995	$45,000	$62,983	$93,607	$53,812
Income distribution	4.6%	10.4%	16.7%	23.4%	34.8%	

Source: U.S. Bureau of the Census, Current Population Reports, Series P60-193, *Money Income in the United States: 1995* (with Separate Data on Valuation of Noncash Benefits) (U.S. Government Printing Office, Washington, D.C., 1996), pp. 17, 30, 32.

Note: Using the source data, average income for the quintiles has been calculated in the following way: The total number of individuals and families was divided in quintiles. For each income group the midpoint was estimated (for example, for income group $0–$5,000, the midpoint is $2,500). Then, midpoint incomes were multiplied by the total number of people. The percentages in income distribution were calculated using a similar procedure.

shown. These data are not adjusted for the factors discussed above; they therefore understate the income of the aged.

The stereotype of the elderly as a poor group is clearly wrong, although there are certainly many poor elderly. It is the distribution of income among the elderly, not just the average level, that affects the demand for long-term care services. The top 20 percent of elderly families has 40 percent of all elderly disposable income (in excess of $77,570 per family; see table footnotes on how upper quintile was calculated), while the bottom 20 percent has only 6.2 percent (averaging $12,021 per family). While many of the elderly in the top 20 percent of the income distribution could pay for long-term care services and catastrophic nursing home expenses without impoverishing their spouse, this is inconceivable for those in the remaining part of the income distribution. (Asset data are unavailable.) The distribution of income for elderly individuals is similar; however, the averages are lower in each quintile. Only a small fraction of elderly individuals could purchase long-term care services without exhausting their assets. Elderly individuals comprise approximately 53 percent of all the elderly, most of whom are women. This income disparity between sexes is important when considering the potential demand for long-term care services; elderly women represent 75 percent of the institutionalized elderly.

Projections of median family incomes for the aged over the next 30 years indicate improved economic prospects, primarily because of higher private pensions, Social Security, and increased numbers of women who entered the labor force at an earlier age. Those aged 65 to 74 years are expected to have more than a doubling of their incomes, those 75 to 84 almost a doubling of incomes, while those 85 and older only a 17 percent increase in incomes (11).

Empirical studies, such as the one by Scanlon, have found a very large and positive effect of per capita income for private-pay patients; the income elasticity of demand was between 2.27 and 2.83, indicating that for private-pay patients, nursing home care is a normal good. Other studies found that low income increases the chances of institutionalization (12). Thus for Medicaid-eligible people, nursing home care is an inferior good; the amount of noninstitutional services that can be bought by an elderly person rises as income rises, while the amount of Medicaid nursing home care that is used does not rise.

Important for any public policy discussion of long-term is the fact that the elderly vary greatly in their incomes and that many elderly, particularly women, blacks, the disabled, and those living alone, are least able to afford long-term care services.

Private Long-Term Care Insurance

Unlike the demand for acute medical services, private insurance for long-term care is negligible, covering less than 5 percent of long-term care expenses (13). In a well-functioning market for LTC insurance, the aged would insure against the uncertain catastrophic costs of long-term care. The aged appear to be quite risk averse, as evidenced by the high percentage (about 75 percent) that purchase Medi-gap insurance (private insurance supplemental to Medicare). It would therefore be expected that a higher percentage of the aged would purchase LTC insurance. An important issue, therefore, is whether there are imperfections in the LTC insurance market that cause private insurance to be such a small percentage of the total market.

The cost of a long stay in a nursing home can be expensive. The magnitude of the loss can be more than $40,000 a year, and 14 percent of the elderly have to spend down their assets to qualify for Medicaid. Since a small percent of the aged incur a financially catastrophic nursing home expense, such as event should be insurable. The aged should be willing to pay a price for such insurance in excess of the pure premium.

There are several reasons why there has been such a small demand for LTC insurance. First, many aged mistakenly believe that Medicare covers long-term nursing care. A 1985 national survey by the American Association of Retired Persons found that 70 percent of the aged believed that Medicare provides coverage for long stays in a nursing home, regardless of the type of care required (14). In fact, Medicare pays for a limited amount of care in a skilled nursing facility and skilled care is for those patients that can benefit from therapy, as after a stroke. Medi-gap policies are also mistakenly believed to cover long-term care services; instead, such policies often cover the deductibles and cost sharing of a relatively short stay in a skilled nursing facility.

The high price of LTC insurance relative to its pure premium decreases the quantity demanded of such insurance. High marketing and sales costs are required to enroll the aged on an individual basis. The lack of coordination of services to provide LTC care in the least costly manner contributes to a higher insurance expense, hence premium. Certain services, if provided in the home, may substitute for care in a nursing home. Informed patient agents, such as case managers, are needed to search out the appropriate settings to provide chronic long-term services, to contract with different providers, and to monitor the quality of care provided. Unfortunately, case managers are not often used. Instead, when long-term care is required, it is often provided in the most expensive setting, the nursing home.

Adverse selection also increases the pure premium, thereby discouraging healthy aged from buying LTC insurance. Those aged who are most in need of expensive chronic care and nursing home services are more likely to purchase such insurance. Further contributing to a high actuarially fair premium is the problem of moral hazard, particularly with regard to home care. If the price of such a service is reduced as a result of insurance coverage, the quantity demanded will increase by a large amount. Evidence from Medicare's home health benefit indicates that between 1990 and 1996 the number of people served doubled, the total number of visits increased by more than 300 percent, and the number of visits per person served increased by 114 percent (15). The range of activities of daily living—bathing, dressing, feeding, companionship, and other social support services—are "custodial" types of care and the use of such services would be greatly increased as the cost to the patient is decreased. Further, with insurance for home and nursing home care, marketed services are likely to be substituted for care currently provided by family members and friends.

High marketing costs, lack of care coordination, adverse selection, and moral hazard result in premiums that are high in relation to the income of many elderly. It has been estimated that only about 42 percent of the aged can afford to buy a long-term care policy (16).

Insurance companies have developed several mechanisms to protect themselves against adverse selection and moral hazard. To discourage the newly insured aged from taking immediate advantage of LTC insurance, a large deductible is included or the insurance takes effect only after the person has been in a nursing home for a certain period of time (e.g., forty-five days). Cost sharing is often used to decrease moral hazard; insurance companies will provide indemnity payments, which are less than the actual price per day or per home visit. Other common features of private insurance plans are limiting insurance coverage to services in a nursing home (to limit the moral hazard of home services), limiting coverage in a nursing home for a certain number of years, excluding preexisting conditions, and providing reimbursement only after some prior event, such as hospitalization.

Depending on which of the above benefits are included in a long-term care policy (and whether indemnity payments are inflation-adjusted), the annual premiums for a seventy-five-year-old person (in 1996) could vary between $2,010 to $5,660; for a sixty-five-year-old, from $720 to $1,980 (17). It becomes important for the aged person to fully understand the benefits available for the different premiums.

Low-income aged will not be able to afford large deductibles and cost sharing. Their catastrophic insurance program is Medicaid. Thus most private insurance is directed at the middle-income aged. Those with high incomes may self-insure or buy insurance.

The private long-term care insurance market has been undergoing important changes starting in the latter half of the 1980s. There has been an increase in the number of companies selling LTC insurance, from 75 companies in 1987 to 125 in 1995. The biggest change has been the growth of employer-sponsored LTC insurance plans, which increased from about 20,000 persons in 1988 to over 330,000 (cumulative) in 1995, for an average annual growth rate of 60 percent. The majority of LTC products are still purchased by individuals and group associations (80.1 percent) with the average age of the buyer being 68 years old. Employer-sponsored plans (12.2 percent) and LTC as part of a life insurance policy (7.7 percent) have younger buyers, 43 and 44 years of age, respectively (18).

Growth in the years ahead is likely to come from the employer market. The new tax law extends the employer tax exclusion to long-term care insurance (up to an annual maximum employer contribution), thereby reducing the price of such insurance. A number of employers believe that such policies will increase the productivity of their employees. Employees who are caregivers for parents or in-laws come in late, spend time on the phone, and leave early. Employer plans usually provide coverage for the employee's parents and in-laws in addition to the employee and his family.

In addition to indemnity LTC insurance, there are a limited number of LTC products for the middle- and high-income elderly that combine the insurance and service delivery products. Life-Care Communities charge a large admission fee, from $50,000 to $175,000, which the aged person can pay by selling her home. In return for the initial fee plus a monthly payment, from $600 to $2,500, the person moves into a community that promises to provide care for the rest of her life. As long as the person is able to, she lives independently in a home or an apartment. When she can no longer do so, she moves into an on-site nursing facility. Because of the high initial investment and significant monthly fees, such communities are applicable to only a small percent of the aged.

Home equity conversion has been proposed (although it has not proved very popular) as a means to enable the elderly to pay for their long-term care needs. The aged mortgage their home and receive monthly payments. Approximately two-thirds of the elderly own their own homes. It is psychologically difficult for many aged to mortgage their homes. Should a person do so, the incentive to maintain the home declines (which is a problem for the bank), the person may outlive the mortgage payments, or the payments may be insufficient for the person's long-term care needs. Further, since Medicaid treats a home as a protected asset for the spouse, why should the family deplete the asset? Home equity conversion is more applicable for meeting the elderly's daily living needs rather than long-term care requirements.

While the distribution of nursing home expense is large for a small percent of private-pay patients, which would seemingly make LTC insurance attractive, few of the elderly have such insurance. While LTC insurance is likely to increase, it will be insufficient to assist a large portion of the elderly.

Government Long-Term Care Insurance (Medicaid)

The major payer for nursing home care is Medicaid. To become Medicaid-eligible, an individual must spend down his assets to $2,000. Current law permits a spouse to keep half of the couple's assets, up to a maximum of $70,000, inflation-adjusted, including a private home. The institutionalized elderly under Medicaid must also turn over almost all of their income. Couples married for many years may divorce so that the partner entering the nursing home will not impoverish the other partner. Covert transfers of assets to children occur when a parent has to enter a nursing home.

While Medicaid also pays for some noninstitutional LTC services, it is small in comparison with its expenditures on nursing home care. Medicaid subsidization of nursing home care, but not of alternatives to such care, creates a distortion in prices facing the elderly person which favors institutionalization.

The other source of government funding for long-term care services is Medicare, which does not, however, cover chronic long-term care services. The $11.7 billion spent by Medicare in 1996 for nursing homes was for postacute nursing home services in skilled nursing facilities. Similarly, Medicare spent $18.3 billion in 1996 (up sharply from $3.9 billion in 1990) for postacute home care visits (19). The Medicare home health benefit is for short-term, part-time, or intermittent skilled care, and is to enable patients to regain their independent functioning.

Preadmission Screening for Medicaid Nursing Homes

Preadmission screening is yet another factor affecting the demand for long-term care and its components. Preadmission screening programs can also increase equity among Medicaid recipients; a more disabled patient would have a better chance of entering a nursing home than would a less disabled Medicaid recipient. Screening programs may counteract, in part, the tendency of nursing home operators to choose light-care over heavy-care Medicaid-eligible patients. Nursing home operators, however, cannot be forced to admit heavy-care patients. One additional problem with such preadmission programs is that they are not effective in screening all Medicaid nursing home patients since many private-pay patients in a nursing home eventually spend down to become Medicaid-eligible.

Consumer Ignorance, Search Costs, and Uncertainty

The demand side of the market for long-term care services is characterized by a large amount of consumer ignorance and uncertainty. The ignorance is due to a variety of factors. An elderly person's cognitive or affective functioning may be impaired, thereby reducing her capacity to make utility-maximizing decisions. At times decisions must be made by someone other than the person involved, usually a family member or a friend, and periodically by a physician. A person's functioning level, or degree of dependence, may change quickly or her support system may alter drastically due to the changed functioning level of the spouse. As a result, a whole new set of consumption choices have to be evaluated.

The financing and delivery of services provided by government agencies compound the problem—it is often difficult to figure out what services are available at what subsidy. All of this increases search costs, as a decision made by a relative for another person consumes the relative's time; each change in condition requires new learning, assessing of needs, and searching for competing providers of possible services; the fragmented social services system can make arranging services extremely difficult. In addition, the instability of the elderly person's condition creates uncertainty about what to do over a period of time.

All these problems can lead consumers and their agents to choose institutional over noninstitutional services.

The market response, both private and public, to high search costs and uncertainty has been case management. The case manager improves efficiency on the demand side by helping elderly people and their families understand what services can be purchased to deal with a disability, how services can substitute for or complement other services, what prices the consumer has to pay, who is eligible for subsidized services, where or how services can be found, and how to combine formal services with informal care. To the extent that the case manager is familiar with the probable course of the disability, future consumption of services can be predicted. The net result of case management is that noninstitutional care for an older person can become more feasible than was previously the case.

Case management is not yet widely available, and where it does exist, most people are not aware of its availability. A few large firms provide their employees with information on case management firms. When their employees suddenly have to assist their elderly parents in another part of the country, the employee does not have to take a leave of absence to make arrangements for his parents. Case management as a market response to high search costs is likely to develop more in coming years.

Currently, however, problems of consumer ignorance, search costs, and uncertainty are important factors in the market for long-term care. The presence of these factors causes deviations in the conditions for efficiency in this market.

Controls on the Number of Nursing Home Beds

Demand for nursing home care is likely to be different from *use* of nursing homes, which refers to the amount actually purchased or consumed. Although demand and use are usually the same, the distinction is relevant in the nursing home market because there are shortages of beds at the prevailing Medicaid price; the demand for beds by Medicaid eligibles exceeds the supply of beds at the Medicaid price. As an attempt to reduce its expenditures for nursing home care, Medicaid limits the number of nursing home beds in the state (certificate of need laws) and then rations access to those beds. Thus this regulatory program, used in approximately half of the states, affects not only the demand for nursing home beds but also the demands for noninstitutional care, both marketed and nonmarketed long-term care services.

The implications of demand being greater than observed utilization are twofold. For private-pay patients, an increase in demand is likely to lead to an increase in observed use, since supply will increase in response to an increase in the private-pay price; nursing home operators preferentially admit private pay-patients, thus the private-pay market is generally in equilibrium (20). Second, with supply constrained, an increase in demand by private-pay patients reduces available supply to Medicaid patients, thereby further increasing excess demand by Medicaid patients. An increase in the number of Medicaid patients would similarly increase the divergence between demand and use by Medicaid patients.

Empirical studies have found that the availability of nursing home beds did not affect demand by private-pay patients but it did affect demand by Medicaid patients. Thus the hypothesis that there is excess demand by Medicaid patients is supported.

To sum up studies on the demand for nursing home care, both private-pay and Medicaid patient demand for institutional services will increase with an increase in the aging of the population, higher disability levels, and a decrease in the level of informal support and would decrease with an increase in the price of noninstitutional substitutes.

Concluding Comments on the Demand for Long-Term Care

A number of factors cause inefficiencies to occur on the demand side. For example, when Medicaid subsidizes the price of nursing homes but not the prices of other long-term care services, a greater-than-optimal amount of nursing home care is demanded. Further, given the excess demand for nursing homes by Medicaid eligibles, those patients selected by the nursing homes may not be those most in need of nursing home care; Medicaid nursing home expenditures may therefore be allocated inefficiently. Perhaps the most important cause of inefficiency for both private-pay and Medicaid patients is their lack of knowledge of alternative suppliers, their relevant prices, and how the different types of care can be substituted for, or complemented with, each other. Without this information, consumers are not in a position to evaluate marginal benefits or relative prices; perceived benefits and prices differ from the actual benefits and prices. The development of case management systems would be a means of enhancing efficiency on the demand side.

The demand for long-term care services is expected to increase in coming years. However, the composition of that demand is likely to change. The aged population is increasing, particularly those most likely to demand long-term care, namely, the old-elderly. The incomes of the aged are also increasing, which is likely to lead to an increase in LTC insurance and in demand for noninstitutional services, since the aged prefer to remain in their own homes as long as possible. Higher-income elderly are also likely to increase the demand for private-pay nursing homes. If limits continue to be placed on the number of nursing home beds in a state, nursing home beds will be shifted toward private-pay patients and away from those serving Medicaid patients.

The divergence among the elderly in their ability to pay for long-term care services is likely to become greater. As the number of elderly and their ability to pay increase, we would expect the supply side to respond, both in terms of quantity of services and in innovative methods of delivering those services. The case management approach is likely to become more prevalent as the ability of the elderly to pay for such services increases and as Medicaid views it as an approach to decreasing nursing home expenditures.

THE SUPPLY OF LONG-TERM CARE SERVICES

Background

The supply of long-term care services consists of marketed and nonmarketed services. The provision of nonmarketed services depends on noneconomic reasons, such as a desire to care for a spouse or a parent, as well as economic factors, such as the price of marketed LTC services, which is a substitute for nonmarketed services. The supply of marketed LTC services depends on the price paid for such services, the cost of inputs for producing such services, and government regulation. (Technology is assumed to be held constant.) As the price paid for LTC services increases, so does its supply; an increase in the price of inputs used in producing long-term care will lead to a smaller supply of such services. And regulations limiting the number of nursing home beds will limit the supply of nursing home services.

The supply of marketed long-term care services consists of institutional care (i.e., nursing homes) and noninstitutional care that is generally provided in the recipient's home. There is a spectrum of long-term care services available for the elderly in between the nursing home and home care. There are, for example, 40,000 board and care homes that provide for 550,000 elderly (21). Residents in these homes vary from a few to large numbers; they typically need assistance with daily activities but not for skilled care. This growing industry varies in the quality of services provided. In some states these homes are regulated while in others they are not. Board and care homes are a potential lower-cost substitute for nursing homes.

Similar in concept but generally for those with higher incomes are congregate housing arrangements. An example of such an arrangement is a housing unit, which may be privately or governmentally funded, and which provides primarily nonmedical services to frail elderly, such as meals and social activities. These institutions provide supportive services to enable the elderly to remain independent. There are, in addition, life care communities, in which individuals live independently; as they require additional services they receive assisted living services as well as nursing home care when needed. And lastly, there is life care at home, whereby the elderly can purchase varying levels of services to enable them to remain in their home as long as possible.

Medicare also pays for services provided in the home; however, these services are *not* considered to be long-term care services. A physician is responsible for establishing and periodically reviewing the services provided, and the services are generally provided for a short duration. Medicaid provides for home-based services that include non-nursing care, such as homemaker-type services. In 1996 there were about 10,000 Medicare-certified home health agencies (up from 5,800 in 1990). The number of agencies providing homemaker-type services, meals, adult day care, and congregate housing for the elderly has been increasing.

The following analysis of the supply of long-term care services, however, emphasizes nursing homes, which receive between 80 and 90 percent of all long-term care expenditures. Further, the nursing home industry is subject to a great deal of government regulation; state agencies establish limits on the number of nursing home beds, establish standards of care in those facilities, and determine reimbursement for nursing home services. Nursing homes are also the most expensive element of long-term care, to the government as a payer under Medicaid and to private-pay patients.

As shown in Table 19.6, the rise in expenditures for nursing homes has been very rapid, from $1.5 billion in 1965 to $8.7 billion in 1975 to $30.6 billion in 1985 to $78 billion in 1995. The rapid growth in this industry makes it suitable for analysis in terms of its efficiency and equity.

As of 1996 there were 16,800 nursing homes that contained 1.8 million beds. Occupancy rates for nursing homes are high, generally 90 percent, and there were almost 1.6 million nursing home residents in 1996 (22). Within the category of nursing homes, 66 percent are for-profit; the remainder are nonprofit (26 percent) and government-controlled (8 percent). Fifty-two percent of all nursing homes were part of a chain. Most

TABLE 19.6 Expenditures for Nursing Home Care, 1960–95

Year	Total (in millions)	Annual Percent Increase
1960	$848	
1965	1,471	14.7%
1970	4,217	37.3
1975	8,668	21.1
1980	17,649	20.7
1985	30,679	14.8
1990	50,928	13.2
1995	77,877	9.0

Source: U.S. Department of Health and Human Services, Health Care Financing Administration, unpublished data, 1996.

nursing homes are certified by Medicare and Medicaid as either skilled nursing facilities (SNFs) or as intermediate care facilities (ICFs); the remainder, 25 percent, are not certified. SNFs generally provide a higher level of care than do ICFs. The average bed size of a nursing home is less than one hundred beds.

The picture that emerges from this description of the nursing home industry is that it is predominately for-profit, operates at high occupancy rates, and is heavily dependent on Medicaid for payment.

Determinants of Nursing Home Costs

The government is a large purchaser, a monopsonist, in the market for nursing home care. Researchers have attempted to estimate the determinants of nursing home average costs, which governments could then use as a basis for reimbursing nursing home firms. Appropriate nursing home reimbursement incentives can be established to achieve efficiency and equity. For example, if larger-scale facilities have lower average costs than those of smaller-scale facilities, payments to nursing homes could be based on the average cost of larger homes. Similarly, to increase access by the most disabled Medicaid patient, cost studies have tried to estimate how much it costs nursing homes to provide care for the more disabled patients. State governments could then establish payment incentives that reward firms for caring for the more disabled elderly.

The major limitation to cost function studies is the ability to separate the nursing home's product (i.e., the type of patient it serves and the quality of care provided) from other factors affecting the cost of care in that home. For example, if nonprofit facilities treat higher-cost, more disabled patients than those treated by for-profit facilities, then ownership status also becomes a proxy for disability status. Yet facilities may also differ as to their efficiency; the incentives for cost minimization facing a for-profit and a nonprofit facility are different. Thus ownership status may also be a proxy for efficiency incentives. Determining the most efficient average cost curve for each type of patient for purposes of government reimbursement is difficult when each of the factors affecting costs cannot be estimated separately. The public policy usefulness of the results is thereby reduced.

Patient characteristics and quality of care are crucial to an analysis of the determinants of nursing home costs because the product produced by a firm with low quality and a lightly disabled patient population is very different from that produced by a firm with high quality and a severely disabled patient population. Each firm would be on a separate average cost curve, reflecting product differences.

Data limitations in measuring product characteristics make it difficult to set reimbursement rates that help control (or encourage) provider behavior to achieve two potentially important government policy goals: adequate access to nursing home care by heavy-care Medicaid-pay patients, and a desired level of quality—that is, the desired supply volume of a nursing home product of a particular type.

Following is a brief summary of the results of nursing home cost studies (23).

1. Size. Studies indicate that there are no large economies of scale (holding occupancy rates constant).

2. Occupancy rates. Most studies show that average costs per patient day decline as occupancy rates increase (holding size and other variables constant). This indicates that marginal costs per patient day tend to be below average costs until all beds are either filled or almost completely filled.

3. Ownership type. Virtually every study has shown that for-profit facilities have lower average costs per patient day than do nonprofit or government facilities. For-profits also have lower RN staffing ratios. There are several possible explanations for these findings: differences in efficiency; a philanthropic wage policy, whereby nonprofits pay higher wage rates to their employees or to family members of the managers; and nonprofit homes' purchase of services from manager-owned suppliers. (Hospital-based nursing home facilities have substantially greater average costs than those of free standing [not hospital-related] nursing homes.)

4. Nursing home location. Nursing homes that face higher input prices because of their location (rather than incentives for efficiency) are expected to be on higher average cost curves. Most studies that include location or input prices as a market characteristic conclude that either location of the facility or level of wages in the area or both significantly affect average cost per patient day.

5. Percent of Medicaid-pay patients. A higher percent of Medicaid patients in the nursing home is an indication both of the state's purchasing power over the nursing home to hold down costs and staffing as well as the degree of competition faced by the home. The lower the percentage of private-pay patients, the lower the competition facing the home.

6. Construction moratoriums and CON. Limits on nursing home bed supplies result in excess demand for the home. The effect is likely to be lower nursing home costs, hence lower quality of care. Greater competition among nursing homes is likely to result in the homes taking patients with heavy care needs and higher staffing ratios.

7. Patient characteristics and quality. Many studies have used some indicator of patient condition, such as case mix and "activities of daily living" (ADL) measures, aggregated to the facility level. Quality is difficult to measure, although some studies have used patients with ulcerations, urinary tract infections, and restraint rates (24). These studies showed a positive and significant relationship between severity of patient condition and costs.

One study, in estimating the effect of different Medicaid payment systems (flat rate and cost-based payment) on quality of nursing home care, measured quality in the following way: estimating the determinants of staff intensity and then the effect of staff intensity on patient outcomes, to determine whether more intensive staffing results in better outcomes (25). Since patient care is so individualized, more intensive staffing could be a quality measure by itself. Staff intensity was measured as the number of RNs.

An important public policy implication of cost studies is that since case mix is an important determinant of cost, reimbursement systems should adjust payment to providers to account for case-mix differences, to avoid nursing home discrimination against heavy-care patients. The measurement of quality, its relationship to cost, along with methods of quality validation remain important issues for designing and monitoring Medicaid payment systems.

Analysis of the Supply of Nursing Home Services

To predict nursing home behavior in response to changes in the market and to government policies, a model of the nursing home as a firm is necessary (26). Nursing homes are assumed to act as though they were profit maximizers. This model of the nursing home is shown in Figure 19.2.

There are two types of patients, private-pay and Medicaid-pay; further, the Medicaid reimbursement price is below the private-pay price and is a flat-rate price; nursing homes can have as many Medicaid patients as they want at the flat-rate price, shown by the horizontal line *MP*. The nursing home faces a demand curve *DD* for private-pay patients which is downward-sloping since each firm differs somewhat from other nursing homes in terms of its location, level of care, and quality. (Location is a particularly important factor to consumers of nursing homes since five of six nursing home residents live in a

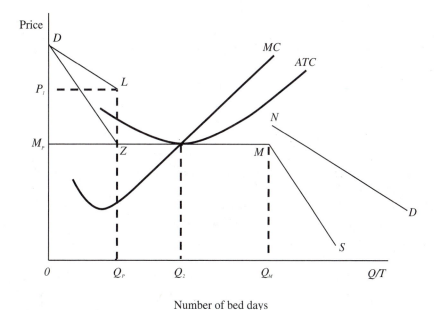

Number of bed days

FIGURE 19.2 • A model of pricing and output for private-pay and Medicaid patients by a proprietary nursing home.

nursing home located less than twenty-five miles from their home [27].) Associated with the demand curve is a marginal revenue curve *MR,* which shows the marginal revenue received by the firm for each bed day supplied. The average costs of the typical firm is shown by *AC* and the marginal costs of producing an additional bed day is shown by *MC.*

If the nursing home were to accept only private-pay patients, the firm's profit-maximizing strategy would be to set price at that point where its marginal cost equals its marginal revenue; that point would also determine the number of private-pay patients the firm will accept. A firm that accepts both private-pay and Medicaid-pay patients faces a demand curve that has three segments: *DL, ZM,* and *ND.* For segments *DL* and *ND,* the firm is a price setter; for *ZM,* which is the Medicaid price, the firm is a price taker. At Q_p, where the Medicaid price equals marginal revenue from private-pay patients, the original private-pay demand curve is shifted to the right by the amount *ZM* or by the $Q_p Q_m$ Medicaid patients who demand care.

At each point along *ZM,* marginal revenue from Medicaid patients exceeds that which can be obtained from more than Q_p private-pay patients. To the right of Q_m, private-pay demand is once again relevant, since marginal revenue from Medicaid-pay patients becomes zero to the right of Q_m. For the profit-maximizing firm the relevant marginal revenue curve becomes *DZMS.*

The typical nursing home faces the situation shown in Figure 19.2; the firm's marginal revenue equals its marginal cost at a point to the right of *Z* and to the left of *M.* The profit-maximizing firm will produce $0Q_2$ units of output. The firm acts as a price discriminator. It sets marginal cost equal to marginal revenue for each type of patient, and sells different quantities at different prices in each market. The firm sells $0Q_p$ bed days for private-pay patients at price P_1 and $Q_p Q_m$ at the Medicaid price M_p. Unless the marginal revenues for each type of patient were equal, the firm could increase profits by reducing output in the market where marginal revenue was lower and increasing output where marginal revenue was higher.

At the Medicaid price of M_p, $Q_2 Q_m$ Medicaid patients who demand nursing home care do not receive it. Thus excess demand by Medicaid patients can exist in an equilibrium situation. The consequence is a waiting list for Medicaid patients and difficulty by hospitals in discharging their Medicaid patients to a nursing home.

When excess demand by Medicaid patients exists, the firm is also able to discriminate according to the type of Medicaid patient it will accept. If the Medicaid price is the same for all types of Medicaid patients, the firm has an incentive to choose less costly patients—those requiring the fewest services. Given excess demand at the single Medicaid price, even if it is profitable at the existing reimbursement price to accept a heavy-care person on Medicaid, it is more profitable for the firm to accept a light-care person. With a larger bed supply, firms would serve both types of persons. But faced with excess demand in equilibrium, profit-maximizing firms would discriminate against heavy-care patients if they are to maximize their profits.

GOVERNMENT POLICY AND THE NURSING HOME INDUSTRY

Since state governments purchase the majority of nursing home services on behalf of Medicaid patients, they are monopsonist buyers in a market with many small suppliers. The government's monopsony power allows it to set nursing home rates that are different from private-pay prices. The government's potential power is enormous since it is also the regulator of nursing home services. As both the largest purchaser and chief regulator of nursing homes, government via its policies affects the performance of this industry. To understand the performance of this industry, it is therefore important to understand the government's objectives.

Ideally, the government should be interested in setting prices so that each nursing home will attempt to be internally efficient as well as to take advantage of economies of scale; that is, the home should be of a size that is at the lowest point on the long-run average-cost curve. Annual rates of increase in the government's price should reflect relative increases in input prices. Further, government payment should reflect both the quality level desired by government and the type of patient cared for in the home (i.e., light- or heavy-care patients). Finally, since nursing homes are but one input in the production of LTC services, government payment should attempt to minimize the cost of producing LTC services; that is, lower-cost substitutes, such as home care services, should be used whenever it is both medically and socially possible.

Observed government behavior is such as to question whether government payment and regulatory policies are intended to achieve the objectives noted above. By examining actual government reimbursement and regulatory policies, it may be possible to infer intended rather than stated government objectives with respect to nursing homes.

By 1979 almost all states enacted CON regulations affecting nursing homes. By controlling the number of nursing home beds in the state, the government can indirectly control the number of Medicaid patients and therefore Medicaid expenditures. Since CON limits entry into the nursing home industry, existing nursing homes can charge higher prices to private-pay patients (and have the option of providing lower-quality care) than would be the case without CON regulations. In the earlier discussion on the demand for nursing home care, it was shown that demand for nursing home beds is increasing over time. With a limited supply of beds, an increased demand, both by private-pay and Medicaid-pay patients, will result in the for-profit nursing home increasing prices to private-pay patients and admitting more private-pay patients relative to Medicaid-pay patients (28).

With reference to Figure 19.3, an increase in demand by private-pay patients will shift their demand to the right, causing the new marginal revenue line, DZ', to intersect the horizontal Medicaid price at some point to the right of its current location (Z' instead of Z). When the nursing home operator again equates marginal revenue in each of the two separate markets to marginal cost, the number of private-pay bed days will increase (from

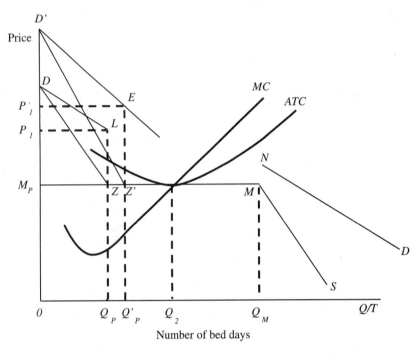

FIGURE 19.3 • An increase in private-pay demand in a nursing home serving private-pay and Medicaid patients.

Q_p to Q_p'), fewer bed days will be available for Medicaid patients, and the private-pay price will increase (from P_1 to P_1') to that point on the new demand curve above the intersection of the new marginal revenue curve and the Medicaid price.

CON barriers decrease both efficiency and equity. Because nursing homes can charge higher prices to private-pay patients, nursing homes that are internally inefficient or that have obsolete facilities can survive and even prosper. Access by Medicaid patients has been reduced, particularly for heavy-care Medicaid patients, and excess Medicaid demand has increased, since total Medicaid demand is also growing over time. As a result of supply constraints, the government spends less on nursing home care; however, an additional burden has been imposed on the Medicaid patient unable to enter the nursing home and on family and friends to care for that person.

A redistribution of income occurs as a result of CON, from private-pay patients (who pay higher prices) to nursing homes. Economic profits to the nursing home are increased (the difference between the private-pay price and the firm's average total cost curve multiplied by its number of private-pay patients). These additional profits are unable to induce entry into the industry since entry is restricted by CON. As would be expected, anecdotal evidence suggests that nursing homes favor CON restrictions. After conducting interviews in eight states, Feder and Scanlon concluded: "In every state we visited, they [the nursing home operators] recognized the advantages of restricting entry. . . . In California, for example, a spokesman for the nursing home association described his members as 'happy as clams' with entry restrictions, and anxious to ensure that they covered all possible competitive threats, including reclassification of hospital beds to nursing home status" (29).

As a monopsonist, the reimbursement system can also be used by government to achieve certain policy objectives. States have substantial discretion in the design of their nursing home reimbursement systems. The different reimbursement systems that states can choose between are retrospective payment of costs or a prospective flat rate. Under retrospective systems, states give each nursing home an interim rate based on the home's previous costs and then pay the home a final amount after the firm's actual costs have been incurred and reported. A ceiling is usually set at some dollar amount or at some percentile (e.g., 75th) of all the nursing home's costs. If a state uses a prospective payment system, a flat rate is established and all facilities are paid one rate regardless of an individual facility's costs. The flat rate may be determined through negotiation with the nursing home association or be based on the cost experience of a grouping of nursing homes.

These payment systems may be modified by adjusting payment for characteristics of the nursing home's patient population; attempts to do so, however, are limited by appropriate patient classification systems. Unless adjustments for patient care requirements are made, there is a disincentive for for-profit homes to admit heavy-care patients, particularly under a prospective or flat-rate payment system.

The various payment systems provide differing incentives for efficiency and for the type of patient to be admitted. Nursing homes are able to react to payment policies by becoming more efficient, changing their size, selecting a different case mix of Medicaid patients, changing the level of quality provided to Medicaid patients, and varying the number of Medicaid patients admitted. Any payment system must evaluate its effects on each of the outcomes noted above. For example, under a retrospective system, as long as a home is under a ceiling, there is no incentive to be efficient, since they will collect whatever costs they report. In fact, the nursing home has an incentive to spend more funds so as to increase their cost base for future reimbursement increases.

Prospective flat-rate systems provide efficiency incentives if the home can keep the difference between its costs and the payment. However, under a prospective system the home can make a greater profit by not admitting patients requiring a great amount of care. It therefore becomes crucial in all payment systems to base payment on a patient case-mix measure that reflects the costs of caring for those patients. However, unless the case-mix payment accurately reflects patient costs, incentives and disincentives are created to care for certain types of patients and not others.

A recent study examined how accurately Minnesota's case-mix payment system reflected the costs of caring for those patients. The authors found that because actual costs were different from the case-mix payments, some patients were more profitable than others. The payment system was not profit-neutral. The nursing homes responded to these profitability differences by increasing their percent of profitable patients and decreasing the less profitable ones (30).

One additional concern of policymakers is the extent to which a payment system creates fraud incentives. A retrospective cost-based system with a high ceiling offers the greatest fraud incentives. Rather than necessarily admitting heavy-care patients, a firm could produce efficiently and achieve economic profits by buying overpriced services from a firm owned by the owner or by hiring and paying high salaries to family members or friends.

The Regulation of Quality in the Nursing Home Industry

Although quality in non-nursing home settings is also a concern, almost all past attention has focused on nursing homes. Quality of nursing home care is multidimensional. However, two major areas can be identified: quality of care and quality of life.

Quality-of-care issues include how well a nursing home assesses the care needs of a resident patient, develops a care plan for that resident, and implements that plan.

Quality-of-life issues are quite varied; they include the degree to which residents have privacy, independence, personal control over daily activities, the ability to keep personal belongings, input into care planning, and personal safety and security of possessions. They also include the ability to eat decent food and to engage in varied social activities. On a more basic level, they include protection from physical and psychological abuse.

Quality-of-life issues are relevant because, unlike an acute care setting, a nursing home is a total living situation for a long-term patient—a home as well as a place to receive medical and personal care services.

There are very wide variations in the quality of care provided by nursing homes. While there are many firms that provide good or very good quality nursing home services, other firms provide care that a 1986 Institute of Medicine report has called "shockingly deficient." Reflecting on the regulatory system and the persistence of serious problems in the quality of nursing home services, the same report observed: "There is broad consensus that government regulation of nursing homes, as it now functions, is not satisfactory because it allows too many marginal or substandard facilities to continue in operation. . . . The apparent inability of the current regulatory system either to force substandard facilities to improve their performance or to eliminate them is the underlying circumstance that prompted this study" (31).

These observations are certainly not new. Why has the regulatory system allowed substandard facilities to continue to operate despite the eruption of periodically highly publicized scandals on nursing home quality?

Many elderly patients requiring long-term care are ill informed as to both the type of care needed and the quality of nursing homes. Problems of consumer choice are compounded by the cognitive impairment of substantial numbers of prospective patients. Given the limits placed on the number of nursing home beds in most states, the difficulties of finding a nursing home bed are particularly troublesome when finding a bed is medically urgent. Moreover, once in a nursing home, patients are often restricted from moving, both because of the difficulty of finding another bed and because of the trauma often associated with transfer. The regulation of quality by government agencies developed because of these limited abilities of prospective patients to make appropriate choices. Why, then, has government regulation of quality consistently failed?

To understand government policies toward nursing homes it is important to determine whether the government itself has a particular interest in the outcome rather than considering the government's role as merely trying to achieve the ideal objectives of economic efficiency and increased equity. Attributing a motivation to the government beyond that of an ideal regulator provides a more accurate explanation as to why efficiency and equity in the provision of nursing home services are rarely, if ever, achieved.

Limiting the increase in Medicaid expenditures, which is the fastest-growing component of state expenditures, has become an overriding concern of government Medicaid agencies. There are many competing constituencies within a state for these state taxes, such as public schools and state colleges. State legislators, desiring reelection, are reluctant to vote for increased taxes. Yet to be able to respond to competing demands (and receive political support) from various constituencies for state funding, legislators must make trade-offs as to how limited state funds are allocated. The cost to legislators of increased Medicaid funding is the forgone political support they would receive by allocating those funds to other constituencies. Thus constraining the increase in Medicaid expenditures is a policy objective of government.

When attempting to limit Medicaid expenditures, however, government agencies (which are assumed to adhere to the preferences of the legislature) face another constraint. Too little funding for nursing home care would result in nursing homes refusing to provide such services and threatening to transfer patients, or the level of quality would be so low that there would be a major scandal, with adverse publicity to the regulatory agency. Thus the regulatory agency must also consider the preferences of the nursing home association, which also has a concentrated interest in funding for nursing homes. As a monopsonist, the state's payment and regulatory policies have a major effect on the profitability of nursing homes. It is therefore in the interest of the nursing home industry to represent their interests (and provide political support) to legislators so as to receive favorable payment and regulatory policies.

Patients and their families are a third group with an interest in Medicaid funding and regulatory policies. Unfortunately, this group has not been successful in organizing themselves, representing their interests before the legislature, and providing political support (votes).

Thus the outcome of Medicaid policy within a state appears to be a compromise between the interests of the government, seeking to constrain its expenditures, and the nursing home industry, seeking increased profitability. The resulting policy has usually been for the government to constrain Medicaid expenditures by limiting the rise in payments to nursing homes, limiting the number of nursing home beds, and providing minimal regulation of the quality of care provided by the nursing home. The net effect of these policies is to create both inefficiencies and inequities in the supply of nursing home care.

These government policies are satisfactory to the nursing home industry. By limiting entry, CON regulations reduce competition among firms, allowing firms to raise private-pay prices, and permit the firms to be more selective in the Medicaid patients they admit, decreasing access to heavy-care patients.

Nursing homes do not have to compete for Medicaid patients. Why should they incur the additional expense of improving quality if they can attract as many Medicaid patients as they want? Increased quality to Medicaid patients adds to production costs but not to revenues. The incentive for nursing homes to provide poor quality to Medicaid patients remains as long as government policies encourage excess demand for Medicaid beds (32). Even if the Medicaid rate were to increase so as to enable the homes to increase quality, it is not necessary for the nursing homes to do so as long as they have excess demand for their beds.

It is not surprising that regulatory agencies are lax in setting, monitoring, and enforcing high standards of quality, given the government's objective of limiting Medicaid expenditures. Enforcement of high-quality standards can be quite costly to the government.

Government's primary objective with respect to nursing homes has been containment of the growth of its Medicaid payments. Certificate of need regulation and Medicaid rate-setting policies have been able to limit the rise in government expenditures, but they have had a negative impact on quality. When there is competition among firms, a firm producing a poor-quality product runs the risk of losing market share to other firms producing higher-quality services for the same price. Limits on the number of nursing home beds, however, have created excess demand for those beds by Medicaid patients.

Since quality assurance is not a high priority of a regulatory agency, the quality criteria for licensure and certification of facilities permit firms great latitude in the quality of care they provide. Quality criteria can be divided into those that pertain to structure, process, and outcomes of the provision of nursing home services (33). Structural criteria include the resources available to provide care—the credentials or training of the staff, the ratio of staff to patients, the safety features in the facility, and the equipment available to be used. Process criteria include the type and method of provision, as well as quantity of services actually delivered to the residents. Outcome criteria include changes in the functional, physical, and mental status of the residents.

Government regulations have tended to focus on structural criteria of quality, despite the fact that they simply measure the capacity to deliver appropriate services—not whether the services were actually delivered or whether they had any impact on the outcomes of residents. Although these criteria are relatively objective and easy to measure relative to other criteria, there is little evidence of consistent associations between these measures and process of care or outcome measures.

Even the best quality criteria are useless without active monitoring and enforcement of sanctions (or incentives) to promote desired firm behavior. The only federal enforcement sanction available has been decertification—denying a facility the ability to receive Medicaid-pay or Medicare-pay patients. This is a drastic action, both for the firm and for the residents of the facility, who may have great difficulty finding another bed in another home, and who can suffer from "transfer trauma." It has seldom been used.

Recently, many states have used their capacity to license facilities to institute "intermediate" or less drastic sanctions. These sanctions include fines, suspension of admissions, and receiverships. The extent of available sanctions and the degree to which they are used varies greatly from state to state. Referring to this interstate variation, the Institute of Medicine report concludes that "Despite extensive government regulation for more than 10 years, some nursing homes can be found in every state that provide seriously inadequate quality of care and quality of life. . . . Tolerance of inadequate care also appears to be widespread" (34).

The Institute of Medicine made several recommendations to improve the quality of nursing home services, several of which emphasized improved regulatory quality criteria focusing on residents and outcomes, more federal involvement in quality issues, and improved state monitoring and enforcement procedures.

It is worthwhile to keep in mind that *the solution is not to just come up with new regulatory criteria, but to provide an incentive for the regulatory agency to actually do something to improve the quality of care.* According to the economic theory of regulation, public policy changes will occur only if nursing home residents and their advocates can form a more effective concentrated interest—to raise the political costs of inaction to the regulatory agency and legislators to the point where it is worth their while to pursue more rigorously the elimination of substandard nursing home care.

The following proposals attempt to improve the efficiency of the market:

1. Remove CON restrictions. Entry of new firms into the marketplace would create the conditions for greater price and nonprice (quality) competition. Allowing Medicaid-pay patients a choice of nursing homes would force producers of low-quality Medicaid-pay nursing homes to either upgrade their care or lose market share to producers of higher-quality care. Different approaches should be used to achieve government cost containment objectives and the elimination of inappropriate placement of patients in nursing homes. For example, strict mandatory pre-nursing home screening programs should be used, not only for people eligible for Medicaid at the point of entry into a nursing home, but also for people likely to spend down to Medicaid status while in the nursing home. No longer would an inefficient or low-quality home be protected by excess demand.

2. Increase funding for noninstitutional alternatives to nursing home care. Medicaid should view long-term care for the Medicaid population as a continuum, from in-home services to congregate living arrangements to nursing homes. To determine the appropriate setting for patients with different care needs, Medicaid should use case managers to evaluate patients' needs and have the necessary funding to pay for noninstitutional long-term care services for persons eligible to enter nursing homes. Medicaid case managers facing

a budget constraint for providing long-term care for the Medicaid population would improve the functioning of the market; they would be similar to informed consumers facing prices for different long-term care services.

3. Create incentives for quality care. Regulatory approaches that emphasize facility characteristics as indicators of quality are inadequate. The emphasis on quality should instead be shifted to the patient rather than the facility. Payments should be based on the types of patients cared for in the home, thereby eliminating the home's incentive to select lighter-care patients. If anything, there should be a financial incentive for the home to select the heavy-care patients. Similar to positive cash incentives for improved quality, there should be negative financial incentives for poor quality. Closure of a home is too drastic a measure and is therefore seldom used. Graduated financial penalties and placing the home in receivership would be less harmful to the home's residents. A receiver could operate the home until the deficiencies are improved or until the home is sold.

Quality is more likely to improve once there is greater market competition for patients. Similar to other areas of the economy, such as hotel services, universities, and automobiles, improved quality results from market competition, not from government regulation. Relying solely on government agencies to improve the quality of nursing home services would be to repeat past mistakes and we should expect to be continually shocked at revelations of the poor quality of our nursing homes.

FINANCING LONG-TERM CARE

Government financing of long-term care has been an important political issue. Medicaid pays for nursing home services and home care for those who are chronically ill. However, to be eligible for Medicaid, patients must spend down their assets. Medicare was designed to provide care for those aged who are ill but it was not intended to serve as a LTC financing program. And, as previously discussed, a very small percent of the aged have private LTC insurance. There are thus important gaps in coverage for the middle-class aged who need LTC services. The fear by middle-class aged of having to deplete their assets should they or their spouse require extended LTC services has resulted in political pressure for a government program to finance long-term care.

To evaluate government policies for financing long-term care, it is necessary to determine both the effects on equity and economic efficiency of each of the various proposals. Equity considerations are twofold: first, are like people treated similarly and, second, if it is desired to redistribute resources, do lower-income groups receive proportionately more benefits relative to their costs than those in higher-income groups? To determine the equity of various proposals it becomes important to determine which elderly receive government benefits and the method used to finance those benefits. Economic efficiency involves two considerations: are the benefits greater than (or at least equal to) the costs of producing those benefits, and is the least-cost combination of benefits provided?

The concerns by the aged with regard to their LTC needs are as follows: First, most aged would prefer to stay out of a nursing home and be treated in their own home as long as possible. Thus the aged would like LTC benefits to include coverage for services in their home. Second, if a person has to enter a nursing home, it should be a good-quality facility. Given the shortage of nursing homes as a result of supply restrictions, access to a good quality nursing home is a major reason why elderly join life care communities. Third, elderly with assets desire to protect their estates, either for spouses or for children (35). Related to this concern is the desire not to impoverish a spouse by entering a nursing home or to spend down assets to go on Medicaid. There are a number of instances where the aged have had to divorce to protect the financial security of the spouse when one member had to qualify for Medicaid.

Private LTC insurance, while likely to increase, will be insufficient to assist a large portion of the elderly. Insurance will still be too expensive for many aged and adverse selection, the purchase of insurance by those who are at high risk for institutionalization, will further increase the cost of such insurance. Thus alternative public financing approaches need to be considered.

The first issue in discussing government financing of long-term care is eligibility. Should public subsidies be used to assist those in financial distress, or should the program be universal and assist all aged regardless of income level? Currently, low-income aged must rely on Medicaid when they can no longer be cared for in their homes; it is difficult for these aged to gain entry into a nursing home (because of supply controls) and, when they do, the quality of their care is suspect. A financing program to achieve the objective of assisting low-income aged would be based on an income ("means") and asset test.

The second motivation underlying government intervention in long-term care is to assist the middle-class elderly. The elderly do not want to deplete their assets if they require long-term care in a home. They want to retain funds for their spouse and they want to be able to leave their assets to their children. To ensure that the middle-class aged benefit from a government-subsidized program, eligibility would not be based on a means test.

It is with regard to the latter group of the aged that government intervention becomes controversial. Should the middle- and upper-income aged be subsidized so as to be able to retain their assets? (36).

Universal, non-means- and non-asset-tested programs that have been proposed provide either "front-end" or "back-end" coverage for nursing homes. The front-end approach would subsidize all the aged for their first three months or first two years in a nursing home ("first dollar" coverage). After that period the aged would be responsible for any remaining nursing home expense. Front-end coverage would be quite expensive and would benefit those aged who would otherwise have spent down their assets (see Figure 19.1). It would also benefit many aged who could afford to pay for such care. Insurance is typically purchased to prevent a catastrophic loss. Front-end coverage would not serve this purpose for many aged, who would be at risk for a longer lifetime use of the nursing home.

"Back-end" coverage subsidizes the use of the nursing home after a large deductible has been met, for example, the first three months or two years of nursing home use. Back-end coverage would benefit the middle- and high-income aged who can afford to pay the large front-end deductible. By providing a government subsidy for their catastrophic expense, middle- and high-income aged would no longer have purchase private LTC insurance.

How a program is financed will determine who benefits and bears the cost. To the extent that the nonpoor aged are subsidized in their use of LTC services, their costs must be financed by imposing a tax on other population groups. Medicare and Social Security are financed by imposing a tax on the working population. This tax is borne by both low- and high-income employees. It is inequitable to tax a low-income employee to provide a subsidy to an aged person with higher income and greater assets. The effect of such a subsidy is a redistribution of wealth, from low-wage employees to higher-income aged and their children who will inherit their assets. The aged currently receive huge subsidies from Medicare and Social Security; another wage-related tax would provide them with yet another large subsidy.

If the aged were to be subsidized for LTC, it would be more equitable to finance this new benefit from general income tax revenues rather than an increase in payroll taxes. However, the aged would still gain a large subsidy for which they would pay little of the cost.

A more equitable approach for financing a new benefit to the aged would be to tax Social Security payments. This approach would not worsen intergenerational equity, as would the above financing approaches. Higher-income aged, who would be the beneficiaries, would pay the cost of it.

Proposals that rely on income and asset-tested programs, such as an improved Medicaid program, also seek to expand the role of the private sector. For example, treating the purchase of LTC insurance similar to employer-paid health insurance would lower its price and increase the quantity demanded. (This approach was included in the 1997 tax law changes.) Another approach is to allow individuals to invest pretax dollars for an individual LTC account. These approaches, which provide an implicit subsidy, would again benefit those who could afford to purchase such insurance. Government subsidies would still be needed for those who could not afford the above private approaches. And the government would have to continue to subsidize current low-income elderly (37).

Unless government-funded long-term care programs specifically target those aged with the lowest incomes and assets and are financed by an income tax, such programs will be more expensive, are unlikely to be equitable, would involve further intergenerational wealth transfers, and should be viewed more as asset protection programs for middle- and high-income elderly. To the extent that legislation is enacted to protect the aged against the costs of long-term care, *regardless of their income levels,* the redistribution of incomes resulting from government programs will be worsened. The working population, including low-income workers, will bear an increased burden for providing new health benefits to the aged, some of whom have greater incomes and assets than themselves.

Long-term care programs should be designed to minimize the cost of long-term care. Even though care in a nursing home can be a financially catastrophic event, any long-term care program should also provide coverage for services in the home. Current approaches for financing long-term care create a distortion in demand for nursing home care. To ensure that home health services are used as a substitute for nursing home care, a case management system, used in conjunction with long-term care coverage, would provide incentives for minimizing the cost of long-term care to the elderly.

SUMMARY

The age structure of the population is changing. The number of persons sixty-five years of age and older is increasing, in both absolute and relative terms, particularly the old-aged. The need for long-term care is directly related to the aging of the population, particularly for those in the eighty-five and older age group, one of the fastest-growing age groups. The increasing number of dependent elderly will demand both institutional and noninstitutional long-term care services. The current method of financing long-term care, largely out-of-pocket payments and Medicaid, is considered to be inadequate. Private long-term care insurance is a minor payer. There is a large disparity among the aged in their ability to pay for long-term care. Those aged least able to pay for long-term care are also those who will be in the oldest age groups and who are more likely to need such services.

There have been a number of imperfections in the long-term care market; in particular, the nursing home industry's performance has been far from optimal. Government regulation limiting the supply of nursing homes has resulted in excess demand and reduced access to care by Medicaid patients with heavy care needs. Government payment systems have not adequately adjusted payments according to patient case mix, thereby providing nursing homes with extra profits while decreasing access by those patients most in need of such care. And quality of care has not been adequately monitored, together with appropriate sanctions for poor quality of service.

Unless Medicaid agencies design accurate case-mix-related payment systems, together with appropriate quality indicators, nursing homes will have little incentive to take heavy-care patients and provide high quality. In addition, case managers are needed in the Medicaid market to act as informed agents and make decisions based on the needs of the patient and the relative prices of different long-term care services. Unless these actions are undertaken, the most severely disabled aged and lighter-care patients will not be in the most appropriate settings.

Patients and their family are not well informed as to patients' care needs, appropriate settings for the patients, and identifying when care needs change. The use of case managers as informed purchasers of LTC services for both private as well as Medicaid patients would improve the functioning of this market. Unfortunately, case management is not readily available and is expensive for private patients. The growth of private insurance will continue but will be more likely to benefit the young-aged. Many old-aged are unlikely to be able afford such insurance. Medicaid is likely to remain as the long-term care insurance for the low-income aged.

The growth of the population of the aged, in addition to increasing the demand for long-term care, is important for another reason. The aged are becoming an increasing portion of the population. Previously this age group has received enormous intergenerational subsidies from Medicare and Social Security. However, as the relative size of the working population begins to shrink, it becomes more expensive per employee to continue to provide these huge subsidies. Thus the likelihood of providing additional intergenerational subsidies in the form of a universal LTC insurance program to protect their assets is less likely. In the future, government subsidies for LTC are likely to be for low-income aged. Current middle- and high-income aged, as well as future aged, will have to rely on their private means for their LTC needs.

Until the decreasing financial capacity of the working population to subsidize additional benefits to the aged become obvious to politicians, there will continue to be pressure by the aged for a universal LTC subsidy. However, any government policy to assure access to long-term care for the aged should be evaluated in terms of efficiency (whether the cost of achieving that objective is least costly) and equity (are the benefits directed toward those with low incomes and financed by those with higher incomes, regardless of age level?).

Key Terms and Concepts

- Demographic trends
- Dependency ratio
- LTC demand determinants
- Nonmarket caregiving

- Case-mix payment systems
- CON and nursing homes
- For-profit nursing homes and the allocation of beds
- "Front-end" and "back-end" subsidies
- Government as a monopsonist purchaser
- Income and asset eligibility tests

Review Questions

1. What are the demographic and economic trends affecting the outlook for long-term care?
2. Why has the private market for long-term care insurance grown so slowly?
3. Why does private long-term care insurance, when sold to the aged, have such a high loading charge relative to the pure premium?

4. Evaluate the redistributive effects of "front-end" and "back-end" government subsidies for long-term care.

5. Evaluate the redistributive effects of income-related refundable tax credits for private long-term care insurance and also the use of individual retirement accounts.

6. How would a for-profit nursing home allocate its beds between private-pay and Medicaid patients? (Use diagrams as part of your answer.)

7. How would the allocation of beds in a for-profit nursing home between private-pay and Medicaid patients change if the following occurred:
    a. The Medicaid price for nursing home patients increased
    b. The demand for nursing homes by private patients increased

REFERENCES

1. Bruce Vladek, Nancy Miller, and Steven Clauser, "The Changing Face of Long Term Care," *Health Care Financing Review,* 14(4), Summer 1993: 5–22; and William J. Scanlon, "A Perspective on Long-Term Care for the Elderly," *Health Care Financing Review,* 1988 Annual Supplement: 7–16.

2. Achintya Dey, "Characteristics of Elderly Nursing Home Residents: Data from the 1995 National Nursing Home Survey," *Advance Data,* 289 (Hyattsville, Md.: National Center for Health Statistics, 1997).

3. Scanlon, *op. cit.,* p. 9.

4. See James D. Reschovsky, "Demand for and Access to Institutional Long Term Care: The Role of Medicaid in Nursing Home Markets," *Inquiry,* 33(1), Spring 1996: 15–29.

5. William J. Scanlon, "A Theory of the Nursing Home Market," *Inquiry* 17(1), Spring 1980: 25.

6. John A. Nyman, "The Private Demand for Nursing Home Care," *Journal of Health Economics,* 8, 1989: 209–231.

7. Susan L. Ettner, "The Effect of the Medicaid Home Care Benefit on Long-Term Care Choices of the Elderly," *Economic Inquiry,* 32(1), January 1994: 103–127.

8. Stephen Crystal, "Measuring Income and Inequality Among the Elderly," *The Gerontologist,* 26(1), February 1986: 56.

9. Karen Holden and Timothy Smeeding, "The Insecure Elderly Caught Inbetween," *Milbank Quarterly,* 68(2), 1990: 205.

10. Crystal, *op. cit.*

11. Alice Rivlin and Joshua Wiener, *Caring for the Disabled Elderly: Who Will Pay?* (Washington, D.C.: The Brookings Institution, 1988), Tables 2.2 and 2.3.

12. See U.S. General Accounting Office, *Medicaid and Nursing Home Care: Cost Increases and the Need for Services Are Creating Problems for the States and the Elderly* (Washington, D.C.: U.S. Government Printing Office, October 21, 1983).

13. Marc A. Cohen and A. K. Nanda Kumar, "The Changing Face of Long Term Care Insurance in 1994: Profiles and Innovations in a Dynamic Market," *Inquiry,* 34(1), Spring 1997.

14. Jay N. Greenberg, Don S. Westwater, and Walter N. Leutz, "Long-Term Care Insurance: How Will It Sell?" *Business and Health,* November 1986: 21.

15. *Medicare and the American Health Care System: Report to the Congress, op. cit.,* p. 111.

16. M. Cohen et al., "The Financial Capacity of the Elderly to Insure for Long Term Care," *The Gerontologist,* 27(4), 1987: 494–502.

17. "Your Needs, Plus Your Budget, Equals What to Pay on Long-Term-Care Policy," *The Wall Street Journal,* March 21, 1997, p. C1.

18. Susan Coronel and Michelle Kitchman, *Long Term Care Insurance in 1995* (Washington, D.C.: Health Insurance Association of America, May 1997).

19. *Medicare and the American Health Care System: Report to the Congress* (Washington, D.C.: Prospective Payment Assessment Commission, June 1997), p. 137.

20. Susan L. Ettner, "Do Elderly Medicaid Patients Experience Reduced Access to Nursing Home Care?" *Journal of Health Economics,* 12(3), October 1993: 259–280.

21. *Board and Care: Insufficient Assurance That Residents' Needs Are Identified and Met* (Washington, D.C.: U.S. General Accounting Office, GAO/HRD-89-50, February, 1989).

22. *Nursing Home Update—1996,* Medical Expenditure Panel Survey Highlights (Rockville, Md.: Agency for Health Care Policy and Research, AHCPR Pub. No. 97-0036, July 1997).

23. The following is a partial list of nursing home cost studies: William Scanlon and William Weissert, "Nursing Home Cost Function Analysis: A Critique,"*Health Services Research,* 18(3), Fall 1983: 387–391; and John Nyman, "The Marginal Cost of Nursing Home Care," *Journal of Health Economics,* 7, 1988: 393–412.

24. Robert E. Schlenker, "Nursing Home Costs, Medicaid Rates, and Profits under Alternative Medicaid Payment Systems," *Health Services Research,* 26(5), December 1991: 624–649.

25. Joel W. Cohen and William D. Spector, "The Effect of Medicaid Reimbursement on Quality of Care in Nursing Homes," *Journal of Health Economics,* 15(1), February 1996: 23–48.

26. This discussion is based on William J. Scanlon, "A Theory of the Nursing Home Market," *Inquiry,* 17, Spring 1980: 25–41. Also see Christine Bishop, "Competition in the Market for Nursing Home Care," *Journal of Health Politics, Policy and Law,* 13(2), Summer 1988: 341–360.

27. Ronald J. Vogel, "The Industrial Organization of the Nursing Home Industry," in Ronald Vogel and Hans C. Palmer, eds., *Long Term Care: Perspectives from Research and Demonstrations* (Washington, D.C.: Health Care Financing Administration, 1983).

28. John A. Nyman, "The Effects of Market Concentration and Excess Demand on the Price of Nursing Home Care," *Journal of Industrial Economics,* 42(2), June 1994: 193–204.

29. Judith Feder and William Scanlon, "Regulating the Bed Supply in Nursing Homes," *Milbank Memorial Fund Quarterly,* 58(1), 1980: 54.

30. John A. Nyman and Robert A. Connor, "Do Case-Mix Adjusted Nursing Home Reimbursements Actually Reflect Costs? Minnesota's Experience," *Journal of Health Economics,* 13(2), July 1994: 145–162.

31. Institute of Medicine, Committee on Nursing Home Regulation, *Improving the Quality of Care in Nursing Homes* (Washington, D.C.: National Academy Press, 1986), pp. 2–3. For a review of the literature on quality, see Mark Davis, "Nursing Home Quality: A Review and Analysis," *Medical Care Review,* 48(2), Summer 1991: 129–166.

32. For a more complete discussion of the effect of excess demand on quality of care, see John A.

Nyman, "Prospective and 'Cost-Plus' Medicaid Reimbursement, Excess Medicaid Demand and the Quality of Nursing Home Care," *Journal of Health Economics,* 4, 1985: 237–259.

33. Avedis Donabedian, "Evaluating the Quality of Medical Care," *Milbank Memorial Fund Quarterly,* 44, 1966: 166–206; Avedis Donabedian, *Exploration in Quality Assessment and Monitoring,* vol. 1, *The Definition of Quality and Approaches to Its Assessment* (Ann Arbor, Mich.: Health Administration Press, 1980).

34. Institute of Medicine, *op. cit.,* p. 13. See also John Nyman and Cynthia Geyer, "Promoting the Quality of Life in Nursing Homes: Can Regulation Succeed?" *Journal of Health Politics, Policy and Law,* 14(4), Winter 1989: 797–816.

35. Pauly explains the lack of long-term care insurance as a rational decision on the part of risk-averse nonpoor aged. See Mark V. Pauly, "The Rational Nonpurchase of Long-Term Care Insurance," *Journal of Political Economy,* 98(1), February 1990: 153–168.

36. Other countries use various approaches for financing LTC for their aged. Some use income tests, others have a universal insurance program but require cost sharing from the beneficiary's pension. See *Long Term Care: Other Countries Tighten Budgets While Seeking Better Access* (Washington, D.C.: U.S. General Accounting Office, GAO/HEHS-94-154, August 1994).

37. For additional readings on financing long term care, see William J. Scanlon, "Possible Reforms for Financing Long-Term Care," *Journal of Economic Perspectives,* 6(3), Summer 1992: 43–58; *Policy Choices for Long-Term Care* (Washington, D.C.: Congressional Budget Office, June 1991); and Edward C. Norton and Joseph P. Newhouse, "Policy Options for Public Long-term Care Insurance," *Journal of the American Medical Association,* 271(19), May 18, 1994: 1520–1524.

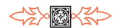

CHAPTER

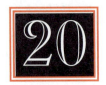

Concluding Comments on the Economics of Medical Care

The purpose of this book has been to demonstrate how the tools of economics can be applied to the study of medical care issues. Economic concepts define and clarify the different aspects of medical care, making them more susceptible to analysis. Differences in values among persons on particular issues can be separated from differences in the efficiency with which various approaches can achieve a specified set of values. In addition, economics offers criteria for determining whether particular policies increase or decrease *efficiency* and *equity* in medical care. Of course, economic analysis cannot resolve all of the concerns that health professionals and the public have with regard to medical care—different problems require different training and analytical expertise. Particularly suited to economic analysis are problems that relate to issues of scarcity. Economics can illustrate the choices a society can make when its resources are insufficient to achieve everything it desires.

The two economic tools used throughout this book are marginal analysis, which underlies all optimization problems, and supply and demand analysis, which is used for predicting new equilibrium situations. These two tools are interrelated in that supply and demand analysis assumes that individuals or firms are attempting to maximize some goal (e.g., utility or profits) subject to certain budget constraints. The welfare criteria we have been concerned with are the effects on equity as a result of different policies, both government and private, and the implications of different market structures, such as competitive and monopolistic markets.

The use of our economic tools may lead to outcomes that turn out to be different than what we predict. One such example is that high rates of return to a medical education should have led to an increase in the supply of physicians during the 1960s. When predictions differ from what we observe (there were very small increases in the supply of physicians during the 1960s), it does not mean that the theory is wrong or not useful. Instead, it is an indication that one or more of the assumptions underlying the theory have been violated. In the physician example cited above, the assumption of free entry in medical education was incorrect. When the underlying assumptions are different from what is expected, there is a possible role for public policy.

There are a number of assumptions with respect to medical care that cause it to be different from other industries. Lack of consumer information, uncertainty of a medical expense and the outcome of a treatment, the dual role of the physician as the patient's agent and the supplier of a service, the large number of not-for-profit firms, payment of providers (in the past) on a cost basis, limitations on entry into the professions and on tasks that different professionals may perform, and the desire by society to provide all its members with a minimum level of medical care are some of the characteristics of this market. Although many of these characteristics might exist in other sectors, together they give medical care a certain uniqueness.

Important policy differences occur with respect to this set of unique characteristics. Should the medical care sector be made to conform to more traditional economic markets (e.g., competitive pricing with its attendant incentives) or should medical care be insulated from traditional market forces? Public policy regarding the organization of medical services has changed over time.

Public policy has been directed at three types of issues. These issues are the three basic questions that any economic system or industry must resolve.

One decision any society must make is how much of its limited resources to spend on medical care. It should be recognized that the choice in question is *not* how much to spend on health, but how much to spend on medical services. People do not desire increased health at any cost, as evidenced by their refusal to stop smoking, wear seat belts, and change their personal health habits. Medical services expenditures serve, to some extent, as a substitute for undertaking other activities to enhance health; part of the costs of neglecting these activities is borne by the population at large through taxes and higher medical care prices. While the decision of how much to spend on health may be more relevant, the emphasis of the U.S. medical care system and government financing is to provide more medical services. Increasing medical services is only one approach, and perhaps one of the most costly, for improving health.

Before it can be determined how much should be spent on medical care, it must be decided whether consumers or government will make the necessary decisions. It should again be recognized that this basic decision, which will determine the size and growth of the medical sector, depends on resolving the issue of whose values are to dominate medical care. Are consumers to determine how much of their income is to be allocated to medical care, or is that decision to be made by a government agency? The answer will determine whether the consumer's or agency's preferences will dominate.

A market approach for allocating resources to different goods and services maximizes the consumer's preferences. Opponents of consumer decision making in medical care argue that medical care is a special case in which a market approach may not be applicable; first, because consumers may not be aware of their medical needs; second, because they may not spend as much as some persons believe they should on their medical needs; and third, because they do not have sufficient information with which to judge different providers. Under such circumstances, opponents of a market approach propose substituting another mechanism for making the necessary allocation choices in medical care, but they do not explicitly state the criteria by which such a system of decision making should be judged. The proponents of relying on consumer preferences recognize the limitations of the current medical system and how they affect consumer ability to make choices, and seek to improve the consumer's decision-making process.

The amount, type, and quality of medical services provided have not represented either consumer or third-party preferences. Consumer demands for medical care have been distorted both by their excess health coverage resulting from tax subsidies for the purchase of health insurance and by the lack of information on which to base their choices. The most knowledgeable purchaser in the medical market—the patient's physician—lacked the fiscal responsibility to be concerned with medical costs and also had a financial interest in the service that she provides. These distortions in the medical care market resulted in the provision of either too many or too few of certain types of services. Public and private policy, starting in the 1980s, sought to improve the consumers' ability to make choices, make consumers bear more of the costs of their choices, and change the incentives facing the providers. In the private sector employees pay higher premiums for more costly health plans and there are increased deductibles and cost sharing in the indemnity plan. Both Medicare and Medicaid are increasing their use of managed care programs. Consumers are being given financial incentives to limit their use of medical services or choose more restrictive plans for a lower premium.

The second basic decision to be made in any medical system is how medical services should be produced to ensure that output is provided at lowest cost. Rapidly increasing medical costs, duplication of expensive facilities and services, provision of unnecessary services, excessive testing, and unnecessary use of expensive settings were all indications that the efficiency with which medical care was provided could be improved. The alternatives were to rely on greater regulation and controls implemented by government agencies, or reliance on competitive market pressures to achieve greater efficiency.

Many people have a basic distrust of a market system; many are also concerned that the patient would not be adequately protected when providers are motivated by profits. This concern for consumer protection resulted in many restrictions, which were promoted by health associations. However, restrictions on who can perform certain tasks, who may enter the health professions, and who may be reimbursed for providing medical services did not eliminate the public's concern that unnecessary services were being performed and that unethical health providers practiced medicine. What these restrictions achieved, however, was the reduction of competition in the provision of medical services.

The movement to a price-competitive market in medical care started in the early 1980s. The Supreme Court ruled in 1982 that anti-trust laws were applicable to the health professions. As anticompetitive restrictions, such as prohibitions on advertising and provider boycotts of insurers promoting cost containment methods, were eliminated and efficiency incentives increased, the health sector underwent a major restructuring. Under the pressure by business and government to reduce their medical expenditures, providers began to take advantage of economies of scale in the provision of services; hospitals merged and the number of hospitals in large multihospital systems increased. Physicians joined group practices so as to take advantage of economies of scale, to be able to market their services as PPOs to businesses, and to bargain with insurance companies. The number of managed care systems increased, as insurance companies and the government found that providers have better incentives to minimize the cost of care when they are placed at financial risk.

A great deal of regulation still exists in medical care. Many states rely on CON laws. Both hospital and physician prices are regulated under Medicare. And there are still many state restrictions on tasks that different professionals may perform. The current trend, however, is away from a regulatory approach for organizing the delivery system and toward a more price-competitive system. As the incentives facing providers change, so does the structure of the medical system. The organization of medical services will begin to reflect the most efficient methods of delivery.

The concern with efficiency in supply and containment of increasing medical expenditures are important public policy issues. Unless ways are found to limit the rise in medical expenditures, benefits and beneficiaries of current public programs will be reduced and new programs are unlikely to be initiated. There is limited political interest in raising taxes to continue funding existing programs for the poor or for funding new programs. Thus efficiency issues, how to provide medical services, affect society's choices regarding equity and access, which is the third basic decision that must be made in medical care.

Equity concerns, namely, how much medical care should be redistributed to different population groups and by what mechanisms, is the other major public policy issue in health care today. The choice of how much medical care to provide to particular population groups is affected by the costs of such programs. Proposals to change Medicare and Medicaid are more often justified by their ability to contain costs than for their success in redistributing medical services.

All health policy has redistributive effects. Explicit redistributive programs, such as Medicare, Medicaid, care for the uninsured, tax subsidies for the purchase of health insurance, and financing medical (and other health professional) education, involve raising funds and distributing benefits. However, some types of taxes and some methods of distributing benefits result in greater equity than others. If low-income persons pay more in taxes than they receive in benefits, they are worse off as a result of that policy. Similarly, when high-income groups receive more in benefits than they pay in taxes, they are made better off. Both types of situations exist in medical care. Unless the costs and benefits of public programs, including tax policies, by income group can be directly measured, such perverse redistributive situations are likely to continue.

While increased efficiency, concern over the rise in medical expenditures, and greater equity in financing medical services are major health policy issues today, it is important to remember that each of these policies has its own redistributive effects. There will be winners and losers, depending on how each of these policy issues are resolved. The uninsured can be provided for by shifting their costs to employers, raising taxes on the middle class to provide them with a voucher for an HMO, or by paying hospitals for uncompensated care. Limiting the rise in medical expenditures can be achieved by increasing patient sensitivity to prices and premiums or by establishing expenditure limits on hospitals and physicians (as is done under Medicare). And increased efficiency can be achieved by moving toward a competitive medical market or by government-mandated standards for medical procedures. Each of these alternative approaches for achieving equity, efficiency, and expenditure limits will impose burdens and provide benefits to different groups. As such, the policy mix is as likely to be guided by the benefits and burdens imposed on politically influential groups as it is by the efficiency and equity of specific approaches.

How efficiently each of the current (and proposed) subsidy programs redistributes medical services to those least able to afford them is questionable. Tax subsidy programs generally benefit those with higher incomes. Given a choice, many of those who receive care in government hospitals would prefer to receive their care in community hospitals. The large majority of the subsidies to health professional education are received by those who come from higher-income families and who subsequently enter those professions whose incomes are among the highest in the country. Recognizing the redistributive benefits that these huge subsidy programs provide to different income groups is the first step in deciding whether the resulting redistributive effects are desirable. It should then be determined whether such subsidies could be provided more efficiently so that they are received by those in greatest financial need.

Implementing redistributive programs involves providing benefits (in excess of their costs) to one group by imposing costs (in excess of the benefits they receive) on other groups. To anticipate which groups will receive net benefits and which groups are likely to bear those costs requires a theory of legislation. According to the economic theory of legislation, legislation is provided in return for political support. Within such a framework, it is unlikely that redistributive legislation will be provided or financed in as equitable a manner as possible unless those groups able to offer the greatest amount of political support are favorably disposed toward that approach.

Funding for redistributive programs could be reduced if government subsidies were targeted directly to desired beneficiary groups. However, the political feasibility of achieving an efficient strategy for redistribution is questionable. Each subsidy program creates a distinct constituency. Attempts to change the current distribution of subsidies will encounter strong political opposition from those who benefit from current subsidies. The potential beneficiaries of a more direct subsidy system, the poor, are not as well organized to engage in the political process, as is indicated by the very fact of their need for such subsidies. Economic analysis of current, as well as of proposed, subsidy programs can indicate who is likely to receive such subsidies and whether the stated objectives of such subsidies can be achieved in a more efficient manner. Such information is an input into the political process and raises the political costs to those who might otherwise benefit from less efficient subsidy schemes.

Medical care is different from other industries. Yet economic analysis is useful in many ways: it offers a perspective by which medical care issues can be viewed and analyzed; the effects of legislation, both current and proposed, affecting the demand and supply sides of the medical markets can be evaluated; and economics can be used to perform such traditional tasks, such as planning and forecasting, which are required in any industry. In addition to its tools—the prediction of changes in prices, quantities, and total expenditures, and the formulation of rules for cost minimization—economics provides a set of criteria for evaluating whether various policies achieve greater efficiency and equity in medical care. The application of these tools and criteria should increase our understanding of medical care issues, enable us to separate differences in values from differences in approaches to achieving a given set of values, and provide us with the ability to evaluate the costs and benefits of different choices in medical care.

GLOSSARY

Actual versus list prices—Actual prices are the fees collected or paid for a particular good or service. The difference between actual and list prices are provider discounts, which vary by type of payer.

Actuarially fair insurance—The expected insurance payments (benefits) are equivalent to the premiums paid by beneficiaries (plus a competitive loading charge).

Adverse selection—This occurs when high-risk individuals have more information on their health status than the insurer and are thus able to buy insurance at a premium based on a lower-risk group.

Ambulatory surgical center (ASC)—A freestanding outpatient facility that performs certain types of procedures.

American Medical Association (AMA)—A national organization established in 1897 to represent the collective interests of physicians.

Anti-trust laws—A body of legislation that promotes competition in the U.S. economy.

Any willing provider laws—Laws that permit the participation of any physician in an insurer's provider panel, thereby negating providers' incentive to compete on price to be included in the panel.

Assignment/participation—An agreement whereby the provider accepts the approved fee from the third-party payer and is not permitted to change the patient more, except for the appropriate co-payment fees.

"Back end" long-term care subsidies—A proposed long-term care insurance plan that would subsidize patients' use of a nursing home after they have paid a large deductible or have financed the first year themselves.

Balance billing—When the physician collects from the patient the difference between the third-party payer's approved fee and the physician's fee.

Barriers to entry—Barriers that may be legal, for example, licensing laws and patents, or economic, that is, economies of scale, that limit entry into an industry.

Benefit/premium ratio—The percent of the total premium paid out in benefits to each insured group divided by the price of insurance.

Blue Cross/Blue Shield—Nonprofit health insurers that provide insurance for hospital (Blue Cross) and physician (Blue Shield) services.

Canadian-type health system—A form of national health insurance in which medical services are free to everyone and the providers are paid by the government. Expenditure limits are used to restrict the growth in medical use and costs.

Capitation incentives—The provider becomes concerned with the coordination of all medical services, providing care in the least costly manner, monitoring the cost of enrollee's hospital use, increasing physician productivity, prescribing less costly drugs, and being innovative in the delivery of medical services. Conversely, the provider has an incentive to reduce use of services and decrease patient access.

Captitation payment—A risk-sharing arrangement in which the provider group receives a predetermined fixed payment per member per month (PMPM) in return for providing all of the contracted services.

Case-mix index—A measure of the relative complexity of the patient mix treated in a given medical care setting.

Certificate of need (CON) laws—State laws requiring health care providers to receive prior approval from a state agency for capital expenditures exceeding certain predetermined levels. CON laws are an entry barrier.

Charity hypothesis of physician pricing—Physicians charge higher prices to those with higher incomes and thereby claim that they are able to charge lower prices to those with lower incomes.

Co-insurance/Co-payment—A fixed percentage of the medical provider's fee made by the insurance beneficiary at the point of service.

Community rating—The insurance premium is the same to all of the insured, regardless of their claims experience or risk group.

Comparable worth-based wages—Wages and salaries are based on an evaluation of each position, including skill required, effort involved, working conditions, and level of responsibility, rather than by supply and demand conditions for that position.

Competitive markets—The interaction between a large number of buyers and suppliers, where no single seller or buyer can influence the market price.

Concentrated interests—When some regulation or legislation has a sufficiently large effect on a group to make it worthwhile for that group to invest resources to either forestall or promote that effect.

Consumer expenditure survey—Conducted as part of the consumer price index, it is a survey of spending patterns for a specified period of time. It consists of two components: an interview survey to determine expenditures on those items (and quantity) that people purchase and a diary or record-keeping survey in which individuals are asked to record small, frequently purchased items.

Consumer price index—Calculated by the Bureau of Labor Statistics, it is used as a measure of the rate of inflation or the rate at which a family's income would have to increase to keep up with rising prices.

Consumer sovereignty—Consumers, rather than health professionals or government, choose the goods and services they can purchase with their incomes.

Cost containment programs—Approaches used to reduce health care costs, such as utilization review and deductibles.

Cost of treatment price index—An index of the price of medical care based on how the price of a treatment for a particular diagnosis changes over time.

Cost shifting—The belief that providers charge a higher price to privately insured patients because some payers, such as Medicaid or the uninsured, do not pay their full costs.

Cost-effectiveness analysis—Determining which programs or inputs are least costly for achieving a given objective.

Criteria for cost minimization—The combination of services and inputs used to provide medical care that is both technically and economically efficient.

Declining marginal productivity of health inputs—The additional contribution to output of a health input declines as more of that input is used.

Decreasing marginal utility of wealth—The marginal utility of money decreases as the person's income or wealth increases.

Deductible—Consumers pay a flat dollar amount for medical services before their insurance picks up all or part of the remainder of the price of that service.

Demand shift (or an increase in demand)—Changes in factors affecting demand, other than the price of the service.

Derived demand—Demand for the particular service or input is based on the demand for the service for which it is an input.

Determinants of firm's demand for employees—Based on the employee's wage relative to other inputs, their employees' marginal productivity, the demand for the firm's product, and the price at which the firm's product is sold.

Diagnosis-related group (DRG)—A method of reimbursement established under Medicare to pay hospitals based on a fixed price per admission, according to diagnostic-related groupings.

Diffuse costs—When the burden of a tax or program is spread over a large population and is relatively small per person so that the per person costs of opposing such a burden exceeds the actual size of the burden on the person.

Direct subsidies—Financial aid targeted to a specific group.

Dynamic shortages—Occurs when demand is increasing more rapidly than supply so that an equilibrium price has not yet been established.

Economic shortage—Occurs when the quantity demanded exceeds the quantity supplied at a given price.

Economic efficiency—The optimal rate of output occurs when all marginal benefits equal all marginal costs.

Economic theory of government—A theory of legislative and regulatory outcomes that assumes political markets are no different from economic markets, in that organized groups seek to further their self-interests.

Economies of scale—The relationship between long-run average total cost (LRATC) and size of firm; as firm size increases, LRATC falls, reaches a minimum, and eventually rises. In a competitive market each firm operates at that size that is at the lowest point on the LRATC curve.

For a given size market, the larger the firm size required to achieve the minimum costs of production, the fewer the number of firms that will be able to compete.

Employee Retirement Income Security Act (ERISA) of 1974—A federal law that applies to employee welfare plans and preempts all state laws with regard to reporting and disclosure policies. Applicable to self-funded plans.

Employer-mandated health insurance—Under this health reform plan all employers are required to provide medical insurance to their employees.

Equal financial access—A value judgment underlying national health insurance in which the financial barriers to medical care would be the same for all.

Equal treatment for equal needs—A value judgment underlying national health insurance in which everyone should have equal consumption of medical services, regardless of economic or other factors affecting utilization.

Expected utility—The weighted sum of the utilities of each outcome, with the weights being the probabilities of each outcome. With regard to the demand for health insurance, expected utility has a linear relationship.

Experience rating—Insurance premiums are based on the claims experience or risk level, such as age, of each insured group.

Externalities—Occur when an action undertaken by an individual (or firm) has secondary effects on others and these effects are not taken into account by the normal operations of the price system.

Fee-for-service payment—A method of payment for medical care services in which payment is made for each unit of service provided.

Flexner Report—Published in 1910, it was a highly critical report evaluating the medical training of physicians in the United States and Canada. This report led to the restructuring of the education and training of physicians and the eventual closure of many medical schools.

Food and Drug Administration (FDA)—A government agency that regulates entry into the U.S. market of all drugs and relevant medical devices, requiring manufacturing firms to demonstrate that their products are safe and efficacious.

Formulary—A list of prescription drugs reimbursed under a managed care plan.

Foundations for medical care (FMCs)—Nonprofit organizations that own plant, property, and equipment associated with medical practice and employ nonphysician employees. The foundation, in turn, contracts with the medical group on a mutually exclusive basis to see all of the foundation's patients. The foundation controls the contracts with payers, owns the medical records, and distributes a negotiated share to the medical group.

"Free choice of provider"—Included in the original Medicare and Medicaid legislation, all beneficiaries had to have access to all providers. Precluded closed provider panels and capitated HMOs. This provision is considered by economists to be anticompetitive in that it limits competition; beneficiaries could not choose a closed provider panel in return for lower prices or increased benefits.

"Front end" long-term care subsidies—A proposed long-term care insurance plan that would subsidize the first part of a nursing home stay (e.g., the first three months or first two years), after which the aged would be responsible for any remaining nursing home expense.

Gatekeeper—In many HMOs the primary care physician, or "gatekeeper," is responsible for the administration of the patient's treatment, and must coordinate and authorize all medical services, laboratory studies, specialty referrals, and hospitalizations.

Geographic market definition—Used in anti-trust analysis to determine the relevant market in which a health care provider competes. The broader the geographic market, the greater the number of substitutes available to the purchaser—hence the smaller the market share of merging firms.

Government policy instruments—The use of tax policy, expenditures, and regulation available to government to achieve its policy objectives.

Government policy objectives—According to public interest theory, government has two policy objectives: improve market efficiency and improve equity and redistribute resources (based on a societal value judgment).

Guaranteed issue—Health insurers have to offer health insurance to those willing to purchase it.

Guaranteed renewal—Requires health insurers to renew all health insurance policies within standard rate bands, thereby precluding insurers from dropping individuals or groups who incur high medical costs.

Health Care Financing Administration (HCFA)—Part of the U.S. Department of Health and Human Services and responsible for administering Medicare and the federal aspect of state Medicaid programs.

Health inputs—The resources that are used to produce a specific output referred to as "good health."

Health maintenance organization (HMO)—A type of managed care plan that offers prepaid comprehensive health care coverage for hospital and physician services, relying on its medical providers to minimize the cost of providing medical services. HMOs contract with or directly employ participating health care providers. Enrollees must pay the full cost of receiving service from non-network providers.

Health manpower surplus—Occurs when physicians (or other health professionals) are earning a below-normal rate of return (price would be below the average total cost curve).

Health production function—Describes the technical relationship between each of the health inputs and their effect (marginal productivity) on health.

HHI (Herfindahl-Hirschman) index—The measure of concentration used by the Department of Justice in its merger guidelines. This index, by summing the square of each provider's market share, makes it sensitive to both the number of firms and their relative sizes.

Horizontal merger—When two or more firms from the same market merge to form one firm.

Hospital collusion—Competing hospitals in the same market agree on price, output, and wage policies.

Incidence of the payroll tax—The extent to which the payroll tax is borne by employers or employees is determined by the elasticity of demand and supply curves for labor.

Income contingent loan repayment plans—A student loan program to cover both tuition and living expenses that would be repaid by paying a fixed percent of adjusted gross income. The fixed percent would be based on the amount borrowed.

Indemnity insurance—Medical insurance that pays the provider or the patient a predetermined amount for the medical service provided.

Independent provider association (IPA)—A physician-owned and -controlled contracting organization comprised of solo and small groups of physicians (on a nonexclusive basis) that enables the physicians to contract with payers on a unified basis.

Indirect subsidies—Financial aid not targeted to a specific group or recipient, available to all users of the subsidized service.

Individual mandate—A proposed national health insurance plan under which individuals are required to buy a minimum level of health insurance. Refundable tax credits are provided to those having incomes below a certain level.

Inferior good—An increase in income leads to a decrease in consumption of that good or service.

Inframarginal externalities—Even though there may be external benefits, the private market produces the optimal quantity (e.g., physicians).

In-kind subsidies—Noncash subsidies provided to specific beneficiary groups based on the donor's (middle class's) preferences.

Insurance premium—Consists of two parts: the expected medical expense of the insured group and the loading charge, which includes administrative expenses and profit.

Integrated delivery system (IDS)—A health care delivery system that includes or contracts with all the health care providers to provide coordinated medical services to the patient. An IDS also views itself as being responsible for the health status of its enrolled population.

Law of demand—The lower the price, the greater the quantity demanded.

Law of supply—The higher the price, the greater is the quantity firms are willing to produce.

Loading charge—That portion of the health insurance premium that is added to the pure (actuarially fair) premium, to include administrative expense and profit.

Managed care organization (MCO)—An organization that controls medical care costs and quality through utilization management, drug formularies, and profiling participating providers according to their appropriate use of medical services.

Mandated benefits—According to state insurance laws, specific medical services, providers, and population groups must be included in health insurance policies.

Marginal benefits—The change in total benefits from purchasing one additional unit.

Marginal contribution of medical care to health—The increase in health status resulting from an additional increment of medical services.

Marginal costs—The change in total costs from producing one additional unit.

Market equilibrium—When the independent actions of buyers and suppliers cause quantity demanded to equal quantity supplied. The result is an equilibrium price and quantity.

Market failure—May occur when there are market imperfections so that price-competitive markets will not produce the optimal amount of output, which is defined as price equaling marginal cost.

Market imperfections—Occur as a result of lack of information by consumers regarding their medical diagnoses, treatment needs, the quality of different providers, and prices charged by different providers. Additional imperfections are tax-free employer-paid health insurance, restrictions on entry and on tasks, and externalities.

Market performance—An indication of the economic efficiency of the market. Economic efficiency occurs when the market price equals marginal cost. When there are no positive or negative externalities, the resulting rate of output is optimal. The marginal benefit (as indicated by market price) equals the marginal cost of producing that last unit.

Market power—An indication of the degree of monopoly power possessed by the firm. It is measured by the ratio of the firm's price to its marginal cost. The higher the price relative to its cost, the greater the firm's market power.

Market structure—The number of suppliers within the market, which is determined by the extent of economies of scale in relation to the size of the market and entry barriers, usually defines the competitiveness of the market.

Medicaid—A health insurance program financed by federal and state governments and administered by the states for qualifying segments of those with low incomes.

Medicaid risk contracts—A Medicaid managed care program in which an HMO contracts to provide medical services in return for a capitation premium.

Medical care price index—Calculated by the Bureau of Labor Statistics and included as part of the consumer price index, it is used as a measure of the rate of inflation in medical care prices.

Medical group—A group of physicians who coordinate their activities in one or more group facilities and who share common overhead expenses, medical records, and professional, technical, and administrative staffs.

Medical savings accounts (MSAs)—A form of national health insurance in which a person can annually contribute, tax free, an amount into his MSA equal to 75 percent of his deductible. The unused portion of the MSA can accumulate over time.

Medicare—A federally sponsored and supervised health insurance plan for the elderly. Part A—provides hospital insurance for inpatient care, home health agency visits, hospice, and skilled nursing facility. The aged are responsible for a deductible but do not have to pay an annual premium. Part B—provides payments for physician services, physician-ordered supplies and services, and outpatient hospital services. Part B is voluntary and the aged pay an annual premium that is 25 percent of the cost of the program in addition to having to pay a deductible and co-payment.

Medicare risk contract—Federally qualified HMOs receive from the government a monthly capitated fee for each enrolled Medicare beneficiary (in addition to the Part B beneficiary premium) and in return provide both Part A and Part B services, plus additional services, such as prescription drugs, as determined by the HMO. Enrollees using non-HMO participating providers are responsible for the full charges of such providers.

Medigap insurance policies—Privately purchased insurance policy by the elderly to supplement Medicare coverage by covering deductibles and co-payments.

Monopolistic competition—A market structure that is characterized by many competing firms, each producing a slightly differentiated product that is a close substitute to the products produced by competing firms.

Monopoly—A market structure in which there is a single seller of a product that has no close substitutes.

Monopoly model of physician pricing—Physicians face a downward sloping demand curve for their services and set prices according to where marginal revenue equals marginal costs.

Monopsony—A market structure characterized by a single purchaser.

Moral hazard—A situation where the individual alters her behavior when she has acquired insurance. Since insurance lowers the price of medical care, the insured will consume more care than if they had to pay the full price themselves.

Mortality rate—For a given population, the ratio of number of individuals who die divided by the average size of the population.

Multihospital system—A system in which a corporation owns, leases, or manages two or more acute care hospitals.

Multilayer system—A system in which reimbursement for medical services is made by multiple third-party payers.

Negative prices—A negative price is when a person or beneficiary group is paid to use a service. When the time and travel costs of a beneficiary group are lowered (e.g., locating facilities closer to the beneficiaries), these may also be considered to be negative prices.

Network health maintenance organization—A type of HMO that signs contracts with a number of group practices to provide medical services.

Nonmarket caregiving—Medical or nursing care provided by the patient's spouse or family without pay.

Nonprice hospital competition—Hospitals compete on the basis of their facilities and services and the latest technology, rather than on price.

Normal good—An increase in income leads to greater consumption.

Normative judgment of a shortage—A noneconomic definition of a health manpower shortage. Estimates of such a shortage are based on a determination of "need" in the population or on some professional estimate of health manpower requirements.

Not-for-profit—An institution that is not allowed to disburse its profits.

Nurse participation rates—The percentage of trained nurses who are employed.

Oligopoly—A market structure characterized by few firms, with each firm considering the actions of the other firms when making price and output decisions (interdependence among firms).

Omnibus Budget Reconciliation Act of 1989—Congressional passage of this legislation resulted in restructuring of physician reimbursement under the Medicare program.

Opportunity costs—Relevant costs for economic decision making, they include explicit as well as implicit costs. For example the opportunity costs of a medical education include the foregone income the student could have earned had she not gone to medical school.

Optimal rate of output—Occurs when the marginal benefit of the last unit equals the price of that unit, which in turn equals the marginal cost of producing the last unit.

Optimization techniques (marginal analysis)—Specify the appropriate criteria to be used when allocating scarce resources so as to minimize the cost of producing a given output or, similarly, maximize output, subject to a budget constraint. For example, costs are minimized when the ratio of the marginal product of each input divided by its cost is equal.

Out-of-pocket price—The amount that the beneficiary must pay after all other payments have been considered by the health plan.

Over-the-counter drug—A drug that is available for public purchase and self-directed use without a prescription.

Patient dumping—A situation where high-cost patients are not admitted to or are discharged early from a hospital because they either have no insurance or because the amount reimbursed by the third-party payer will be less than the cost of caring for these patients.

Per diem payments—A method of payment to institutional providers that is based on a fixed daily amount and does not differ according to the level of service provided.

Periodic reexamination—Would require physicians to maintain their qualifications by requiring them to undergo periodic testing for relicensure.

Physician/agency relationships—The physician acts on behalf of the patient. Agency relationships may be perfect or imperfect and method of physician payment, fee-for-service or capitation, would produce different behavioral responses among imperfect physician agents.

Physician control model of the hospital—The hospital's behavior, pricing, cost control, and investments are expected to be determined according to the medical staff's economic interests.

Physician hospital organization (PHO)—An organization where hospitals and their medical staffs develop new types of group practice arrangements that will allow the hospitals to seek contracts from HMOs and other carriers on behalf of physicians and the hospitals together.

Physician market entry barriers—Licensure, graduation from an approved medical school, and continual increases in training times cause the supply of physicians to be smaller than if such barriers did not exist. The ostensible reasons for such barriers, namely, a high-quality workforce, could be achieved more directly.

Physician/population ratio—The number of physicians per one hundred thousand population has often been used as an indicator of a shortage or surplus of physicians. These ratios do not consider changes in demands for physicians or increases in physician productivity, nor do differences in these ratios over time indicate the importance, in terms of physician fees, of shortages or surpluses using this approach.

Play or pay—Under this form of national health insurgence (also referred to as an employer mandate) employers are required to either provide some basic level of medical insurance to their employees ("play") or pay a certain amount per employee into a government pool that would provide the employee with insurance.

Point-of-service—A plan that allows the beneficiary to select from participating providers (the HMO) or use nonparticipating providers and pay a high co-payment.

Portability—Included as part of health insurance reform that enables the insured to change jobs without losing their insurance or having to be liable for another preexisting exclusion period.

Preexisting exclusion—To protect themselves against adverse selection by new enrollees, insurers use a preexisting exclusion clause that excludes treatment for any or specified illnesses that have been diagnosed within the previous (usually) twelve months.

Preferred provider organization (PPO)—An arrangement between a panel of health care providers and purchasers of health care services in which a closed panel of providers agree to supply services to a defined group of patients on a discounted fee-for-service basis. This type of plan offers a limited number of physicians and hospitals, negotiated fee schedules, utilization review, and consumer incentives to use PPO participating providers.

Preferred risk selection—Occurs when insurers receive the same premium for everyone in an insured group and try to attract only those with lower risks, whose expected medical costs would be less than the group's average premium.

Prepaid group practice (PGP)—A type of practice where the providers are reimbursed a capitated amount per enrollee for a stipulated length of time.

Prescription drug—A drug that can be obtained only with a physician's prescription.

Prestige maximization goal—Not-for-profit providers (hospitals and medical schools) whose pricing and investment behavior is directed so as to increase the prestige of the institution rather than the rate of return on their investments.

Price discrimination—An indication of monopoly power by a provider. The provider is able to charge different purchasers different prices, according to the purchaser's elasticity of demand (willingness to pay), for the same or similar service.

Price fixing—Occurs when competing firms agree to set prices so as to increase profits. The competing firms act like a monopolist in that they use the industry demand curve, which is less price elastic, to establish their prices. Such actions are considered to be a per se violation of anti-trust laws.

Price of legislation—Is the political support an organized group can offer to legislators, namely, campaign contributions, volunteer time, and votes.

Primary care physician (PCP)—A physician who coordinates all of the routine medical care needs of an individual. Typically, this type of physician specializes in family practice, internal medicine, pediatrics, or obstetrics/gynecology.

Process measures of quality—A type of quality assessment that evaluates process of care by measuring the specific way in which care is provided or, with respect to health manpower, training requirements.

Producer legislation—May be categorized into five types: demand-increasing, secure the highest method of payment, reduce the price or increase the quantity of complements, decrease the availability or increase the price of substitutes, and limit increases in supply.

Product market definition—Used in anti-trust cases to determine whether the product or service in question has close substitutes, which depends on the willingness of purchasers to use other services if their relative prices change. The closer the substitutes, the smaller the market share of the product being examined.

Production possibilities curve—Shows the different combinations (trade-off) of two different goods or outputs that can be produced with a fixed amount of resources.

Professional licensure—A prerequisite that requires health professionals, such as physicians, who want to practice to obtain a license from the government.

Profit-maximizing model of hospital behavior—Not-for-profit hospitals act as though they tried to maximize profits by setting price at that point on their demand curve where marginal revenue equals marginal cost. Further, such hospitals would invest so as to receive the highest rate of return on their assets. Any "profits" generated would be internally invested rather than paid out to shareholders.

Prospective payment—A method of payment for medical services in which providers are paid based on a predetermined rate for the services rendered, regardless of the actual costs of care incurred. Medicare uses a prospective payment system for hospital care based on a fixed price per hospital admission (by diagnosis).

Public interest theory of government—Assumes that legislation is enacted to serve the public interest. The two basic objectives of government according to this theory are to improve market efficiency and, based on a societal value judgment, redistribute income.

Pure premium—Is the expected claims experience for an insured group, exclusive of the loading charge. As described in the text, the pure premium for an individual is calculated by multiplying the size of the loss by the probability the loss will occur.

Rate of return to a professional education—Is calculated by estimating the costs of an investment in a medical education, including both explicit and implicit (opportunity) costs and the expected higher financial returns as a result of that investment. More precisely, the internal rate of return is that discount rate which, when applied to the future earnings stream, will make its present value equal to the cost of the investment in a medical education.

Rational behavior—Assumes that the decision maker chooses that course of action offering the highest ratio of marginal benefits to marginal costs.

Redistribution—Is based on society's value judgment that those with higher incomes should be taxed to provide for those with lower incomes.

Refundable tax credits—A proposal for national health insurance under which individuals are given a tax credit to purchase health insurance. The tax credit may be income-related, that is, declining at higher levels of income. Persons whose tax credit exceeded their tax liabilities would receive a refund for the difference. For those with little or no tax liability, the tax credit is essentially a voucher for a health plan.

Regressive taxes—When those with lower incomes pay a higher portion of their income for that tax than do those with higher incomes.

Report cards—Standardized data, representing both process and outcome measures of quality, and collected by independent organizations, to enable purchasers to make more informed choices of health plans and their participating providers.

Resource-based relative value scale (RBRVS)—The current Medicare fee for service payment system for physicians, initiated in 1992, under which each physician service is assigned a relative value, based on the presumed resource costs of performing that service. The relative value for each service is then multiplied by a conversion factor (in dollars) to arrive at the physician's fee.

Risk-adjusted premiums—The employer adjusts the insurance premium to reflect the risk levels of the employees enrolled with different insurers.

Risk aversion—Preferring an assured outcome to a more risky alternative.

Risk pool—Represents a population group that is defined by its expected claim experience.

Risk selection—Occurs when insurers attempt to attract a more favorable risk group than the average risk group, which was the basis for the group's premium (preferred risk selection). Similarly, enrollees may seek to join a health plan at a premium that reflects a lower level of risk than their own (adverse selection).

"Rule of reason"—Used in anti-trust cases to determine whether the anticompetitive harm caused by a particular activity (e.g., merger) exceeds the procompetitive benefits of not permitting the particular activity.

Scarce resources—A basic assumption underlying economic analysis that there are insufficient resources, that is, time or money, to satisfy all wants.

Second opinions—A utilization review approach in which decisions to initiate a medical intervention are typically reviewed by two physicians.

Self-funding self-insurance—A health care program in which employers fund benefit plans from their own resources without purchasing insurance. Self-funded plans may be self-administered, or the employer may contract with an outside administrator for an administrative service only (ASO) arrangement. Employers who self-fund can limit their liability via stop-loss insurance.

Shadow pricing—A practice previously engaged in by HMOs to set their premiums just below those charged by traditional insurers.

Sherman Anti-trust Act—Anti-trust legislation established in 1890 to prevent anticompetitive behavior.

Shift in supply—Caused by changes in input prices or a technology, which would change the marginal productivity of inputs.

Single payer—A form of national health insurance in which a single third-party payer, usually government, pays the health care providers and the entire population has free choice of all providers at zero (or little) out-of-pocket expense.

Skilled nursing facility (SNF)—A long-term care facility that provides inpatient skilled nursing care and rehabilitation services.

Specialty HMOs—A type of HMO that offers one or more limited health care benefits, such as pharmacy, vision, and dental.

Specialty PPOs—A type of PPO that offers one or more limited health care services or benefits, such as anesthesia, vision, and dental services.

Staff-model health maintenance organization—A type of HMO that hires salaried physicians to provide health care services on an exclusive basis to the HMO's enrollees.

Static economic shortage—A situation in which demand exceeds supply at the market price. May occur because price is set below the equilibrium level by government or because of barriers to entry. In the case of entry barriers, the market price or wage is greater than if entry were permitted; the effect is to cause those in the industry to earn excess profits, which is an indication of a long-run shortage.

Stop-loss insurance—Insurance coverage providing protection from losses resulting from claims greater than a specific dollar amount (equivalent to a large deductible).

Structural quality measures—Measures of the quality of care that focus on the context of the environment within which medical services are provided. At the institutional level these measures can include facility licensure, compliance with health and safety codes, and medical staff appointments.

Sunk costs—Costs that have already been incurred and should be ignored for economic decision making.

Supplier-induced demand—When physicians modify their diagnosis and treatment to favorably affect their own economic well-being.

Supply and demand analysis—Used for predicting new equilibrium situations; for example, predicting the effect of a change in demand for a service or in its cost of production on the price and quantity of that service.

Surplus—When the quantity supplied exceeds the quantity demanded at the market price. With respect to health professionals, a surplus occurs when the profession, on average, earns a below normal rate of return.

Survivor analysis—An approach for estimating economies of scale by examining the size distribution of firms in an industry to determine which size of firms become more numerous.

Target-income hypothesis—A model of supplier-induced demand that assumes physicians will induce demand only to the extent they will achieve a target income, which is determined by the local income distribution, particularly with respect to the relative incomes of other physicians and professionals in the area.

Task licensure—Task or specific purpose licenses would recognize that physicians are not always qualified to do all the tasks for which they are licensed to perform. Task licensure would ensure that only those qualified for a particular task would be permitted to perform that task.

Tax Equity and Fiscal Responsibility Act (TEFRA) of 1982—Legislation that set limits on Medicare reimbursements on a per case basis for hospital costs (DRGs) and limited the annual rates of increase in DRG payments.

Tax-exempt employer-paid health insurance—Health insurance purchased by the employer on behalf of employees is not considered to be taxable income to the employee. By lowering the price of insurance, the quantity demanded is increased (as well as its comprehensiveness). The major beneficiaries are those who are in higher income tax brackets.

Technical efficiency—The inputs used in a production function produce the maximum output for a given time period.

Tertiary care—This type of care includes the most complex services, such as transplantation, open heart surgery, and burn treatment, provided in inpatient hospital settings.

Third-party administrator (TPA)—An independent entity that provides administrative services, such as the processing of claims, to a company that self-insures. A TPA does not underwrite the risk.

Third-party payer—An organization, such as an HMO, insurance company, or government agency, that pays for all or part of the insured's medical services.

Triple option health plan—A type of health plan in which employees may choose from an HMO, PPO, or indemnity plan, depending on how much they are willing to contribute.

Uncompensated care—Services rendered by the provider without reimbursement, as in the case of charity care and bad debts.

Universal coverage—When the entire population is eligible for medical services or health insurance.

Usual, customary, and reasonable fees (UCR)—A method of reimbursement in which the fee is 'usual' in that physician's office, 'customary' in that community, and 'reasonable' in terms of the distribution of all physician charges for that service in the community.

Utility-maximizing model of hospital behavior—The nonprofit hospital's pricing and investment policies are assumed to be undertaken for the purpose of maximizing the utility of the hospital's decision makers, namely, the management and trustees of the hospital. These decision makers prefer a large, high-quality prestigious institution.

Utilization review organization (URO)—An organization that conducts utilization reviews to determine whether specific health care service(s) are medically necessary and delivered at an appropriate cost and quality. These organizations provide their services to various health plans, employers, and insurers.

Vacancy rates—The percent of a hospital's budgeted registered nursing positions that are unfilled.

Value judgment of minimum provision—A value judgment underlying national health insurance in which all persons should receive a minimum quantity of medical services.

Vertical integration—The organization of a delivery system that provides an entire range of services, to include inpatient care, ambulatory care clinics, outpatient surgery, and home care.

Vertical merger—A merger between two firms that have a supplier–relationship.

Virtual integration—The organization of a delivery system that relies on contractual relationships, rather than complete ownership, to provide all medical services required by the patient.

Voluntary performance standard—An expenditure target adopted by the Medicare program to limit the rate of increase in its expenditures for physician's services.

Welfare criteria—Economics relies on a set of welfare criteria to determine whether someone is made better or worse off as a result of a policy change.

INDEX

A

Academic Health Center (AHC), 415
activities of daily living (ADL), 563, 580
administrative services only (ASO), 177
adverse selection, 137–139, 140, 572
advertising, and the health professions, 208, 262–266, 383, 394, 495
AFL-CIO, 553
American Academy of Family Practitioners, 499
American Association of Retired Persons, 571
American Dental Association (ADA), 492–493, 497, 505
   Council on Dental Education, 384
   and dental hygienists, 503
   and denturists, 502–503
   and foreign dental education, 504
American Hospital Association (AHA), 494, 497–498, 500
   and surgicenters, 503–504
American Medical Association (AMA), 214, 381, 409, 500
   Council on Medical Education, 382
   and entry barriers to medicine, 384–386
   and Medicare Part B, 205, 502, 553
   and national health insurance, 492
   and nurse practitioners, 499
   and osteopaths, 502
   political positions, 319–320, 552
   "Principles of Medical Ethics," 394
   and relicensure, 396
American Nurses' Association (ANA), 442n. 3, 449, 493–494, 497
   and educational requirements, 450, 505–506
   and educational subsidies, 447–448
   and foreign nurses, 503
   and unionization, 446
American Optometric Association, 505
anti-trust laws, 187, 197, 199, 327, 329–330, 495, 601
   and competition, 213–217
   enforcement, 213–217
"any willing provider" laws, 234, 255, 496–497, 508

Arrow, Kenneth J., 160–161, 323, 352
Association of American Dental Schools, 504
Association of American Medical Colleges (AAMC), 494
Association of American Medical Schools, 372
Auster-Leveson-Sarachek (ALS) study, 27
average area per capita cost (AAPCC), 533

B

balance billing, 277, 279, 283–285, 394
Bane Report, 359
Barr, Nicholas, 511
Barzel, Yoram, 72
benefit design, 154–159
Benham, Alexandra, 28–29
Benham, Lee, 28–29
Blair, Roger D., 179–180
Blue Cross, 121–122, 199–200, 494, 500–501
   and favorable tax treatment, 180–181, 199
   and hospital discount, 181–183, 199, 498
   service benefit policy, 121–122, 149–152
Blue Cross and Blue Shield (BCBS) plans, 176, 177, 393–394
Blue Shield, 495–496, 502
brand name recognition, 226
Brown, Douglas M., 244–245
Buerhaus, Peter, 442
Bureau of Labor Statistics (BLS), 54–61, 67–71, 75, 78
Burge, Russell T., 244

C

California, and hospital competition, 328
Canadian–type health system, 538–540
capitation, 111, 149, 152, 218–219, 535
   capitation-based system, 134
   and physician agency, 262, 287–288
   versus fee-for-service, 221–224
Capron, William M., 352
Carnegie Commission, 382, 407n. 2, 416, 420
Carter, Jimmy, 207, 540
catastrophic case management, 218

certificate of need (CON) legislation, 205, 297, 504, 508, 583, 585, 588
  1979 amendments, 210–211
charity hypothesis, 390, 392
Civil Rights Act (1964), 453
Civilian Health and Medical Program for Uniformed Services (CHAMPUS), 531
Clinton, Bill, 540
Clinton health reform proposal, 194, 207, 544–545
closed panels, 234
co-insurance, 120, 145
  effect on demand for medical care, 111–113
collusion, 165, 166
Columbia/HCA, 307
Commission on the Cost of Medical Care, 210
Commission on Graduate Medical Education (COGME), 373, 374
comparable worth, 453–456
competition, 4, 166
  and anti-trust laws, 213–217
  effect on quality, 224–228
  emergence in medical care, 205–209
  federal initiatives, 209–212
  private-sector initiatives, 212–213
  and quality, 224–233
Congressional Budget Office (CBO), 231
Consultant Group on Nursing, 447–448
consumer choice, 225–226
Consumer Expenditure (CE) Survey, 56, 57, 61, 62–65
consumer price index (CPI)
  CPI-U, 55, 61
  CPI-W, 55, 61
  index measures, 53–55
  medical care component (MCPI), 60–65
    accuracy of measured prices, 65–69
    cost-of-treatment approach, 74–78
    input versus treatment approach, 71–74
    and new products, 69–71
    and quality changes, 69–71
  and new products, 58–60
  population coverage, 55
  and quality changes, 58–60
  sampling problems, 55–57
  and substitution bias, 57–58
consumer protection, 4, 13, 466, 472

consumer sovereignty, 85–86
Cook, Francis, 33
Corman, Hope, 31
cost containment, 40, 490
  unavailability, 195–197
cost/benefit analysis, 413, 471
cost-of-living index, 54, 74–77
cost-of-treatment index, 72–78
cost sharing, 104–105
cost shifting, 279, 330–333
Crandall, Robert, 543–544
crowding theory, 454–455
Cutler, David, 534

D
deductibles, 118–120, 144–145
demand
  and annual changes in personal medical expenditures, 105–108
  determinants, 87–88
  faced by the firm, 108–110
  factors affecting, 88–94
  for health insurance, 122–137
  for medical care, 86–87
  versus need, 83–86
  role of physician in, 94–96
  selected studies of, 95–105
demand analysis, 82
demand-inducement hypothesis, 96, 274
demand policy, 44–48
dental services, 65
Department of Justice (DOJ), 298, 300–301
diagnosis-related grouping (DRG), 212, 308–309, 315, 327–328, 337
Dranove, David, 67

E
economic boycott, 215
economic efficiency, 163, 175–176
Economic Stabilization Program (ESP), 3, 206–207, 267, 269n. 9, 281, 335
Economic Theory of Regulation, 487
economics
  applicability to study of medical care, 12–13
  contribution to health policy, 4–6
economies of scale, 165, 179–180, 298
  informational, 246–248

in medical practice, 242–246

Edgren, John, 449

Employee Retirement and Security Act (ERISA), 132

Enthoven, Alain C., 211

equal access, 517–519

Evans, Robert, 258n. 6

externalities, 4, 412–413, 469–473, 471n. 4, 485

F

Feder, Judith, 585

Federal Trade Commission (FTC), 214–215, 265, 298, 299, 394

fee splitting, 495, 512

fee-for-service, 43, 95, 217, 221–224, 226–227, 229–230

    inefficiencies, 281

Feldstein, Paul J., 231, 300n. 2

FHP International, 310

Financial Accounting Standards Board (FASB), 555

first-dollar coverage, 131

Flexner Report, 382, 407n. 2

Ford, Gerald, 440

for-profit status, 225, 311

foreign medical graduates (FMGs), 365–366, 365–366n. 4, 409, 410

Frech, H. E., 203

free care plans, 104–105

"free choice of provider," 508

free riding, 515

Friedman, Milton, 123, 378, 387n. 1

Fuchs, Victor, 29–30, 258

G

Gaynor, Martin, 248

generic drugs, 68–69

Gertler, Paul, 248

Getzen, Thomas E., 246

Gies Report, 384

Goldman, Lee, 33

government

    and consumer protection, 466, 472

    imperfections, 464–468

    and in-kind subsidies, 473–481

    market failure, 468–474

Graduate Medical Education National Advisory Committee (GMENAC), 356–357, 371, 372

Grossman, Michael, 28, 31–33, 87

Group Health Association, 210

Group Health Insurance (GHI), 259

Gruber, Jonathan, 534

H

Haas-Wilson, Deborah, 291

Hadley, Jack, 28

Hansen, W. Lee, 362, 362n. 3, 417–418

Harris, Jeffrey E., 343

health insurance, 92

    and additional benefits, 154–159

    appropriateness, 117–118

    and the benefit/premium ratio, 187–189

    catastrophic, 474

    and community rating, 191–195

    and competitive behavior, 183–185, 187–189

    and cost containment programs, 186, 195–197

    demand schedule, 130

    demand side, 176–179

    determinants of premiums, 186–187

    and economic efficiency, 175–176

    employer-paid, 206, 465–466, 535–537

    fallback plan, 550

    and federal legislation, 197–198

    as fringe benefit, 153–154

    group policies, 132, 178n. 1

    guaranteed issue, 197

    guaranteed renewal, 197

    individual policies, 178, 178n. 1, 179

    limits, 120–121

    maximums, 120–121

    and moral hazard, 141–146

    multiple-option plan, 216

    portability, 197

    and preexisting exclusions, 197–198

    and state regulation, 198

    supply side, 179–183

    switching costs, 189–191

    tax treatment, 131, 148, 198, 465–466, 535–537

    theory of demand, 122–137

    waiting period, 197–198

Health Insurance Plan of Greater New York (HIP), 259
health maintenance organization (HMO), 19, 43, 176–177, 210, 218–221
  and the aged, 140, 185
  and anti-trust laws, 213–217
  and the chronically ill, 228
  effect on medical expenditures, 228–233
  federal act establishing, 210
  minimal growth of, 207–209
  organized medicine's opposition to, 392–393
  and preferred risk selection, 185
  and shadow pricing, 183–185, 230
health manpower shortages/surpluses
  conflicting estimates, 369–372
  correction of imbalances, 372–375
  empirical estimates, 362–369
  professional determination, 356–357
  and the rate-of-return approach, 360–363, 376
  and the ratio technique, 357–360, 369–371, 376
  relative income approach to, 362n. 2
  shortage
    dynamic, 352
    economic definitions, 349–354
    noneconomic definitions, 347–349
    static, 353–354
  surplus, definitions of, 355
Health Plan Employer Data Information Set (HEDIS), 227
Health Planning Act, 210
health production function, 20–25
Health Professions Educational Assistance Act (HPEA) (1965), 209, 368, 409–410
hedonic technique, 59n. 5
Hellinger, Fred J. 229–230
Herfindahl-Hirschman Index (HHI), 300–301, 301n. 3, 328–329
Hill-Burton program, 83, 324, 463, 481, 500
Hofer, Timothy P., 561
home health care services (HHC), 155–159, 567
hospital services
  background, 294–297
  case-mix studies, 303–304
  charity care, 325–326
  and competition, 326–330
  cross-subsidization of services, 318

  economies of scale, 298–304
  extent of markets, 305–306
  for-profit, 318, 325–326
  hospital performance, 333–339
  mergers, 298–301
  multihospital systems, 306–307
  nonprofit, 314, 318, 323–326
  physician-control model, 319–323, 324
  profit-maximizing model, 312–315
  and substitute product lines, 339
  survivor analyses, 304
  utility-maximizing model, 315–319
  vertical integration, 306–311
Hsiao, William C., 282–283

I

Immigration Act (1965), 365, 365–366n. 4
Immigration Nurse Relief Act (1989), 441
incentives, 144, 152. *See also* co-insurance; deductibles
income contingent loan repayment plan (ICLRP), 421–422, 426
income elasticity, 90, 102–103, 110
indemnity, 121–122, 149, 231
Independent Practice Association (IPA), 218
Indian Health Services, 531
innovation, 224, 311, 507–508
Institute of Medicine, 586, 589
integrated delivery system (IDS), 308–309
interest groups, 552

J

Johnson, Lyndon, 267
Jones, Lewis, 83, 347, 356

K

Kaiser Foundation, 208, 210, 310
Kassenbaum-Kennedy bill, 197
Katz, Steven J., 561
Keeler, Emmett B., 547
Kessel, Reuben, 391, 392, 394, 407n. 2
Kuznets, Simon, 378

L

Laspeyres index, 54, 54n. 1, 58n. 3, 76
law of diminishing returns. *See* law of variable proportions
law of variable proportions, 170, 321

Lee, Roger, 83, 347, 356
Lees, Dennis, 160–161
legislation
  and complements, 499–501
  demand-increasing, 492–494
  economic theory of, 486–491
  public interest view of, 484–486
  and reimbursement, 495–499
  and substitutes, 501–504
  and supply increases, 504–506
Liaison Committee on Medical Education
    (LCME), 408, 465
licensed practical nurses (LPNs), 428, 429,
    493–494
life care communities, 573, 577
lifestyle variables, 27, 30
Lindsay, Cotton M., 378
linking, 58–59, 58n. 4, 68–69, 69n. 6
loading charge, 128, 130, 186, 188
Long, Millard F., 300n. 2
long run, 170–171
long-term care (LTC), 556. See also nursing
    homes
  background, 577–579
  and case management, 572, 575, 576–577,
    590, 593–594
  and consumer ignorance/uncertainty,
    374–375
  demographics, 562–566
  and elderly's incomes, 568–571
  financing, 590–593
  government insurance for, 574
  in other countries, 597
  price, 566–568
  private insurance for, 571–574
Luft, Harold S., 227–228, 230, 327

M
McCarthy, Thomas R., 260, 287
malpractice, 397
  insurance, 255n. 5, 270, 500
managed care, 72, 177, 272–273. See also fee-
    for-service; HMO; PPO
  characteristics of plans, 217–221
  effect on medical expenditures, 228–233
  and hospital costs, 328–329
  and medical schools, 415–416
Marder, William D., 245

marginal analysis, 5, 7–9, 23, 598
marginal benefits, 71, 86
marginal costs, 86, 467
marginal productivity, 169–170
marginal utility, 467
market efficiency, 4
market performance, 167–168
market power, 167–168, 248–250, 299
market structure, 165–166
  competitive, 165–166
  monopolistic, 165–166
  monopsonistic, 182
  oligopolistic, 165
mastectomies, outpatient, 235
maternity stays, 235
Medicaid, 3, 131, 205–207, 241, 533–535,
    551, 554–555
  beneficiaries, 475–477
  and long-term care, 587–588
medical care
  and allocation of resources, 20–25
  definition, 52–53
  expenditures on, 2, 37–41
  as input to health, 18–19
  interrelationship of markets, 41–44
  as output of the medical services industry,
    18–19
  uniqueness, 599
medical education, 240–241, 382
  accreditation of schools, 408, 423
  applicant/acceptance ratio, 367–368
  competitive system in, 402–404, 422–423,
    424
  costs, 425
  curriculum, 415–416
  economic efficiency, 401–416
  equity of financing, 416–423
  and government subsidies, 405, 413–414,
    416–422, 498–499
  Harvard, 405–407
  Johns Hopkins, 405–407
  performance, 401
  prestige maximization, 405–407
  quality-assurance mechanisms, 241n. 1
  rate-of-return approach to, 360–361
  reform, 408
  tuition, 402–404, 404–405, 414–415, 423
medical expenditures, trends in, 1–4

medical savings account (MSA), 546–547
medical services
  and cultural-demographic factors, 89
  determination of output, 6–9
  distribution, 11–12
  and economic factors, 89–90
  production, 9–11
  public policy and, 599–603
  quantity-quality trade-off, 13–15
  redistribution, 146n. 2
medical societies, 324–325, 390–393
Medicare, 3, 205–206, 241, 475–477, 531–533,
    554–555
  and baby boomers, 532
  cost-based system of, 180
  effect on hospital performance, 333–339
  fee index, 207
  and long-term care, 571–572, 575, 578
  Part A, 180
  Part B, 280–281, 285
  payments to hospitals, 66
  physician payment system, 272, 276–286, 496
  and residencies, 373
  and risk selection, 230
  trust fund, 206, 532
Medi-gap policies, 285–286, 571, 572
Melnick, Glenn, 328
metropolitan statistical area (MSA), 305
microanalysis, 26
middle class, 556–557
Miller, Robert H., 227–228, 230
minimum provision, 515–517
misallocation, 152
monopoly, 165, 251–255, 468–469, 485, 488
moral hazard, 122, 141–146, 162, 572
mortality rates, 26–30
  and heart disease, 33
  infant, 29–30, 29n. 5, 30–33
Mundt resolution, 391
Musgrave, Peggy B. 483
Musgrave, Richard A., 483

N

National Federation of Independent Business,
    544
National Health Accounts (NHAs), 62–65
national health insurance (NHI), 474
  beneficiaries, 525–526
  Canadian-type system, 538–540
  concentrated interests, 554–547
  conflicting goals, 551–554
  employer-mandated, 540–545
  equitable financing, 526–530
  evidence from Medicare, 521–525
  incentives for efficiency, 526
  legislative developments, 557–559
  tax credits, 547–551
  theoretical framework, 515–521
National Health Planning and Resource
    Development Act. *See* certificate of need
    legislation
National Labor Relations Act, 445
National League for Nursing (NLN), 449–450
National Medical Care Expenditure Survey
    (NMCES), 115, 259–260
need, as basis for public policy, 83–86
Nelson, Philip, 263n. 7
New York, and community rating, 194
Nixon, Richard, 206–207, 210, 267, 440, 540
nonprofit status, 225, 311
nurse practitioners, 497, 499
Nurse Shortage Reduction Act (1988), 441
Nurse Training Act (NTA) (1964), 437, 448,
    458, 462, 500
nursing homes, 309
  analysis of services, 581–583
  and back-end subsidies, 592
  controls on bed number, 575–576
  decertification, 589
  determinants of costs, 579–581
  and front-end subsidies, 591–592
  government policy and, 583–586
  intermediate care facilities (ICFs), 599
  preadmission screening, 574
  private insurance for, 571–575
  regulation of quality, 586–590
  skilled nursing facilities (SNFs), 566
Nyman, John A., 567

O

oligopoly, 165, 306
optimization, 5, 16. *See also* marginal analysis;
    supply and demand analysis; welfare
    criteria

Oregon, and cost containment measures, 196–197, 214

outpatient services, 295, 322, 338

P

Paasche index, 58n. 3, 69

Pacific Business Group on Health (PBGH), 226, 227

Palo Alto Medical Clinic (PAMC), 73

patient weighted price index (PWPI), 76

Pauly, Mark V., 144, 161, 162, 260–261

payroll taxes, 488–489, 527–530

Pennsylvania Dental Association (PDA), 497

Pepper Commission, 540, 543

PEW Commission, 373

physician
    as patient's agent, 94–96, 110, 256, 262
    as supplier of medical services, 94–96, 256

physician assistants (PAs), 244–245, 244n. 2, 384, 494, 500

physician manpower
    and assurance of quality, 396–398
    board certification, 385
    citizenship requirements, 386
    disciplinary actions and, 397–398
    educational requirements, 382, 396
    entry restrictions, 380–381
    licensure, 381–382, 395–396
    and price-discriminating monopoly, 387–395
    reexamination, 384–385, 396
    relicensure, 384–385, 396
    training, 383, 396

physician profiling, 262

physician services market
    and demand, 239
    group practice, 242–250, 286
    market conduct, 250–266
    payment under Medicare, 276–286
    performance, 266–276
    physician expenditures, 267–271
    physician fees, 267–271
    physician incomes, 271–273
    solo practice, 242–246
    structure, 242–250
    survivor analysis, 245–246
    and use of aides, 240, 244–245
    visits to physicians, 267–271

physician/population ratio, 95, 258–262, 347, 357–360, 364–369, 376, 489–490

physicians, increased supply of, 209

point-of-purchase survey, 56–57

point-of-service (POS) plan, 176, 219

Pope, Gregory C., 244

preauthorization, 262

preexisting condition, 121

preferred provider organization (PPO), 66, 177, 217–218, 272–273

preferred risk selection, 139–141, 185, 194, 230

prescription drugs, 68–69, 224

preventive care, 147n. 3, 222, 224

price competition, 230, 234, 495, 601

price discrimination, 166, 332, 387–395, 495–499

price elasticity, 90–93, 98–105, 110, 164

price fixing, 215

price/cost ratio, 167

price-of-insurance index, 79–80

primary care physicians (PCPs), 272, 370

probability sampling, 56

producer price index (PPI), 68

production functions
    characteristics, 169–171
    law of variable proportions, 171
    marginal productivity, 169–170
    and the medical sector at large, 172–173
    returns to scale, 170–171
    short versus long run, 170
    substitutability, 169, 171
    technical change, 171
    underlying assumptions, 171–172

professional standards review organization (PSRO), 386

Prospective Payment Reform Commission, 279

provider networks, 327, 328

provider panels, 187

public policy, 6, 168–169, 599–603

Q

quality bias, 59

quality review, 225

quality-quantity trade-off, 13–15, 233, 316–319. *See also* hospital services, utility-maximizing model

R

RAND Health Insurance Experiment, 29, 98, 103–105, 229
Reagan, Ronald, 212
Reder, Melvin, 79
redistribution, 4, 163–164, 337, 485–486, 491, 601–603
registered nurses (RNs)
    education, 449–450
    employment, 443–447
    and hospital collusion, 438–439, 454, 458
    licensure, 442n. 3, 450
    and managed care, 442, 458–459
    measures of market performance, 427–432
    before Medicare/Medicaid, 432–438
    in the post–Medicare period, 439–443
    training, 447–452
    unionization, 445
    wages, 443–447, 453–457
regression analysis, 59n. 5
regulation, of medical practice, 558, 601
Reinhardt, Uwe, 243, 244, 260
resource-based relative value scales, 241, 281–283, 285. *See also* Medicare
retiree benefits, 555
Rice, Robert, 160–161
Rice, Thomas H., 258
risk, 311
risk, reduction of, 248
risk aversion, 128, 130
risk-adjusted premiums, 185, 233–234
Rizzo, John A., 265n. 8
Robinson, James C., 310, 327
Rossiter, Louis F., 259–260

S

salary continuation, 121
Satterthwaite, Mark A., 260–261
Savage, L., 123
Scanlon, William J., 567, 571, 585
scarcity, 5
Schwartz, William B., 371
Scitovsky, Anne, 72, 73
search costs, 252–253, 252n. 4, 261, 263
self-insurance, 123, 132, 177, 474
service benefits, 121–122
service price index, 74–77

Sherman Anti-Trust Act, 393
short run, 170–171
Silver, M., 26n. 1
single-payer system. *See* Canadian-type health system
Sloan, Frank A., 378
Social Security tax, 527–530, 554
specialists, 272, 370–372
spending down, 556
spillover effect, 229, 231
Staiger, Douglas, 337, 442
state mandates, 132, 161
state practice acts, 494, 499
stop loss levels, 120–121
student loan programs, 421–422, 422n. 3
substitution, 10, 58, 88, 151, 169, 171, 299
substitution bias, 59
supplier-induced demand (SID), 255–262, 287
supply
    determinants, 163–165
    elasticity, 46–48, 164–165
    policy, 48–49
    subsidy, 48–49
supply and demand analysis, 5, 16, 598
Svorny, Shirley, 367

T

Taft-Hartley Act, 446
target-income hypothesis, 256–257
tax exemption, 148, 343, 466
technology, 132–134, 232–233, 295, 296
third-party administrator (TPA), 177
time costs, 92–94, 97
transaction cost, 66, 161, 308
Truman, Harry S., 492
tying arrangements, 215

U

uncertainty, reduction of, 248
unions, 211, 545, 553, 555–556
U.S. medical graduates (USMGs), 240, 366, 369
U.S. Public Health Service, 447
"usual, customary, and reasonable" (UCR) fee, 255
utilization review, 95, 98, 144, 152, 195, 207, 213, 262

utility, 7, 123–126

V

Veterans Administration (VA) medical system, 472n. 5, 478–479, 531
"virtual" integration, 309–310
Vogel, Ronald J., 179–180
volume-performance standard (VPS), 279, 283–285
vouchers, 235

W

Washington State, and waiting period elimination, 198
Weiner, Jonathan P., 369–370

Weisbrod, Burton, 323–324, 417–418
welfare criteria, 5–6, 11–12, 16, 134–135
Weller, Charles D., 181–182
Wennberg, John, 273–274
Wickizer, Thomas M., 231
Wilensky, Gail, 259–260
work-loss rates, 26n. 1

Y

Yett, Donald E., 433n. 2, 439

Z

Zeckhauser, Richard J., 265n. 8
Zuckerman, Stephen, 245
Zwanziger, Jack, 328